IMMUNOLOGY
A Short Course

FOURTH EDITION

Eli Benjamini
Professor Emeritus
Department of Medical Microbiology and Immunology
University of California School of Medicine
Davis, California

Richard Coico
Professor and Chairman
Department of Microbiology and Immunology
City University of New York Medical School
New York, New York

Geoffrey Sunshine
Staff Scientist
Health Effects Institute
Cambridge, Massachusetts
and
Lecturer, Department of Pathology
Tufts University School of Medicine
Boston, Massachusetts

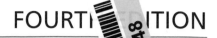

WILEY-LISS

A JOHN WILEY & SONS, INC., PUBLICATION

New York • Chichester • Weinheim • Brisbane • Singapore • Toronto

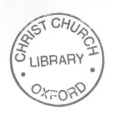

This book is printed on acid-free paper. ⊗

While the authors, editors, and publisher believe that drug selection and dosage and the specification and usage of equipment and devices, as set forth in this book, are in accord with current recommendation and practice at the time of publication, they accept no legal responsibility for any errors or omission, and make no warranty, express or implied, with respect to material contained herein. In view of ongoing research, equipment modifications, changes in governmental regulation, and the constant flow of information relating to drug therapy, drug reactions, and the use of equipment and devices, the reader is urged to review and evaluate the information provided in the package inset or instructions for each drug, piece of equipment, or device for, among other things, any changes in instruction or indication of dosage or usage and for added warnings and precautions.

For ordering and customer service, call 1-800-CALL-WILEY.

Library of Congress Cataloging-in-Publication Data:

Library of Congress Cataloging-in-Publication Data is available.
0-471-34890-2

Printed in the United States of America.

10 9 8 7 6 5 4 3 2 1

To
Lisa, Jonathan, and Jennifer
R.C.

To
Ilene, Caroline, Alex, and Pearl
G.S.

ABOUT THE AUTHORS

Eli Benjamini is a professor emeritus of immunology in the Department of Medical Microbiology and Immunology at the School of Medicine of the University of California at Davis. Dr. Benjamini has taught immunology to undergraduate, graduate, and medical students, as well as having served for 10 years as Chairman of the Graduate Program of Immunology on the Davis campus—a program which he was instrumental in forming. His research interests include the immunobiology of protein antigens, mechanisms of immune regulation, and principles of synthetic vaccine.

Richard Coico is a professor and chairman of the Department of Microbiology and Immunology at the City University of New York Medical School (http://med.cuny.edu). For the past six years, he has directed the Microbiology and Immunology course taught to medical students, and also participates in the teaching of immunology to graduate students and physician assistant students at CUNY. He is a member of the Education Committee of the Association of Medical School Microbiology and Immunology Chairs (AMSMIC) and currently serves as program chair of a biannual meeting sponsored by AMSMIC entitled, Educational Strategies Workshop for Microbiology and Immunology. His research interests include studies of the regulation of antibody responses and germinal center formation, mechanisms of T cell-mediated B cell activation, and the physiologic role of IgD in the immune system.

Geoffrey Sunshine is a staff scientist at the Health Effects Institute in Cambridge, Massachusetts where he reviews research on the biological effects of air pollutants. He is also a lecturer in the Department of Pathology at Tufts University School of Medicine. For several years, he has directed a course in immunology for graduate dental students at Tufts University Dental School, and previously directed a course for veterinary students at Tufts University Veterinary School. He was also a member of the Sackler School of Graduate Biomedical Sciences at Tufts University, doing research in antigen presentation and teaching immunology to medical, graduate, and undergraduate students.

CONTENTS

6 THE GENETIC BASIS OF ANTIBODY STRUCTURE   117

7 BIOLOGY OF THE B LYMPHOCYTE   135

8 THE ROLE OF THE MAJOR HISTOCOMPATIBILITY COMPLEX IN THE IMMUNE RESPONSE   147

9 BIOLOGY OF THE T LYMPHOCYTE   169

10 ACTIVATION AND FUNCTION OF T AND B CELLS 187

11 CONTROL MECHANISMS IN THE IMMUNE RESPONSE 211

20 TUMOR IMMUNOLOGY 401

21 RESISTANCE AND IMMUNIZATION TO INFECTIOUS DISEASES — 421

PREFACE AND ACKNOWLEDGMENTS

Since the last edition, significant developments in biomedical research have helped to refine and, in some cases, redefine our understanding of many aspects of the immune system. As a result, every chapter published in the fourth edition has been either updated or rewritten to incorporate new findings and to delete information that no longer reflects current thinking. In addition, several new chapters have been added to the book, including one on cytokines and another on resistance and immunization to infectious diseases. Finally, a new section on experimental systems has been added to Chapter 5. Describing how and why biomedical scientists utilize various experimental tools to investigate the complexities of the immune system is essential to a student's understanding of the subject of immunology.

As in the first three editions, we remain committed to the motto "less is more." Therefore, our objective in creating this edition has been to present what we consider to be the most pertinent material in a concise, palatable, and easily digestible fashion to the introductory student of immunology. Additional supportive material for students and course instructors can also now be found on a Web site (see below).

We are deeply indebted to Dr. Susan Gottesman, who contributed the chapter entitled, "Immunodeficiency and Other Disorders of the Immune System." We also thank Dr. Karen Yamaga, who updated the autoimmunity chapter. The important contributions of Dr. Patricia Giclas, who updated the complement chapter, and Dr. Arturo Casedeval, who added the new final chapter on resistance and immunization to infectious diseases, are also gratefully acknowledged.

Richard Coico would like to acknowledge the loving support of his family during the writing of this book. Their fortitude, inspiration, and enduring patience helped make the job an enjoyable adventure. Special thanks is extended to the following list of colleagues who generously provided their insightful scientific expertise and many helpful suggestions for the Fourth Edition: Drs. Ethan Shevach (NIH), David Margulies (NIH), Lloyd Mayer (Mount Sinai School of Medicine), Lakshmi Tamma (CUNY Medical School), Linda Spatz (CUNY Medical School), Laurel Eckhardt (Hunter College), Kathleen Barnes (Johns Hopkins School of Medicine), Soldano Ferrone (Roswell Park Memorial Institute), and Harriet Robinson (Emory University). Finally, he would like to thank his mentors, Drs. Ronald Curley, Susan Krown, Robert A. Good, and G. Jeanette Thorbecke, each of whom has greatly influenced his commitment and passion to the road taken.

Geoffrey Sunshine would like to thank Peter Brodeur (Tufts University Medical School) and Cindy Theodos (Tufts University Veterinary School) for their unstinting help during the preparation of his section of the current edition; they reviewed chapters in both the Third and Fourth Editions, and offered suggestions for making the material relevant and accessible to introductory readers. He is also grateful to the many friends and colleagues who answered questions about their areas of expertise, especially Mark Exley, Susan Kalled, and Paula Hochman. In addition, he would like to thank his family for their continued support and understanding during the writing.

The authors wish to express their appreciation to the staff members of John Wiley and Sons, Inc., who helped to bring the Fourth Edition to publication and did so with skill, patience, and good humor. Special thanks to our co-workers, including secretaries, office assistants, and other staff members, who helped with the preparation of the manuscript.

Finally, we wish to acknowledge the important contributions made by Dr. Sidney Leskowitz to the earlier editions of this book. The Hypersensitivity chapters are dedicated to his memory.

IMMUNOLOGY: A SHORT COURSE ON THE WEB

The Web site is designed as an additional resource for students and educators who adopt the book for use in their courses (http://www.wiley.com/immuno-short course.com). The site uses WebCT, a versatile online course management tool. The following features are included in the Web site:

- Table of contents
- Information about the authors
- Sample chapter
- All figures and tables published in the 4th edition
- Icon page with downloadable clip art images
- Embellished and regularly updated CD Antigens and Cytokine tables
- Embellished and regularly updated Glossary
- Embellished and regularly updated Review Questions and Answers section
- Links to other useful Web sites

The authors chose to use the WebCT course management tool because it is the undisputed e-learning leader in higher education. The Web site and its WebCT backbone allow those who adopt the 4th edition of **Immunology: A Short Course** to teach *their* courses *their* way.

We remain committed to updating the Web site regularly with the goal of facilitating the teaching efforts of instructors and, of course, student e-learning. First and foremost, our commitment in maintaining this Web site will be to provide an immunology-related educational resource that presents appropriate current information in a clear, concise, and student-friendly manner.

PREFACE AND ACKNOWLEDGMENTS TO THE THIRD EDITION

Since the last edition, the intense efforts of research scientists around the world have produced significant new findings that have reshaped our understanding of many aspects of the immune system. As a result, every chapter in the current edition has been either updated or rewritten to incorporate new findings and to delete information that no longer reflects current thinking.

As in the first and second editions, we remain committed to the motto "less is more." Our task has been to present what we consider the most relevant material in a concise, palatable, and easily digestible fashion to the introductory student. That reader will be the best judge of whether we have succeeded.

We are deeply indebted to Dr. Demosthenes Pappagianis, who contributed the chapter on immunoprophylaxis and immunotherapy, and Dr. Karen Yamaga, who contributed the chapter on control mechanisms in the immune response and on autoimmunity. We wish to thank the many co-workers and students who contributed to the first and second editions and those who were helpful in the preparation of the third edition, in particular, Dr. Robert J. Scibienski of the School of Medicine, University of California at Davis, and Dr. Donna M. Rennick, DNA Research Institute, Palo Alto, California. Geoffrey Sunshine would like to thank the many friends who patiently answered his questions during the writing of the third edition, in particular, Peter Brodeur, Mark Exley, and Paula Hochman. He would also like to thank his family for their continued support: Ilene, for her encouragement and dedication to the cause, and Alex and Caroline, for their optimism. His sections are dedicated to his father Harry, who did not live to see the new edition.

PREFACE TO THE SECOND EDITION

An anxiety common to authors of textbooks in rapidly developing fields is the necessity of relatively frequent revisions to include material that, in the previous edition, was in the "twilight zone," between fact and fancy but that since has gained the status of important fact. Indeed, the rapidly developing field of immunology requires continuous revisions; hence, the present edition.

In this second edition, various concepts and findings have been updated and expanded; new information has been added on such diverse topics as the molecular biology and genes controlling antibody synthesis and isotype switch, T-cell differentiation and the T-cell receptor, antigen processing and presentation, cytokines and lymphokines, new therapeutic approaches for immunodeficiency disorders and tumors, and new aspects of prophylaxis and immunotherapy of infectious diseases. In addition, we have added a section on AIDS and several techniques such as Western blots and fluorescence-activated cell sorting. We have also expanded the glossary and added review questions as well as several clinical correlates.

Although we have deleted and shortened some sections, the expanded and added material increased somewhat the size of the book. We can, however, assure the readers that with this second edition, as with the first edition, we remain committed to the motto "less is more" and have attempted to present the principles of immunology in a concise, palatable, and easily digestible form.

Revision and change is the constant burden that authors writing about a dynamically changing field have to carry. Students, too, have to partake of that burden and must prepare themselves with the realization that science is not static and they must continually move on to new levels of understanding. Good luck to us both.

PREFACE TO THE FIRST EDITION

Why was this book written? At a time when so many excellent, extensive, and beautifully illustrated texts flood the bookstores, why offer another one? The reasons are fairly simple and rather unsophisticated. In our collective 40 some-odd years of teaching all kinds of students, we have become convinced that most texts fail their purpose because they overshoot the mark.

Anyone coming into contact with these students year after year cannot fail to appreciate the burden under which they operate. If they are to graduate, they must learn an enormous amount of material on an exceptionally diverse series of subjects, each increasing in scope yearly. As any student can tell you, every faculty lecturer considers his/her particular topic absolutely essential for future graduates, and so the pile of required "essentials" grows and grows. This is a manifestly untenable approach to curriculum.

A second cruel observaton arises from long years of questioning students: many of them are not really that interested in immunology! As exciting, dynamic, and all-encompassing in its passion that we practitioners of immunology find it to be, the students have many other interests and concerns, one of which is to pass the five or six other subjects usually taken simultaneously with immunology.

This book was therefore conceived along the lines of the noted architect Mies van der Rohe's dictum, "less is more." We have devised this text to present the bare essentials of immunology in a palatable form that will enable most students to grasp the essential principles of immunology sufficiently to pass their course. For those developing a deeper interest in the field, numerous advanced and more complete texts exist to further their interests.

The book follows the outlines of most immunology courses and is divided into chapters that mostly approximate the length of an average lecture reading assignment. A short introduction setting the stage precedes the main text of each chapter, the end of each chapter contains a summary, and a series of study questions appears at the very end. The questions are designed to enable students to evaluate their own progress and comprehension; the appended answers are meant as a further learning experience. As new terms or concepts are introduced, they are highlighted in italics and boldface and defined for easy recognition and recall.

It is our hope that students using this text will avoid that choking sensation so common in a course in immunology and even conceive a curiosity about the subject that will lead to further study.

ACKNOWLEDGMENTS TO THE FIRST AND SECOND EDITIONS

The authors are deeply indebted to a number of colleagues and students for valuable contributions to the first and/or second edition of the book.

Dr. Demosthenes Pappagianis of the University of California School of Medicine at Davis contributed the chapter on immunoprophylaxis and immunotherapy, which provides useful, practical insights into the application of immunology to the prevention and therapy of infectious diseases.

Dr. Geoffrey Sunshine of Tufts University Veterinary School was deeply involved in the revision of many chapters of the second edition. His valuable and major contributions to the second edition are gratefully acknowledged.

Drs. Linda Werner and Jacqueline Maisonnave of the University of California School of Medicine at Davis and Drs. Peter Brodeur, Arthur Rabson, and Lanny Rosenwasser of Tufts University School of Medicine were most helpful in reading and contributing valuable suggestions to portions of the first edition. Many other colleagues reviewed portions of the text, and we are grateful for their criticisms and comments. These colleagues include Drs. James R. Carlson, Robert S. Chang, Allan C. Enders, Kent L. Erickson, Paul Luciw, Claramae H. Miller, and Robert J. Scibienski of the University of California School of Medicine, Davis; Drs. Dov Michaeli and Patricia R. Salber of the University of California School of Medicine, San Francisco; Dr. Shoshana Levy, Stanford University School of Medicine; Dr. Henry N. Claman, University of Colorado School of Medicine; Dr. Patricia Kongshavn, McGill University School of Medicine; and Dr. Karen M. Yamaga, University of Hawaii School of Medicine. Our apologies to other colleagues whose names have been unintentionally omitted.

Finally, we applaud the forbearance of our wives, Joy and Thelma, who continued to tolerate our irritability and whining during the writing of this book.

1

INTRODUCTION AND OVERVIEW

INTRODUCTION

The story is told about a man who visited a wise old rabbi. The man challenged the rabbi to teach him the essentials of his religion while the man stood on one foot. The rabbi, accepting the challenge, answered, "The essence of my religion is do not do unto others that which is hateful unto you; all the rest is commentary, now go and study."

The essence of immunology can be similarly stated while standing on one foot. Immunology deals with understanding how the body distinguishes between what is self and what is nonself; all the rest is technical detail.

In his penetrating essays, scientist-author Lewis Thomas, discussing parasitism and symbiosis, described the forces that would drive all living matter into one huge ball of protoplasm were it not for recognition mechanisms that kept self and nonself apart. The origins of these recognition mechanisms go far back in evolutionary history, and many, in fact, originated as markers for allowing cells to recognize each other to set up symbiotic households. Genetically related sponge colonies that are placed close to each other, for example, will tend to grow toward each other and fuse into one large colony. Unrelated colonies, however, will react in a different way, destroying cells that come in contact and leaving a zone of rejection between the colonies.

In the plant kingdom, similar types of recognition occur. In self-pollinating species, a pollen grain landing on the stigma of a genetically related flower will send a pollen tubule down the style to the ovary for fertilization. A pollen grain from a genetically distinct plant either will not germinate or the pollen tubule, once formed, will disintegrate in the style. The opposite occurs in cross-pollinating species: self-marked pollen grains disintegrate, while nonself grains germinate and fertilize.

The nature of these primitive recognition mechanisms has not been completely worked out, but almost certainly involves cell surface molecules that are able to specifically bind and adhere to other molecules on opposing cell surfaces. This simple method of molecular recognition has evolved over time into the very complex system of the immune response, which, however, still retains as its essential feature the ability of a protein molecule to recognize and bind specifically to a particular shaped structure on another molecule. Such molecular recognition is the underlying principle involved in the discrimination between self and nonself by the immune response. It is the purpose of this book to describe how the fully mature immune response that has evolved from this simple beginning makes use of this principle of recognition in increasingly complex and sophisticated ways.

The study of immunology as a science or subspecialty of biology has gone through several periods of quiescence and active development, usually succeeding the introduction of a new technique or a changed paradigm for thinking about the subject. Perhaps the biggest catalyst for progress in this and many other biomedical areas has been the advent of molecular biologic techniques. It is important to acknowledge, however, that certain technological advances in the field of molecular biology were made possible by earlier progress in the field of immunology. For example, the importance of immunologic methods used to purify proteins as well as identify specific cDNA clones cannot be understated. These advances have been greatly facilitated by the pioneering studies of Kohler and Milstein (1975), who developed a method for producing monoclonal antibodies. Their achievement was rewarded with the Nobel Prize in Medicine. It revolutionized research efforts in virtually all areas of biomedical science. Some monoclonal antibodies produced against so-called tumor-specific antigens have now been approved by the Food and Drug Administration for use in patients to treat certain malignancies. Monoclonal antibody technology is, perhaps, an excellent example of how the science of immunology has transformed not only the field of medicine but also fields ranging from agriculture to the food science industry.

Given the rapid advances occurring in immunology and the many other biologic sciences, every textbook runs a considerable risk of being outdated before it appears in print. Nevertheless, we take solace from the observation that new formulations generally build on and expand the old rather than replacing or negating them completely.

OVERVIEW

Innate and Acquired Immunity

The Latin term *immunis*, meaning "exempt," gave rise to the English word *immunity*, which refers to all the mechanisms used by the body as protection against environmental agents that are foreign to the body. These agents may be microorganisms or their products, foods, chemicals, drugs, pollen, or animal hair and dander. Immunity may be innate or acquired.

Innate Immunity. Innate immunity is conferred by all those elements with which an individual is born and which are always present and available at very short notice to protect the individual from challenges by foreign invaders. These elements include body surfaces and internal components, such as the skin, the mucous membranes, and the cough reflex, which present effective barriers to environmental agents. Chemical influences such as pH and secreted fatty acids constitute effective barriers against invasion by many microorganisms.

Numerous internal components are also features of innate immunity: fever, interferons, and other substances released by leukocytes, as well as a variety of serum proteins such as beta-lysin, the enzyme lysozyme, polyamines, and the kinins, among others. All of these elements either affect pathogenic invaders directly or enhance the effectiveness of host reactions to them. Other internal elements of innate immunity include phagocytic cells such as granulocytes, macrophages, and microglial cells of the central nervous system, which participate in the destruction and elimination of foreign material that has penetrated the physical and chemical barriers.

Acquired Immunity. Acquired immunity is more specialized than innate immunity, and it supplements the protection provided by innate immunity. Acquired immunity came into play relatively late, in evolutionary terms, and is present only in vertebrates.

Although an individual is born with the capacity to mount an immune response to a foreign invader, immunity is acquired by contact with the invader and is specific to that invader only, hence the term *acquired immunity*. The initial contact with the foreign agent (*immunization*) triggers a chain of events that leads to the activation of certain cells (*lymphocytes*) and the synthesis of proteins, some of which exhibit specific reactivity against the foreign agent. By this process, the individual acquires the immunity to withstand and resist a subsequent attack by, or exposure to, the same offending agent.

The discovery of acquired immunity predates many of the concepts of modern medicine. It has been recognized for centuries that people who did not die from such life-threatening diseases as bubonic plague or smallpox were subsequently more resistant to the disease than were people who had never been exposed to it. The rediscovery of acquired immunity is credited to the English physician Edward Jenner, who, in the late eighteenth century, experimentally induced immunity to smallpox. If Jenner performed his experiment today, his medical license would be revoked, and he would be the defendant in a sensational malpractice lawsuit: he inoculated a young boy with pus from a lesion of a dairy maid who had cowpox, a relatively benign disease that is related to smallpox. He then deliberately exposed the boy to smallpox. This exposure failed to cause disease! Because of the protective effect of inoculation with cowpox (*vaccinia*, from the Latin word *vacca*, meaning cow), the process of inducing acquired immunity has been termed *vaccination*.

The concept of vaccination or immunization was expanded by Louis Pasteur and Paul Ehrlich almost 100 years after Jenner's experiment. By the year 1900, it had become apparent that immunity could be induced against not only microorganisms but also their products. We now know that immunity can be induced against thousands of natural and synthetic compounds, which include metals, chemicals of relatively low molecular weight, carbohydrates, proteins, and nucleotides.

The compound to which the acquired immune response is induced is termed an *antigen*.

Active, Passive, and Adoptive Immunization

Acquired immunity is induced by immunization, which can be achieved in several ways:

1. *Active immunization* refers to immunization of an individual by administration of an antigen.
2. *Passive immunization* refers to immunization through the transfer of specific antibody from an immunized individual to a nonimmunized individual.
3. *Adoptive transfer* (immunization) refers to the transfer of immunity by the transfer of immune cells.

Characteristics of the Immune Response

The acquired immune response has several generalized features that characterize it and serve to distinguish it from other physiologic systems, such as circulation, respiration, or reproduction. These features are as follows:

Specificity: The ability to discriminate among different molecular entities presented to it and to respond only to those uniquely required, rather than making a random, undifferentiated response.

Adaptiveness: The ability to respond to previously unseen molecules that may in fact never have existed before on earth.

Discrimination between "self" and "nonself": A cardinal feature of the specificity of the immune response is its ability to recognize and respond to molecules that are foreign or nonself and avoid making a response to those molecules that are self. This distinction, and the recognition of antigen, is conferred by specialized cells, namely, lymphocytes, which bear on their surface receptors specific for antigen. Moreover, as different lymphocytes bear different receptors specific for different antigens, each cell also bears identical receptors specific for an identical antigen or a portion of the antigen.

Memory: A property shared with the nervous system is the ability to recall previous contact with a foreign molecule and respond to it in a learned manner, that is, a more rapid and larger response. The term used to describe immunologic memory is *anamnestic response*.

When you reach the end of this book you should understand the cellular and molecular bases of these properties of the immune response.

Cells Involved in the Acquired Immune Response

For many years immunology remained an empirical subject in which the effects of injecting various substances into hosts were studied primarily in terms of the products elicited. Most progress came in the form of more quantitative methods for detecting these products of the immune response. A major change in emphasis came in the 1950s with the recognition that *lymphocytes* were the major cellular players in the immune response, and the field of *cellular immunology* came to life.

It is now firmly established that there are three major cell types involved in acquired immunity and that complex interactions among these cell types are required for the expression of the full range of immune responses. Two of these cell types come from a common lymphoid precursor cell but differentiate along different developmental lines. One line matures in the thymus and is referred to as **T cell**; the other matures in the bone marrow and is referred to as **B cell**. Cells of the B and T lymphocyte series differ in many functional aspects but share one of the important properties of the immune response, namely, they exhibit specificity toward an antigen. Thus the major recognition and reaction functions of the immune response are contained within the lymphocytes.

Antigen-presenting cells (APC) such as macrophages and dendritic cells, constitute the third cell type that participate in the acquired immune response. Although these cells do not have antigen-specific receptors as do the lymphocytes, their important function is to process and present the antigen to the specific receptors (T cell receptors [TCR]) on T lymphocytes. The antigen-presenting cells have on their surface two types of special molecules that function in antigen presentation. These molecules, called **MHC class I** and **MHC class II molecules**, are encoded by a set of genes that is also responsible for the rejection or acceptance of transplanted tissue. This set of genes is referred to as the major histocompatibility complex (MHC). The processed antigen is noncovalently bound to MHC class I or class II molecules (or both) and is thus presented to the antigen-specific receptors on the T cell. Antigen presented on MHC class I molecules is presented to and participates in activation of one T cell subpopulation (cytotoxic T cells), while antigen processed and expressed on APCs in the context of MHC class II molecules results in activation of another subpopulation (helper T cells)

In addition, other cell types such as neutrophils and mast cells participate in immune responses. In fact, they participate in both innate immunity and acquired immunity. They are involved primarily in the effector phases of the response. These cells have no specific antigen recognition properties and are activated by various substances, collectively termed **cytokines**, which are released by various cells, including activated antigen-specific lymphocytes.

Clonal Selection Theory

A turning point in immunology came in the 1950s with the introduction of a Darwinian view of the cellular basis of specificity in the immune response. This was the now universally accepted **clonal selection theory** proposed and developed by Jerne and Burnet (both Nobel Prize winners) and by Talmage. The essential postulates of this theory are summarized below.

The specificity of the immune response is based on the ability of its components (namely, antigen-specific T and B lymphocytes) to recognize particular foreign molecules (antigens) and respond to them in order to eliminate them. Inherent in this theory is the need to clonally delete lymphocytes that may be self- or autoreactive. If such a mechanism were absent, autoimmune responses might occur routinely. Fortunately, lymphocytes with receptors that bind to self-antigens are eliminated during the early phases of lymphocyte development, thus ensuring **tolerance** of self (Figure 1.1).

Since, as we have already stated, the immune response is capable of recognizing literally thousands of foreign antigens, how is the response to any one accomplished? In addition to the now-proven postulate that self-reactive clones of lymphocytes are normally deleted, the clonal selection theory proposed that:

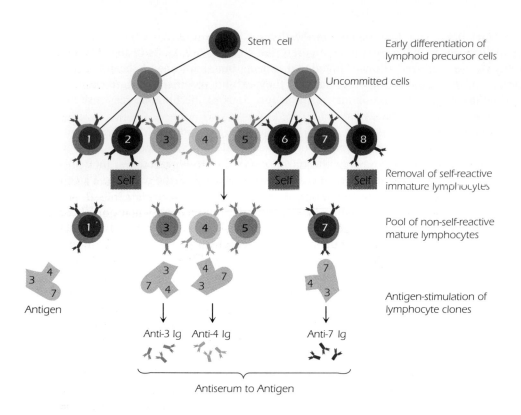

Figure 1.1. Representation of the clonal selection theory of B cells leading to antibody production.

1. T and B lymphocytes of myriad specificities exist before there is any contact with the foreign antigen.

2. The lymphocytes participating in the immune response have ***antigen-specific*** receptors on their surface membranes. As a consequence of antigen binding to the lymphocyte, the cell is activated and releases various products. In the case of B lymphocytes, the receptors are molecules (antibodies) bearing the same specificity as the antibody that the cell will subsequently produce and secrete. T cells have complex receptors denoted as ***T cell receptors*** (TCRs). Unlike the B cell, the T cell products are not the same as their surface receptors but are other protein molecules called cytokines that participate in elimination of the antigen by regulating the many cells needed to mount an effective immune response.

3. Each lymphocyte carries on its surface receptor molecules of only a single specificity as demonstrated in Figure 1.1 for B cells, and holds true also for T cells.

These three postulates describe the existence of a large ***repertoire*** of possible specificities formed by cellular multiplication and differentiation *before* there is any contact with the foreign substance to which the response is to be made.

The introduction of the foreign antigen then selects from among all the available specificities those with specificity for the antigen enabling binding to occur (Figure 1.1). Again, the scheme shown in Figure 1.1 for B cells also applies to T cells. However, T cells have receptors that are not antibodies and secrete molecules other than antibodies.

The remaining postulates of the clonal selection theory account for this process of selection by the antigen from among all the available cells in the repertoire.

4. Immunocompetent lymphocytes combine with the foreign antigen, or a portion of it, termed *epitope*, by virtue of their surface receptors. They are stimulated under appropriate conditions to proliferate and differentiate into clones of cells with the corresponding identical receptors to the particular portion of the antigen, termed ***antigenic determinant*** or ***epitope***. With B cell clones this will lead to the synthesis of antibodies having precisely the same specificity. Collectively, the clonally secreted antibodies constitute the polyclonal antiserum, which is capable of interacting with the multiple epitopes expressed by the antigen. T cells will be similarly selected by appropriate antigens or portions thereof. Each selected T cell will be activated to divide and produce clones of the same specificity. Thus, the clonal response to the antigen will be amplified; the cells will release various ***cytokines***, and subsequent exposure to the same antigen would now result in the activation of many cells or clones of that specificity. Instead of synthesizing and releasing antibodies like the B cells, the T cells synthesize and release cytokines. These cytokines, which are soluble mediators, exert their effect on other cells to grow or become activated and eventually eliminate the antigen. Several distinct regions of an antigen (epitopes) can be recognized: Several different clones of B cells will be stimulated to produce antibody, whose sum total is an antigen-specific antiserum that comprises antibodies of differing specificity (Figure 1.1); all the T cell clones that recognize various epitopes on the same antigen will be activated to perform their function.

A final postulate was added to account for the ability to recognize self-antigens without making a response:

5. Circulating self-antigens that reach the developing lymphoid system before some undesignated maturational step will serve to shut off those cells that recognize it specifically, and no subsequent immune response will be induced.

This formulation of the immune response had a truly revolutionary effect on the field and changed forever our way of looking at and studying immunology. The immune system is, therefore, programmed to induce tolerance to self-antigens using one of several mechanisms discussed in subsequent chapters of this book.

Humoral and Cellular Immunity

There are two arms (branches) of acquired immunity that have different sets of participants and different sets of purposes but with one common aim: to eliminate the antigen. As we shall see later, these two arms interact with each other and collaborate to achieve the final goal of eliminating the antigen. Of these two arms of the acquired immune response, one is mediated mainly by B cells and circulating antibodies, a form of immunity referred to as *humoral* (the word "humors" was formerly used to define body fluids). The other is mediated by T cells that, as we stated before, do not synthesize antibodies but instead synthesize and release various cytokines that affect other cells. Hence this arm of the acquired immune response is termed *cellular* or *cell-mediated immunity*.

Humoral Immunity. Humoral immunity is mediated by serum antibodies, which are the proteins secreted by the B cell compartment of the immune response. B cells are initially activated to secrete antibodies after the binding of antigens to specific membrane *immunoglobulin* (Ig) molecules (*B cell receptors* [BCR]), which are expressed by these cells. It has been estimated that each B cell expresses $\sim 10^5$ BCR of exactly the same specificity. Once ligated, the B cell receives signals to begin making the secreted form of this Ig, a process that initiates the full-blown antibody response whose purpose is to eliminate the antigen from the host. Antibodies are a heterogeneous mixture of serum globulins, all of which share the ability to bind individually to specific antigens. All serum globulins with antibody activity are referred to as immunoglobulins.

All immunoglobulin molecules have common structural features, which enable them to do two things: (1) recognize and bind specifically to a unique structural entity on an antigen, namely, the epitope, and (2) perform a common biologic function after combining with the antigen. Basically, each immunoglobulin molecule consists of two identical light (L) chains and two identical heavy (H) chains linked by disulfide bridges. The resultant structure can be represented schematically as shown below.

The portion of the molecule that binds antigen consists of an area composed of the amino-terminal regions of both H and L chains. Thus, each immunoglobulin molecule is symmetric and is capable of binding two identical eptitopes present on the same antigen molecule or on different molecules.

In addition to differences in the antigen-binding portion of different immunoglobulin molecules, there are other differences, the most important of which are those in the H chains. There are five major classes of H chains (termed γ, μ, α, ε, and δ). On the basis of differences in their H chains, immunoglobulin molecules are divided into five major classes—IgG, IgM, IgA, IgE, and IgD—each of which has several unique biologic properties. For example, IgG is the only class of immunoglobulin that crosses the placenta, conferring the mother's immunity on the fetus, and IgA is the major antibody found in secretions such as tears and saliva. It is important to remember that antibodies in all five classes may possess precisely the

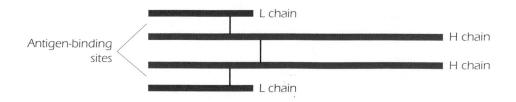

Figure 1.2. Typical antibody molecule composed of two heavy (H) and two light (L) chains. Arrows point to antigen-binding sites.

same specificity against an antigen (antigen-combining regions), while at the same time having different functional (biologic effector) properties.

The binding between antigen and antibody is not covalent but depends on many relatively weak forces, such as hydrogen bonds, van der Waals forces, and hydrophobic interactions. Since these forces are weak, successful binding between antigen and antibody depends on a very close fit over a sizable area, much like the contacts between a lock and a key.

Another important element involved in humoral immunity is the **complement** system. The reaction between antigen and antibody serves to activate this system, which consists of a series of serum enzymes, the end result of which is lysis of the target or enhanced phagocytosis (ingestion of the antigen) by phagocytic cells. The activation of complement (see Chapter 13) also results in the recruitment of highly **phagocytic polymorphonuclear** (PMN) **cells**, which constitute part of the innate immune system. These activities maximize the effective response made by the humoral arm of immunity against invading agents.

Cell-Mediated Immunity. The antigen-specific arm of ***cell-mediated immunity*** consists of the ***T lymphocytes***. Unlike B cells, which produce soluble antibody that circulates to bind its specific antigens, each T cell, bearing many identical antigen receptors ($\sim 10^5$/cell) called ***T cell receptors*** (TCR), circulates directly to the site of antigen and performs its function when interacting with antigen.

There are several subpopulations of T cells, each of which may have the same specificity for an antigenic determinant (i.e., epitope), although each subpopulation may perform different functions. This is analogous to the different classes of immunoglobulin molecules that may have identical specificity but different biologic functions. The functions ascribed to the various subsets of T cells include:

1. **Cooperation with B cells to enhance the production of antibodies.** Such T cells are called ***T helper cells*** (T_H) and function by releasing cytokines that provide various activation signals for the B cells. As mentioned earlier, cytokines are soluble substances or mediators released by cells; such mediators

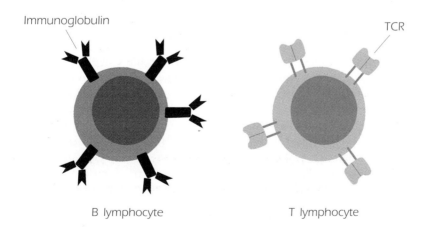

Immunoglobulin

TCR

B lymphocyte

T lymphocyte

Figure 1.3. Antigen receptors expressed as transmembrane molecules on B and T lymphocytes.

released by lymphocytes are also termed lymphokines. A group of low-molecular-weight cytokines has been given the name chemokines. These play a role in inflammatory response as discussed below. Additional information about cytokines is presented in Chapter 12.

2. **Inflammatory effects.** On activation, a certain T cell subpopulation releases cytokines that induce the migration and activation of monocytes and mac-rophages, leading to the so-called *delayed-type hypersensitivity* inflammatory reactions (Chapter 16). Some term this subpopulation of T cells T_{DTH}, for T cells participating in delayed-type hypersensitivity, and others term this sub-population simply T_H.

3. **Cytotoxic effects.** The T cells in this subset become cytotoxic killer cells that on contact with their target, are able to deliver a lethal hit, leading to the death of the target cells. These T cells are termed *T cytotoxic* cells (T_C).

4. **Regulatory effects.** Helper T cells can be divided into different functional subsets which are defined by the cytokines they release. As you will learn in subsequent chapters, these subsets (T_H1, T_H2) have distinct regulatory prop-erties which are mediated by the cytokines they release. Moreover, T_H1 cells can negatively cross-regulate T_H2 cells and vice versa. Similarly, cytokines released by a particular T_H subset can also suppress other effector cells of the immune system leading to a downward modulation or a shutoff in reactivity of those cells. Previously, these suppressor activities were attributed to a third subpopulation of T cells known as T suppressor cells This designation (T suppressor cells) is no longer used to define such cells given our knowledge of the cytokine-mediated regulatory properties of T_H subsets.

5. **Signal via cytokines.** T cells and other cells within the immune system (e.g., macrophages) exert numerous effects on many cells, lymphoid and nonlym-phoid, through many different cytokines that they release. Thus, directly or indirectly T cells communicate and collaborate with many cell types.

For many years immunologists have recognized that cells activated by antigen manifest a variety of effector phenomena. It is only in the last decade or so that they began to appreciate the complexity of events that take place in activation by antigen and communication with other cells. We know today that just mere contact of the T cell receptor with antigen is not sufficient to activate the cell. In fact, at least two signals must be delivered to the antigen-specific T cell for activation to occur: Signal 1 involves the binding of the TCR to antigen, which must be presented in the ap-propriate manner by antigen-presenting cells. Signal 2 involves the ligation of *co-stimulatory molecules* expressed on T cells and antigen-presenting cells. Once this has been achieved, a series of complicated events take place and the activated cell synthesizes and releases cytokines. In turn, these cytokines come in contact with appropriate receptors on different cells and exert their effect on these cells.

Although both the humoral and cellular arms of the immune response have been considered as separate and distinct components, it is important to understand that the response to any particular pathogen may involve a complex interaction between both, as well as the components of innate immunity. All this with the purpose to ensure maximal survival advantage for the host, in eliminating the antigen, and, as we shall see, in protecting the host from mounting an immune response against self.

Generation of Diversity in the Immune Response

The most recent tidal surge in immunologic research represents a triumph of the marriage of molecular biology and immunology. While cellular immunology had delineated the cellular basis for the existence of a large and diverse repertoire of responses, as well as the nature of the exquisite specificity that could be achieved, arguments abounded on the exact genetic mechanisms that enabled all these specificities to become part of the repertoire in every individual of the species.

Briefly, the arguments were as follows:

1. By various calculations the number of antigenic specificities toward which an immune response can be generated could range upward of $10^6 - 10^7$.
2. If every specific response, in the form of either antibodies or T cell receptors, were to be encoded by a single gene, did this mean that over 10^7 genes (one for each specific antibody) would be required in every individual? How was this massive amount of DNA carried intact from individual to individual?

The pioneering studies of Tonegawa (a Nobel laureate) and Leder, using molecular biologic techniques, finally addressed these issues by describing a unique genetic mechanism by which immunologic receptors (BCR) of enormous diversity could be produced with a modest amount of DNA reserved for this purpose.

The technique evolved by nature was one of ***genetic recombination*** in which a protein could be encoded by a DNA molecule composed of a set of recombined minigenes that made up a complete gene. Given small sets of these minigenes, which could be randomly combined to make the complete gene, it was possible to produce an enormous repertoire of specificities from a limited number of gene fragments. (This is discussed in detail in Chapter 6.)

Although this mechanism was first elucidated to explain the enormous diversity of antibodies that are not only released by B cells but that in fact constitute the antigen- or epitope-specific receptors on B cells (BCR), it was subsequently established that the same mechanisms operate in generating diversity of the antigen-specific T cell receptor (TCR). Mechanisms operating in generating diversity of B cell receptors and antibodies are discussed in Chapter 6. Those operating in generating diversity of TCR are discussed in Chapter 9. Suffice it to say at this point that various techniques of molecular biology that not only permit genes to be analyzed, but also to be moved around at will from one cell to another, have continued to provide impetus to the onrushing tide of immunologic progress.

Benefits of Immunology

While we have thus far discussed the theoretical aspects of immunology, its practical applications are of paramount importance for survival and must be part of the education of students of medicine.

The field of immunology has been in the public limelight since the late 1960s, when successful transplantation of the human kidney was achieved. More recently, the spectacular transplantation of the human heart and other major organs, such as the liver, has been the focus of much publicity. Public interest in immunology was intensified by the potential application of the immune response to the detection and management of cancer, and in the 1980s the general public became familiar with some aspects of immunology because of the alarming spread of acquired immune deficiency syndrome (AIDS).

The innate and acquired immune systems play an integral role in the prevention of and recovery from infectious diseases and are, without question, essential to the survival of the individual. Metchnikoff was the first to propose in the 1800s that phagocytic cells formed the first line of defense against infection and that the inflammatory response could actually subserve a protective function for the host. Indeed, innate immune responses are responsible for the detection and rapid destruction of most infectious agents that are encountered in the daily life of most individuals. We now know that innate immune responses operate in concert with adaptive immune responses to generate antigen-specific effector mechanisms that lead to the death and elimination of the invading pathogen. Chapter 21 presents information concerning how our immune systems respond to microorganisms and how methods developed to exploit these mechanisms are used as immunoprophylaxis. Vaccination against infectious diseases has been an effective form of prophylaxis. Immunoprophylaxis against the virus that causes poliomyelitis has reduced this dreadful disease to relative insignificance in many parts of the world and, for the first time, a previously widespread disease, smallpox, has been eliminated from the face of the earth. Recent developments in immunology hold the promise of immunoprophylaxis against malaria and several other parasitic diseases that plague many parts of the world and affect billions of people. Vaccination against diseases of domestic animals promises to increase the production of meat in developing countries, while vaccination against various substances that play roles in the reproductive processes in mammals offers the possibility of long-term contraception in humans and companion animals such as cats and dogs.

Damaging Effects of the Immune Response

The enormous survival value of the immune response is self-evident. Acquired immunity directed against a foreign material has as its ultimate goal the elimination of the invading substance. In the process some tissue damage may occur as the result of the accumulation of components with nonspecific effects. This damage is generally temporary. As soon as the invader is eliminated, the situation at that site reverts to normal.

There are instances in which the power of the immune response, although directed against innocuous foreign substances such as some medications, inhaled pollen particles, or substances deposited by insect bites, produces a response that may result in severe pathologic consequences and even death. These responses are known collectively as *hypersensitivity* reactions or *allergic reactions*. An understanding of the basic mechanisms underlying these disease processes has been fundamental in their treatment and control, but in addition has contributed much to our knowledge of the normal immune response. The latter is true because both use essentially identical mechanisms, but, in hypersensitivity, these mechanisms are misdirected or out of control.

Hypersensitivity reactions are divided into two major categories depending on the effectors involved. The first category is antibody-mediated and, as the term implies, may be passively transferred to another individual by the appropriate amount and type of antibody in serum. This group is, in turn, divided into three classes, depending on the specific underlying mechanisms involving either mast cells or complement and neutrophils. These reactions have in common a rapidity of response that can range from minutes to a few hours following the exposure to antigen and are therefore generally grouped as *immediate hypersensitivity reactions*.

The second major category of hypersensitivity reactions is mediated largely by T cells with consequent involvement of monocytes and is appropriately termed *cell-mediated immunity* (CMI). These responses are much more delayed in appearance, generally taking approximately 18-24 hours to reach their full expression, and have been traditionally referred to as *delayed-type hypersensitivity* (DTH). Unlike antibody-mediated hypersensitivity, which can be transferred from a sensitive individual to a nonsensitive individual via serum, DTH may be transferred not by serum but by T cells.

It should be reemphasized that all these hypersensitivity reactions have a normal counterpart in that the same mechanisms may operate to protect the host from invading organisms. It is only when the consequences of these responses are misplaced or exaggerated that deleterious effects to the host occur, and we call them hypersensitivity reactions.

Regulation of the Immune Response

Given the complexity of the immune response and its potential for inducing damage, it is self-evident that it must operate under carefully regulated conditions, as does any other physiologic system. These controls are multiple and include feedback inhibition by soluble products as well as cell–cell interactions of many types that may either heighten or reduce the response. The net result is to maintain a state of *homeostasis* such that when the system is perturbed by a foreign invader, enough response is generated to control the invader, and then the system returns to equilibrium; in other words, the immune response is shut down. However, its memory of that particular invader is retained so that a more rapid and heightened response will occur should the invader return.

Disturbances in these regulatory mechanisms may be caused by conditions such as congenital defect, hormonal imbalance, or infection, any of which may have disastrous consequences. AIDS may serve as a timely example; it is associated with an infection of T lymphocytes that participate in regulating the immune response. As a result of infection with the human immunodeficiency virus (HIV), which causes AIDS, there is a decrease in occurrence and function of one vital subpopulation of T cells that leads to immunologic deficiency, which renders the patient powerless to resist infections by microorganisms that are normally benign.

An important form of regulation concerns the prevention of immune responses against self-antigens. For various reasons, this regulation may be defective, thus causing an immune response against "self" to be mounted. This type of immune response is termed *autoimmunity* and is the cause of diseases such as some forms of arthritis, thyroiditis, and diabetes that are very difficult to treat.

The Future of Immunology

A peek into the world of the future for the student of immunology suggests many exciting areas in which the application of molecular biologic techniques promises significant dividends. To cite just a few examples, we may take vaccine development and control of the immune response. In the former, rather than the laborious, empirical search for an attenuated virus or bacterium for use in immunization, it is now possible to obtain the nucleotide sequence of the DNA that encodes the component of the invading organism that accounts for the protective immune response. Educated guesses can be made from these sequences about the segment of the encoded protein most likely to be responsible for inducing immunity. Such segments can be readily synthesized and tested for use as a vaccine. Alternatively, the recent advent of DNA vaccines (currently experimental) which involve the injection of DNA vectors that encode immunizing proteins, may revolutionize vaccination protocols in the not-too-distant future. The identification of various genes and the proteins that they are encoding makes it possible to design vaccines against a wide spectrum of biologically important compounds. For example, there are already clinical trials to evaluate the efficacy of antifertility vaccines [anti-HCG (human chorionic gonadotropin)] and other gonadotropic hormones.

Another area of great promise is the characterization and synthesis of various cytokines that enhance and control the activation of various cells associated with the immune response as well as with other functions of the body. Techniques of gene isolation, clonal reproduction, the polymerase chain reaction and biosynthesis have contributed to rapid progress. Powerful and important modulators have been synthesized by the methods of recombinant DNA technology and are being tested for their therapeutic efficacy in a variety of diseases, including many different cancers. In some cases, cytokine research efforts have already moved from the bench to the bedside with the development of therapeutic agents used to treat patients.

Finally, and probably one of the most exciting areas, is the technology to genetically engineer various cells and even whole animals, such as mice, that lack one or more specific trait (gene knockout) or carry a specific trait (transgenic). These, and other immune-based experimental systems are the subject of Chapter 5. They allow the immunologist to study the effects of these traits on the immune system and on the body as a whole with the aim of understanding the intricate regulation, expression, and function of the immune response and with the ultimate aim of controlling the trait to the benefit of the individual. Thus, our burgeoning understanding of the functioning of the immune system, combined with the recently acquired ability to alter and manipulate its components, carries enormous implications for the future of humankind.

In the following chapters we attempt a more detailed account of the workings of the immune system, beginning with its cellular components, followed by a description of the structure of the reactants and the general methodology for measuring their reactions. This is followed by chapters describing the formation and activation of the cellular and molecular components of the immune apparatus required to generate a response. A discussion of the control mechanisms that regulate the scope and intensity of the immune response completes the description of the basic nature of immunity. Included in this section of the book is a chapter on cytokines B, the soluble mediators that regulate immune responses and play a significant role in hematopoiesis. Next are chapters that deal with the great variety of diseases involving immunologic components. These vary from ineffective or absent immune response (immunodeficiency) to those produced by aberrant immune responses (hypersensitivity) to responses to self-antigens (autoimmunity). This is followed by chapters that describe the role of the immune response in transplantation, and antitumor reactions. A final chapter discusses the spectrum of microorganisms that challenge the immune system and how immune responses are mounted in a vigilant, orchestrated crusade to protect the host from infectious diseases. Included is a discussion of immunopro-phylaxis using vaccines that protect us from variety of pathogenic organisms. With-out question, the successful use of vaccines helped to revolutionize the field of medicine in the twentieth century. What lies ahead as we begin the twenty-first century are research efforts related to the development of crucial new vaccines to protect mankind from pathogenic viruses and microorganisms that have either just begun to plague us (most notably, HIV) or have yet to be identified.

With the enormous scope of the subject and the extraordinary richness of detail available, we have made every effort to adhere to fundamental elements and basic concepts required to achieve an integrated, if not extensive, understanding of the immune response. If the reader's interest has been aroused, many current books, articles, and reviews, and growing numbers of educational Internet sites, including the one that supports this textbook (see Forward section for URL), are available to flesh out the details on the scaffolding provided by this book.

2

ELEMENTS OF INNATE AND ACQUIRED IMMUNITY

● INTRODUCTION

Every living organism is confronted by continual intrusions from its environment. Our immune systems are equipped with a network of mechanisms to safeguard us from infectious microorganisms that would otherwise take advantage of our bodies for their own survival. In short, the immune system has evolved as a surveillance system poised to initiate and maintain protective responses against virtually any harmful foreign elements we might encounter. These defenses range from physical barriers, such as a cell wall, to highly sophisticated systems, such as the acquired immune response. This chapter describes the defense systems: the elements that constitute the defense, the participating cells and organs, and the action of the participants in the immune response to foreign substances that invade the body.

In vertebrates, immunity against microorganisms and their products, or against other foreign substances that may invade the body, is divided into two major categories: *innate* or *nonspecific immunity* (sometimes referred to as *natural immunity*) and *acquired immunity*. These two types of immunity and their origins, components, and interrelationships are discussed in the present chapter.

● INNATE (NONSPECIFIC) IMMUNITY

Innate immunity is present from birth and consists of many factors that are relatively nonspecific; that is, they operate against almost any substance that threatens the body. Some of the important nonspecific factors that are part of innate immunity are given below.

Physiologic and Chemical Barriers (Skin and Mucous Membranes)

Most organisms and foreign substances cannot penetrate intact skin, but can enter the body if the skin is damaged. Some microorganisms can enter through sebaceous glands and hair follicles. However, the *acid pH* of sweat and sebaceous secretions and the presence of various fatty acids and hydrolytic enzymes (e.g., lysozymes) all have some antimicrobial effect, therefore minimizing the importance of this route of infection. In addition, soluble proteins, including the *interferons* and certain members of the *complement system* found in the serum, contribute to nonspecific immunity. Interferons are a group of proteins made by cells in response to virus infection, which essentially induce a generalized antiviral state in surrounding cells. Activation of complement components in response to certain microorganisms results in a controlled enzymatic cascade, which targets the membrane of pathogenic organisms and leads to their destruction. Additional information about interferons and complement is included in Chapters 12 and 13, respectively.

An important innate mechanism involved in the protection of many areas of the body, including the respiratory and gastrointestinal tracks, involves the simple fact that surfaces in these areas are covered with mucous. In these areas, the *mucous-membrane barrier* traps microorganisms, which are then swept away, by ciliated epithelial cells, toward the external openings. The hairs in the nostrils and the cough reflex are also helpful in preventing organisms from infecting the respiratory tract. Alcohol consumption, cigarette smoking, and narcotics suppress this entire defense system.

The elimination of microorganisms from the respiratory tract is aided by pulmonary or alveolar macrophages, which, as we shall see later, are phagocytic cells able to engulf and destroy some microorganisms. Other microorganisms that have penetrated the mucous-membrane barrier can be picked up by macrophages or otherwise transported to lymph nodes, where many are destroyed.

The environment of the gastrointestinal tract is made hostile to many microorganisms by other innate mechanisms, including the *hydrolytic enzymes in saliva*, the low pH of the stomach, and the *proteolytic enzymes and bile* in the small intestine. The low pH of the vagina serves a similar function.

Cellular Defenses

Once an invading microorganism has penetrated the various physiologic and chemical barriers, the next line of defense consists of various specialized cells whose purpose is to destroy the invader. There are several cell types that fulfill this function. The developmental pathways of hematopoietic cells and interrelationship between the various cell types that will be discussed in this and subsequent chapters is shown diagrammatically in Figure 2.1.

Phagocytosis and Extracellular Killing

As part of its innate immunity, the body has developed defenses mediated by specialized cells that destroy the invading microorganism by first ingesting and then destroying it (phagocytosis), or by killing it extracellularly (without ingesting it).

Endocytosis and Phagocytosis. Two innate immune mechanisms result in the internalization of foreign macromolecules and cells and can lead to their intra-

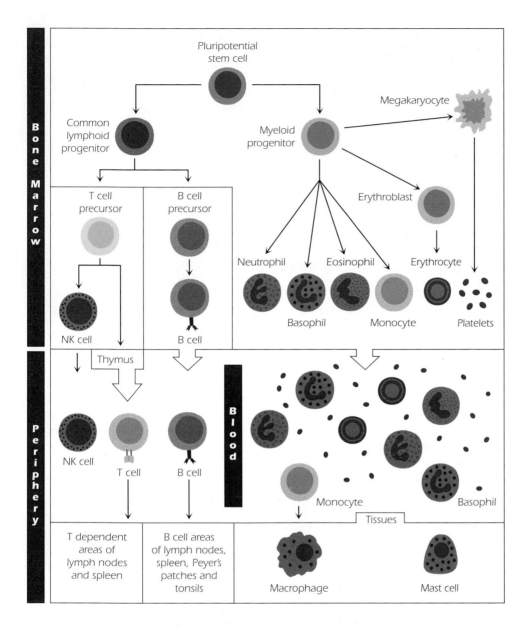

Figure 2.1. The developmental pathway of various cell types from pluripotential bone marrow stem cells.

cellular destruction and elimination. These involve processes called endocytosis and phagocytosis.

ENDOCYTOSIS. *Endocytosis* is the process whereby macromolecules present in extracellular tissue fluid are ingested by cells. This can occur either by *pinocytosis*, which involves nonspecific membrane invagination, or *receptor-mediated endocytosis*, a process involving the selective binding of macromolecules to specific membrane receptors. In both cases, ingestion of the foreign macromolecules generates endocytic vesicles filled with the foreign material, which then fuse with acidic compartments called **endosomes**. Edosomes then fuse with **lysosomes** containing degradative enzymes (e.g., nucleases, lipases, proteases) to reduce the ingested macromolecules to small breakdown products, including nucleotides, sugars, and peptides (Figure 2.2).

PHAGOCYTOSIS. **Phagocytosis** is the ingestion and destruction by individual cells of invading foreign particles, such as bacteria. Many microorganisms release substances that attract phagocytic cells. Phagocytosis may be enhanced by a variety of factors that make the foreign particle an easier target. These factors, collectively referred to as **opsonins** (Greek "prepare food for," consist of antibodies and various serum components of complement (see Chapter 13). After ingestion, the foreign particle is entrapped in a phagocytic vacuole (phagosome) that fuses with lysosomes (Figure 2.2). The latter release their powerful enzymes that digest the particle.

The phagocytic cells consist of certain types of polymorphonuclear leukocytes, phagocytic monocytes (i.e., macrophages), and fixed macrophages of the reticuloendothelial system. On activation, all these cells release soluble substances called cytokines, which have different effects on various cells (see Chapter 12).

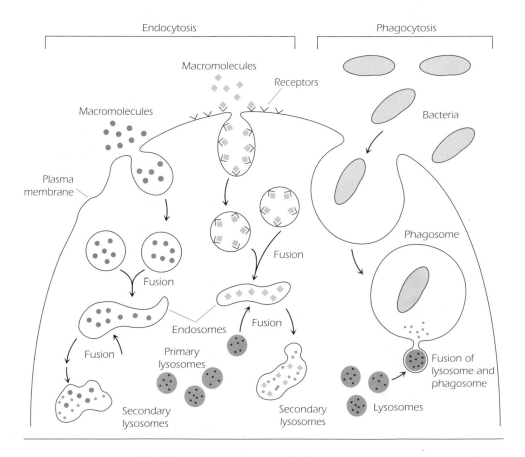

Figure 2.2. Endocytosis and phagocytosis by macrophages.

Polymorphonuclear Leukocytes. **Polymorphonuclear leukocytes** (PMN) are a population of cells also referred to as **granulocytes**. These include the basophils, mast cells, eosinophils, and neutrophils. Granulocytes are short-lived phagocytic cells that containing the enzyme-rich lysosomes, which can facilitate destruction of infectious microorganisms (Figure 2.3). They also produce peroxide and superoxide radicals that are toxic to many microorganisms. Some lysosomes also contain bactericidal proteins such as lactoferrin. PMN play a major role in protection against infection. Defects in PMN function are accompanied by chronic or recurrent infection.

Macrophages. **Macrophages** (see Figure 2.4) are phagocytes derived from blood monocytes. The monocyte itself is a small, spherical cell with few projections, abundant cytoplasm, little endoplasmic reticulum, and many granules. Following migration of monocytes from the blood to various tissues, they undergo further differentiation into a variety of histologic forms, all of which play a role in phagocytosis. These include the following:

Kupffer cells in the liver; large cells with many cytoplasmic projections
Alveolar macrophages, in the lung
Splenic macrophages, in the white pulp

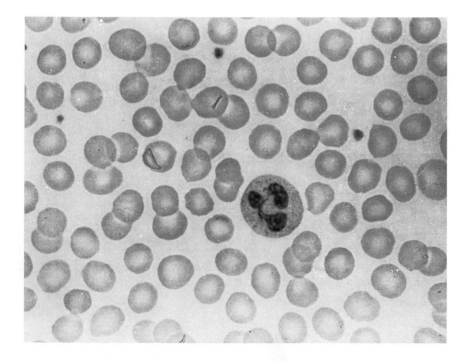

Figure 2.3. A polymorphonuclear leukocyte (surrounded by erythrocytes in a blood smear) with a trilobed nucleus and cytoplasmic granules. ×950. (Photograph courtesy of Dr. A. C. Enders, School of Medicine, University of California, Davis).

Peritoneal macrophages, free-floating in peritoneal fluid

Microglial cells, in the central nervous tissue

Reticuloendothelial System. Each of these macrophage populations is included in the ***reticuloendothelial system*** (RES), which is widely distributed throughout the body. The major function of the RES is to phagocytize microorganisms and foreign substances that are in the bloodstream and in various tissues. The RES also functions in the destruction of aged and imperfect cells, such as erythrocytes.

Although associated with diverse names and locations, many of these cells share common features, such as the ability to bind and engulf particulate materials and antigens. Because of their location along capillaries, these cells are most likely to make first contact with invading pathogens and antigens, and, as we shall see later, play a large part in the success of innate as well as acquired immunity.

In general, cells of the macrophage series have two major functions. One of their functions, as their name ("large eater") implies, is to engulf and, with the aid of all the degradative enzymes in their lysosomal granules, break down trapped materials into simple amino acids, sugars, and other substances for excretion or reutilization. Thus, these cells play a key role in the removal of bacteria and parasites from the blood. As we shall see in later chapters, the second major function of the macrophages is to take up antigens, process them by denaturation or by partial digestion, and present them, on their surfaces, to specific T cells. Thus ***macrophages also function as antigen-presenting cells***.

Dendritic cells in spleen and lymph nodes, interdigitating cells of the thymus, and Langerhans cells in the skin are derived from the same hematopoietic precursor cells as monocytes. Although these cells are not very phagocytic, they are potent antigen-presenting cells.

From this outline, it can be seen that monocytes play a central role in innate immunity. They also play a key role in the afferent or induction limb of the acquired immune response (by initiating T-cell responses). Finally, the macrophages play a role in the efferent or effector limb of the acquired immune response as the end cells that become activated by T-cell-released cytokines that enhance their killing of pathogens.

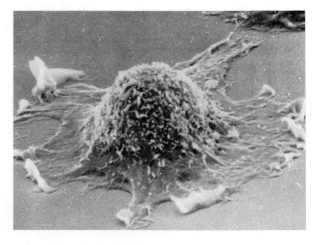

Figure 2.4. A scanning electron micrograph of a macrophage with ruffled membranes and a surface covered with microvilli. ×5200. (Photograph courtesy of Dr. K. L. Erickson, School of Medicine, University of California, Davis; reproduced with permission from Lippincott/ Harper and Row).

Extracellular Killing. Altered features of the membranes of abnormal cells, such as those found on virus-infected or cancer cells, are recognized by cytotoxic or killer cells that destroy the target cell not by phagocytosis but by releasing biologically potent molecules that, within a very short time, kill the target cell. Such killer cells include the antigen-specific ***cytotoxic T lymphocytes***, which constitute an arm of the acquired immune response (discussed in more detail in Chapter 10), and the ***natural-killer*** (NK) ***cells***, a component of the innate immune system.

NK cells probably play a role in the early stages of viral infection or tumorogenesis, before the cytotoxic T lymphocytes of the acquired immune response increase in numbers. NK cells are large granular lymphocytes that are able to lyse certain virus-infected cells and tumor cells without prior stimulation. Unlike cytotoxic T lymphocytes, which recognize antigen-bearing target cells via their Tcell receptors (TCRs), NK cells lack antigen-specific TCRs. How, then, do they seek and destroy their targets? They do this by using a mechanism involving cell–cell contact, which allows them to determine whether a potential target cell has lost a particular self-antigen (major histocompatibility complex [MHC] class I). MHC class I is expressed on virtually all normal nucleated cells. NK cells express non-TCR-related receptors called ***killer-cell inhibitory receptors*** (KIR), which bind to class I MHC antigen. When ligated, KIRs protect the target from being killed by NK cells. Virus-infected or transformed (tumor) cells have reduced class I MHC antigen on their surfaces. Thus, when such cells encounter NK cells, they fail to effectively engage these killer cell inhibitory receptors and therefore become susceptible to NK cell-mediated cytotoxicity (Figure 2.5)

Killing is achieved by the release of various cytotoxic molecules. Some of these molecules cause the formation of pores in the membrane of the target cell leading to its lysis. Other molecules enter the target cell and cause ***apoptosis*** (programmed cell death) of the target cell by enhanced fragmentation of its nuclear DNA. The activity of NK cells is highly increased by soluble mediators such as interleukin-2

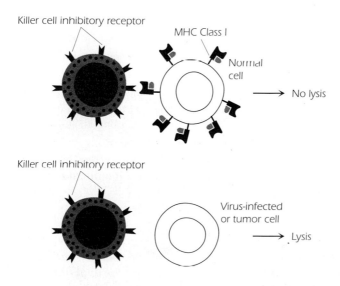

Figure 2.5. Schematic representation of NK cell inhibitory receptors and killing.

(IL-2), IL-12, and interferons. As discussed in Chapter 12, interferons α and β are antiviral proteins synthesized and released by leukocytes, fibroblasts, and virally infected cells; IL-2 and interferon γ are released by activated T lymphocytes.

Inflammation

An important function of phagocytic cells and phagocytosis is their participation in inflammation, a major component of the body's defense mechanism. The important aspects of inflammation are summarized below.

Inflammation is a complex process initiated by tissue damage caused by endogenous factors (such as tissue necrosis or bone fracture) as well as exogenous factors. These include various types of damage such as mechanical injury (e.g., cut), physical injury (e.g., burn), chemical injury (e.g., exposure to a corrosive chemical), biologic injury (e.g., infection by microorganisms; see Chapter 21), and immunologic injury (e.g., hypersensitivity reactions; see Chapters 14–16). The inflammatory response constitutes an important part of both innate and acquired immunity. It has evolved as a protective response against injury and infection. Although in certain cases, such as hypersensitivity, inflammation becomes the problem rather than the solution to a problem such as infection, by and large the inflammatory response is protective; it is one of the major responses to injury and constitutes a process aimed at bringing the injured tissue back to its normal state.

The hallmark signs of inflammation, described almost 2000 years ago, are *swelling* (*tumor*), redness (*rubor*), heat (*calor*), pain (*dolor*), and loss of function of the inflamed area. Within minutes after injury, the inflammatory process begins with the activation and increased concentration of pharmacologically powerful substances such as a group of proteins known as *acute-phase proteins*. The acute phase response induces both localized and systemic responses. *Localized inflammatory responses* are generated, in part, due to the *activation of the clotting, kinin-forming, and fibrolytic pathways.*

The *kinins* have several important effects:

1. They act directly on local smooth muscle and cause muscle contraction.
2. They act on axons to block nervous impulses, leading to a distal muscle relaxation.
3. Most importantly, they act on vascular endothelial cells, causing them to contract, leading to increase in vascular permeability, and to express endothelial cell adhesion molecules (ECAMs), leading to leukocyte adhesion and extravasation.
4. Kinins are very potent nerve stimulators and are the molecules most responsible for pain (and itching) associated with inflammation.

Kinins are rapidly inactivated following their activation by proteases that are generated during these localized responses.

The *systemic inflammatory response* includes the induction of *fever* (discussed below), *increased white blood cell production, increased synthesis of hydrocortisone and adrenocorticotropic hormone (ACTH), and production of the acute-phase proteins* (also see Chapter 12). An important member of the acute-phase proteins is the C-reactive protein. This protein binds to the membrane of certain microorganisms and activates the complement system (Chapter 13). This results in the lysis of the microorganism or its enhanced phagocytosis by phagocytic cells, as well as other important biologic functions, as we shall see later.

Cytokines play a key role in the inflammatory response. Interleukin-1 and interleukin-6 (IL-1, IL-6), and *tumor necrosis factor* α (TNF-α) (Chapter 12) are among the most important cytokines involved. These cytokines released by activated macrophages induce adhesion molecules on the walls of vascular endothelial cells to which neutrophils, monocytes, and lymphocytes adhere before moving out of the vessel through a process called *extravasation*, to the affected tissue. These cytokines also induce coagulation and increased vascular permeability. Other cytokines, including IL-8 and interferon-γ, exert additional effects such as increased chemotaxis for leukocytes and increased phagocytosis. All these effects result in the ***accumulation of fluid (edema) and leukocytic cells in the injured areas***. These, in turn, amplify the response further since additional biologically active compounds are transported in the fluid and also are released from the accumulated cells, attracting and activating still more cells.

Most of the cells involved in the inflammatory response are phagocytic cells, first consisting mainly of the ***polymorphonuclear leukocytes***, which accumulate within 30–60 minutes, phagocytize the intruder or damaged tissue, and release their lysosomal enzymes in an attempt to destroy the intruder. If the cause of the inflammatory response persists beyond this point, within 56 hours the area will be infiltrated by mononuclear cells, which include macrophages and lymphocytes. The macrophages supplement the phagocytic activity of the polymorphonuclear cells, thus adding to the defense of the area. Moreover, the macrophages participate in the processing and presentation of antigen to lymphocytes, which respond to the foreign antigens of the invader by inducing the acquired immune response specific to those antigens.

If the injury or the invasion by microorganisms continues, the inflammatory response will be supplemented and augmented by elements of acquired immunity that include antibodies and cell-mediated immunity. The antibody response initiates the complement cascade in which pharmacologically active compounds are activated and released. These include substances that increase vascular permeability and capillary dilatation, as well as chemotactic substances that attract and activate additional polymorphonuclear cells and antigen-specific lymphocytes. The lymphocytes themselves are capable of destroying some foreign invaders. More importantly, they release cytokines that activate macrophages and other cells to participate in destroying and removing the invaders.

Many substances activated during the inflammatory process participate in repairing the injury. During this remarkable process many cells, including leukocytes, are being destroyed. The macrophages that are present in the area phagocytize the debris and the inflammation subsides; the tissue may be restored to its normal state, or scar tissue may be formed.

Sometimes it is difficult or impossible to remove the causes of inflammation. This results in chronic inflammation, which occurs in situations of chronic infection such as tuberculosis or chronic activation of the immune response, exemplified by rheumatoid arthritis or glomerulonephritis. In these cases the inflammatory response continues and can be only temporarily modified by the administration of antiinflammatory agents such as aspirin, ibuprofen, or cortisone. These and other drugs act on several of the metabolic pathways involved in the elaboration and activation of some of the pharmacologic mediators of inflammation. However, they do not affect the root cause of the inflammation, and so when withdrawn, the symptoms may return.

Fever

Although fever is one of the most common manifestations of infection and inflammation, there is still limited information about the significance of fever in the course of infection in mammals. Fever is caused by many bacterial products, most notably the endotoxins of gram-negative bacteria, generally as the result of the release of endogenous **pyrogens** that derive from monocytes and macrophages and include **interleukin-1** (IL-1) and **certain interferons**.

Biologically Active Substances

Many tissues synthesize substances that are harmful to microorganisms. Examples are **degradative enzymes, toxic free radicals, acids, inhibitors of growth, and, as noted above, acute-phase proteins, and interferons**. Thus, depending on their ability to synthesize these substances, certain tissues may have a heightened resistance to infection by some microorganisms.

Innate (nonspecific) immunity is related to many attributes of the individual that are determined genetically. Differences in innate immunity among various people may, in addition, be attributed to age, race, and the hormonal and metabolic conditions of the individual.

 ## ACQUIRED IMMUNITY

In contrast to innate immunity, which is an attribute of every living organism, acquired immunity is a more specialized form of immunity. It developed late in evolution and is found only in vertebrates. The various elements that participate in innate immunity do not exhibit specificity against the foreign agents they encounter; by contrast, acquired immunity always exhibits such specificity. As its name implies, acquired immunity is a consequence of an encounter with a foreign substance. The first encounter with a foreign substance that has penetrated the body triggers a chain of events that induces an immune response with specificity against that foreign substance.

Although an individual is genetically endowed with the capacity to mount an immune response against a certain substance, acquired immunity is usually exhibited only after an initial encounter with the substance. Thus, acquired immunity develops only after exposure to, or immunization with, a given substance.

There are two major types of cells that participate in acquired immunity: B lymphocytes (so named because they originate in the bone marrow), and T lymphocytes (named for their differentiation in the thymus). B lymphocytes and T lymphocytes are responsible for the specificity exhibited by the acquired immune response. B lymphocytes synthesize and secrete into the bloodstream antibodies with specificity against the foreign substance. This is termed **humoral immunity**. The T lymphocytes, which also exhibit specificity against the foreign substance by virtue of their receptors (TCR), do not make antibodies, but perform various effector functions when APCs bring antigens into the secondary lymphoid organs. T lymphocytes also interact with B cells and help the latter make antibodies; they activate macrophages, and they have a central role in the development and regulation of acquired immunity (see Chapter 10). Acquired immunity mediated by T lymphocytes is termed *cellular immunity* or *cell-mediated immunity* (CMI). As we have seen, macrophages are phagocytic cells; they do not exhibit specificity against a given substance, but they are involved in the processing and presentation of foreign substances to T lymphocytes and activation of T lymphocytes (see Chapters 9 and 10).

CELLS INVOLVED IN THE IMMUNE RESPONSE

In mammalian species, circulating blood cells have their common origin in a small cluster of cells that move from the primitive yolk sac to the fetal liver, and finally to the bone marrow, where they take up permanent residence. These cells are the *hematopoietic stem cells*, so called because they are the undifferentiated cells from which all the other specialized cells in blood develop (Figure 2.1).

The undifferentiated stem cells are characterized by an ability to proliferate throughout life as a self- renewing reservoir that replenishes the pool of more mature cells as they are used up during normal activity. These early stem cells are considered to be *pluripotent*; that is, they are capable of developing into any of the more differentiated lines of cells, under the influence of a variety of soluble factors that control both the extent and the direction of maturation. Isolation and characterization of these earliest hematopoietic and pluripotent stem cells have been facilitated by the recent identification on their surface of a molecule referred to as CD34. The "CD" nomenclature is discussed in Chapter 5. Expression of CD34 is quite specific for early progenitor cells (as well as endothelial cells). Once differentiation in any direction has occurred, the cells become committed to make only a single type of cell lineage; that is, they become *unipotent* and CD34 expression decreases. One pathway of differentiation (*myeloid differentiation*) starts from a bone marrow stem cell that gives rise to differentiated precursors and culminates with erythrocytes, thrombocytes (platelets), and the various granule- containing cells of the granulocyte-monocyte series. The other pathway of differentiation (*lymphocytic differentiation*) leads to two distinct cell types called B and T lymphocytes.

Lymphatic Organs

The lymphatic organs are those organs in which lymphocyte maturation, differentiation, and proliferation take place. They are generally divided into two categories. The primary or central lymphoid organs are those in which the maturation of T and B lymphocytes into antigen-recognizing lymphocytes occurs. As we shall see in subsequent chapters, developing T and B cells acquire their antigen-specific receptors in primary lymphoid organs. Mature B and T lymphocytes migrate from the bone marrow and thymus, respectively, through the bloodstream to the peripheral lymphoid tissues, including the lymph nodes, spleen, and gut-associated lymphoid tissues such as the tonsils. These secondary (peripheral) lymphoid organs are those organs in which antigen-driven proliferation and differentiation take place (Figure 2.6).

Primary Lymphoid Organs. There are two major primary lymphoid organs, one in which the T cells develop and the other in which the B cells develop.

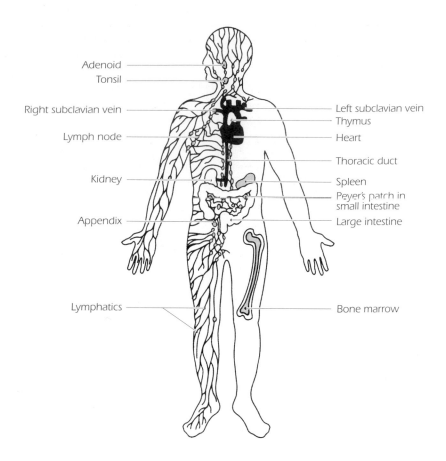

Adenoid
Tonsil
Right subclavian vein
Lymph node
Kidney
Appendix
Lymphatics

Left subclavian vein
Thymus
Heart
Thoracic duct
Spleen
Peyer's patch in small intestine
Large intestine
Bone marrow

Figure 2.6. The distribution of lymphoid tissues in the body. (Reproduced with permission from F. S. Rosen and R. S. Geha, *Case Studies in Immunology*, Garland Publishing, Inc.)

THYMUS GLAND. Progenitor cells from the bone marrow migrate to the primary lymphoid organ, the thymus gland, where they differentiate into T lymphocytes. The thymus gland (Figure 2.7) is a bilobed structure, derived from the endoderm of the third and fourth pharyngeal pouches. During fetal development, the size of the thymus increases. The growth continues until puberty. Thereafter, the thymus undergoes atrophy with aging.

The thymus is a *lymphoepithelial* organ and consists of epithelial cells organized into cortical (outer) and medullary (central) areas that are infiltrated with lymphoid cells (*thymocytes*). The cortex is densely populated with lymphocytes of various sizes, most of which are immature, and scattered macrophages involved in clearing apoptotic thymocytes. T lymphocytes mature in the cortex and migrate to the medulla, where they encounter macrophages and dendritic cells. Here they undergo thymic selection, which results in the development of mature, functional T cells, which then leave to enter the peripheral blood circulation, through which they are transported to the secondary lymphoid organs (T-cell development is discussed in detail in Chapter 9). It is in these secondary lymphoid organs that the T cells encounter and respond to foreign antigens.

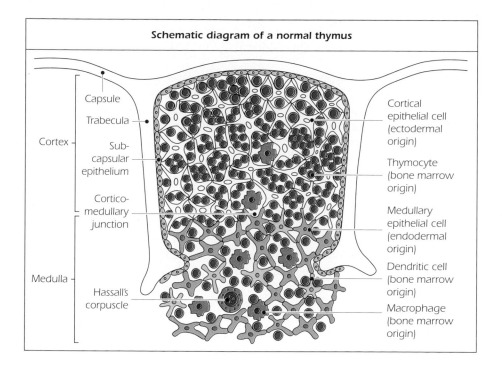

Figure 2.7. The cellular organization of the thymus. (Reproduced with permission from F. S. Rosen and R. S. Geha, *Case Studies in Immunology*, Garland Publishing, Inc.)

Maturation of the T lymphocyte involves the commitment of a given T cell to recognize and respond to a given determinant or *epitope* of a foreign antigen. This recognition is achieved by a specific receptor on the T cell (TCR), which is acquired during differentiation in the thymus (Chapter 9). Mature T lymphocytes in the medulla are capable of responding to foreign antigens in the same way that they would respond in the secondary lymphoid organs. However, the thymus is considered to be a primary lymphoid organ because it is the site where T cells differentiate to express TCR.

The maturation of T lymphocytes occurs mainly during fetal development and for a short time after birth. In mice, removal of the thymus gland from a neonate results in a severe reduction in the quantity and quality of T lymphocytes and produces a potentially lethal wasting disease. Removal of the thymus from an adult generally has little effect on the quantity and quality of the T lymphocytes, which have already matured and populated the secondary lymphoid organs. However, adult thymectomy could, in time, result in a deficiency of T cells if there is acute death of the T cells that originally populated the secondary lymphoid organs (such as following whole-body irradiation). Without the thymus there would be no mechanism for repopulation of the secondary organs with new T lymphocytes.

Only 5–10% of maturing lymphocytes survive and eventually leave the thymus; 90–95% of all thymocytes die in the thymus. It is clear that the lymphocytes that die have developed specificity to self-structures or have failed to make functional receptors and therefore, are eliminated. The lymphocytes that survive develop specificity against foreign antigens. This is discussed in detail in Chapter 9.

BURSA OF FABRICIUS AND BONE MARROW. A primary lymphoid organ was first discovered in birds. In birds, B cells undergo maturation in the bursa of Fabricius. This organ, situated near the cloaca, consists of lymphoid centers that contain epithelial cells and lymphocytes. Unlike the lymphocytes in the thymus, these lymphocytes consist solely of antibody-producing B cells (see Chapter 7).

Mammals do not have a bursa of Fabricius. Consequently, much work has been directed toward the identification of a mammalian equivalent of the primary lymphoid organ in which B cells develop and mature. It is now clear that in embryonic life, B cells differentiate from hematopoietic stem cells in the fetal liver. After birth and for the life of the individual this function moves to the bone marrow, a structure that is considered to be a primary lymphoid organ with functions equivalent to that of the avian bursa. Each mature B lymphocyte bears antigen-specific receptors that have a structure and specificity identical to the antibody later synthesized by that B cell. The mature B cells are transported by the circulating blood to the secondary lymphoid organs, where they encounter and respond to foreign antigens.

Secondary Lymphoid Organs. The **secondary lymphoid organs** consist of certain structures in which mature, antigen-committed lymphocytes are stimulated by antigen to undergo further division and differentiation. The major secondary lymphoid organs are the spleen and the lymph nodes. In addition, tonsils, appendix, clusters of lymphocytes distributed in the lining of the small intestine (Peyer's patches), and lymphoid aggregates spread throughout mucosal tissue are considered secondary lymphoid organs. These secondary lymphoid organs comprise various areas of the body, such as the linings of the digestive tract, the respiratory and genitourinary tracts, the conjunctiva, and the salivary glands, where mature lymphocytes interact with antigen and differentiate to synthesize specific antibodies. These mucosal secondary lymphoid organs have been given the name **mucosa-associated lymphoid tissue** (MALT). Those lymphoid tissues associated with the gut are **gut-associated lymphoid tissue** (GALT); those associated with the bronchial tree are termed **bronchus-associated lymphoid tissue** (BALT).

The secondary lymphoid organs have two major functions: they are highly efficient in trapping and concentrating foreign substances, and they are the main sites of production of antibodies and the induction of antigen-specific T lymphocytes.

THE SPLEEN. The spleen (Figure 2.8) is the largest of the secondary lymphoid organs. It is highly efficient in trapping and concentrating foreign substances carried in the blood. It is the major organ in the body in which antibodies are synthesized and from which they are released into the circulation. The spleen is composed of **white pulp**, rich in lymphoid cells, and **red pulp**, which contains many sinuses as well as large quantities of erythrocytes and macrophages, some lymphocytes, and a few other cells.

The areas of white pulp are located mainly around small arterioles, the peripheral regions of which are rich in T cells, with B cells present mainly in **germinal centers**. Approximately 50% of spleen cells are B lymphocytes; 30–40% are T lymphocytes. Following antigenic stimulation, the germinal centers contain large numbers of B cells and **plasma cells**. These cells synthesize and release antibodies.

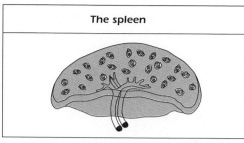

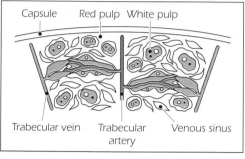

 Figure 2.8. Schematic views and light micrograph of a section of spleen. (Reproduced with permission from F. S. Rosen and R. S. Geha, *Case Studies in Immunology*, Garland Publishing, Inc.)

LYMPH NODES. Lymph nodes (Figure 2.9A,B) are small ovoid structures (normally less than 1 cm in diameter) found in various regions throughout the body. They are close to major junctions of the lymphatic channels (see Figure 2.9A,B), which are connected to the thoracic duct. The thoracic duct transports lymph and lymphocytes to the vena cava, the vessel that carries blood to the right side of the heart (see Figure 2.10) from where it is redistributed throughout the body.

The lymph nodes are composed of a medulla with many sinuses and a cortex, which is surrounded by a capsule of connective tissue (Figure 2.9A). The *cortical region contains primary lymphoid follicles*. Following antigenic stimulation, these structures enlarge to form secondary lymphoid follicles with germinal centers that contain dense populations of lymphocytes (mostly B cells) that are undergoing mitosis. In response to antigen stimulation, antigen-specific B cells proliferate within these germinal centers also undergo a process known as *affinity maturation* to generate clones of cells with higher affinity receptors (antibody) for the antigenic epitope that triggered the initial response (see Chapter 7). The remaining antigen–nonspecific B cells are pushed to the outside to form the *mantle zone*. The *deep cortical area or paracortical region contains T cells and dendritic cells*. Antigens are brought into these areas by dendritic cells which present antigen fragments to T cells, events that result in activation of the T cells. The medullary area of the lymph node contains antibody-secreting plasma cells that have traveled from the cortex to the medulla via lymphatic vessels.

Lymph nodes are highly efficient in trapping antigen that enters through the afferent lymphatic vessels. In the node, the antigen interacts with macrophages, T cells, and B cells, and that interaction brings about an immune response, manifested by the generation of antibodies and antigen-specific T cells. Lymph, antibodies, and cells leave the lymph node through the efferent lymphatic vessel, which is just below the medullary region.

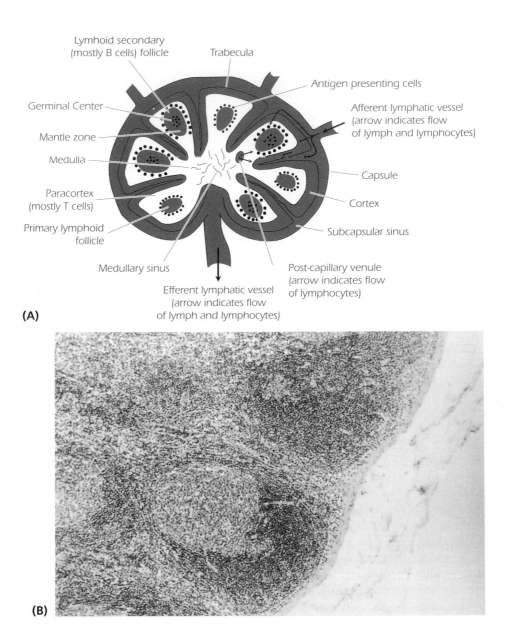

(A)

(B)

Figure 2.9. **(A)** A diagrammatic representation of a section of a lymph node. **(B)** A section through a lymph node showing the capsule, the subcapsular sinus, the medulla (**upper left**), and the cortex with secondary follicles containing germinal centers. Also shown (**upper right**) is a follicle without a germinal center. ×140. (Photograph courtesy of Dr. A. C. Ender, School of Medicine, University of California, Davis).

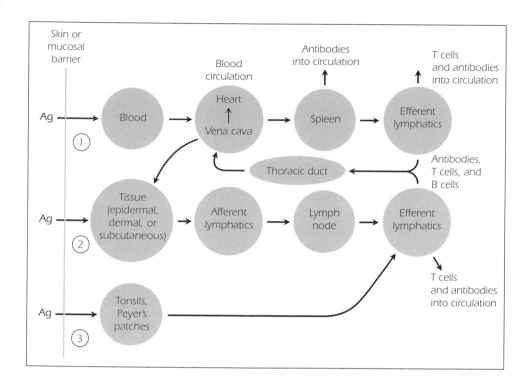

Figure 2.10. Circulation of lymph and fate of antigen following penetration through (1) the bloodstream, (2) the skin, and (3) the gastrointestinal or respiratory track.

LYMPHOCYTE RECIRCULATION

Blood lymphocytes enter the lymph nodes through **postcapillary venules** and leave the lymph nodes through efferent lymphatic vessels that eventually converge in the thoracic duct. This duct empties into the vena cava, the vessel that returns the blood to the heart, thus providing for the continual recirculation of lymphocytes.

The spleen functions in a similar manner. Arterial blood lymphocytes enter the spleen through the hilus and pass into the **trabecular artery**, which along its course becomes narrow and branched. At the farthest branches of the trabecular artery, capillaries lead to lymphoid nodules. Ultimately, the lymphocytes return to the venous circulation through the **trabecular vein**. Like lymph nodes, the spleen contains efferent lymphatic vessels through which lymph empties into the lymphatics from which the cells continue their recirculation through the body and back to the afferent vessels.

The migration of lymphocytes between various lymphoid and nonlymphoid tissue and their homing to a particular site is highly regulated by means of various **cell-surface adhesion molecules** (CAMs) and receptors to these molecules. Thus, except in the spleen where small arterioles end in the parenchyma, allowing access to blood lymphocytes, blood lymphocytes must generally cross the endothelial vascular lining of postcapillary vascular sites termed **high endothelial venules** (HEVs).

This process is called **extravasation**. Recirculating lymphocytes selectively bind to specific receptors on the HEV of lymphoid tissue or inflammatory tissue spaces and appear to completely ignore other vascular endothelium. Moreover, it appears that a selective binding of finer specificity operates between the HEV and various distinct subsets of lymphocytes, further regulating the migration of lymphocytes into the various lymphoid and nonlymphoid tissue. Recirculating monocytes and granulocytes also express adhesion molecule receptors and migrate to tissue sites using a similar mechanism.

The traffic of lymphocytes between lymphoid and nonlymphoid tissue ensures that on exposure to an antigen, the antigen and the lymphocytes specific to that antigen are sequestered in the lymphoid tissue, where the lymphocytes undergo proliferation and differentiation. The differentiated cells (memory cells) leave the lymphoid organ and are disseminated in the body to reconcentrate at the site where antigen persists and, at that place, exert their protective function.

⬤ THE FATE OF ANTIGEN AFTER PENETRATION

The reticuloendothelial system is designed to trap foreign antigens that have penetrated the body and to subject them to ingestion and degradation by the phagocytic cells of the system. Also, there is constant movement of lymphocytes throughout the body, and this movement permits deposition of lymphocytes in strategic places along the lymphatic vessels. The system not only traps antigens but also provides loci (the secondary lymphoid organs) where antigen, macrophages, T cells, and B cells can interact within a very small area to initiate an immune response.

The fate of an antigen that has penetrated the physical barriers and the cellular and antibody components of the ensuing immune response are shown in Figure 2.10. Three major routes may be followed by an antigen after it has penetrated the interior of the body:

1. The antigen may enter the body through the **bloodstream**. In this case, it is carried to the spleen, where it interacts with **antigen-presenting cells** (APC), such as dendritic cells, and macrophages. B cells also serve as APCs, although their major role is to produce antibodies in response to the antigenic stimulus. APCs are essential in the activation of antigen-specific T cells. The interactions between APCs and T cells ultimately leads to activation of B and T cell and hence, the immune response. The spleen then releases the antibodies directly into the circulation. Lymphocytes also leave the spleen through the efferent lymphatics, to reenter the circulation via the thoracic duct.

2. The antigen may lodge in the **epidermal, dermal, or subcutaneous tissue**, where it may cause an inflammatory response. From these tissues the antigen, either free or trapped by antigen-presenting cells, is transported through the afferent lymphatic channels into the regional draining lymph node. In the lymph node, the antigen, macrophages, dendritic cells, T cells, and B cells interact to generate the immune response. Eventually, antigen-specific T cells and antibodies, which have been synthesized in the lymph node, enter the circulation and are transported to the various tissues. Antigen-specific T cells, B cells, and antibodies also enter the circulation via the thoracic duct.

3. The antigen may enter the **gastrointestinal or respiratory tract**, where it lodges in the mucosa-associated lymphoid tissue (MALT). There it will interact with macrophages and lymphocytes. Antibodies synthesized in these organs are deposited in the local tissue. In addition, lymphocytes entering the efferent lymphatics are carried through the **thoracic duct** to the circulation and are thereby redistributed to various tissue.

The induction of an acquired immune response necessitates the interaction of the foreign antigen with lymphocytes that recognize that specific antigen. It has been estimated that in a naive (nonimmunized) animal, only one in every 10^3-10^5 lymphocytes is capable of recognizing a typical antigen. Therefore, the probability that an antigen will encounter these cells is very low. The problem is compounded by the fact that, for synthesis of antibody to ensue, two different kinds of lymphocyte, the T lymphocyte and B lymphocyte, each with specificity against this particular antigen, must interact.

Statistically, the chances for the interaction of specific T lymphocytes with their particular antigen, and then with B lymphocytes specific for the same antigen, are very low. However, nature has devised an ingenious mechanism for bringing these cells into contact with antigen: the antigen is carried via the draining lymphatics to the secondary lymphoid organs. In these organs, the antigen is exposed on the surface of fixed specialized cells. Because both T and B lymphocytes circulate at a rather rapid rate, making the rounds every several days, some circulating lymphocytes with specificity for the particular antigen should pass by the antigen within a relatively short time. When these lymphocytes encounter the antigen for which they are specific, the lymphocytes become activated, and the acquired immune response, with specificity against this antigen, is triggered.

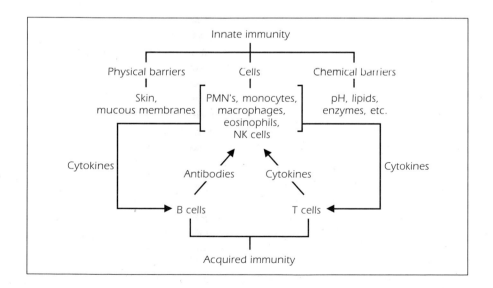

Figure 2.11. The interrelationship between innate and acquired immunity.

INTERRELATIONSHIP BETWEEN INNATE AND ACQUIRED IMMUNITY

The innate and acquired arms of the immune system have developed a beautiful interrelationship. The intricate and ingenious communication system through the various cytokines and cell adhesion molecules allows components of innate and acquired immunity to interact, send each other signals, activate each other, and work in concert toward the final goal of destroying and eliminating the invading microorganism and its products. The interrelationship between innate and acquired immunity is shown in Figure 2.11.

SUMMARY

1. There are two forms of immunity: (*a*) innate, or nonspecific, and (*b*) acquired.

2. Many elements participate in innate immunity; these include various physical barriers, chemical barriers, and cellular components.

3. Two major types of cells participate in acquired immunity: (*a*) B lymphocytes and (*b*) T lymphocytes.

4. Macrophages constitute an essential part of the reticuloendothelial system and function to trap, process, and present antigen to T lymphocytes, thus assuming an important function in both innate and acquired immunity.

5. B and T lymphocytes have receptors that are specific for particular antigens and, thus, constitute the components of acquired immunity that are responsible for antigenic specificity.

6. B and T lymphocytes develop in primary lymphoid organs. B cells differentiate within the bone marrow and exit as functional cells; T cells differentiate partly within the bone marrow and ultimately mature to become functional cells in the thymus before migrating to the peripheral lymphoid organs.

7. Mature B and T lymphocytes differentiate and proliferate in response to antigenic stimulation. These events generally take place in secondary lymphoid organs.

8. B lymphocytes synthesize and secrete antibodies; but T lymphocytes do not. However, T lymphocytes participate in cell-mediated immunity; they help B cells make antibodies by providing them with soluble growth and differentiation factors (cytokines) needed for B cell activation. They also participate in various other regulatory aspects of the immune response by releasing cytokines.

9. Lymphocytes continuously recirculate between the blood, lymph, lymphoid organs, and tissues. Receptors on lymphocytes interact with cell adhesion molecules (CAMs) located on specialized high endothelial venules (HEVs) facilitating extravasation to tissue sites where immune-cell activation occurs.

REFERENCES

Gallatin M, St John TP, Siegelman M, Reichert R, Butcher CE, Weissman I (1986): Lymphocyte homing receptors. *Cell* 44:673.

Lanier, LL (1998): NK cell receptors. *Annu Rev Immunol* 16:359.

Mackay CR, Imhof BA (1993): Cell adhesion in the immune system. *Immunol Today* 14:99.

Miller JFAP (1993): The role of the thymus in immunity: thirty years of progress. *Immunologist* 1:9.

Stekel, DJ, Parker, CE, Nowak, MA (1997): A model for lymphocyte recirculation. *Immunol Today* 18:216.

 # REVIEW QUESTIONS

For each question, choose the ONE BEST answer or completion.

1. Which of the following generally does not apply to bone marrow (a primary lymphoid organ) and secondary lymphoid organs?
   A) cellular proliferation
   B) differentiation of lymphocytes
   C) cellular interaction
   D) antigen-dependent response
   E) None of the above.

2. Which of the following apply uniquely to secondary lymphoid organs?
   A) presence of precursor B and T cells
   B) circulation of lymphocytes
   C) terminal differentiation
   D) cellular proliferation
   E) All of the above.

3. Which of the following does not apply to "innate" immune mechanisms?
   A) absence of specificity
   B) activation by a stimulus
   C) involvement of multiple cell types
   D) a memory component

4. Which of the following is the major function of the lymphoid system?
   A) innate immunity
   B) inflammation
   C) phagocytosis
   D) acquired immunity
   E) None of the above.

5. Removal of the bursa of Fabricius from a chicken results in
   A) a markedly decreased number of circulating T lymphocytes.
   B) anemia.
   C) delayed rejection of skin graft.
   D) low serum levels of antibodies in serum.
   E) all of the above.
   F) none of the above.

6. The germinal centers found in the cortical region of lymph nodes and the peripheral region of splenic periarteriolar lymphatic tissue
   A) support the development of immature B and T cells.
   B) function in the removal of damaged erythrocytes from the circulation.
   C) act as the major source of stem cells and thus help to maintain hematopoiesis.
   D) provide an infrastructure that on antigenic stimulation contains large populations of B lymphocytes and plasma cells.
   E) are the sites of NK-cell differentiation.

7. Which of the following is correct?
   A) NK cells proliferate in response to antigen.
   B) NK cells kill their target cells by phagocytosis and intracellular digestion.
   C) NK cells are a subset of polymorphonuclear cells.
   D) NK-cell killing is extracellular.
   E) NK cells are particularly effective against certain bacteria.

Answers to Review Questions

1. *D* Cellular proliferation, differentiation of lymphocyte, and cellular interactions can take place in bone marrow (or bursa of Fabricius). However, antigen-dependent responses occur in the secondary lymphoid organs, such as the spleen and lymph nodes.

2. *C* Terminal differentiation of B cells into plasma cells occurs only in secondary lymphoid organs, such as the spleen and lymph nodes. Circulation of lymphocytes and cellular proliferation (but not antigen-dependent responses of terminal differentiation) also take place in the primary lymphoid organs, such as the bursa of Fabricius, or its equivalent, and the thymus. The bone marrow is the site where pluripotential stem cells differentiate into precursor B and T cells.

3. *D* Innate immunity has none of the antigenic specificity exhibited by acquired immunity. It is activated by such stimuli as the invasion of the foreign particles into the body. Innate immunity involves multiple cell types, such as those of the monocytic series (macrophages) and those of the granulocytic series (neutrophils, eosinophils, etc.).

4. *D* The major function of the lymphoid system is the recognition of foreign antigen by lymphocytes, which leads to the acquired immune response. Functions such as phagocytosis and inflammation do not necessarily require the lymphoid system, and they constitute part of innate immunity.

5. *D* Removal of the bursa of Fabricius from a chicken results in low levels of antibodies in serum, since this organ serves as a primary lymphoid organ in which B lymphocytes (which eventually synthesize and secrete antibodies) undergo maturation. The removal of the organ will not result in a marked decrease in the number of circulating T lymphocytes, nor will it result in anemia, characterized by a marked decrease in erythrocyte count, since erythrocytes undergo maturation outside the bursa. Bursectomy has no effect on rejection of skin grafts.

6. *D* On antigenic stimulation, the germinal centers contain large populations of B lymphocytes undergoing mitosis and plasma cells secreting antibodies. Virgin immunocompetent lymphocytes are developed in the primary lymphoid organs, not in the secondary lymphoid organs, such as the spleen and lymph nodes. Germinal centers do not participate in the removal of damaged erythrocytes, nor are they a source of stem cells; the latter are found in the bone marrow.

7. *D* NK cells are large granular lymphocytes. Their number does not increase in response to antigen. Their killing is extracellular, and their target cells are virus-infected cells or tumor cells. They are not particularly effective against bacterial cells.

3

IMMUNOGENS AND ANTIGENS

● INTRODUCTION

Acquired immune responses arise as a result of exposure to foreign stimuli. The compound that evokes the response is referred to either as "antigen" or as "immunogen." The distinction between these terms is functional. An *antigen* is any agent capable of binding specifically to components of the immune response, such as lymphocytes and antibodies. By contrast, an *immunogen* is any agent capable of inducing an immune response. The distinction between the terms is necessary because there are many compounds that are incapable of inducing an immune response, yet they are capable of binding with components of the immune system that have been induced specifically against them. Thus, all immunogens are antigens, but not all antigens need be immunogens. This difference becomes obvious in the case of low-molecular-weight compounds, a group of substances that includes many antibiotics and drugs. By themselves, these compounds are incapable of inducing an immune response, but when they are coupled with much larger entities, such as proteins, the resultant conjugate induces an immune response that is directed against various parts of the conjugate, including the low-molecular-weight compound. When manipulated in this manner, the low-molecular-weight compound is referred to as a *hapten* (from the Greek *hapten*, which means "to grasp"); the high-molecular-weight compound to which the hapten is conjugated is referred to as a *carrier*. Thus, a hapten is a compound that, by itself, is incapable of inducing an immune response, but against which an immune response can be induced by immunization with the hapten conjugated to a carrier.

In this chapter we deal with some attributes of compounds that render them immunogenic and antigenic.

REQUIREMENTS FOR IMMUNOGENICITY

A substance must possess the following characteristics to be immunogenic: (*a*) **foreignness**, (*b*) **high molecular weight**, (*c*) chemical complexity, and, in most cases, (*d*) **degradability**.

Foreignness

Animals normally do not respond immunologically to "self." Thus, for example, if a rabbit is injected with its own serum albumin, it will not mount an immune response; it recognizes the albumin as self. By contrast, if rabbit serum albumin is injected into a guinea pig, the guinea pig recognizes the rabbit serum albumin as "foreign" and mounts an immune response against it. To prove that the rabbit, which did not respond to its own serum albumin, is immunologically competent, it can be injected with guinea pig albumin. The competent rabbit will mount an immune response to guinea pig serum albumin because it recognizes the substance as foreign. Thus, the first requirement for a compound to be immunogenic is foreignness. The more foreign the substance, the more immunogenic it is.

In general, compounds that are part of self are not immunogenic to the individual. However, there are exceptional cases in which an individual mounts an immune response against his or her own tissues. This condition is termed **autoimmunity** (see Chapter 17).

High Molecular Weight

The second requirement that determines whether a compound is immunogenic is that it must have a certain minimal molecular weight. In general, compounds that have a molecular weight less than 1000 Da (e.g., penicillin, progesterone, aspirin) are not immunogenic; those of molecular weight between 1000 and 6000 Da (e.g., insulin, adrenocorticotropic hormone [ACTH]) may or may not be immunogenic; and those of molecular weight **greater than 6000 Da** (e.g., albumin, tetanus toxin) **are generally immunogenic**.

Chemical Complexity

The third characteristic necessary for a compound to be immunogenic is a certain degree of physicochemical complexity. Thus, for example, various homopolymers of amino acids, such as a polymer of lysine of molecular weight 30,000 Da, are seldom good immunogens. Similarly, a homopolymer of poly-γ-D-glutamic acid (the capsular material of *Bacillus anthracis*) of molecular weight 50,000 Da is not immunogenic. This absence of immunogenicity is because these compounds, although of high molecular weight, are not sufficiently chemically complex. However, if the complexity is increased by the attachment of various moieties, such as dinitrophenol or other low-molecular-weight compounds, which, by themselves, are not immunogenic, to the epsilon amino group of polylysine, the entire macromolecule becomes immunogenic. The resulting immune response is directed not only against the coupled low-molecular-weight compounds but also against the high-molecular-weight homopolymer. In general, an increase in the chemical complexity of a compound is accompanied by an increase in its immunogenicity. Thus, copolymers of several amino acids such as polyglutamic, alanine, and lysine (poly-GAT) tend to be highly immunogenic.

Because many immunogens are proteins, it is important to understand the structural features of these molecules. Each of the four levels of protein contribute to their immunogenicity. The acquired immune response recognizes many structural features and chemical properties of compounds. For example, antibodies can recognize various structural features of a protein, such as its **primary structure** (the amino acid sequence), **secondary structures** (the structure of the backbone of the polypeptide chain, such as an α-helix or β-pleated sheet), and **tertiary structures** (formed by the three-dimensional configuration of the protein, which is conferred by the folding of the polypeptide chain and held by disulfide bridges, hydrogen bonds, hydrophobic interactions, etc.) (Figure 3.1A). They can also recognize **quaternary structures** (formed by the juxtaposition of separate parts if the molecule is composed of more than one protein subunit) (Figure 3.1B).

Degradability

In order for most antigens to stimulate immune responses (B- or T-cell-mediated), interactions between antigen-presenting cells (APC) and helper T cells must occur. APCs must first degrade the antigen through a process known as **antigen processing** (enzymatic degradation of antigen) before they can express antigenic epitopes on their surface and stimulate antigen-specific helper T cells. The antigen-presenting cells have structures referred to as major histocompatibility complex (MHC) proteins to which "processed" fragments of the protein can bind noncovalently. This complex is then "presented" to receptors on T cells that in turn are activated. This mechanism is discussed in detail in Chapters 8 and 10. Regarding susceptibility to enzymatic degradation, on one hand the substance has to be sufficiently stable so that it can reach the site of interaction with B cells or T cells necessary for the immune response; on the other hand—and this is particularly true for proteins—the substance must be susceptible to partial enzymatic degradation that takes place during antigen "processing" by presenting cells such as macrophages. Indeed, it has been repeatedly demonstrated that peptides composed of D-amino acids, which are resistant to enzymatic degradation, are not immunogenic, whereas their L-isomers are susceptible to enzymes and are immunogenic. These observations are of particular importance with respect to proteins. By contrast, carbohydrates are not processed or presented and are thus unable to activate T cells, although they can activate B cells.

In general, a substance must have all four of these characteristics to be immunogenic; it must be foreign to the individual to whom it is administered, have a relatively high molecular weight, possess a certain degree of chemical complexity, and be degradable.

Haptens

Substances called **haptens** fail to induce immune responses in their native form due to their low-molecular-weight and their chemical simplicity. These compounds are not immunogenic unless they are **conjugated** to high-molecular-weight, physiochemically complex **carriers**. Thus, an immune response can be evoked to thousands of chemical compounds—those of high molecular weight and those of low molecular weight provided the latter is conjugated to high molecular weight complex carriers.

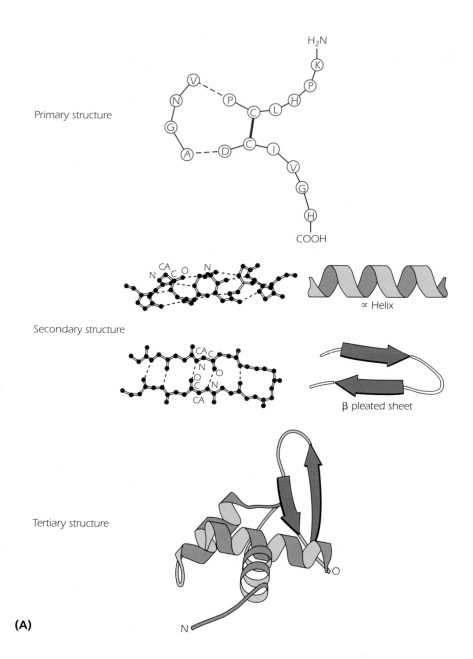

Primary structure

Secondary structure

Tertiary structure

(A)

Figure 3.1A. Levels of protein organizational structure. The primary structure is indicated by the linear arrangement of amino acids (using single letter code) and includes any intrachain disulfide bonds as shown. The secondary structure derives from the folding of the polypeptide chain into α helices and β pleated sheets. The tertiary structure, shown as a ribbon diagram, is formed by the folding of regions between secondary features.

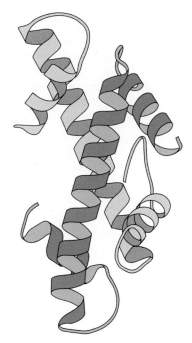

(B) Quaternary structure

Figure 3.1B. The quaternary structure results from the association of two or more polypeptide chains, which form a polymeric protein. [Adapted from P. Sun and J.C. Boyington (1998): Current Protocols in Protein Science. New York: Wiley, with permission.]

Immune responses have been demonstrated against all the known biochemical families of compounds—carbohydrates, lipids, proteins, and nucleic acids—as well as to drugs, antibiotics, food additives, cosmetics, and small synthetic peptides.

Further Requirements for Immunogenicity

Several other factors play roles in determining whether a substance is immunogenic. The ***genetic makeup*** (genotype) of the immunized individual plays an important role in determining whether a given substance will stimulate an immune response. Genetic control of immune responsiveness is largely ***controlled by genes mapping within the MHC***. Another factor that plays a crucial role in the immunogenicity of substances relates to the B and T cell repertoires of an individual. Acquired immune responses are triggered following the binding of antigenic epitopes to antigen-specific receptors on B and T lymphocytes. If an individual lacks a particular clone of lymphocytes consisting of cells bearing the identical antigen-specific receptor needed to respond to the stimulus, an immune response to that antigen will not take place. Finally, practical issues such as the ***dosage and route of administration*** of antigens play a role in determining whether the substance is immunogenic. Insufficient doses of antigen may not stimulate an immune response either because the amount administered fails to activate enough lymphocytes or because such a dose renders the responding cells unresponsive. The latter phenomenon induces a state of tolerance to that antigen (discussed further in Chapter 11). Aside from the need to administer a threshold amount of antigen to induce an immune response, the **number of doses administered** also affects the outcome of the immune response generated. As discussed below, repeated administration of antigen is required to stimulate a strong immune response. Finally, the route of administration can affect the outcome of the immunization strategy because this determines which organs and cell populations will be involved in the response. Intravenously administered antigens are carried first to the spleen, whereas those administered using the subcutaneous route travel to the local or draining lymph nodes. Since immune responses depend upon multiple cellular interactions, the type and extent of the immune response is affected by the cells populating the organ in which the antigen is ultimately delivered.

The stringent requirements given above constitute a portion of the delicate control mechanisms, expanded and elaborated in subsequent chapters, which, on one hand, trigger the acquired immune response and, on the other hand, protect the individual from responding to substances in cases where such responses are detrimental.

 ## PRIMARY AND SECONDARY RESPONSES

The first exposure of an individual to an immunogen is referred to as the **priming immunization**. As we shall see in subsequent chapters, many events take place during this primary immunization—cells "process" antigen, triggering antigen-specific lymphocytes to proliferate and differentiate. T lymphocyte subsets interact with other subsets and induce the latter to differentiate into T lymphocytes with specialized function. T lymphocytes also interact with B lymphocytes, inducing them to synthesize and secrete antibodies. The first measurable immune response is called the **primary response**.

A second exposure to the same immunogen results in a **secondary response**. This second exposure may occur after the response to the first immune event has leveled off or has totally subsided (within weeks or even years). The secondary response differs from the primary response in many respects. Most notably and biologically relevant is the much **quicker onset** and the much **higher magnitude** of the response. In a sense, this secondary (and subsequent) exposure behaves as if the body "remembers" that it had been previously exposed to that same immunogen. In fact, secondary and subsequent responses exploit the expanded number of antigen-specific lymphocytes generated in response to the primary immune response. Thus, the increased arsenal of responding lymphocytes accounts, in part, for the magnitude of the response observed. The secondary response is also called the **memory** or **anamnestic** response and the B and T lymphocytes that participate in the memory response are termed **memory cells**. The kinetics of antibody production following immunization are given in detail in Chapter 4 and Figure 4.13.

 ## ANTIGENICITY AND ANTIGEN-BINDING SITE

An immune response induced by an antigen generates antibodies or lymphocytes that react specifically with the antigen. The antigen-binding site of an antibody or a receptor on a lymphocyte has a unique structure that allows a complementary "fit"

to some structural aspect of the specific antigen. The portion of the immunoglobulin that specifically binds to the antigenic determinant or epitope is concentrated in several **hypervariable regions** of the molecule that forms the **complementarity-determining region** (CDR). Additional structural features of the immunoglobulin molecule are described in Chapter 4.

Various studies indicate that the size of an epitope that combines with the CDR on a given antibody is approximately equivalent to 5–7 amino acids. These dimensions were calculated from experiments that involved the binding of antibodies to polysaccharides, as well as to peptide epitopes. Such dimensions would also be expected to correspond roughly to the size of the complementary antibody-combining site, termed **paratope**, and indeed this expectation has been confirmed by X-ray crystallography.

The size of an epitope that binds to a specific T cell is somewhat larger since it contains an area that binds to the MHC proteins of the antigen-presenting cell (an area referred to as **agretope**) and an area that binds to the specific receptor on the T cell, forming a trimolecular complex (TCR–antigen–MHC). Thus the size of the epitope (including the agretope) is approximately equivalent to 8–15 amino acid residues.

EPITOPES RECOGNIZED BY B CELLS AND T CELLS

It was demonstrated over 25 years ago that when the peptide glucagon (a pancreatic hormone used as a model antigen) was used to immunize an inbred strain of guinea pigs, the antibody response was directed to the N-terminal half and the T cell response was directed to the C-terminal half of the peptide, implying that B and T cells recognize different epitopes. However, when the same peptide was used to immunize guinea pigs of different inbred strains, the recognition was reversed, implying that there really were not different physicochemical attributes that distinguished the interaction with B or T cells. Other examples show that B cells and T cells can recognize the same epitope. These examples notwithstanding, there is a large body of evidence pointing out that the properties of many epitopes recognized by B cells differ from those recognized by T cells (Table 3.1).

 T A B L E 3.1. Antigen Recognition by B and T Cells

Characteristic	B cells	T cells
Antigen interaction	B-cell receptor (membrane Ig) binds Ag	T-cell receptor binds Ag + MHC
Nature of antigens	Protein, polysaccharide, lipid	Peptide
Binding soluble antigens	Yes	No
Epitopes recognized	Accessible, sequential, or nonsequential	Internal linear peptides produced by antigen processing (proteolytic degradation)

In general, membrane-bound antibody (epitope receptors) present on **B cells** recognizes and ***binds free antigen in solution***. Thus, the epitopes on the antigen are on the "outside" of the molecule, accessible for interaction with the B cell receptor. Terminal side chains of polysaccharides and hydrophilic portions on protein molecules generally constitute B-cell epitopes. Such ***epitopes may be composed of sequential*** (Figure 3.2) or ***nonsequential amino acids*** (Figure 3.3). Noncontiguous residues along a polypeptide chain can be brought together by the folded conformation of the protein as shown in Figure 3.3. Such nonsequential B-cell epitopes are also called conformational determinants.

In contrast to B cells, ***T cells are unable to bind soluble antigen***. The interaction of an epitope with the T-cell receptor requires prior "processing" of the antigen, and the association of an area of the processed antigen with MHC molecules present on the surface of the antigen-presenting cell. Figure 3.4 illustrates the structural organization of a class I MHC bound to an antigenic peptide. Generally such "processed" epitopes are internal denatured linear hydrophobic areas of proteins. Polysaccharides do not yield such areas and indeed are not known to bind or activate T cells. By contrast, such areas are obtained following processing of proteins. Thus polysaccharides contain solely B cell recognizable epitopes, whereas proteins contain both B and T cell recognizable epitopes (Table 3.1).

Antigenic epitopes may have the characteristics shown schematically in Figure 3.5. Thus, they may consist of a single epitope (hapten) or have varying numbers of the same epitope on the same molecule (e.g., polysaccharides). The most common antigens (proteins) have varying numbers of different epitopes on the same molecule.

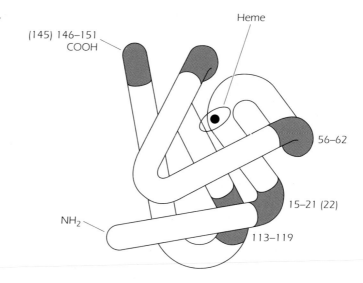

Figure 3.2. An example of an antigen (sperm whale myoglobin) containing five sequential B-cell epitopes shown in red.

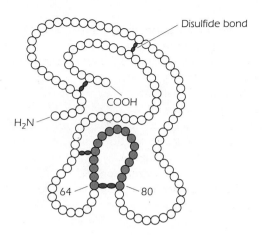

Figure 3.3. Diagram of an antigen showing amino acid residues (circles), which form a nonsequential epitope "loop" shown in blue resulting from a disulfide bond between residues 64 and 80.

MAJOR CLASSES OF ANTIGENS

The following major chemical families may be antigenic:

1. ***Carbohydrates (polysaccharides).*** Polysaccharides are potentially, but not always, immunogenic. Normally, polysaccharides, which form part of more complex molecules such as cell-surface ***glycoproteins***, elicit an immune response, part of which is directed specifically against the polysaccharide moiety of the molecule. An immune response, consisting primarily of antibodies, can be induced against many kinds of polysaccharide molecules, such as components of microorganisms and of eukaryotic cells. An excellent example of antigenicity of polysaccharides is the immune response associated with the ***ABO blood groups***, which are polysaccharides on the surface of the red blood cells.

2. ***Lipids.*** Lipids are rarely immunogenic, but an immune response to lipids may be induced if the lipids are conjugated to protein carriers. Thus, in a sense, lipids may be regarded as haptens. Immune responses to ***glycolipids*** and to ***sphingolipids*** have also been demonstrated.

3. ***Nucleic acids.*** Nucleic acids are poor immunogens by themselves, but they become immunogenic when they are conjugated to protein carriers. DNA, in its native helical state, is usually nonimmunogenic in normal animals. However, immune responses to nucleic acids have been reported in many instances. One important example in clinical medicine is the appearance of anti-DNA antibodies in patients with ***systemic lupus erythematosus*** (discussed in detail in Chapter 17).

4. ***Proteins.*** Virtually all proteins are immunogenic. Thus, the most common immune responses are those to proteins. Furthermore, the greater the degree

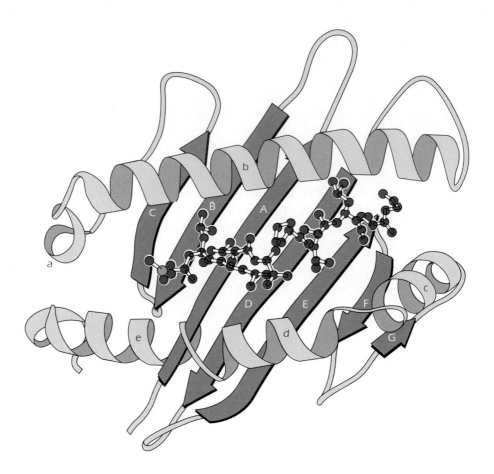

Figure 3.4. Structure of class I MHC complex (ribbon diagram) with an antigenic peptide (ball-and-stick model).

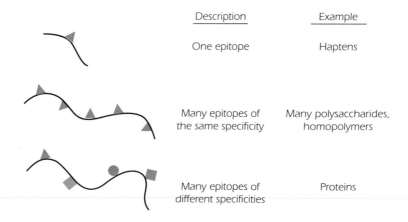

Figure 3.5. Representation of some possible antigenic structures containing single or multiple epitopes.

of complexity of the protein, the more vigorous will be the immune response to that protein. In general, proteins are **multideterminant** (*multiepitope*) **antigens**.

 ## BINDING OF ANTIGEN WITH ANTIGEN-SPECIFIC ANTIBODIES OR T CELLS

The binding between antigen and antibodies is discussed in detail in Chapter 5. The interactions of antigen with both B and T cells and subsequent activation events are discussed in Chapter 10. At this point, it is important to emphasize only that the binding of antigen with antibodies or immunocompetent cells does not involve covalent bonds. The binding may involve **electrostatic interactions, hydrophobic interactions, hydrogen bonds, and van der Waals forces**. Since these interactive forces are relatively weak, the "fit" between antigen and its complementary site on the antigen receptor must occur over an area large enough to allow the summation of all the possible available interactions. This requirement is the basis for the exquisite specificity observed in immunologic interactions.

 ## CROSS-REACTIVITY

Since macromolecular antigens contain several distinct epitopes, some of these macromolecules can be altered without totally changing the immunogenic and antigenic structure of the entire molecule. This concept is important in relation to immunization against highly pathogenic microorganisms or highly toxic compounds. For example, a lethal dose of tetanus toxin for mice is measured in picograms (10^{-12} g), while a dose required for immunization is measured in micrograms (10^{-6} g). Obviously, immunization with the toxin is unwise. However, it is possible to destroy the biologic activity of this and a broad variety of other toxins (e.g., bacterial toxins and snake venoms) without appreciably affecting their antigenicity or immunogenicity. A toxin that has been modified to the extent that it is no longer toxic but still maintains some of its immunochemical characteristics is called a **toxoid**. Thus we can say that a toxoid **cross-reacts** immunologically with the toxin. Accordingly, it is possible to immunize individuals with the toxoid and thereby induce immune responses to some of the epitopes that the toxoid still shares with the native toxin because these epitopes have not been destroyed by the modification. Although the molecules of toxin and toxoid differ in many physicochemical and biologic respects, they nevertheless cross-react immunologically: they share enough epitopes to allow the immune response to the toxoid to mount an effective defense against the toxin itself. An immunologic reaction in which the immune components, either cells or antibodies, react with two molecules that share epitopes, but are otherwise dissimilar, is called a **cross-reaction**. When two compounds cross-react immunologically, the compounds will have one or more epitopes in common and the immune response to one of the compounds will recognize one or more of the same epitope(s) on the other compound and react with it. Another form of cross-reactivity is seen when antibodies or cells with specificity to one epitope bind, usually more weakly, to another epitope that is not quite identical, but has a structural resemblance, to the first epitope. To denote that the antigen used for immunization is different from the one with which the induced immune components are then allowed to react, the terms homologous and heterologous are used. **Homologous** denotes that the antigen and the immunogen are the same; **heterologous** denotes that the substance used to induce the immune response is different from the substance that is then used to react with the products of the induced response. In the latter case, the heterologous antigen may or may not react with the immune components. If reaction does take place, it may be concluded that the heterologous and homologous antigens exhibit **immunologic cross-reactivity**.

Although the hallmark of immunology is specificity, immunologic cross-reactivity has been observed on many levels. This does not mean that the immunologic specificity has been diminished, but rather that the substances that cross-react share antigenic determinants. In cases of cross-reactivity, the antigenic determinants of the cross-reacting substances may have identical chemical structures, or they may be composed of similar but not identical physicochemical configurations. In the example described above, a toxin and its corresponding toxoid represent two molecules, the toxin being the **native** molecule and the toxoid being a **modified** molecule that cross-reacts with the native molecule.

There are other examples of immunologic cross-reactivity, wherein the two cross-reacting substances are unrelated to each other except that they have one or more epitopes in common, specifically, one or more areas that have similar three-dimensional characteristics. These substances are referred to as **heterophile antigens**. For example, human blood group A antigen reacts with antiserum raised against pneumococcal capsular polysaccharide (type XIV). Similarly, human blood group B antigen reacts with antibodies to certain strains of *Escherichia coli*. In these examples of cross-reactivity, the antigens of the microorganisms are referred to as the heterophile antigens (with respect to the blood group antigen).

IMMUNOLOGIC ADJUVANTS

To enhance the immune response to a given immunogen, various additives or vehicles are often used. An **adjuvant** (from the Latin, *adjuvare*, "to help") is a substance that, when mixed with an immunogen, enhances the immune response against the immunogen. It is important to distinguish between a carrier for a hapten and an adjuvant. A hapten will become immunogenic when conjugated covalently to a carrier; it will not become immunogenic if mixed with an adjuvant. Thus, an adjuvant enhances the immune response to immunogens but does not confer immunogenicity on haptens.

Adjuvants have been used to augment immune responses to antigens for more than 70 years. Interest in vaccine adjuvants is growing because many new vaccine candidates lack sufficient immunogenicity. While many adjuvants have been developed in animal models and tested experimentally in humans, only one has been accepted for routine vaccination. Currently, aluminum potassium sulfate (**alum**) is the only adjuvant used for licensed human vaccines in the United States. Alum increases the immunogenicity of immunogens by causing the antigen to precipitate. When injected, the precipitated antigen is released more slowly than antigen alone at the injection site. Moreover, the increased "size" of the antigen, which occurs as a consequence of precipitation, increases the probability that the macromolecule will be phagocytized.

Many adjuvants have been used in animals. One such adjuvant is ***Freund's complete adjuvant*** (FCA), which consists of a water-in-oil emulsion and killed *Mycobacterium tuberculosis* or *M. butyricum*. The antigen is contained in the water phase. Other microorganisms used as adjuvants are ***bacille Calmette-Guerin*** (BCG) (an attenuated *Mycobacterium*), *Corynebacterium parvum*, and *Bordetella pertussis*. These adjuvants are presumed to release antigen slowly but continuously and to stimulate macrophages to take up, process, and present antigen to T lymphocytes as well as upregulation of expression of costimulatory molecules (discussed in detail in Chapter 10), which are essential for T-cell activation. Other adjuvants used are bacterial endotoxins consisting of ***lipopolysaccharide*** (LPS), and still others contain a synthetic ***muramyldipeptide*** [*N*-acetylmuramyl-L-alanyl-D-isoglutamine (MDP)]. In the mouse, LPS enhances the antibody response by stimulating B cells, while muramyl dipeptide, the effective constituent of mycobacterial cell walls, stimulates macrophages and T cells.

SUMMARY

1. ***Immunogenicity*** is the capacity of a compound to induce an immune response. Immunogenicity requires that a compound (i) be foreign to the immunized individual, (ii) possesses a certain minimal molecular weight, (iii) possesses a certain degree of chemical complexity, and (iv) be degradable or susceptible to antigen processing and presentation.

2. ***Antigenicity*** refers to the ability of a compound to bind with antibodies or with cells of the immune system. This binding is highly specific; the immune components are capable of recognizing various physicochemical aspects of the compound. The binding between antigen and immune components involves several weak forces operating over short distances (van der Waals forces, electrostatic interactions, hydrophobic interactions, and hydrogen bonds); it does not involve covalent bonds.

3. The smallest unit of antigen that is capable of binding with antibodies is called an ***antigenic determinant*** or ***epitope***. Compounds may have one or more epitopes capable of reacting with immune components. The immune response against these compounds involves the production of antibodies or the generation of cells with specificities directed against most or all of the epitopes.

4. B cell membrane Ig or secreted antibody tend to recognize amino acid sequences that are accessible, usually hydrophobic and mobile. These can be contiguous, or noncontiguous amino acids (conformational determinants), which are brought into proximity by the three-dimensional folding of the protein. B cell membrane Ig and antibody are capable of recognizing polysaccharides and lipids.

5. T cells recognize internal amino acid sequences of proteins in the context of class I or class II MHC molecules. Peptide fragments of protein antigens are generated by antigen processing (proteolysis) thus allowing them to associate with MHC molecules.

6. Immunologic *cross-reactivity* denotes a situation in which two or more substances, which may have various degrees of dissimilarity, share epitopes and would, therefore, react with the immune components induced against any one of these substances. Thus, a toxoid, which is a modified form of toxin, may have one or more epitopes in common with the toxin. Immunization with the toxoid leads to an immune response capable of reacting not only with the toxoid but also with the native toxin.

REFFRENCES

Atassi MZ (1977): Immunochemistry of Proteins, Vols 1 and 2. New York: Plenum.

Benjamin DC, Berzofsky JA, East IJ, Gurd FRN, Hannum C, Leach SJ, Margoliash E, Michael JG, Miller A, Prager EM, Reichlin M, Sercarz EE, Smith-Gill SJ, Todd PE, Wilson AC (1984): The antigenic structure of proteins: a reappraisal. *Annu Rev Immunol* 2:67.

Berzofsky JA, Berkower IJ (1998): Immunogenicity and antigen structure. In Paul WE (ed): Fundamental Immunology, 4th ed. New York: Lippincott-Raven.

Berzofsky JA, Cease KB, Cornette JL, Spouge JL, Margalit H, Berkower IJ, Good FM, Miller LH, DeLisi C (1987): Protein antigenic structures recognized by T cells: potential applications to vaccine design. *Immunol Rev* 98:9.

Davis, MM, Boniface, JJ, Reich, Z, Lyons, D, Hampl, J, Arden, B, Chien, Y. (1998): Ligand recognition by $\alpha\beta$ T cell receptors. *Annu Rev Immunol* 16:523.

Hopp TP, Woods KR (1981): Prediction of protein antigenic determinants from amino acid sequences. *Proc Natl Acad Sci USA* 78:3824.

Novotny J, Handschumacher H, Bruccoleri RE (1987): Protein antigenicity: a static surface property. *Immunol Today* 8:26.

Rothbard JB, Gefter ML (1991): Interactions between immunogenic peptides and MHC proteins. *Annu Rev Immunol* 9:527.

Sercarz EE, Berzofsky A (eds) (1987): Immunogenicity of Protein Antigens: Repertoire and Regulation. Boca Raton, FL: CRC Press.

Watts, C (1997): Capture and processing of exogenous antigens for presentation on MHC molecules. *Annu Rev Immunol* 15:821.

REVIEW QUESTIONS

For each question, choose the ONE BEST answer or completion.

1. The following properties render a substance immunogenic:
   A) high molecular weight
   B) chemical complexity
   C) sufficient stability and persistence after injection
   D) All of the above.
   E) All of the above are essential but not sufficient.

2. The protection against smallpox afforded by prior infection with cowpox represents
   A) antigenic specificity.
   B) antigenic cross-reactivity.

C) enhanced viral uptake by macrophages.

D) innate immunity.

E) passive protection.

3. Converting a toxin to a toxoid

A) makes the toxin more immunogenic.

B) reduces the pharmacologic activity of the toxin.

C) enhances binding with antitoxin.

D) induces only innate immunity.

E) increases phagocytosis.

4. Haptens

A) require carrier molecules to be immunogenic.

B) react with specific antibodies when homologous carriers are not employed.

C) interact with specific antibody even if the hapten is monovalent.

D) cannot stimulate secondary antibody responses without carriers.

E) all of the above.

5. An immunologic adjuvant is a substance that

A) reduces the toxicity of the immunogen.

B) enhances the immunogenicity of haptens.

C) enhances hematopoiesis.

D) enhances the immune response against the immunogen.

E) enchances immunologic cross-reactivity.

6. An antibody made against the antigen tetanus toxoid (TT) reacts with it even when the TT is denatured by disrupting all disulfide bonds. Another antibody against TT fails to react when the TT is similarly denatured. The most likely explanation can be stated as follows:

A) The first antibody is specific for several epitopes expressed by TT.

B) The first antibody is specific for the primary amino acid sequence of TT, whereas the second is specific for conformational determinants.

C) The second antibody is specific for disulfide bonds.

D) The first antibody has a higher affinity for TT.

Answers To Review Questions

1. *E* All of the properties are essential but not sufficient, since, for immunogenicity, the substance must be foreign to the immunized individual.

2. *B* The protection against smallpox provided by prior infection with cowpox is an example of antigenic cross-reactivity. Immunization with cowpox leads to the production of antibodies capable of reacting with smallpox because the two viruses share several identical, or structurally similar, determinants.

3. *B* Conversion of a toxin to a toxoid is performed in order to reduce the pharmacologic activity of the toxin, so that sufficient toxoid can be injected to induce an immune response.

4. *E* Haptens are substances, usually of low molecular weight and univalent, that, by themselves, cannot induce immune responses (primary or secondary), but can do so if conjugated to high-molecular-weight carriers. The haptens can and do interact with the induced antibodies, without it being necessary that they be conjugated to the carrier.

5. D An immunologic adjuvant is a substance that, when mixed with an immunogen, enhances the immune response against that immunogen. It does not enhance cross-reactivity, nor does it enhance hematopoiesis. An adjuvant does not enhance the immune response against a hapten, which requires its conjugation to an immunogenic carrier to induce a response against the hapten. The adjuvant has no relevance to possible toxicity of an immunogen.

6. B Antibodies can recognize single epitopes formed by primary sequence structures or secondary, tertiary, and quaternary conformational structures. Denaturing a protein by disrupting disulfide bonds generally destroys conformational determinants. Therefore it is likely that the first antibody reacts with a primary amino acid sequence determinant that is present on both native and denatured TT, while the second antibody sees a conformational determinant only on native TT.

4

ANTIBODY STRUCTURE AND FUNCTION

 INTRODUCTION

One of the major functions of the immune system is the production of soluble proteins that circulate freely and exhibit properties that contribute specifically to immunity and protection against foreign material. These soluble proteins are the *antibodies*, which belong to the class of proteins called *globulins* because of their globular structure. Initially, owing to their migratory properties in an electrophoretic field, they were called γ-globulins (in relation to the more rapidly migrating albumin, α-globulin, and β-globulin); today they are known collectively as *immunoglobulins* (Ig).

Immunoglobulins are expressed as secreted and membrane-bound forms. Secreted antibodies are produced by plasma cells—the terminally differentiated B cells that serve as antibody factories housed largely within the bone marrow. Membrane-bound antibody is present on the surface of B cells where it serves as the antigen-specific receptor. *The membrane-bound form of antibody is associated with a heterodimer called Igα/Igβ* to form the B cell receptor (BCR). As will be discussed in Chapter 7, the Igα/Igβ heterodimer mediates the intracellular signaling mechanisms associated with B-cell activation.

The structure of immunoglobulins incorporates several features essential for their participation in the immune response. The two most important of these features are specificity and biologic activity. As discussed later in this chapter, *specificity* is attributed to a defined region of the antibody molecule containing the hypervariable or *complementarity-determining region* (CDR). This restricts the antibody to combine only with those substances that contain one particular antigenic structure. The existence of a vast array of potential antigenic determinants or epitopes (see Chapter 3) has necessitated the evolution of a system for producing a repertoire of antibody molecules, each of which is capable of combining with a particular antigenic structure. Thus, antibodies collectively exhibit great diversity, in terms of the types of molecular structure with which they are capable of reacting, but individually they exhibit a high degree of specificity, since each is able to react with only one particular antigenic structure.

Despite the large numbers of different specific individual antibodies capable of reacting with many different structural entities, the biologic effects of such reactions are rather few in number. These include neutralization of toxins, immobilization of microorganisms, neutralization of viral activity, agglutination (clumping together) of microorganisms or of antigenic particles (see Chapter 5), binding with soluble antigen leading to the formation of precipitates (which are readily phagocytized and destroyed by phagocytic cells; see Chapter 2), and activating serum complement to facilitate the lysis of microorganisms (see Chapter 13) or their phagocytosis and destruction either by phagocytic cells or by killer lymphocytes. Still another important biologic function of antibodies is their ability to cross the placenta from the mother to the fetus. Not all antibody molecules are equal in the performance of all of these biologic tasks.

The differences in the various **biologic activities** of antibodies are attributed to their **isotypic (class)** structure. While one part of the antibody molecule must be adaptable to allow the accommodation of a large number of epitopes, another part of the antibody molecule must be adaptable to allow the antibody molecule to participate in biologic activities common to many antibodies. The determination of the structure of antibody, the establishment of the relationship between this structure and function, and the elucidation of the genetic organization of the Ig molecule have led to an understanding of the evolution of a sophisticated, highly specialized system in which diverse structures (immunoglobulins) all recognize the same antigen, but in which combination of immunoglobulin with antigen leads to an array of diverse biologic effects. This chapter deals with these structural and biologic properties of immunoglobulins.

 ## ISOLATION AND CHARACTERIZATION

Serum is the antibody-containing component of blood left when it has clotted and the clot, which contains cells and clotting factors, is removed. When serum is subjected to electrophoresis (separation in an electrical field) at slightly alkaline pH (8.2), five major components can normally be visualized (see Figure 4.1). The slowest, in terms of migration toward the anode, called γ-globulin, was shown by Kabat and Tiselius in 1939 to contain antibody. This demonstration entailed the simple comparison of the electrophoretic pattern of antiserum from a hyperimmune rabbit before and after the specific antibody had been removed by precipitation with the antigen. Only the size of the γ-globulin fraction was diminished by this procedure. Analysis showed that when this fraction was collected separately, all measurable antibodies were contained within it. Later it was shown that antibody activity is present not only in the γ-globulin fraction but also in a slightly more anodic area. Consequently, all globular proteins with antibody activity are generically referred to as immunoglobulins (Ig), as exemplified by the γ peak (see Figure 4.1).

From the broad electrophoretic peaks, it is clear that a heterogeneous collection of immunoglobulin molecules with slightly different charges is present. This hetero-

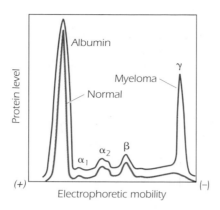

Figure 4.1. Electrophoretic mobility of serum proteins obtained from a normal individual (lower tracing in blue) and from a patient with IgG myeloma (upper tracing in red). (Courtesy of Dr. C. Miller, School of Medicine, University of California, Davis).

geneity was one of the early obstacles in attempts to determine the structure of antibodies, since analytical chemistry requires homogeneous, crystallizable compounds as starting material. This problem was solved, in part, by the discovery of *myeloma proteins*, which are homogeneous immunoglobulins produced by the progeny of a single plasma cell that has become neoplastic in the malignant disease called *multiple myeloma*. This is clearly demonstrated by the γ-globulin spike in the electrophoretic pattern of serum proteins of a patient with multiple myeloma (see Figure 4.1). When it became clear that some myeloma proteins bound antigen, it also became apparent that they could be dealt with as typical immunoglobulin molecules.

Another aid to structural studies of antibodies was the discovery of *Bence Jones proteins* in the urine. These homogeneous proteins, produced in large quantities by some patients with multiple myeloma, are *dimers of immunoglobulin κ or λ light chains*. They were very useful in the determination of the structure of this portion of the immunoglobulin molecule. Today, the powerful technique of cell–cell hybridization (hybridomas) permits the production of large quantities of homogeneous preparations of monoclonal antibody of virtually any specificity (see Chapter 5).

STRUCTURE OF LIGHT AND HEAVY CHAINS

Analysis of the structural characteristics of antibody molecules really began in 1959 with two discoveries that, for the first time, revealed that the molecule could be separated into analyzable parts suitable for further study. In England, Porter found that proteolytic treatment with the enzyme papain split the immunoglobulin molecule (molecular weight 150,000 Da) into three fragments of about equal size (see Figure 4.2). Two of these fragments were found to retain the antibody's ability to bind antigen specifically, although, unlike the intact molecule, they could no longer precipitate the antigen from solution. These two fragments are referred to as *Fab* (fragment antigen binding) fragments and are considered to be univalent, possessing one binding site each and being in every way identical to each other. The third fragment

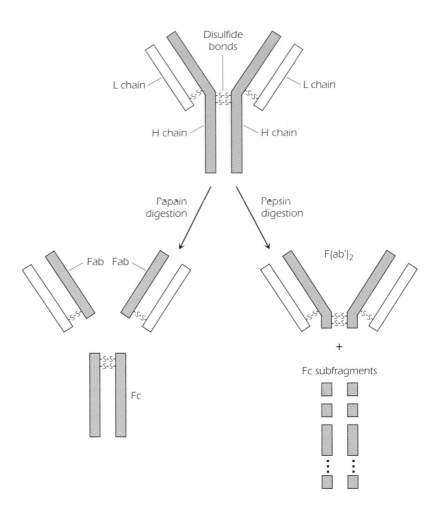

Figure 4.2. Proteolytic digestion of immunoglobulin using papain and pepsin.

could be crystallized out of solution, a property indicative of its apparent homogeneity. This fragment is called **Fc** (fragment-crystallizable). It cannot bind antigen, but, as was subsequently shown, it is responsible for the biologic functions of the antibody molecule after antigen has been bound to the Fab part of the intact molecule.

At about the same time, Edelman in the United States discovered that when γ-globulin was extensively reduced by treatment with mercaptoethanol (a reagent that breaks SS bonds), the molecule fell apart into four chains: two identical chains with a molecular weight of about 53,000 Da each and two others of about 22,000 Da each. The larger chains were designated heavy (H) and the smaller ones, light (L). On the basis of these results, the structure of immunoglobulin molecules, as depicted in Figure 4.2, was proposed. This model was subsequently shown to be essentially correct, and Porter and Edelman shared the Nobel Prize for the elucidation of antibody structure. Thus, all immunoglobulin molecules consist of a basic unit of four polypeptide chains, two identical H chains and two identical L chains, held together by a number of disulfide bonds. It should be noted that *papain digestion* of the immunoglobulin molecule results in cleavage N-terminally to the disulfide bridge between the heavy chains at the hinge region, yielding *two monovalent Fab fragments and an Fc fragment*. On the other hand, *pepsin digestion* results in cleavage C-terminally to the disulfide bridge, resulting in a *divalent fragment referred to as F(ab')2*, consisting of two Fab fragments joined by the disulfide bond and *several Fc subfragments*. A more detailed diagram of a generic immunoglobulin molecule, consisting of two glycosylated heavy (H) chains and two light (L) chains, is shown in Figure 4.3. Note that in addition to the interchain disulfide bonds that hold the chains together, the H and L chains each contain intrachain disulfide bonds to create the *immunoglobulin-fold domains* to create the antiparallel beta-pleated sheet structure characteristic of antibody molecules. As discussed later in this chapter, other molecules belonging to the so-called *immunoglobulin superfamily* share this structural feature.

As is the case with other proteins, immunoglobulins of one species are immunogenic in another species. The use of immunoglobulins of a given species as immunogens in another species allowed the production of a variety of antisera that could distinguish between features of different immunoglobulin chains. By a combination of biochemical and serologic (utilizing serum antibodies) techniques, it was shown that almost all species studied have *two major classes of L chains*, called κ and λ. Any one individual of a species produces both types of L chain, but the ratio of κ chains to λ chains varies with the species (mouse: 95% κ; human: 60% κ). However, in any one immunoglobulin molecule, the L chains are always either both κ or both λ, never one of each. While there are two types of L chains, the immunoglobulins of virtually all species have been shown to consist of *five different classes (isotypes)* that differ in the structure of their *H chains*. These H chains differ

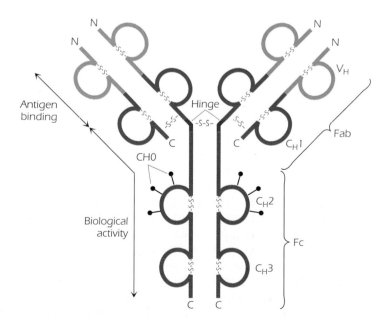

Figure 4.3. Schematic representation of an immunoglobulin molecule showing immunoglobulin-fold domains formed by intrachain disulfide bonds.

as antigens (serologically), in carbohydrate content, and in size. Most importantly, they confer different biologic functions on each isotype. The H chains, whose constant regions are derived from Ig heavy chain genes (discussed in detail in Chapter 6) are designated with Greek letters as shown below:

Immunoglobulin class (isotype)	Heavy chain
IgM	μ
IgD	δ
IgG	γ
IgA	α
IgE	ε

The genes encoding the constant regions of the heavy chains are similarly designated. Therefore, the genes encoding the constant (C) regions responsible for the γ, δ, γ, α, and ε heavy chains are called Cγ, Cδ, Cγ, Cα, and Cε, respectively.

Any individual of a species makes all H chains, in proportions characteristic of the species, but in any one antibody molecule both H chains are identical (i.e., 2γ or 2ε, etc.). Thus, an antibody molecule of the IgG class could have the structure $\kappa2\gamma2$ or $\lambda2\gamma2$, while an antibody of the IgE class could have the structure $\kappa2\varepsilon2$ or $\lambda2\varepsilon2$. In each case, it is the nature of the H chains that confers on the molecule its unique biologic properties, such as its half-life in the circulation, its ability to bind to certain receptors, and its ability to activate enzymes (see Chapter 13) on combination with antigen.

Further characterization of these isotypes by specific antisera has led to the designation of several *subclasses* that have more subtle differences among themselves. Thus, the major class of ***human IgG*** can be subdivided into the subclasses *IgG₁, IgG₂, IgG₃, and IgG₄*. IgA has been divided similarly into two subclasses, ***IgA₁ and IgA₂***. The subclasses differ from one another in numbers and arrangement of interchain disulfide bonds, as well as by alterations in other structural features. These alterations, in turn, produce some changes in functional properties that will be discussed later.

 DOMAINS

Early in the study of the structure of immunoglobulins, it became apparent that, in addition to interchain disulfide bonds that hold together L and H chains, as well as H and H chains, ***intrachain disulfide bonds exist that form loops within the chain***. The globular structure of immunoglobulins, and the ability of enzymes to cleave these molecules at very restricted positions into large entities instead of degrading them to oligopeptides and amino acids, is indicative of a very compact structure. Furthermore, the presence of intrachain disulfide bonds at regular, approximately equal intervals of about 100–110 amino acids leads to the prediction that each loop in the peptide chains should form a compactly folded ***globular domain***. In fact, L chains have two domains each, and H chains have four or five domains, separated by a short unfolded stretch (see Figure 4.3). These configurations have been confirmed by direct observation and by genetic analysis (see Chapter 6).

Immunoglobulin molecules are assemblies of separate domains, each centered on a disulfide bond, and each having so much homology with the others as to suggest that they evolved from a single ancestral gene, which duplicated itself several times and then changed its amino acid sequence to enable the resultant different domains to fulfill different functions. Each domain is designated by a letter that indicates whether it is on an L chain or an H chain and a number that indicates its position. As we shall soon discuss in more detail, the first domain on L and H chains is highly variable, in terms of amino acid sequence, from one antibody to the next, and it is designated V_L or V_H accordingly (see Figure 4.3). The second and subsequent domains on both chains are much more constant in amino acid sequence and are designated C_L or C_H1, C_H2, and C_H3 (Figure 4.3). In addition to their interchain disulfide bonding, the globular domains bind to each other in homologous pairs, largely by hydrophobic interactions, as follows: V_HV_L, C_H1C_L, C_H2C_H2, and C_H3C_H3.

HINGE REGION

In the immunoglobulins (with the possible exception of IgM and IgE), the *hinge region* is composed of a short segment of amino acids and is found between the C_H1 and C_H2 regions of the H chains (see Figure 4.3). This segment is made up predominantly of cysteine and proline residues. The cysteines are involved in formation of interchain disulfide bonds, and the proline residues prevent folding in a globular structure. This region of the H chain provides an important structural characteristic of immunoglobulins. It permits *flexibility between the two Fab arms* of the Y-shaped antibody molecule. It allows the two Fab arms to open and close *to accommodate binding to two epitopes*, separated by a fixed distance, as might be found on the surface of a bacterium. Additionally, since this stretch of amino acids is open and as accessible as any other nonfolded peptide, it can be cleaved by proteases, such as papain, to generate the Fab and Fc fragments described above (see Figure 4.2).

VARIABLE REGION

The biologic functions of the antibody molecule derive from the properties of a constant region, which is identical for antibodies of all specificities within a particular class. It is the *variable region* that constitutes the part of the molecule that *binds to the epitope*. A major problem for immunologists was to determine how so many individual specificities, which are required to meet the enormous variety of antigenic challenges, are generated from the variable region. As we shall see in Chapter 6, this issue has been largely resolved.

When the amino acid sequences of proteins of sufficient homogeneity (e.g., myeloma proteins, monoclonal antibodies, Bence Jones proteins) were determined, it was found that the greatest variability in sequence existed in the *N-terminal 110 amino acids of both the L and H chains*. Kabat and Wu compared the amino acid sequences of many different V_L and V_H regions. They plotted the variability in the amino acids at each position in the chain and showed that the *greatest amount of variability* (defined as the ratio of the number of different amino acids at a given position to the frequency of the most common amino acid at that position) occurred in three regions of the L and H chains. These regions are called *hypervariable*

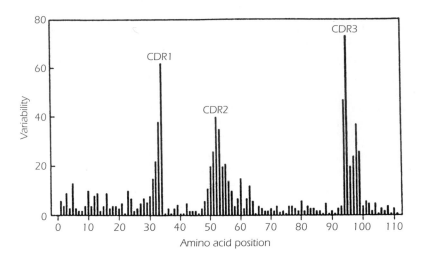

Figure 4.4. Variability of amino acids representing the N-terminal residues of V_H in a representative immunoglobulin molecule.

regions. The less variable stretches, which occur between these hypervariable regions, are called framework regions. It is now clear that the hypervariable regions participate in the binding with antigen and form the region complementary in structure to the antigen epitope. Consequently, ***hypervariability regions are termed complementarity-determining regions*** (CDRs) of the L and H chains: CDR1, CDR2, and CDR3 (see Figure 4.4)

The hypervariable regions, although separated in the linear, two-dimensional model of the peptide chains, are actually brought together in the folded form of the intact antibody molecule, and together they constitute the combining site, which is complementary to the epitope (Figure 4.5). The variability in these CDRs provides the diversity in the shape of the combining site that is required for the function of antibodies of different specificities. All the known ***forces involved in antigen–antibody interactions are weak, noncovalent interactions*** (e.g., ionic, hydrogen-bonding, and hydrophobic interactions) (see Chapter 5). It is therefore necessary that there be a close fit between antigen and antibody over a sufficiently large region to allow a total binding force that is adequate for stable interaction. Contributions to this binding interaction by both H and L chains are involved in the overall association between epitope and antibody.

It should now be apparent that two antibody molecules with different antigenic specificities must have different amino acid sequences in their hypervariable regions and that those with similar sequences will generally have similar specificities. However, it is possible for two antibodies with different amino acid sequences to have specificity to the same epitope. In this case, the binding affinities of the antibodies with the epitope will probably be different because there will be differences in the number and types of binding forces available to bind identical antigens to the different binding sites of the two antibodies.

An additional source of variability involves the size of the combining site on the antibody, which is usually (but not always) considered to take the form of a depression or cleft. In some instances, especially when small, hydrophobic haptens

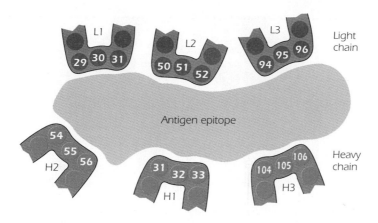

Figure 4.5. A schematic representation of the complementarity between an epitope and the antibody-combining site consisting of the hypervariable areas of the L and H chains. Numbered letters denote CDR of H and L chains; circled numbers denote the number of the amino acid residue in the CDRs.

are involved, the epitopes do not occupy the entire combining site, yet they achieve sufficient affinity of binding. It has been shown that antibodies specific for such a small hapten may, in fact, react with other antigens that have no obvious similarity to the hapten (e.g., dinitrophenol and sheep red cells). These large, dissimilar antigens bind either to a larger area or to a different area of the combining site on the antibody (see Figure 4.6). Thus, a particular antibody combining site may have the ability to combine with two (or more) apparently diverse epitopes, a property called ***redundancy***. The ability of a single antibody molecule to cross-react with an unknown number of epitopes may reduce the number of different antibodies needed to defend an individual against the range of antigenic challenges.

IMMUNOGLOBULIN VARIANTS

Isotypes of Immunoglobulins

Thus far we have described the features common to all immunoglobulin molecules, such as the four-chain unit and the structural domains. In its defense against invading foreign substances, the body has evolved a variety of mechanisms, each dependent on a somewhat different property or function of an immunoglobulin molecule. Thus, when a specific antibody molecule combines with a specific antigen or a pathogen, several different effector mechanisms come into play. These different mechanisms derive from the different classes of ***immunoglobulin (isotypes)***, each of which may combine with the same epitope but each of which triggers a different response. These differences result from structural variations in H chains, which have generated domains that mediate a variety of functions. The structural features are discussed here. A summary of the properties of the immunoglobulin classes is given in Tables 4.1 and 4.2.

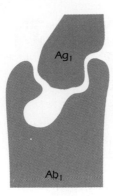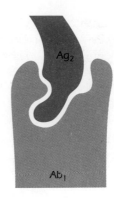

Figure 4.6. A representation of how an antibody of a given specificity (Ab) can exhibit binding with two different epitopes (Ag₁ and Ag₂).

Allotypes

Another form of variation in the structure of immunoglobulins is **allotypy**. It is based on genetic differences between individuals. It depends on the existence of allelic forms (allotypes) of the same protein, as a result of the presence of different forms of the same gene at a given locus. As a result of allotypy, a heavy or light chain constituent of any immunoglobulin can be present in some members of a species and absent in others. This situation contrasts with that of immunoglobulin classes or subclasses, which are present in all members of a species.

Allotypic differences at known loci usually involve changes in only one or two amino acids in the constant region of a chain. With a few exceptions, the presence of allotypic differences in two identical immunoglobulin molecules does not generally affect binding with antigen, but it serves as an important marker for analysis of Mendelian inheritance.

Some known allotype markers constitute a group on the γ-chain of human IgG (called Gm for IgG markers), a group on the κ chain (formerly called InV, now called Km), and a group on the α chain (called Am).

Allotypic markers have been found in the immunoglobulins of several species, usually by the use of antisera generated by immunization of one member of a species with antibody from another member of the same species. As with other allelic systems, allotypes are inherited as dominant Mendelian traits. The genes encoding the markers are expressed codominantly, so that an individual may be homozygous or heterozygous for a given marker.

Idiotypes

As we have seen, the combining site of a specific antibody molecule is made up of a unique combination of amino acids in the variable regions of the L and H chains. Since this combination is not present in other antibody molecules, it should, theoretically, be immunogenic and capable of stimulating an immunologic response against itself in an animal of the same species. Such was actually found to be the case by Oudin and Kunkel, who, in the early 1960s, showed independently that experimental immunization with a particular antibody or myeloma protein could

● TABLE 4.1. The Most Important Features of Immunoglobulin Isotopes

	Isotype				
	IgG	IgA	IgM	IgD	IgE
Molecular weight	150,000	160,000 for monomer	900,000	180,000	200,000
Additional protein subunits	—	J and S	J	—	—
Approximate concentration in serum (mg/ml)	12	1.8	1	0–0.04	0.00002
Percent of total Ig	80	13	6	0.2	0.002
Distribution	~Equal: intravascular and extravascular	Intravascular and secretions	Mostly intravascular	Present on lymphocyte surface	On basophils and mast cells present in saliva and nasal secretions
Half-life (days)	23	5.5	5	2.8	2.0
Placental passage	+	—	—	—	—
Presence in secretion	—	++	—	—	—
Presence in milk	+	+	0 to trace	—	—
Activation of complement	+	—	+++	—	—
Binding to Fc receptors on macrophages, polymorphonuclear cells, and NK[1] cells	++	—	—	—	—
Relative agglutinating capacity	+	++	+++	—	—
Antiviral activity	+++	+++	+	—	—
Antibacterial activity (gram-negative)	+++	++ (with lysozyme)	+++ (with complement)	—	—
Antitoxin activity	+++	—	—	—	—
Allergic activity	—	—	—	—	++

[1]Natural killer.

● T A B L E 4.2. Important Differences Between Human IgG Subclasses

	IgG_1	IgG_2	IgG_3	IgG
Occurrence (% of total IgG)	70	20	7	3
Half-life	23	23	7	23
Complement binding	+	+	+++	—
Placental passage	++	±	++	++
Binding of monocytes	+++	+	+++	±

produce an antiserum specific only for the antibody that was used to induce the response and for no other immunoglobulin of the species. These antisera contain populations of antibodies specific for several epitopes, called *idiotopes*, which are present in the variable region of the antibody used for inoculation. The collection of all idiotopes on the inoculated antibody molecule is called the *idiotype* (Id). In some cases, anti-idiotypic sera prevent binding of the antibody with its antigen, in which event the idiotypic determinant is considered to be in or very near the combining site itself. Anti-idiotypic sera, which do not block binding of antibody with antigen, are probably directed against variable determinants of the framework area, outside the combining site (see Figure 4.7). On theoretical grounds, it is possible to visualize that an anti-idiotypic antibody with a combining site complementary to that of the idiotype resembles the epitope, which is also complementary to the idiotypes combining site. Thus, *the anti-idiotype may represent a facsimile or an internal image of the nominal epitope*. Indeed, there are examples of immunization of experimental animals using anti-idiotypic internal images as immunogens (Chapter 21). Such immunogens induce antibodies capable of reacting with the antigen that carries the epitope to which the original idiotype is directed. Such antibodies are induced without the immunized animal ever having seen the original antigen.

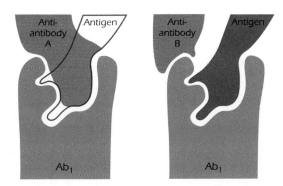

● Figure 4.7. Two anti-idiotypic antibodies to Ab_1. **(A)** The anti-idiotypic antibody on the left is directed to the combining site of Ab_1, preventing binding of Ab_1 with the antigen. **(B)** The anti-idiotypic antibody on the right binds with framework areas of Ab_1 and does not prevent its binding with antigen.

In some instances, especially with inbred animals, antiidiotypic antibodies react with several different antibodies that are directed against the same epitope and share idiotypes. These idiotypes are called *public or cross-reacting idiotypes*, and this term frequently defines families of antibody molecules. By contrast, sera that react with only one particular antibody molecule define *a private idiotype*. As we discuss in Chapter 11, the presence of idiotypic determinants on immunoglobulin molecules may have a role in the control and modulation of the immune response, as envisioned in the Jerne network theory, although this remains controversial.

● STRUCTURAL FEATURES OF IgG

IgG is the predominant immunoglobulin in blood, lymph fluid, cerebrospinal fluid, and peritoneal fluid. The IgG molecule consists of two γ H chains of molecular weight approximately 50,000 Da each and two L chains (either κ or λ) of molecular weight approximately 25,000 Da each, held together by disulfide bonds (Figure 4.8). Thus, the IgG molecule has a molecular weight of approximately 150,000 Da and a sedimentation coefficient of 7S. Electrophoretically, the IgG molecule is the least anodic of all serum proteins, and it migrates to the γ range of serum globulins; hence its earlier designation as γ-globulin or 7S immunoglobulin.

The *IgG* class of immunoglobulins *in humans contains four subclasses designated IgG$_1$, IgG$_2$, IgG$_3$, and IgG$_4$*. Except for their variable regions, all the immunoglobulins within a class (e.g., IgG$_1$ and IgG$_2$) have about 90% homology in their amino acid sequences, but only 60% homology exists between classes (e.g., IgG and IgA). This degree of homology means that an antiserum to IgG may be produced against a determinant that is common to, and specific for, all members of a given class (e.g., all members of the IgG class) while other antisera may be raised that are specific for determinants found in only one of the subclasses (e.g., in IgG$_2$). This variation was first detected antigenically by the use of antibodies against various γ chains. The IgG subclasses differ in their chemical properties and, more importantly, in their biologic properties, which are discussed below.

● BIOLOGIC PROPERTIES OF IgG

IgG present in the serum of human adults represents about 15% of the total protein (other proteins include albumins, globulins, and enzymes). *IgG is distributed approximately equally between the intravascular and extravascular spaces.*

Except for the IgG$_3$ subclass, which has a rapid turnover, with a half-life of 7 days, *the half-life of IgG (i.e., IgG$_1$, IgG$_2$, and IgG$_4$) is approximately 23 days*, which is the longest half-life of all Ig isotypes. This persistence in the serum makes IgG the most suitable for passive immunization by transfer of antibodies. Interestingly, as the concentration of IgG in the serum increases (as in cases of multiple myeloma or after the transfer of very high concentrations of IgG), the rate of catabolism of IgG increases, and the half-life of IgG decreases to 15–20 days or even less. Recent studies have provided a clear explanation for the prolonged survival of IgG relative to other serum proteins and why its half-life decreases at high concentrations. A saturable IgG protection receptor (FcRp, also called the Brambell receptor)

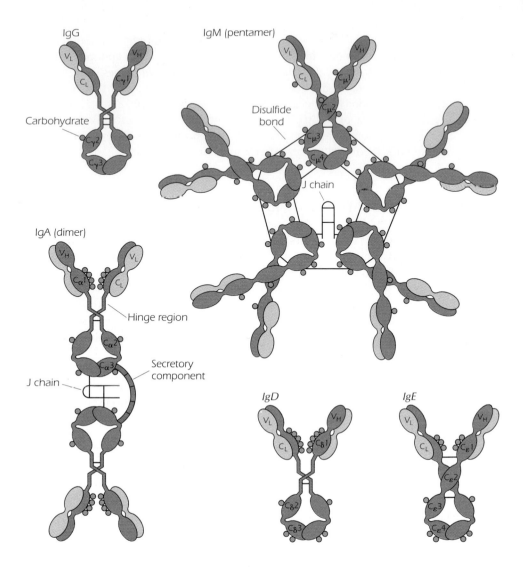

Figure 4.8. Structures of the five major classes of secreted antibody. Light chains are shown in green; heavy chains are shown in blue. Orange circles denote areas of glycosylation. The polymeric IgM and IgA molecules contain a polypeptide known as the J chain. The dimeric IgA molecule shown includes the secretory component (red).

has been identified and shown to bind to the Fc region of this isotype. This receptor is found in cellular endosomes and selectively recycles endocytized IgG (e.g., following endocytosis of antigen–antibody immune complexes) back to the circulation. Figure 4.9 illustrates how this mechanism operates to "cleanse" IgG antibody of antigen and harvest antigen for presentation without antibody destruction. Conditions associated with high IgG levels saturate the FcRp receptors rendering the catabolism of excess IgG indistinguishable from albumin or other Ig isotypes.

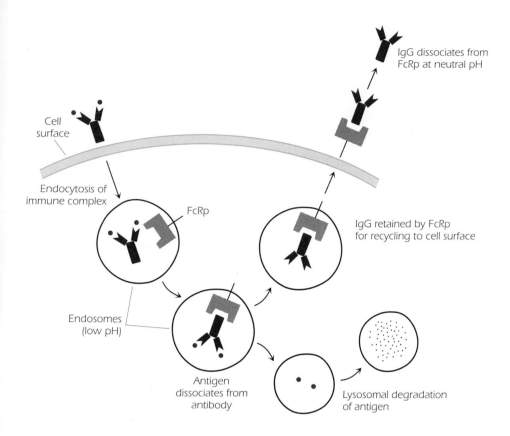

Figure 4.9. Recycling of IgG utilizing the protector receptor (FcRp). Circulating monomeric IgG plus antigen (immune complex) enters an antigen- presenting cell through the process of endocytosis. Within the endosome, the complex binds FcRp; IgG and Ag dissociate allowing the IgG to be directed to the cell surface for recycling. Antigen undergoes lysosomal degredation (antigen processing), and its proteolytic fragments are ultimately expressed on the cell surface in the context of MHC class II molecules.

Agglutination and Formation of Precipitate

IgG molecules can cause the ***agglutination*** or clumping of particulate (insoluble) antigens such as microorganisms. The reaction of IgG with soluble, multivalent antigens can generate ***precipitates*** (see Chapter 5). This property of IgG is undoubtedly of considerable survival value since insoluble antigen–antibody complexes are easily phagocytized and destroyed by phagocytic cells.

IgG molecules may be made to ***aggregate*** by a variety of procedures. For example, precipitation with alcohol, a method employed in the purification of IgG, or heating at 56°C for 10 minutes, a method used to inactivate complement (see Chapter 13), cause aggregation. Aggregated IgG can still combine with antigen.

Many of the properties that are attributed to antigen–antibody complexes are exhibited by aggregated IgG (without antigen) for example, attachment to phagocytic cells, as well as the activation of complement and other biologically active substances that may be harmful to the body. Such activation is attributable to the juxtaposition of Fc domains by the aggregation process in a way analogous to that produced by antigen-induced immune complex formation. It is therefore imperative that no aggregated IgG be present in passively administered IgG.

Passage Through the Placenta and Absorption in Neonates

The IgG isotype (except for subclass IgG_2) is the only class of immunoglobulin that can pass through the placenta, enabling the mother to transfer her immunity to the fetus. Placental transfer is facilitated by expression of an IgG protection receptor (FcRn) expressed on placental cells. FcRn was recently shown to be identical to the IgG protection receptor (FcRp) found in the cellular endosomes. Analysis of fetal immunoglobulins (see Figure 21.2) shows that, at the third or fourth month of pregnancy, there is a rapid increase in the concentration of IgG. This IgG must be of maternal origin, since the fetus is unable to synthesize immunoglobulins at this age. Then, during the fifth month of pregnancy, the fetus begins to synthesize IgM and trace amounts of IgA. It is not until 3 or 4 months after birth, when the level of inherited maternal IgG drops as a result of catabolism (the half-life of IgG is 23 days), that the infant begins to synthesize its own IgG antibodies. Thus, the resistance of the fetus and the neonate to infection is conferred almost entirely by the mother's IgG, which passes across the placenta. It has been established that passage across the placenta is mediated by the Fc portion of the IgG molecule; $F(ab')_2$ or Fab fragments of IgG do not pass through the placenta. It is of interest to note that the IgG protection receptor (FcRn) expressed on placental cells is transiently superexpressed in the intestinal tissue of neonates. Absorption of maternal IgG contained in the colostrum of nursing mothers is achieved by its binding to these high density receptors in intestinal tissue. FcRn are downregulated in intestinal tissue at 2 weeks of age.

While passage of IgG molecules across the placenta confers immunity to infection on the fetus, it may also be responsible for hemolytic disease of the newborn (erythroblastosis fetalis) (see Chapter 15). This is caused by maternal antibodies to fetal red blood cells. The maternal IgG antibodies, produced by an Rh mother, to Rh antigen pass across the placenta and attack the fetal red blood cells that express Rh antigens (Rh^+).

Opsonization

IgG is an opsonizing antibody (from the Greek *opsonin*, which means to prepare for eating). It reacts with epitopes on microorganisms via its Fab portions, but it is the Fc portion that confers the opsonizing property. Many phagocytic cells, including macrophages and polymorphonuclear phagocytes, bear receptors for the Fc portion of the IgG molecule. These cells adhere to the antibody-coated bacteria by virtue of their receptors for Fc. The net effect is a zipperlike closure of the surface membrane of the phagocytic cell around the organism, as receptors for Fc and the Fc regions on the antibodies continue to combine, leading to the final engulfing and destruction of the microorganism (see Figure 4.10).

Antibody-Dependent, Cell-Mediated Cytotoxicity

The IgG molecule plays an important role in *antibody-dependent, cell-mediated cytotoxicity* (ADCC). In this form of cytotoxicity, the Fab portion binds with the

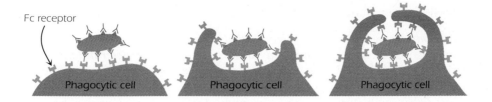

Figure 4.10. A diagrammatic representation of phagocytosis of a particle coated with antibodies.

target cell, whether it is a microorganism or a tumor cell, and the Fc portion binds with specific receptors for Fc that are found on certain large granular lymphocytic cells called **natural killer** (NK) cells (see Chapter 2). By this mechanism, the IgG molecule focuses the killer cells on their target, and the **killer cells destroy the target**, not by phagocytosis but with the various substances that they release.

Activation of Complement

The IgG molecule can activate the complement system (see Chapter 12). Activation of complement results in the release of several important biologically active molecules and leads to lysis if the antibody is bound to antigen on the surface of a cell. Some of the **complement components are also opsonins**; they bind to the target antigen and thereby direct phagocytes, which carry receptors specific for these opsonins, to focus their phagocytic activity on the target antigen. Other components from the activation of complement are chemotactic; specifically, they attract phagocytic cells. All in all, the activation of complement by IgG has profound biologic effects on the host and on the target antigen, whether it is a live cell, a microorganism, or a tumor cell.

Neutralization of Toxin

The **IgG molecule is an excellent antibody for the neutralization of such toxins as tetanus and botulinus**, or for the inactivation of, for example, snake and scorpion venoms. Because of its ability to neutralize such poisons (mostly by blocking their active sites) and because of its long half-life, compared to that of other isotypes, the **IgG molecule is the isotype of choice for passive immunization (i.e., the transfer of antibodies) against toxins and venoms**.

Immobilization of Bacteria

IgG molecules are efficient in immobilizing various motile bacteria. Reaction of antibodies specific for the flagella and cilia of certain microorganisms causes them to clump, thereby arresting their movement and preventing their ability to spread or invade tissue.

Neutralization of Viruses

IgG antibody is an efficient virus-neutralizing antibody. One mechanism of neutralization is that in which the *antibody binds with antigenic determinants* present on various portions of the virus coat, among which is the region *used by the virus for attachment to the target cell.* Inhibition of viral attachment effectively arrests infection. Other antibodies are thought to inhibit viral penetration or shedding of the viral coat required for release of the viral DNA or RNA needed to induce infection.

The versatility in function of the IgG molecule makes it a very important molecule in the immune response. Its importance is underscored in those immune deficiency disorders in which an individual is unable to synthesize IgG molecules (see Chapter 18). Such individuals are prone to infections that may result in toxemias and death.

 ## STRUCTURAL FEATURES OF IgM

As we shall see later in this chapter, *IgM is the first immunoglobulin produced following immunization.* Its name derives from its initial description as a macroglobulin (M) of high molecular weight (900,000 Da). It has a sedimentation coefficient of 19S, and it *has an extra C_H domain.* In comparison to the IgG molecule, which consists of one four-chain structure, IgM is a *pentameric molecule* composed of five such units, each of which consists of two L and two H chains, all joined together by additional disulfide bonds between their Fc portions and by a polypeptide chain termed the *J chain* (see Figure 4.8). The J chain, which, like L and H chains, is synthesized in the B cell or plasma cell, has a molecular weight of 15,000 Da. This pentameric ensemble of IgM, which is held together by disulfide bonds, comes apart after mild treatment with reducing agents such as mercaptoethanol.

Surprisingly, each pentameric IgM molecule appears to have a valence of 5 (i.e., five antigen combining sites), instead of the expected valence of 10 predicted by the 10 Fab segments contained in the pentamer. This apparent reduction in valence is probably the result of conformational constraints imposed by the polymerization. It is known that pentameric IgM has a planar configuration, such that each of its 10 Fab portions cannot open fully with respect to the adjacent Fab, when it combines with antigen, as is possible in the case of IgG. Thus, any large antigen bound to one Fab may block a neighboring site from binding with antigen, making the molecule appear pentavalent (or of even lesser valence).

 ## BIOLOGIC PROPERTIES OF IgM

IgM present in adult human serum is found predominantly in the intravascular spaces. The half-life of the IgM molecule is approximately 5 days. *IgM is also found on the surface of mature B cells together with IgD* (see below), *where it serves as an antigen-specific B cell receptor* (BCR). Once the B cell is activated by antigen following ligation of the BCR, it may undergo class switching (see Chapter 6) and begin to secrete and express other membrane Ig isotypes (e.g., IgG).

IgM antibodies do not pass through the placenta; however, since this is the only class of immunoglobulins that is synthesized by the fetus beginning at approximately 5 months of gestation, elevated levels of IgM in the fetus are indicative of congenital or perinatal infection.

IgM is the isotype synthesized by children and adults in appreciable amounts after immunization or exposure to T-independent antigens, and it is the first isotype that is synthesized after immunization with T-dependent antigens (see Figure 4.11). Thus, *elevated levels of IgM usually indicate either recent infection or recent exposure to antigen*.

Agglutination

IgM molecules are efficient agglutinating antibodies. Because of their pentameric form, IgM antibodies can form macromolecular bridges between epitopes on molecules that may be too distant from each other to be bridged by the smaller IgG antibodies. Furthermore, because of their pentameric form and multiple valence, the IgM antibodies are particularly well suited to combine with antigens that contain repeated patterns of the same antigenic determinant, as in the case of polysaccharide antigens or cellular antigens, which are multiply expressed on cell surfaces.

Isohemagglutinins

The IgM antibodies include the so-called natural isohemagglutinins—the naturally occurring antibodies against the red blood cell antigens of the ABO blood groups. These antibodies are presumed to arise as a result of immunization by bacteria in the gastrointestinal and respiratory tracts, which bear determinants similar to the oligosaccharides of the ABO blood groups. Thus, without known prior immunization, people with the type O blood group have isohemagglutinins to the A and B antigens; those with the type A blood group have antibodies to the B antigens; and those with the B antigen have antibodies to the A antigen. An individual of the AB group has neither anti-A nor anti-B antibodies. Fortunately, the IgM isohemagglutinins do not pass through the placenta, so incompatibility of the ABO groups

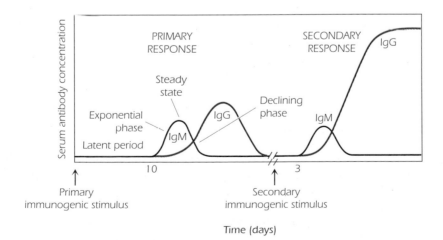

Figure 4.11. The kinetics of an antibody response.

between mother and fetus poses no danger to the fetus. However, transfusion reactions, which arise as a result of ABO incompatibility, and in which the recipient's isohemagglutinins react with the donor's red blood cells, may have disastrous consequences.

Activation of Complement

Because of its pentameric form, *IgM is an excellent complement-fixing or complement-activating antibody*. Unlike other classes of immunoglobulins, a single molecule of IgM, on binding to antigen with at least two of its Fab arms, can initiate the complement sequence, making it the most efficient immunoglobulin as an initiator of the complement-mediated lysis of microorganisms and other cells. This ability, taken together with the appearance of *IgM as the first class of antibodies generated after immunization or infection, makes IgM antibodies very important as providers of an early line of immunologic defense against bacterial infections.*

In contrast to IgG, the *IgM antibodies are not very versatile; they are poor toxin-neutralizing antibodies, and they are not efficient in the neutralization of viruses.*

STRUCTURAL AND BIOLOGIC PROPERTIES OF IgA

IgA is the major immunoglobulin in external secretions such as saliva, mucus, sweat, gastric fluid, and tears. It is, moreover, the major immunoglobulin of colostrum and milk, and it may provide the neonate with a major source of intestinal protection against pathogens. The IgA molecule consists of either two κ chains or two λ chains and two H α chains. The α chain is somewhat larger than the γ chain. The molecular weight of monomeric IgA is approximately 165,000 Da, and its sedimentation coefficient is 7S. Electrophoretically it migrates to the slow β or fast γ region of serum globulins. Dimeric IgA has a molecular weight of 400,000 Da.

The IgA class of immunoglobulins contains two subclasses: IgA$_1$ (93%) and IgA$_2$ (7%). It is interesting to note that if all production of IgA on mucosal surfaces (respiratory, gastrointestinal, and urinary tracts) is taken into account, IgA would be the major immunoglobulin in terms of quantity.

Serum IgA, which has no known biologic function, has a half-life of 5.5 days. *The IgA present in serum is predominantly monomeric (one four-chain unit)* and has presumably been released before dimerization so that it fails to bind to the secretory component. Secretory IgA is very important biologically, but *little is known of any function for serum IgA.*

Most IgA is present not in the serum, but in secretions such as tears, saliva, colostrum, sweat, and mucus, where it serves an important biologic function such *as being part of the mucosa-associated lymphoid tissue* (MALT) as alluded to in Chapter 2. Within mucous secretions, IgA exists as a dimer consisting of two four-chain units linked by the same joining (J) chain found in IgM molecules (see Figure 4.8). *Plasma cells synthesize only the basic IgA molecules and the J chains, which form the dimers.* Such IgA-secreting plasma cells are located predominantly in the connective tissue called *lamina propria* that lies immediately below the basement membrane of many surface epithelia (e.g., in the parotid gland, along the gastrointestinal tract in the intestinal villi, in tear glands, in the lactating breast, or beneath bronchial mucosa). When these dimeric molecules are released from plasma cells, they bind to the **poly-Ig receptor** expressed on the basal membranes of adjacent epithelial cells. This receptor transports the molecules through the epithelial cells and releases them into extracellular fluids (e.g., in the gut or bronchi). Release is facilitated by enzymatic cleavage of the poly-Ig receptor, leaving a large 70,000 Da fragment (i.e., the **secretory component**) of the receptor still attached to the Fc piece of the dimeric IgA molecule (see Figure 4.12). The secretory component may help to protect the dimeric IgA from proteolytic cleavage. It should also be noted that **the secretory component also binds and transports pentameric IgM to mucosal surfaces in small amounts.**

Role in Mucosal Infections

Because of its presence in secretions, such as saliva, urine, and gastric fluid, secretory **IgA is of importance in the primary immunologic defense against local infections in such areas as the respiratory or gastrointestinal tract.** Its protective effect is thought to be due to its ability to prevent the invading organism from attaching to and penetrating the epithelial surface. For example, in the case of cholera, the pathogenic *Vibrio* organism attaches to, but never penetrates beyond, the cells that line

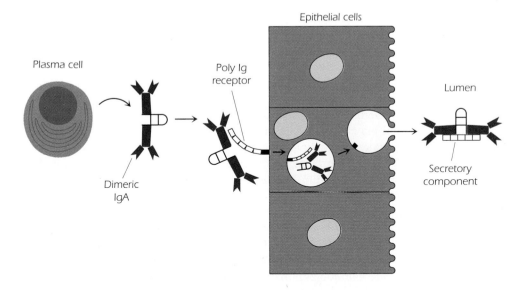

Figure 4.12. Transcytosis of dimeric IgA across epithelia. Plasma cells in close proximity to epithelial basement membranes in the gut, respiratory epithelia, salivary and tear glands, and lactating mammary glands, release dimeric IgA. The IgA binds to the poly-Ig receptor and the complex undergoes transcytosis within vesicles across the cell. The poly-Ig receptor is cleaved from the complex at the apical surface to release the IgA from the cell. After exiting the cell, a pentameric fragment of the poly-Ig receptor known as the secretory component remains attached to the dimeric IgA and is believed to protect the antibody within the lumen of several organs that are in contact with the external environment.

the gastrointestinal tract, where it secretes an exotoxin responsible for all symptoms. IgA antibody, which can prevent attachment of the organism to the cells, provides protection from the pathogen. Thus, for protection against local infections, routes of immunization that result in local production of IgA are much more effective than routes that primarily produce antibodies in serum.

Bactericidal Activity

The IgA molecule does not contain receptors for complement and, thus, *IgA is not a complement-activating or complement-fixing immunoglobulin.* Consequently, it does not induce complement-mediated bacterial lysis. However, *IgA has been shown to possess bactericidal activity against gram-negative organisms, but only in the presence of lysozyme*, which is also present in the same secretions that contain secretory IgA.

Antiviral Activity

Secretory IgA is an efficient antiviral antibody, preventing the viruses from entering host cells. In addition, secretory IgA is an efficient agglutinating antibody.

 STRUCTURAL AND BIOLOGIC PROPERTIES OF IgD

The IgD molecule consists of either two κ or two λ L chains and two H δ-chains (see Figure 4.8). IgD is present as a monomer with a molecular weight of 180,000 Da, it has a sedimentation coefficient of 7S, and it migrates to the fast γ-region of serum globulins. No H-chain allotypes (see below) or subclasses have been reported for the IgD molecule.

IgD is present in serum in very low and variable amounts, probably because it is not secreted by plasma cells and because, among immunoglobulins, it is uniquely susceptible to proteolytic degradation. In addition, following B-cell activation, transcription of the δ heavy chain protein is rapidly downregulated—a phenomenon that also helps to explain the low serum IgD levels.

IgD is coexpressed with IgM on the surface of mature B cells and, like IgM, functions as an antigen-specific BCR. Its presence there serves as a marker of the differentiation of B cells to a more mature form. Thus, during ontogeny of B cells, expression of IgD lags behind that of IgM (see Chapter 7).

While the function of IgD has not been fully elucidated, expression of membrane IgD appears to correlate with the elimination of B cells with the capacity to generate self-reactive antibodies. Furthermore, in mature B cells, binding autoreactive of IgM- and IgD-positive cells to self-antigens results in the loss of surface expression of IgM but not of IgD. Such cells are unable to enter the primary follicles in lymphoid tissues where appropriate T cell help would facilitate the development of autoreactive responses. Therefore, these cells are rendered anergic and are rapidly lost. The removal of self-antigens, however, allows these cells to enter the follicles. This indicates that neither the mere loss of IgM surface expression nor the exclusive expression of IgD (without IgM) can explain the failure of such cells to enter the lymphoid follicles. In addition, studies using transgenic mice lacking IgD suggest that such animals can break B-cell tolerance to self-antigens. Whether IgD has a clear role in the development of B-cell tolerance remains to be seen. If this is so, the major biologic significance of IgD will be in silencing autoreactive B cells during development.

 ## STRUCTURAL AND BIOLOGIC PROPERTIES OF IgE

The IgE molecule consists of two L chains (κ or λ) and two H ε-chains. Like the IgM molecule, IgE has an extra C_H domain (see Figure 4.9). IgE has a molecular weight of approximately 200,000 Da, its sedimentation coefficient is 8S, and it migrates electrophoretically to the fast γ-region of serum globulins. To date, no H-chain allotypes or subclasses of IgE have been reported.

Importance of IgE in Parasitic Infections and Hypersensitivity Reactions

IgE, also termed *reaginic antibody*, has a half-life in serum of 2 days, the shortest half-life of all classes of immunoglobulins. It is *present in serum in the lowest concentration* of all immunoglobulins. These low levels are due in part to a low rate of synthesis and to the unique ability of the Fc portion of IgE containing the extra C_H domain to *bind with very high affinity to receptors (Fcε receptors) found on mast cells and basophils*. Once bound to these high-affinity receptors, IgE may be retained by these cells for weeks or months. When antigen reappears, it combines with the Fab portion of the IgE attached to these cells causing it to be cross-linked. The cells become activated and release the contents of their granules: histamine, heparin, leukotrienes, and other pharmacologically active compounds that trigger the immediate hypersensitivity reactions. These reactions may be mild, as in the case of a mosquito bite, or severe, as in the case of bronchial asthma; they may even result in systemic anaphylaxis, which can cause death within minutes (see Chapter 14).

IgE is not an agglutinating or complement-activating antibody; nevertheless, *it has a role in protection against certain parasites, such as helminths (worms)*, a protection achieved by activation of the same acute inflammatory response seen in a more pathologic form of immediate hypersensitivity responses. Elevated levels of IgE in serum have been shown to occur during infections with ascaris (a roundworm). In fact, immunization with ascaris antigen induces the formation of IgE.

 ## KINETICS OF THE ANTIBODY RESPONSE FOLLOWING IMMUNIZATION

Primary Response

As mentioned in Chapter 3, the first exposure of an individual to a particular immunogen is referred to as the *priming immunization* and the measurable response that ensues is called the *primary response*. As shown in Figure 4.11, the primary antibody response may be divided into several phases, as follows:

1. Latent or lag phase: After initial injection of antigen, a significant amount of time elapses before antibody is detectable in the serum. The length of this

period is generally 12 weeks, depending on the species immunized, the antigen, and other factors that will become apparent in subsequent chapters. The length of the latent period is also greatly dependent on the sensitivity of the assay used to measure the product of the response. As we shall see in more detail in subsequent chapters, *the latent period includes the time taken for T and B cells to make contact with the antigen, to proliferate, and to differentiate*. B cells must also secrete antibody in sufficient quantity so that it can be detected in the serum. The less sensitive the assay used for detection of antibody, the more antibody will be required for detection and the longer the apparent latent period will be.

2. Exponential production phase: During this phase, the *concentration of antibody in the serum increases exponentially*.

3. Steady state: During this period, *production and degradation of antibody are balanced*.

4. Declining phase: Finally, *the immune response begins to shut down*, and the concentration of antibody in serum declines rapidly.

In the primary response, *the first class of antibody detected is generally IgM*, which in some instances may be the only class of immunoglobulin that is made. If production of IgG antibody ensues, its appearance is generally accompanied by a rapid cessation of production of IgM (see Figure 4.11).

Secondary Response

Although production of antibody after a priming contact with antigen may cease entirely within a few weeks (see Figure 4.11), the immunized individual is left with a cellular memory (i.e., long-lasting *memory cells*) of this contact. This memory becomes apparent when a response is triggered by a second injection of the same antigen. After the second injection, *the lag phase is considerably shorter* and antibody may appear in less than half the time required for the primary response. The production of antibody is much greater, and higher concentrations of antibody are detectable in the serum. The *production of antibody may also continue for a longer period*, with persistent levels remaining in serum months, or even years, later.

There is a marked change in the type and quality of antibody produced in the secondary response. There is a shift in class response known as *class switching*, with *IgG* antibodies appearing at higher concentrations, and with greater persistence, than IgM, which may be greatly reduced or disappear altogether. This may be also accompanied by the appearance of *IgA* and *IgE*. In addition, *affinity maturation* occurs, such that the average affinity (binding constant) of the antibodies for the antigen increases as the secondary response develops. The driving force for this increase in affinity may be a selection process during which B cells compete with free antibody to capture a decreasing amount of antigen. Thus, only those B-cell clones with high-affinity Ig receptors on their surfaces will bind enough antigen to ensure that the B cells are triggered to differentiate into plasma cells. These plasma cells, which arise from preferentially selected B cells, synthesize this antibody with high affinity for antigen.

The capacity to make a secondary or *anamnestic* (memory) response may persist for a long time (years in humans), and it provides an obvious selective advantage for an individual that survives the first contact with an invading pathogen. Establishment of this memory for generating a specific response is, of course, the purpose of public health immunization programs.

THE IMMUNOGLOBULIN SUPERFAMILY

The shared structural features of immunoglobulin heavy and light chains which include the *immunoglobulin-fold domains* (see Figures 4.3 and 4.4) *are also seen in a large number of proteins*. Most of these have been found to be membrane-bound glycoproteins. Because of this structural similarity, these proteins are classified as members of the *immunoglobulin superfamily*. The redundant structural characteristic seen in these proteins suggests that the genes that encode them arose from a common primordial gene—one that generated the basic domain structure. Duplication and subsequent divergence of this primordial gene would explain the existence of the large number of membrane proteins that possess one or more regions homologous to the immunoglobulin-fold domain. Genetic and functional analyses of these immunoglobulin superfamily proteins have indicated that these genes have evolved independently, since they do not share genetic linkage or function. Figure 4.13 il-

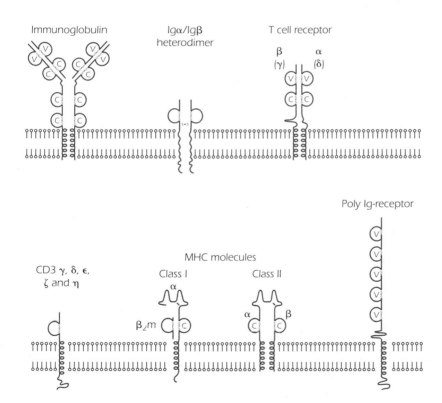

Figure 4.13. Representative members of the immunoglobulin superfamily. The immunoglobulin-fold domains (shown as circular loops in blue) form the common structural features of these molecules. In all cases, the carboxyl-terminal end of the molecules shown are anchored in the membrane.

lustrates some examples of proteins that are members of the immunoglobulin super-family. Numerous other examples are discussed in other chapters. As can be seen, each molecule contains the characteristic Ig-fold structure (loops) formed as a result of intrachain disulfide bonds and consisting of approximately 110 amino acids. These Ig-fold domains are believed to facilitate interactions between membrane proteins (e.g., CD4 molecules on helper T cells and class II MHC molecules on antigen-presenting cells).

SUMMARY

1. Immunoglobulins of all classes have a fundamental four-chain structure, consisting of two identical light (L) and two identical heavy (H) chains. Through disulfide bonds each light chain is linked to a heavy chain and the two heavy chains are linked to each other.

2. In the native state, the chains are coiled into domains, each of which consists of about 110 amino acids, stabilized by an intrachain disulfide bond. A group of other proteins (e.g., TCR, CD4, class I and class II MHC molecules) also contain these immunoglobulin-fold domains making them all members of the immunoglobulin superfamily.

3. Immunoglobulins are expressed in two forms: a membrane-bound antibody present on the surface of B cells and a secreted antibody produced by plasma cells. Membrane-bound antibodies associate with a heterodimer called Igα/Igβ to form the B cell receptor (BCR).

4. The N-terminal domains of both H and L chains are the variable (V) regions and contain the hypervariable regions, also called complementarity-determining regions (CDR), which make up the combining site of the antibody and vary according to the specificity of the antibody.

5. The other domains are the constant (C) regions, and these domains are similar within each class of immunoglobulin molecule.

6. Digestion of the immunoglobulin molecule with papain yields two monovalent Fab fragments and one Fc fragment. Digestion with pepsin yields one divalent F(ab')$_2$ fragment and several peptide fragments from the Fc region.

7. The classes of immunoglobulin molecules differ by virtue of the Fc regions of their H chains, which are responsible for the different biologic functions carried out by each class.

8. Certain genetic markers within the C regions of the H chains, which result from differences in one or two amino acids, are called allotypes and distinguish individuals within a species. By contrast, idiotypic markers are represented by the unique combinations of amino acids that make up the combining site of an antibody molecule and that are unique for that particular antibody.

9. Biologic properties of immunoglobulins (excluding binding with antigen) are conferred on the antibody by the heavy chain. Functional activities are mediated by the Fc portion of the antibody and by the hinge region.

10. IgG is the most versatile class of antibody, capable of carrying out numerous biologic functions that range from neutralization of toxin to activation of complement and opsonization. IgG is the only class of immunoglobulin that passes through the placenta and confers maternal immunity on the fetus. The half-life of IgG (23 days) is the longest of all immunoglobulin classes.

11. IgM is expressed on the surface of mature B cells (as a monomer) and is secreted as a pentameric antibody; of all classes of immunoglobulin it functions as the best agglutinating and complement-activating antibody.

12. IgA antibody is present in monomeric as well as dimeric form. The dimeric IgA found in secretions and referred to as secretory IgA is an important antiviral immunoglobulin.

13. IgD is present on the surface of mature B cells and is coexpressed and shares antigen-specificity with IgM. The functional properties of IgD have not been fully elucidated.

14. IgE, also called reaginic antibody, is of paramount importance in immediate hypersensitivity (allergic) reactions. It also appears to be of importance in protection against parasitic infections. The Fc portion of IgE binds with high affinity to receptors on mast cells and, on contact with antigen, it triggers the degranulation of mast cells, resulting in the release of pharmacologically active substances that mediate the hypersensitivity reactions.

15. Following first immunization, the primary response consists mainly of the production of IgM antibodies. The second exposure to the same antigen results in a secondary or anamnestic (memory) response, which is much quicker than the primary response and in which the response shifts from IgM production to the synthesis of IgG and other isotypes. The secondary response lasts much longer than the primary response.

REFERENCES

Alzari PM, Lascombe MB, Poljak RJ (1988): Three dimensional structure of antibodies. *Annu Rev Immunol* 6:555.

Capra D, Edmundson AB (1977): The antibody combining site. *Sci Am* 236:50.

Carayannopoulos L, Capra JD (1998): Immunoglobulins: structure and function. In Paul WE (ed): Fundamental Immunology, 4th ed. New York: Raven Press.

Davies DR, Metzger H (1983): Structural basis of antibody function. *Annu Rev Immunol* 1: 87.

Jefferis R (1993): What is an idiotype? *Immunol Today* 14:19.

Junghans RP, Anderson CL (1996): The protection receptor for IgG catabolism is the β2-microglobulin-containing neonatal intestinal transport receptor. *Proc Natl Acad Sci USA* 93:5512.

Koshland ME (1985): The coming of age of the immunoglobulin J chain. *Annu Rev Immunol* 3:425.

Mestecky J, McGhee JR (1987): Immunoglobulin A (IgA): Molecular and cellular interactions involved in IgA biosynthesis and immune response. *Adv Immunol* 40:153.

Stanfield RL, Fisher TM, Lerner R, Wilson IA (1990): Crystal structure of an antibody to a peptide and its complex with peptide antigen at 2.8 D. *Science* 248:712.

Tomasi TB (1992): The discovery of secretory IgA and the mucosal immune system. *Immunol Today* 13:416.

Williams AF, Barclay AN (1988): The immunoglobulin superfamily. *Annu Rev Immunol* 6: 381.

 REVIEW QUESTIONS

For each question, choose the ONE BEST answer or completion.

1. The class-specific antigenic determinants (epitopes) of immunoglobulins are associated with
   A) L chains.
   B) J chains.
   C) disulfide bonds.
   D) H chains.
   E) variable regions.

2. The idiotype of an antibody molecule is determined by the amino acid sequence of the
   A) constant region of the L chain.
   B) variable region of the L chain.
   C) constant region of the H chain.
   D) constant regions of the H and L chains.
   E) variable regions of the H and L chains.

3. Injection into rabbits of a preparation of pooled human IgG could stimulate production of
   A) anti-γ heavy-chain antibody.
   B) anti-κ chain antibody.
   C) anti-λ chain antibody.
   D) anti-Fc antibody.
   E) All are correct.

4. A polyclonal antiserum raised against pooled human IgA will react with
   A) human IgM.
   B) κ light chains.
   C) human IgG.
   D) J chain.
   E) All are correct.

5. An individual was found to be heterologous for IgG_1 allotypes 3 and 12. The different possible IgG_1 antibodies produced by this individual will never have
   A) two H chains of allotype 12.
   B) two L chains of either κ or λ.
   C) two H chains of allotype 3.
   D) two H chains, one of allotype 3 and one of allotype 12.

6. Papain digestion of an IgG preparation of antibody specific for the antigen hen egg albumin (HEA) will
   A) lose its antigen specificity.

B) precipitate with HEA.

C) lose all interchain disulfide bonds.

D) produce two Fab molecules and one Fc fragment.

E) None of the above.

7. The first immunoglobulin synthesized by the fetus is

A) IgA.

B) IgE.

C) IgG.

D) IgM.

E) None; the fetus does not synthesize immunoglobulins.

8. The following properties of human IgG are true *except*:

A) It can pass through the placenta.

B) It can be cleaved by pepsin and yet remain divalent.

C) Its half-life is approximately 23 days.

D) It induces the formation of leukocytes.

E) It participates in the activation of complement.

F) It has the longest half-life of all Ig isotopes.

9. The relative level of specific IgM antibodies can be of diagnostic significance because

A) IgM is easier to detect than the other isotypes.

B) viral infection often results in very high IgM responses.

C) IgM antibodies are more often protective against reinfections than are the other isotypes.

D) relatively high levels of IgM often correlate with a first recent exposure to the inducing agent.

10. The primary and secondary antibody responses differ in

A) the predominant isotype generated.

B) the number of lymphocytes responding to antigen.

C) the speed at which antibodies appear in the serum.

D) the biologic functions manifested by the Ig isotypes produced.

E) All of the above.

Answers to Review Questions

1. *D* The five classes of Ig molecules are defined by the H chains (γ, μ, α, λ ε).

2. *E* The idiotype is the antigenic determinant of an Ig molecule, which involves its antigen-combining site, which in turn consists of contributions from the variable regions of both L and H chains.

3. *E* All are correct statements. Since a pool of IgG is injected, it can be assumed that both κ and λ chains will be present and that antibodies will be made against them, as well as against the other determinants (H chain and Fc region) present in all IgG molecules.

4. *E* All are correct statements. Antibody to IgA will have antibody specific for κ and λ light chains, which, of course, will react with IgG and IgM, both of which have κ and λ chains. Antibody will also be present against J chain if the IgA used for immunization was dimeric.

5. *D* In any immunoglobulin produced by a single cell, the two H chains and the two L chains are identical. Therefore, any antibody molecule in this individual would have either allotype 3 H chains or allotype 12 H chains, not a mixture. Similarly, the antibody would have either two κ or two λchains.

6. *D* Papain digestion cleaves the IgG molecules above the hinge region, generating two Fab molecules and an Fc fragment. The Fab fragments can still bind to HEA, but since they are not held together by disulfide binds, they cannot precipitate the antigen. This contrasts with the effects of pepsin treatment of IgG, which cleaves below the hinge region, leaving intact one divalent $F(ab')_2$ molecule capable of precipitating the antigen. Fragments of pepsin-treated HEA-specific antibody will have the same affinity for the antigen as the original Fab regions of the antibody, since the CDR regions of the molecules are preserved.

7. *D* The first (and only) immunoglobulin synthesized by the fetus is IgM. The IgG present in the fetus is maternal IgG that has passed through the placenta. No other immunoglobulins are found in the fetus.

8. *D* Human IgG is the only Ig that passes across the placenta. It has a half-life of 23 days, the longest of all Ig isotypes. It can be cleaved by pepsin to yield a divalent antibody portion $F(ab')_2$, and it participates in the activation of complement. It does not induce the formation of leukocytes. Thus all the statements are true except D.

9. *D* Only the last statement is correct. Relatively high levels of IgM often correlate with first recent exposure to an inducing agent, since IgM is the first isotype synthesized in response to an immunogen. All other statements are not true.

10. *E* All are correct. The statements are self-explanatory.

5

ANTIGEN–ANTIBODY INTERACTIONS, IMMUNE ASSAYS, AND EXPERIMENTAL SYSTEMS

● INTRODUCTION

The utilization of the in vitro reaction between antigen and serum antibodies (*serology*) serves as the basis for many immune assays. Because of the exquisite specificity of the immune response, the interaction between antigen and antibody in vitro is widely used for diagnostic purposes, for the detection and identification of either antigen or antibody. An example of the use of serology for the identification and classification of antigens is the *serotyping* of various microorganisms by the use of specific antisera.

The interaction of antigen with antibodies may result in a variety of consequences, including *precipitation* (if the antigen is soluble), *agglutination* (if the antigen is particulate), and *activation of complement*. All of these outcomes are caused by the interactions between multivalent antigens and antibodies that have at least two combining sites per molecule. The consequences of antigen–antibody interaction listed above do not represent the primary interaction between antibodies and a given epitope but, rather, depend on secondary phenomena, which result from the interactions between multivalent antigens and antibodies. Such phenomena as the formation of precipitate, agglutination, and complement activation would not occur if the antibody with two or more combining sites reacted with a hapten (i.e., a unideterminant, univalent antigen), nor would they occur as a result of the interaction between a univalent fragment of antibody, such as Fab, and an antigen, even if the antigen is multivalent. The reasons for these differences are depicted in Figure 5.1. *Crosslinking* of various antigen molecules by antibody is required for precipitation, agglutination, or complement activation, and it is possible only if the antigen is multivalent and the antibody is divalent [either intact, or F(ab′)$_2$] (see Figure 5.1).

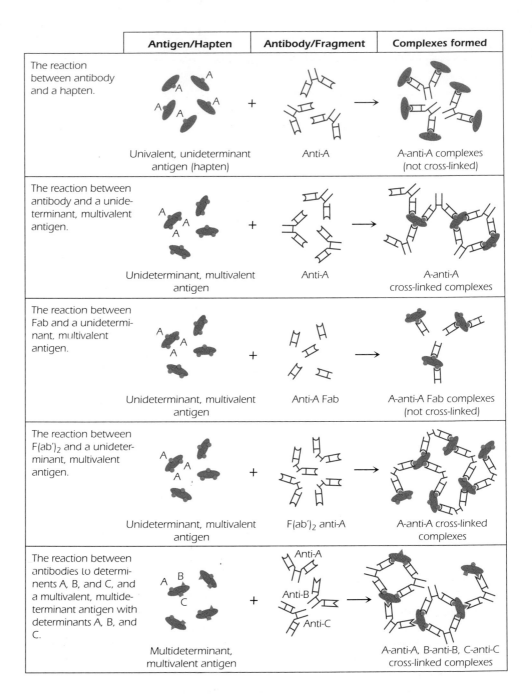

Figure 5.1. Reactions between antibody or antibody fragments and antigens or hapten.

By contrast, no crosslinking is possible if the antigen or the antibody is univalent (Figure 5.1).

There are many serologic reactions that demonstrate the binding between antigen and antibodies. This chapter describes selected reactions that are used in diagnosis; many others, not included here, are mostly variations of the reactions described here.

Other immune assays used in the evaluation and study of the cellular components of the immune system are also described in this chapter. Among these are the routine methods used to measure lymphocyte function. Assays designed to measure responses of B cells to antigenic or mitogenic stimulation are sometimes used clinically to assess humoral immunocompence. In experimental settings, these assays help us to understand the regulatory and molecular mechanisms associated with B-cell activation. Similarly, assays for measuring T-cell function are used both clinically and experimentally to measure T-cell proliferative and effector responses and T-cell and cytokine profiles. T-cell assays have contributed significantly to our understanding of T-cell functional diversity and to the identification of the many cytokines produced by cells belonging to a particular subset.

Several experimental systems have revolutionized our ability to investigate a myriad of questions about the development of the immune system, its functional and regulatory properties, and the pathologic mechanisms associated immunodeficiency and autoimmune diseases. Many of these experimental systems depend upon cell culture methods used to maintain cells in vitro. Cell culture systems have facilitated several major scientific breakthroughs including the development in the 1970s of B cell hybridoma/monoclonal antibody technology by Kohler and Milstein. Knowledge of the growth factors required to maintain lymphoid cells has made it possible to clone and grow functionally competent cells in vitro. Moreover, recombinant DNA techniques have permitted the transfer of genes to cloned cell lines thereby allowing researchers to answer many questions related to the gene under investigation. Similarly, recombinant DNA techniques have made it possible to develop genetically engineered immune molecules and receptors, which can then be transferred into cells that are then used to elucidate the biologic consequences of receptor expression and receptor triggering (e.g., ligand binding). These in vitro systems continue to be used to advance our knowledge of the immune system and, in some cases, to develop new biologic therapies and vaccines for clinical use.

Finally, this chapter will discuss several important in vivo animal models that have been developed with experimental value and clinical payoffs similar to those emerging from the use of the in vitro systems noted above. These in vivo systems rely on the use of inbred mouse strains with a variety of genetic profiles, some of which are genetically engineered. Some inbred stains have an innate predisposition for developing a particular disease (e.g., mammary cancer, leukemia, autoimmune disease, severe combined immunodeficiency disease). Genetically altered animals, on the other hand, have been developed to either express a particular cloned foreign gene (transgenic mice) or by interfering with the expression of targeted genes (knockout mice). Such strains are useful in the study of the expression of a particular transgene or in determining the consequences of gene silencing in knockout mice.

 ## PRIMARY INTERACTIONS BETWEEN ANTIBODY AND ANTIGEN

No covalent bonds are involved in the interaction between antibody and an epitope. Consequently, the binding forces are relatively weak. They consist mainly of *van*

der Waals forces, electrostatic forces, and *hydrophobic forces*, all of which require a very close proximity between the interacting moieties. Thus the interaction requires a very close fit between an epitope and the antibody, a fit that is often compared to that between a lock and a key. Because of the low levels of energy involved in the interaction between antigen and antibody, antigen–antibody complexes can be readily *dissociated* by *low or high pH*, by *high salt concentrations*, or by *chaotropic ions*, such as cyanates, which efficiently interfere with the hydrogen bonding of water molecules.

Association Constant

The reaction between an antibody and an epitope of an antigen is exemplified by the reaction between antibody and a univalent hapten. Because an antibody molecule is symmetric, with two identical Fab antigen combining sites, one antibody molecule binds with two identical monovalent hapten molecules, each Fab binding in an independent fashion with one hapten molecule. The binding of a monovalent antigen (Ag) with each site can be represented by the equation:

$$Ag + Ab \underset{k_{-1}}{\overset{k_1}{\rightleftharpoons}} Ab - Ag$$

where k_1 represents the forward (association) rate constant and k_{-1} represents the reverse (dissociation) rate constant. The ratio of k_1/k_{-1} is the association constant K, a measure of affinity. It can be calculated by determining the ratio of bound AbAg complex to the concentration of unbound antigen and antibody. Thus,

$$K = \frac{k_1}{k_{-1}} = \frac{[Ag - Ag]}{[Ab][Ag]}$$

The association constant (K) is really a measure of the *affinity* of the antibody for the epitope (see below). When all the antibody molecules that bind a given hapten or epitope are identical (as in the case of monoclonal antibodies), then K represents the *intrinsic association constant*. However, because serum antibodies—even those binding to a single epitope—are heterogeneous, an *average association constant* of all the antibodies to the epitope is referred to as K_0. The interaction between antibodies and each epitope of a multivalent antigen follows the same kinetics and energetics as those involved in the interaction between antibodies and haptens because each epitope of the antigen reacts with its corresponding antibody in the same manner as that described above.

The association constant K can be determined using the method of *equilibrium dialysis*. In this procedure, a dialysis chamber is used in which two compartments are separated by a semipermeable membrane allowing the free passage of appropriately sized molecules from one side to the other. Antibody is placed on one side of the semipermeable membrane and cannot pass through due to its size. On the antigen side of the membrane, a known amount of small, permeable, radiolabeled hapten molecules, oligosaccharides, or oligopeptides composing the epitope of the complex carbohydrate or protein is added. At time zero, the hapten or antigenic epitope used (referred to as the "ligand" hereafter) will then diffuse across the membrane and at equilibrium, the concentration of free hapten will be the same on both sides. However, the total amount of hapten will be greater on the Ab-containing side because some of the ligand will be bound to the antibody molecules. The difference in the ligand concentration in the two compartments represents the concentration of the ligand bound to antibody (i.e., the [AgAb] complex). The higher the affinity of the antibody, the more ligand that is bound.

Since the concentration of antibody added to the equilibrium dialysis chamber can be predetermined and kept constant, varying concentrations of ligand can also be used in this analysis. This approach facilitates the so-called ***Scatchard*** analysis of the antibody. This is useful in determining whether a given antibody preparation is homogeneous (e.g., monoclonal antibody) or heterogeneous (e.g., polyclonal antiserum) and in measuring the average affinity constant (K_o).

Affinity and Avidity

As noted above, the intrinsic association constant that characterizes the binding of an antibody with an epitope or a hapten is termed ***affinity***. When the antigen consists of many repeating identical epitopes or when antigens are multivalent, the association between the entire antigen molecule and antibodies depends not only on the affinity between each epitope and its corresponding antibody but also on the sum of the affinities of all the epitopes involved. For example, the affinity of binding of anti-A with multivalent A (shown in Figure 5.1) may be four or five orders of magnitude higher than between the same antibody (i.e., anti-A) and univalent A (Figure 5.1). This is because the pairing of anti-A with A (where A is multivalent) is influenced by the increased number of sites on A with which anti-A can react.

While the term affinity denotes the intrinsic association constant between antibody and a univalent ligand such as a hapten, the term ***avidity*** is used to denote the overall binding energy between antibodies and a multivalent antigen. Thus, in general, IgM antibodies are of higher avidity than IgG antibodies, although the binding of each Fab in the IgM antibody with ligand may be of the same affinity as that of the Fab from IgG.

SECONDARY INTERACTIONS BETWEEN ANTIBODY AND ANTIGEN

Agglutination Reactions

Referring again to the representations given in Figure 5.1, the reactions of antibody with a multivalent antigen that is ***particulate*** (i.e., an insoluble particle) results in the crosslinking of the various antigen particles by the antibodies. This crosslinking eventually results in the clumping or agglutination of the antigen particles by the antibodies.

Titer. The agglutination of an antigen as a result of crosslinking by antibodies is dependent on the correct proportion of antigen to antibody. A method sometimes used to measure the level of serum antibody specific for a particulate antigen is the ***agglutination assay***. More sensitive, quantitative assays (e.g., ELISA, discussed later in this chapter) have largely replaced this approach for measuring antibody levels in serum. Indeed, the agglutinating titer of a certain serum is only a ***semiquantitative*** expression of the antibodies present in the serum; it is not a quantitative measure of the concentration of antibody (weight/volume). The assay is performed by mixing twofold serial dilutions of serum with a fixed concentration of antigen. High dilutions of serum usually do not cause antigen agglutination because at such dilutions there are not enough antibodies to cause appreciable, visible agglutination. The highest dilution of serum that still causes agglutination, but beyond which no agglutination occurs, is termed the *titer*. It is a common observation that agglutination may not occur at high concentrations of antibody, even though it does take place at higher dilutions of serum. The tubes with high concentrations of serum, where agglutination does not occur, represent a *prozone*. In the prozone, antibodies are present in excess. Agglutination may not occur at high ratio of antibody:antigen because every epitope on one particle may bind only to a single antibody molecule, preventing crosslinking between different particles.

Because of the prozone phenomenon, in testing for the presence of agglutinating antibodies to a certain antigen, it is imperative that the antiserum be tested at several dilutions. Testing serum at only one concentration may give misleading conclusions if no agglutination occurs, because the absence of agglutination might reflect either a prozone or a lack of antibody.

Zeta Potential. The surfaces of certain particulate antigens may possess an electrical charge, as, for example, the net negative charge on the surface of red blood cells caused by the presence of sialic acid. When such charged particles are suspended in saline solution, an electrical potential termed the *zeta potential* is created between particles, preventing them from getting very close to each other. This introduces a difficulty in agglutinating charged particles by antibodies, in particular red blood cells by IgG antibodies. The distance between the Fab arms of the IgG molecule, even in its most extended form, is too short to allow effective bridging between two red blood cells across the zeta potential. Thus, although IgG antibodies may be directed against antigens on the charged erythrocyte, agglutination may not occur because of the repulsion by the zeta potential. On the other hand, some of the Fab areas of *IgM pentamers* are far enough apart and can bridge red blood cells separated by the zeta potential. This property of IgM antibodies, together with their pentavalence, is a major reason for their effectiveness as agglutinating antibodies.

Through the years attempts were made to improve agglutination reactions by decreasing the zeta potential in various ways, none of which was universally applicable or effective. However, an ingenious method was devised in the 1950s by Coombs to overcome this problem. This method, described below, facilitates the agglutination of erythrocytes by IgG antibodies specific for erythrocyte antigens. It is also useful for the detection of nonagglutinating antibodies that are present on the surface of erythrocytes.

The Coombs Test. The Coombs test employs antibodies to immunoglobulins (hence it is also called the *anti-immunoglobulin test*). It is based on two important facts: (1) that immunoglobulins of one species (e.g., human) are immunogenic when injected into another species (e.g., rabbit) and lead to the production of antibodies against the immunoglobulins, and (2) that many of the anti-immunoglobulins (e.g., rabbit anti-human Ig) bind with antigenic determinants present on the Fc portion of the antibody, and leave the Fab portions free to react with antigen. Thus, for example, if human IgG antibodies are attached to their respective epitopes on erythrocyte, then the addition of rabbit antibodies to human IgG will result in their binding with the

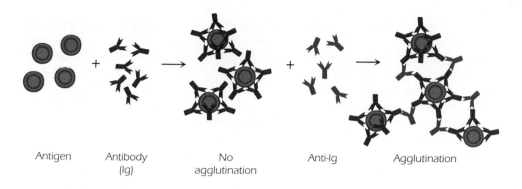

Figure 5.2. A representation of the anti-immunoglobulin (Coombs) test.

Fc portions of the human antibodies bound to the erythrocytes by their Fab portion (see Figure 5.2). These rabbit antibodies not only bind with the human antibodies that are bound to the erythrocyte but also, by so doing, they crosslink (form bridges) between human IgG on relatively distant erythrocytes, across the separation caused by the zeta potential, and cause agglutination. The addition of anti-immunoglobulin brings about agglutination, even if the antibodies directed against the erythrocytes are present at sufficiently high concentrations to cause the prozone phenomenon.

There are two versions of the Coombs test: the *direct Coombs test* and the *indirect Coombs test*. The two versions differ somewhat in the mechanics of the test but both are based on the same principle: using heterologous anti-immunoglobulins to detect a reaction between immunoglobulins and antigen. In the direct Coombs test, anti-immunoglobulins are added to the particles (e.g., red blood cells) that are suspected of having antibodies bound to antigens on their surfaces. For example, a newborn baby is suspected of having hemolytic disease of the newborn caused by maternal anti-Rh IgG antibodies that are bound to the baby's erythrocytes. If that suspicion proved to be correct, the direct Coombs test would have the following results: the addition of anti-immunoglobulin to a suspension of the baby's erythrocytes would result in the binding of the anti-immunoglobulin to the maternal IgG on the surface of the erythrocytes and would cause agglutination. The *indirect Coombs test* is used to detect the presence, *in the serum*, of antibodies specific to antigens on the particle. The serum antibodies, when added to the particles, may fail to cause agglutination because of the zeta potential. The subsequent addition of anti-Ig will cause agglutination. A common application of the indirect Coombs test is in the detection of anti-Rh IgG antibodies in the blood of an Rh-negative woman (see Chapter 15). This consists, first, of the reaction of the woman's serum with Rh^+ erythrocytes, and then the addition of the anti-immunoglobulin reagents (as in the direct Coombs test). Thus, the direct Coombs test measures bound antibody while the indirect test measures serum antibody.

Originally, the Coombs test was used for the detection of human antibodies on the surface of erythrocytes. Today the term is applied to the detection, by the use of anti-immunoglobulin, of any Ig that is bound to antigen.

Passive Agglutination. The agglutination reaction can be used with particulate antigens (e.g., erythrocytes or bacteria) and also with soluble antigens, provided that the soluble antigen can be firmly attached to insoluble particles. For example, the soluble antigen thyroglobulin can be attached to latex particles, so that the addition of antibodies to the thyroglobulin antigen will cause agglutination of the latex particles coated with thyroglobulin. Of course, the addition of soluble antigen to the antibodies before the introduction of the thyroglobulin cortex latex particles will inhibit the agglutination because the antibodies will first combine with the soluble antigen, and if the soluble antigen is present in excess, the antibodies will not be able to bind with the particulate antigen. This latter example is referred to as *agglutination inhibition*. It should be distinguished from agglutination inhibition in which antibodies to certain viruses inhibit the agglutination of red blood cells by the virus. In these cases, the antibodies are directed to the area or areas on the virus that bind with the appropriate virus receptors on the red blood cells.

When the antigen is a natural constituent of a particle, the agglutination reaction is referred to as *direct agglutination*. When the agglutination reaction takes place between antibodies and soluble antigen that had been attached to an insoluble particle, the reaction is referred to as *passive agglutination*.

The agglutination reaction (direct or passive, either employing or not employing the Coombs test) is widely used clinically. In addition to the examples already given, major applications include erythrocyte typing in blood banks, diagnosis of various immunologically mediated hemolytic diseases, such as drug-induced autohemolytic anemia, tests for rheumatoid factor (human IgM anti-human IgG), confirmatory test for syphilis, and the latex test for pregnancy, which involves the detection of human chorionic gonadotropin (HCG) in the urine of pregnant women.

Precipitation Reaction

Reaction in Solutions. In contrast to the agglutination reaction, which takes place between antibodies and particulate antigen, the *precipitation reaction* takes place when antibodies and *soluble antigen* are mixed. As in the case of agglutination, precipitation of antigen–antibody complexes occurs because the divalent antibody molecules crosslink multivalent antigen molecules to form a *lattice*. When it reaches a certain size, this antigen–antibody complex loses its solubility and precipitates out of solution. The phenomenon of precipitation is termed the *precipitin reaction*.

Figure 5.3 depicts a qualitative precipitin reaction. When increasing concentrations of antigen are added to a series of tubes that contain a constant concentration of antibodies, variable amounts of precipitate form. The weight of the precipitate in each tube may be determined by a variety of methods. If the amount of the precipitate is plotted against the amount of antigen added, a precipitin curve like the one shown in Figure 5.3 is obtained.

There are three important areas under the curve shown in Figure 5.3: (1) the *zone of antibody excess*, (2) the *equivalence zone*, and (3) the *zone of antigen excess*. In the equivalence zone, the proportion of antigen to antibody is optimal for maximal precipitation; in the zones of antibody excess or antigen excess, the proportions of the reactants do not lead to efficient crosslinking and formation of precipitate.

It should be emphasized that the zones of the precipitin curve are based on the amount of *antigen–antibody complexes* precipitated. However, the zones of antigen or antibody excess may contain soluble antigen–antibody complexes, particularly the zone of antigen excess where a minimal amount of precipitate is formed, but

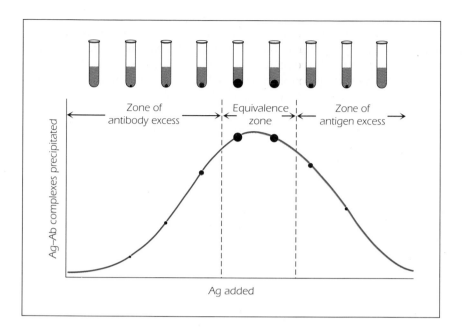

Figure 5.3. A representation of the precipitin reaction.

large amounts of antigen–antibody complexes are present in the supernatant. Thus, the amount of precipitate formed is dependent on the proportions of the reactant antigens and antibodies: the correct proportion of the reactions result in maximal formation of precipitate; excess of antigen (or antibody) results in soluble complexes.

Precipitation Reactions in Gels. Precipitation reactions between soluble antigens and antibodies can take place not only in solution but also in semisolid media such as agar gels. When soluble antigen and antibodies are placed in wells cut in the gel (Figure 5.4A), the reactants diffuse in the gel and form gradients of concen-

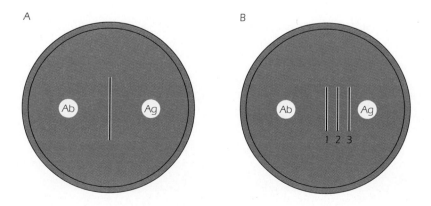

Figure 5.4. Gel diffusion by antibodies and a single antigen **(A)** and antibodies to antigens 1, 2, 3, and their respective antigens **(B)**.

tration, with the highest concentrations closest to the wells. Somewhere between the two wells, the reacting antigen and antibodies will be present at proportions that are optimal for formation of a precipitate.

If the antibody well contains antibodies 1, 2, and 3 specific for antigens 1, 2, and 3, respectively, and if antigens 1, 2, and 3, placed in the antigen well diffuse at different rates (with diffusion rates of 1 > 2 > 3), then three distinct precipitin lines will form. These three precipitin lines form because anti-1, anti-2, and anti-3, which diffuse at the same rate, react independently with antigens 1, 2, and 3, respectively, to form three equivalence zones and thus three separate lines of precipitate (Figure 5.4B). Different rates of diffusion of both antibody and antibody and antigen result from differences in concentration, molecular size, or shape.

This **double-diffusion** method, developed by **Ouchterlony** (a name sometimes used to describe the assay in lieu of double-diffusion), where antigen and antibody diffuse toward each other, is very useful for establishing the antigenic relationship between various substances, as shown in Figure 5.5. Three reaction patterns are seen in gel diffusion, each of which is illustrated in Figure 5.5: patterns of identity, patterns of nonidentity, and patterns of partial identity.

PATTERNS OF IDENTITY. In the example given on the left in Figure 5.5, the central well contains antibodies and the peripheral wells contain identical antigens. The antibodies diffuse from the central well toward the antigens that, since they are identical, form one **continuous, coalescing** precipitin line. This pattern, formed when the two antigens are identical, is termed a **pattern of identity**.

PATTERNS OF NONIDENTITY. In the example in the center of Figure 5.5, the central well contains antibodies to antigen 1 and antibodies to antigen 2, two non-related antigens, and the peripheral wells contain the two nonrelated antigens, antigen 1 and antigen 2. The two antibody (immunoglobulin) populations diffuse toward the peripheral wells. Antigen 1 and antigen 2 diffuse from the two peripheral wells toward the antibodies. Each antigen forms an independent precipitin line with its corresponding antibody at an equivalent point. The precipitin lines cross each other since each antigen diffuses across the band formed by the other antigen until it meets its specific antibody diffusing toward it. A pattern where the precipitin lines **cross each other** denotes **nonidentity** of the two antigens.

PATTERNS OF PARTIAL IDENTITY. The pattern of partial identity is shown in the right-hand portion of Figure 5.5, where the center well contains antibodies to various

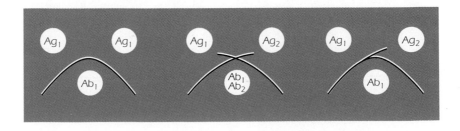

Figure 5.5. Double gel-diffusion patterns showing pattern of identity **(left)**, pattern of nonidentity (center), and pattern of partial identity **(right)**.

epitopes of antigen 1. The reaction of these antibodies with antigen 1 results in a precipitin line. Antigen 2, however, contains some (but not all) of the epitopes present on antigen 1. Thus, some of the antibodies to antigen 1 will also combine with antigen 2. This **partial identity** between the two antigens is responsible for the coalescence of the two lines to give a line of identity. However, antibodies that do not bind with antigen 2 will pass through this line of precipitate, combine with antigen 1 on the other side, and form a spur. This pattern, with the formation of a **spur**, denotes partial identity, signifying that antigen 1 and antigen 2 share epitopes, with antigen 1 having more epitopes (and being able to react with more antibody populations) than antigen 2.

Radial Immunodiffusion. The radial immunodiffusion test, depicted in Figure 5.6, represents a variation of the double-diffusion test. The wells contain antigen at different concentrations, while the antibodies are distributed uniformly in the agar gel. Thus, the precipitin line is replaced by a precipitin ring around the well. The distance the precipitin ring migrates from the center of the antigen well is directly proportional to the concentration of antigen in the well. The relationship between concentration of antigen in a well and the diameter of the precipitin ring can be plotted as shown in Figure 5.6. If wells, such as F and G, contain unknown amounts of the same antigen, the concentration of that antigen in these wells can be determined by comparing the diameter of the precipitin ring with the **diameter** of the ring formed by a known concentration of the antigen.

An important application of radial immunodiffusion is its use clinically to measure concentrations of serum proteins. To do so, antiserum to various serum proteins is incorporated in the gel; concentration of a particular protein in a serum sample is determined by comparing the diameter of the resulting precipitin ring with the diameter obtained by known concentrations of the protein in question.

Immunoelectrophoresis. Immunoelectrophoresis involves separating a mixture of proteins in an electrical field (electrophoresis) followed by their detection with antibodies diffusing into the gel. It is very useful for the analysis of a mixture of antigens by antiserum that contains antibodies to the antigens in the mixture. For

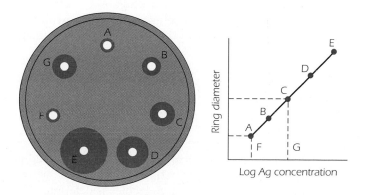

Figure 5.6. Radial diffusion, A, B, C, D, and E represent known concentrations of antigen; F and G represent unknown concentrations that can be determined from the graph.

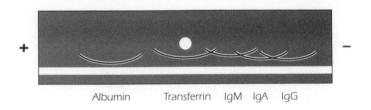

+   Albumin   Transferrin   IgM   IgA   IgG   –

 Figure 5.7. Patterns of immunoelectrophoresis of serum proteins.

example, in the clinical characterization of human serum proteins, a small drop of human serum is placed in a well cut in the center of a slide that is coated with agar gel. The serum is then subjected to electrophoresis, which separates the various components according to their mobilities in the electrical field. After electrophoresis, a trough is cut along the side of the slides, and antibodies to human serum proteins are placed in the trough. The antibodies diffuse in the agar, as do the separated serum proteins. At an optimal antigen:antibody ratio for each antigen and its corresponding antibodies, they form precipitin lines. The result is a pattern similar to that depicted in Figure 5.7. Comparison of the pattern and intensity of lines of normal human serum with the patterns and intensity of lines obtained with sera of patients may reveal an absence, overabundance, or other abnormality of one or more serum proteins. In fact, it was through the use of the immunoelectrophoresis assay that the first antibody-deficiency syndrome was identified in 1952 (Bruton's agammaglobulinemia) (see Chapter 18).

Western Blots (Immunoblots). In the Western blot (immunoblot) technique, antigen (or a mixture of antigens) is first separated in a gel. The separated material is then transferred onto protein-binding sheets (e.g., nitrocellulose) by using an electroblotting method. Antibody, which is then applied to the nitrocellulose sheet, binds with its specific antigen. The antibody may be labeled (e.g., with radioactivity), or a labeled anti-immunoglobulin may be used to localize the antibody and the antigen to which the first antibody is bound. These so-called "Western blots" are used widely in research and clinical laboratories for the detection and characterization of antigens. A particularly useful example is the confirmatory diagnosis of HIV infection by the application of a patient's serum to the nitrocellulose sheets on which HIV antigens are bound. The finding of specific antibody is strong evidence of infection by the virus (Figure 5.8).

IMMUNOASSAYS

Direct Binding Immunoassays

Radioimmunoassay (RIA) employs isotopically labeled molecules and permits measurements of extremely small amounts of antigen, antibody, or antigen–antibody complexes. The concentration of such labeled molecules is determined by measuring their radioactivity, rather than by chemical analysis. The sensitivity of detection is thus increased by several orders of magnitude. For the development of this highly sensitive analytical method that has tremendous application in hormone assays as

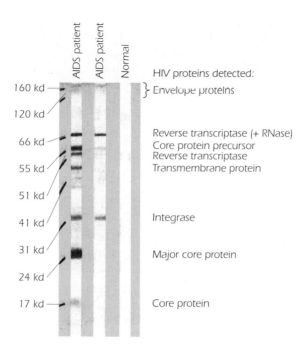

HIV proteins detected:

} Envelope proteins

Reverse transcriptase (+ RNase)
Core protein precursor
Reverse transcriptase
Transmembrane protein

Integrase

Major core protein

Core protein

Figure 5.8. Western blots of serum samples from two HIV-infected individuals and one control subject.

well as assays of other substances found at low levels in biological fluids. Rosalyn Yalow received the Nobel Prize.

The principle of radioimmunoassay is illustrated in Figure 5.9. A known amount of radioactively labeled antigen is reacted with a limited amount of antibody. The solution now contains antibody-bound labeled antigen, as well as some unbound labeled antigen. After separating the antigen bound to antibody from free antigen, the amount of radioactivity bound to antibody is determined. The test continues with performance of a similar procedure in which the same amount of labeled antigen is premixed with unlabeled antigen (Figure 5.10). The mixture is reacted with the same

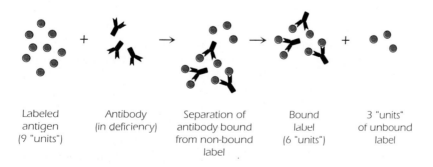

| Labeled antigen (9 "units") | Antibody (in deficiency) | Separation of antibody bound from non-bound label | Bound label (6 "units") | 3 "units" of unbound label |

Figure 5.9. Amount of label bound to antibody after incubation of constant amounts of antibody and labeled antigen.

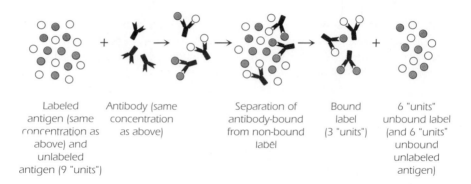

Labeled antigen (same concentration as above) and unlabeled antigen (9 "units") + Antibody (same concentration as above) → Separation of antibody-bound from non-bound label → Bound label (3 "units") + 6 "units" unbound label (and 6 "units" unbound unlabeled antigen)

Figure 5.10. Radioimmunoassay, based on the competition of nonlabeled and labeled antigens for antibody.

amount of antibody as before, and the antibody-bound antigen is separated from the unbound antigen. The unlabeled antigen **competes** with the labeled antigen for the antibody and, as a result, less label is bound to antibody than in the absence of unlabeled antigen. The more unlabeled antigen present in the reaction mixture, the smaller the ratio of antibody-bound, radiolabeled antigen to free, radiolabeled antigen. This ratio can be plotted as a function of the concentration of the unlabeled antigen used for competition.

To determine an unknown concentration of antigen in a solution, a sample of the solution is mixed with predetermined amounts of labeled antigen and antibody. The ratio of **bound/free radioactivity** is compared with that obtained in the absence of unlabeled antigen (the latter value is set at 100%).

An important step in performing a radioimmunoassay, as described above, is the separation of free antigen from that bound to antibody. Depending upon the antigen, this separation can be achieved in a variety of ways, principal among which is the anti-immunoglobulin procedure.

The **anti-immunoglobulin procedure** is based on the fact that antigen (labeled or unlabeled) bound to immunoglobulin will also be precipitated, following the addition of anti-immunoglobulin antibodies, so that only unbound antigen remains in the supernatant. Radioimmunoassays commonly employ rabbit antibodies to the desired antigens. These rabbit antibody–antigen complexes may be precipitated by the addition of goat antibodies raised against rabbit immunoglobulins.

Since the amounts of antigen and antibody required for radioimmunoassay are extremely small, the antigen–antibody complexes reacted with anti-immunoglobulin would form only tiny precipitates. It is difficult, if not impossible, to recover these precipitates quantitatively by conventional means, in order to determine their radioactivity. To overcome this problem, it is customary to add immunoglobulins that are not specific for the antigen in the reaction mixture, thereby increasing the amount of total immunoglobulins to an amount that can easily be precipitated by anti-immunoglobulins and recovered quantitatively. Such precipitates consist mainly of nonspecific immunoglobulins to which radioactive antigen does not bind. However, they also contain the extremely small amount of antigen-specific immunoglobulin and any radioactive antigen bound to it.

An alternative method of separating complexes of antigen bound to antibody from free antigen is based on the fact that immunoglobulins become insoluble and precipitate in a solution containing 33% saturated ammonium sulfate. If the antigen does not precipitate in 33% ammonium sulfate, the addition of ammonium sulfate to 33% will cause the antibody complexed to antigen to precipitate, leaving the free antigen in solution. Here again, the amounts of antibodies reacting with antigen (or free antibodies) are small and unable to form precipitates. As described for the radioimmunoassay where anti-immunoglobulins are used for the separation of antibody-bound antigen from free antigen, a sufficient amount of nonspecific immunoglobulins is added to the mixture; an appreciable precipitate will form at 33% saturation ammonium sulfate to enable the separation of free antigen from antigen bound to antibody.

Solid-Phase Immunoassays

Solid-phase immunoassay is one of the most widely used immunologic techniques. It is now automated and is widely used in clinical medicine for the detection of antigen or antibody. A good example is the use of solid-phase immunoassay for the detection of antibodies to HIV (see Chapter 18).

Solid-phase immunoassays employ the property of various plastics (e.g., polyvinyl or polystyrene) to adsorb monomolecular layers of proteins onto their surface. Although the adsorbed molecules may lose some of their antigenic determinants, enough remain unaltered and can still react with their corresponding antibodies. The presence of these antibodies, bound to antigen adsorbed onto the plastic, may be detected by the use of anti-immunoglobulins (Figure 5.11) labeled with a radioactive tracer or with an enzyme. If the test uses anti-immunoglobulins that are labeled with an enzyme that can be detected by the appearance of a color on addition of substrate, the test is called an ***enzyme-linked immunosorbent assay*** (ELISA).

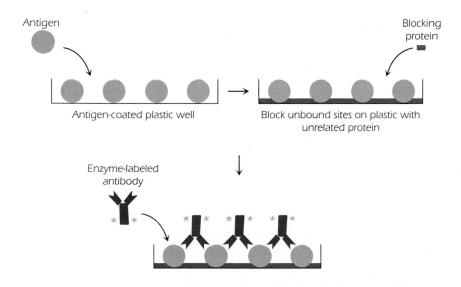

Figure 5.11. A representative ELISA using a well coated directly with antigen.

It should be emphasized that after coating the plastic surface with antigen, it is imperative to "block"any uncoated plastic surface to prevent it from absorbing the other reagents, most importantly the labeled reagent. Such "blocking"is achieved by coating the plastic surface with a high concentration of an unrelated protein, such as gelatin, after the application of the antigen.

Solid-phase immunoassay may be used to detect the presence of antibodies to the antigen that coats the plastic. Since the plastic wells are usually coated with relatively large amounts of antigen, the higher the concentration of antibodies bound with the antigen, the higher the amount of labeled anti-immunoglobulin that can bind to the antibodies. Thus, it is important always to use an excess of labeled anti-immunoglobulin to assure saturation.

Solid-phase immunoassay may be used for the qualitative or quantitative determinations of antigen. Such determinations are performed by mixing the antiserum with varying known amounts of antigen before adding the antiserum to the antigen-coated plastic wells. This preliminary procedure results in the binding of the antibodies with the soluble antigen, decreasing the availability of free antibodies for binding with the antigen that is coating the plastic. The higher the concentration of the soluble antigen that reacts with antibodies before the addition of the antibody to the wells, the lower the number of antibodies that can bind with the antigen on the plate, and the lower the number of labeled anti-immunoglobulin that can bind to these antibodies. The decrease in the amount of bound label as a function of the concentration of antigen used to cause this decrease can be plotted, and the amount of antigen in an unknown solution can then be determined from the graph by a comparison of the decrease in bound label caused by the unknown solution to the decrease caused by known concentrations of pure antigen.

IMMUNOFLUORESCENCE

A fluorescent compound has the property of emitting light of a certain wavelength when it is excited by exposure to light of a shorter wavelength. Immunofluorescence is a method for localizing an antigen by the use of fluorescently labeled antibodies. The procedure, originally described by Coombs, employs antibodies to which fluorescent groups have been covalently linked without any appreciable change in antibody activity.

One fluorescent compound that is widely used in immunology is **fluorescein isothiocyanate** (FITC), which fluoresces with a visible greenish color when excited by ultraviolet light. FITC is easily coupled to free amino groups. Another widely used fluorescent compound is **phycoerythrin** (PE), which fluoresces red and is also easily coupled to free amino groups. Fluorescence microscopes equipped with a UV light source permit visualization of fluorescent antibody on a microscopic specimen, and fluorescent antibodies are widely used to localize antigens on various tissues and microorganisms.

There are two important and related procedures that employ fluorescent antibodies: direct immunofluorescence and indirect immunofluorescence.

Direct Immunofluorescence

Direct immunofluorescence is primarily for detection of antigen and involves reacting the target tissue (or microorganism) with fluorescently labeled specific antibodies. It is widely used clinically for identifying lymphocytic subsets and for demonstrating the presence of specific protein deposition in certain tissues such as kidney and skin in cases of systemic lupus erythematosus (SLE) (see Chapter 17).

Indirect Immunofluorescence

Indirect immunofluorescence involves first reacting the target with unlabeled specific antibodies. This reaction is followed by subsequent reaction with fluorescently labeled anti-immunoglobulin.

The indirect immunofluorescence method is more widely used than the direct method, because a single fluorescent anti-immunoglobulin antibody can be used to localize antibody of many different specificities. Moreover, since the anti-immunoglobulins contain antibodies to many epitopes on the specific immunoglobulin, the use of fluorescent anti-immunoglobulins significantly amplifies the fluorescent signal. An excellent example for the use of indirect immunofluorescence is the screening of patients' sera for antiDNA antibodies in cases of SLE.

 FLUORESCENCE-ACTIVATED CELL-SORTING ANALYSIS

A very powerful tool has been developed around the use of fluorescent antibody specific for cell-surface antigens. This is the technique of fluorescence-activated cell sorting (FACS). A cell suspension labeled with specific fluorescent antibody is passed through an apparatus that forms a stream of small droplets each containing one cell. These droplets are passed between a laser beam of ultraviolet light and a detector for picking up emitted fluorescence when a labeled cell is present in the droplet. This emitted signal is passed to an electrode that charges the droplet, leading to its deflection in an electromagnetic field (Figure 5.12). Thus as all droplets fall past the laser beam they are counted and can be sorted (e.g., unlabeled versus labeled) according to whether they emit a signal. The intensity of fluorescein-staining on each cell, which reflects the density of antigen expressed on the cell, may be determined by sophisticated electronics.

With this type of apparatus it is now possible to rapidly develop a profile of a pool of lymphocytes based on their differential expression of cell-surface molecules, the relative amount of cell-surface molecule expressed on each cell, and the size distribution and numbers of each cell type. It is also possible to use the apparatus to sort a collection of cells stained with five or more different fluorescent labels and obtain a very homogeneous sample of a particular cell type. A variation of this technique uses fluorescent antibodies coupled to magnetic beads to separate cell populations. Cells which bind to the fluorescent antibody can be separated from unstained cells by a magnet. Both FACS and magnetic bead separation methods have resulted in the isolation of very rare cells such as hematopoietic stem cells.

The most common method for phenotyping and sorting cells involves the use of antibodies that react with cell-surface proteins identified as *cluster of differentiation* (CD) *antigens*. The CD nomenclature originates from studies using monoclonal antibodies (discussed later in this chapter) to phenotypically characterize cells. It was found that cell-surface markers (CD antigens) are associated with distinct developmental stages. Moreover, these proteins have important biologic functions required for normal cell physiology. The developmental stages of B and T cells and functional

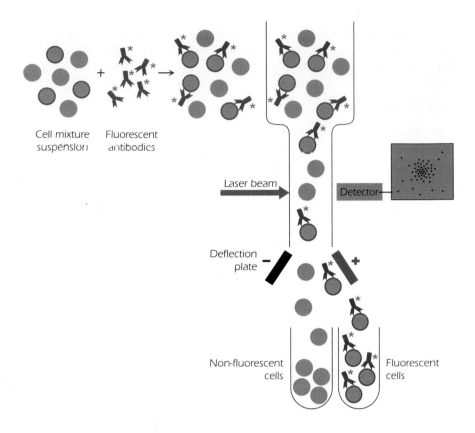

Figure 5.12. A schematic representation of a fluorescence-activated cell sorter (FACS).

subsets of these cells can now be phenotyped based on their expression of CD markers. It is also worth noting, however, that surface expression of a particular molecule may not be specific for just one cell or even for a cell lineage. Nonetheless, cell-surface expression can be exploited for purification, as well as characterization, of cells. For practical purposes, the CD acronym is followed by an arbitrary number that identifies a specific cell-surface protein. CD numbers are assigned by the Nomenclature Committee of the International Union of Immunologic Sciences. A list some of some of the more important CD antigens expressed by B cells, various T-cell subsets, and other cells can be found in the Appendix.

IMMUNOABSORPTION AND IMMUNOADSORPTION

Because of the specific binding between antigen and antibody, it is possible to "trap," or selectively remove, an antigen against which an antibody is directed from a mixture of antigens in solution. Similarly, it is possible to trap or selectively remove the antigen-specific antibodies from a mixture of antibodies, using the specific antigen.

There are two general methods by which this removal can be achieved. The methods are related, but, in one method, the absorption is done with both reagents in solution (***immunoabsorption***); in the second method, it is performed with one reagent attached to an insoluble support (***immunoadsorption***). Immunoadsorption is of particular value because the adsorbed material can be recovered from the complex by careful treatments that dissociate antigen–antibody complexes, such as lowering the pH (HCl-glycine or acetic acid, pH 2–3) or adding chaotropic ions. This enables the effective purification of antigens or antibodies of interest.

 ## ASSAYS TO ASSESS LYMPHOCYTE FUNCTION

Assays used to assess lymphocyte function generally attempt to answer one of the following questions: (1) Do the B or T cells respond normally to mitogenic stimuli that activate cells to undergo a proliferative response?; (2) Does mitogenic or antigen-driven stimulation result in antibody production (for B cells) or cytokine production (for T cells)?; In addition, given the functional heterogeneity of T cells that exist as phenotypically distinct T-cell subsets (e.g., $CD4^+$ helper T cells, $CD8^+$ cytotoxic T cells), T-cell assays can also be used to quantitate the functional properties associated with a particular T-cell subset. In the case of T helper cell assays, the target cell of interest (i.e., the cell population which receives the help) generally determines the functional parameter to be measured. For example, if one were interested in knowing whether T cells provide help for B cell activation in response to antigen stimulation, the assay might quantitate the level of antibody produced. Similarly, if one were interested in knowing whether T cells provide help needed to optimally activate macrophages, the parameters measured would focus on functional properties associated with these phagocytic cells. It is important to note that many of the assays used to assess helper T-cell function also rely upon the measurement of specific cytokines since the cells receiving help (e.g., macrophages) may be activated to produce cytokines themselves. Finally, the cytotoxic activity of antigen-specific $CD8^+$ T cells can be measured using one of several qualitative or quantitative methods. The cytotoxic activity of null lymphocytes called natural killer (NK) cells (i.e., cells which fail to express the membrane molecules that distinguish T and B cells) can also be quantitated employing methods similar to those used for measuring cytotoxic T activity.

B-Cell and T-Cell Proliferation Assays

Mitogen-stimulated lymphocyte activation triggers biochemical signaling pathways that lead to gene expression, protein synthesis, cell proliferation, and differentiation. The proliferative responses generated in response to mitogens are polyclonal in nature. Moreover, mitogens have been identified that selectively stimulate either B- or T-cell populations. Therefore, unlike immunogens that activate only the lymphocyte clones bearing the appropriate antigen receptor, polyclonal activators stimulate many B- or T-cell clones regardless of their antigenic specificity. Mitogens that selectively activate B cells, such as the ***lipopolysaccharide*** (LPS) component of gram-negative bacterial cell walls, will cause polyclonal stimulation of B cells in vitro. The magnitude of cell proliferation in response to mitogenic stimulation can be measured by adding radiolabeled nucleosides (e.g., tritiated thymidine) to the medium during cell culture and then quantitating its incorporation into the DNA of dividing cells using a liquid scintillation counter. Similarly, several sugar-binding proteins called ***lectins*** including **concanavalin A** (Con A) and **phytohemagglutinin** (PHA) are very effective T-cell mitogens. Pokeweed mitogen (PWM) is another example of a lectin with potent mitogenic properties. However, unlike Con A and PHA, **PWM stimulates polyclonal activation of both B and T cells**.

Antibody Production by B Cells

Mitogenic stimulation of B and T cells results in the proliferation and differentiation of many clones of cells. Therefore, in the case of B cells, the polyclonal activators LPS or PWM can be used to assess the ability of a population of B cells to produce antibody. **ELISAs** are the most commonly used quantitative assays for measuring antibody levels. Alternatively, B cells can be stimulated with mitogens or specific antigens in vitro, then temporarily cultured in chambers directly on nitrocellulose membranes in a so-called **ELISPOT** assay. The protein-binding property of nitrocellulose facilitates the capture of secreted antibody by individual B cells. This yields discrete foci of antibody bound to the nitrocellulose that can be detected using a secondary, enzyme-labeled antibody specific for the bound antibody, allowing for the enumeration of antibody-secreting cells.

Effector Cell Assays for T Cells and NK Cells

As noted above, the choice of effector cell assay used depends on the questions that need to be answered. T-cell assays are as varied as the functional diverse T-cell subsets known to exist. Thus, various assays that measure T helper cell function have been developed which focus on helper activity for B cells, macrophage activation, and even other T cells can be used to measure the helper properties of $CD4^+$ T cells. Similarly, several assays which measure cytotoxic activity of $CD8^+$ T cells are available. One such assay (**cytotoxicity assay**) measures the ability of cytotoxic T cells or NK cells to kill radiolabeled target cells expressing the antigen to which the cytotoxic T cells were sensitized. In a related assay, the NK cells are cultured with radiolabeled target cells bound to target cell-specific antibodies. The rationale for this approach is based on the fact that NK cells express membrane Fc receptors that bind to the Fc region of certain immunoglobulin isotypes. This method measures an important functional property of NK cells known as **antibody-dependent cell-mediated cytotoxicity** (ADCC).

 CELL CULTURE SYSTEMS

Primary Cell Cultures and Cloned Lymphoid Cell Lines

As with many other fields of biologic science, cell culture systems have served as an essential investigational tool to facilitate our understanding of many developmental/maturational and physiologic properties of cells. The ability to culture primary lymphoid cells consisting of a heterogeneous populations of T and/or B cells (albeit for limited periods of time) has allowed immunologists to study the biochemical and molecular mechanisms controlling many important biologic features of B and T cells, including gene rearrangement. Advances in cell culture systems have evolved rapidly during the past few decades leading to the development of cell cloning techniques.

Transformation of B and T cells derived from a specific parent cell to generate cloned, immortal cell lines has been achieved using a variety of methods including exposure of cells to certain carcinogens or viruses (e.g., Epstein-Barr virus for the transformation of B cells; human T cell leukemia virus type 1 for the transformation of T cells). It should be noted that many cell lines are derived from tumors arising either spontaneously or experimentally (as a result of administration of carcinogens or virus infection). The major advantage of using cloned cell lines is that large numbers of cells can be generated for investigation. A disadvantage in the use of carcinogen- or virus-transformed cells is that they are, by definition, abnormal. Indeed, many transformed cells have abnormal numbers of chromosomes and often display phenotypic and functional properties not seen in normal cells. A major advance in the generation of cloned lymphoid cells came in the late 1970s with the discovery that nontransformed antigen-specific T-cell lines and antigen-specific T-cell clones could be grown indefinitely when a T cell growth factor (interleukin-2) was included in the culture together with a source of antigen and antigen-presenting cells. This approach offered several advantages over the use of transformed cells since the cells derived from such cultures were, for all intents and purposes, normal. Thus, large numbers of nontransformed antigen-specific T cells could be generated for investigation. Indeed, many of these cloned T-cell lines have been used in the identification and biochemical characterization of cytokines, leading to the ultimate cloning of genes that encode these proteins.

The combined use of cell cloning systems, gene transfer methods, and animal models has led to a growing understanding of how lymphoid cells develop self-tolerance as well as how they can escape tolerance-inducing mechanisms to become disease-causing autoreactive cells. In short, cell culture systems have served as a gateway for research endeavors to shed light on both the physiologic and pathophysiologic properties of lymphoid cells. As will be discussed below, cell culture systems have also been productively exploited with the development of many useful diagnostic and therapeutic reagents, such as monoclonal antibodies.

MONOCLONAL AND GENETICALLY ENGINEERED ANTIBODIES

Monoclonal Antibodies

The specificity of the immune response has served as the basis for serologic reactions in which antibody specificity is used for the qualitative and quantitative determination of antigen. The discriminating power of serum antibody is not without limitations, however, because the immunizing antigen, which usually has many epitopes, leads to production of antisera that contain a mixture of antibodies with varying specificity for all the epitopes. Indeed, even antibodies to a single epitope are usually mixtures of immunoglobulins with different *fine specificities*, and therefore different affinities for the determinant. Furthermore, immunization with an antigen expands various populations of antibody-forming lymphocytes. These cells can be maintained in culture for only a short time (on the order of days), so it is impractical, if not impossible, to grow normal cells and obtain clones that produce antibodies of a single specificity. A quantum leap in the resolution and discriminating power of antibodies took place in the 1970s with the development of methods for the generation of monoclonal antibodies by Milstein and Köhler, who shared the Nobel Prize for this development. *Monoclonal antibodies* are homogeneous populations of antibody molecules, derived from a single antibody-producing cell, in which all antibodies are identical and of the same precise specificity for a given epitope.

Milstein and Köhler took advantage of the properties of malignant plasma cells, which are "immortal" and can be maintained in culture for years. They selected a population of malignant plasma cells unable to secrete immunoglobulin but also deficient in the enzyme hypoxanthine guanine phosphoribosyl transferase (HGPRT) that would die unless HGPRT was provided either in culture or by fusing the cells with HGPRT^{+} cells. The malignant cells were then *fused* (hybridized) with freshly harvested spleen cells from a mouse recently immunized with antigen. Since the antibody-producing splenic B cells are HGPRT^{+}, hybridoma cells consisting of myeloma cells fused with B cells survived in the absence of HGPRT in the culture medium. The biotechnology for the production of *hybridomas*, developed by Köhler and Milstein, is illustrated in Figure 5.13. The fusion is often accomplished by the use of polyethylene glycol (PEG). The nuclei of the hybrids also fuse, and the hybridoma cells then possess both the capacity to manufacture immunoglobulins and the ability to survive in culture in a select medium such as that containing hypoxanthine, aminopterin, and thymidine (HAT). The enzyme deficiency of the malignant cell results in its death in this medium unless that deficiency is corrected by the acquisition of the enzyme-producing cell. Thus, the hybrids can be separated from the contaminating malignant cells, which do not survive, because they have not acquired the enzyme.

Those hybrid cells synthesizing specific antibody are selected by some test for antigen reactivity (e.g., ELISA) and then *cloned* from single cells and propagated in tissue culture, each clone synthesizing antibodies of a *single specificity*. Those highly specific, monoclonal antibodies are used for numerous procedures, ranging from specific diagnostic tests to biologic agents used in immunotherapy of cancer (see Chapter 20). In immunotherapy, various drugs or toxins are conjugated to monoclonal antibodies, which, in turn, "deliver" these substances to the tumor cells against which the antibodies are specifically directed.

T-Cell Hybridomas

It is important to note that hybridoma technology is not limited to the production of monoclonal immunoglobulins. In the late 1970s, methods for producing hybridomas were also developed for T cells, fusing lines of malignant T cells with nonmalignant, antigen-specific T lymphocytes whose populations have been expanded by immunization with antigen. T cell hybridomas have been very useful for studying the relationship between T cells of a single specificity with their corresponding epitope.

GENETICALLY ENGINEERED MOLECULES AND RECEPTORS

To date most of the monoclonal antibodies are made in mouse cells. These are suitable for diagnostic and many other purposes. However, their administration into humans carries the complication that the patient will form antibodies to the mouse immunoglobulins. Attempts to develop in vitro human monoclonal antibodies have, by and large, not been very successful.

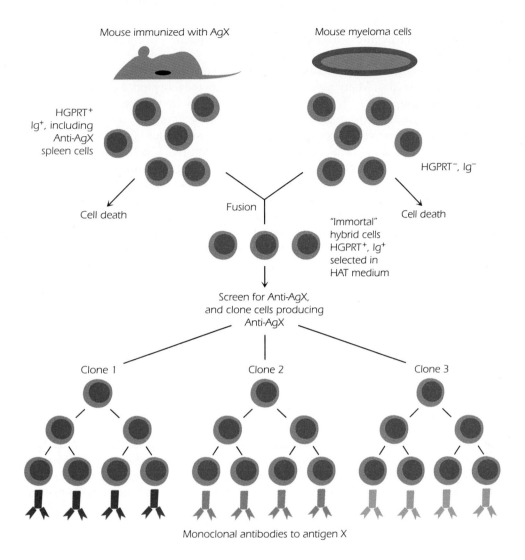

Mouse immunized with AgX

Mouse myeloma cells

HGPRT$^+$
Ig$^+$, including
Anti-AgX
spleen cells

HGPRT$^-$, Ig$^-$

Cell death

Fusion

Cell death

"Immortal"
hybrid cells
HGPRT$^+$, Ig$^+$
selected in
HAT medium

Screen for Anti-AgX,
and clone cells producing
Anti-AgX

Clone 1

Clone 2

Clone 3

Monoclonal antibodies to antigen X

Figure 5.13. A schematic representation of the production of monoclonal antibodies.

Human monoclonal antibodies are currently being produced by genetic engineering utilizing several approaches. One method utilizes the technology of recombinant DNA to produce a chimeric monoclonal antibody. This molecule consists of the constant region of human immunoglobulin and a variable region of a mouse immunoglobulin. A similar method is used to construct humanized antibodies consisting of a human constant region and a variable region containing a mouse hypervariable region and a human framework region. Another method utilizes the polymerase chain reaction (PCR) to generate gene libraries of heavy and light chains from DNA obtained from hybridoma cells or plasma cells, joining at random numerous heavy and light chains and screening the resulting Fab clones for antibody activity against a desired antigen. With this technology it is now possible to produce millions of clones of different specificities, to rapidly screen them for the desired specificity and generate the desired monoclonal Fab constructs without immunization and without the difficulties encountered with the production of monoclonal antibodies, especially human monoclonal antibodies.

Genetic engineering of immune proteins is not limited to the production of monoclonal antibodies. Many genes encoding membrane receptors expressed on lymphoid and nonlymphoid cells have been cloned and, in some cases, genetically engineered to allow for gene transfer to cells that do not normally express these receptors. The expression of certain costimulator molecules facilitates cell–cell interactions (e.g., the physical contact between cytotoxic T cells and target cells, which results in the killing of the latter). The expression, through gene transfer, of such costimulator molecules (e.g., B7) on tumor cells significantly enhances the ability of T cells to recognize and kill these cells. Experimental vaccination strategies (a form of immunotherapy) have demonstrated that immunization of tumor-bearing animals with their own tumor cells, which have been removed and transfected with the B7 gene, can potentiate T cells to recognize and destroy the parent tumor cells. It should be noted that a similar strategy using tumor cells transfected with certain cytokine genes has also been used with some success in animal models. Immunotherapeutic strategies used to treat a variety of diseases are discussed in several chapters of this book (see Chapters 18, 20, and 21).

EXPERIMENTAL ANIMAL MODELS

Inbred Strains

Many of the classic experiments in the field of immunology have been performed using inbred strains of animals such as mice, rats, and guinea pigs. Selective inbreeding of littermates for more than 20 generations usually leads to the production of an inbred strain. All members of inbred strains of animals are genetically identical. Therefore, like identical twins, they are said to be *syngeneic*. Immune responses of inbred strains can be studied in the absence of variables associated with genetic differences between animals. As will be discussed in Chapter 19, organ transplants between members of inbred stains are always accepted since their major histocompatibility complex (MHC) antigens are identical. Indeed, knowledge of the laws of transplantation and the fact that the MHC is the major genetic barrier to transplantation was made possible through the use of inbred strains. Experiments using inbred strains led to the identification of class I and class II MHC genes whose main function is to deliver peptide fragments of antigen to the cell surface thus allowing them to be recognized by antigen-specific T cells. Subsequent chapters will elaborate on the important role of the MHC in (1) the generation of normal immune responses; (2) T-cell development; (3) disease susceptibility; and, (4) organ transplantation.

Adoptive Transfer

Protection against many diseases is conferred through *cell-mediated immunity* as opposed to *antibody-mediated (humoral) immunity*. The distinction between these two arms of the immune response can be readily demonstrated by adoptive transfer of lymphoid cells or by passive administration of antiserum or purified antibodies. *Adoptive transfer* of lymphoid cells is usually performed using genetically identical donor and recipients (e.g., inbred strains) and results in long-term *adoptive immunization* following antigen priming. By contrast, passive transfer of serum containing antibodies can be performed across MHC barriers and is effective as long as the transferred antibodies remain active in the recipient. This type of transfer is therefore called ***passive immunization***.

SCID Mice

Severe combined immunodeficiency disease (SCID) is a disorder in which B and T cells fail to develop, causing the individual to be compromised with respect to lymphoid defense mechanisms. Chapter 18 discusses various causes of SCID in man. In the 1980s, an inbred strain of mice spontaneously developed an autosomal recessive mutation, resulting in SCID in homozygous scid/scid mice. Because of the absence of functional T and B cells, SCID mice are able to accept cells and tissue grafts from other strains of mice or other species. Thus, SCID mice can be successfully engrafted with human hematopoietic stem cells to create SCID-human chimeras. Such chimeric mice develop mature, functional T and B cells derived from the infused human stem-cell precursors. This animal model has become a valuable research tool, since it allows immunologists to manipulate the human immune system in vivo and to investigate the development of various lymphoid cells. Moreover, SCID-human mice can be used to test candidate vaccines, including those that might useful in protecting humans from HIV infection.

Thymectomized and Congenically Athymic (Nude) Mice

The importance of the thymus in the development of mature T cells can be demonstrated by using mice that have been neonatally thymectomized, irradiated, and then reconstituted with syngeneic bone marrow. Such mice fail to develop mature T cells. Similarly, mice homozygous for the recessive nude mutation also fail to develop mature T cells because the mutation results in an athymic (and hairless, hence, the term nude) phenotype. In both situations, T-cell development can be restored by grafting these mice with thymic epithelial tissue. Like SCID mice, these animal models have been useful in the study of T-cell development. They have also been useful for the in vivo propagation of tumor cell lines and fresh tumor explants from other strains and other species due to the absence of T cells required to reject such foreign cells.

TRANSGENIC MICE AND GENE TARGETING

Transgenic Mice

Another significant animal system used extensively in immunologic research is the transgenic mouse. ***Transgenic mice*** are made by injecting a cloned gene (***transgene***) into fertilized mouse eggs. The eggs are then microinjected into pseudopregnant mice (Figure 5.14). The success rate of this technique is rather low with approximately 10% to 30% of the offspring expressing the transgene. Since the transgene is integrated into both somatic and germ-line cells, it is transmitted to the offspring as a Mendelian trait. By constructing a transgene with a particular promoter, it is possible to control the gene's expression. For example, some promoters function only in certain tissues (e.g., the insulin promoter only functions in the pancreas), whereas others function in response to biochemical signals that can be supplied, in some

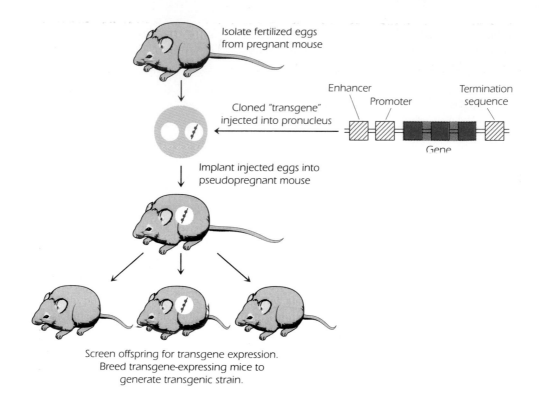

Figure 5.14. A general procedure for producing transgenic mice.

cases, as a dietary supplement (e.g., the metallothionine promoter that functions in response to zinc which can be added to the drinking water). Transgenic mice have been used to study genes that are not usually expressed in vivo (e.g., oncogenes), as well as the effects of transgenes encoding particular immunoglobulin molecules, T cell receptors, MHC class I or class II molecules, and a variety of cytokines. A disadvantage of the transgenic method is that the transgene integrates randomly within the genome. This limitation, together with the fact that it is unphysiologic to express high quantities of transgenes in the wrong tissues, forces investigators to use great care in interpreting results obtained in transgenic mice.

Knockout Mice

Sometimes, it is of interest to determine how the removal of a particular gene product affects the immune system. Using a *gene targeting* method, it is possible to replace a normal gene with one that has been mutated or disrupted to generate so-called *knockout mice*. Thus, unlike the method used to generate transgenic mice, knockout mice express transgenes which integrate at specific endogenous genes through a process known as homologous recombination. Virtually any gene for which a mutated or altered transgene exists can be targeted this way. Knockout mice have been generated by using mutated or altered transgenes that target, and therefore silence, the expression of a variety of important genes, including those encoding particular cytokines and MHC molecules.

SUMMARY

1. The reaction between an antibody and an epitope does not involve covalent forces; it involves weak forces of interaction such as electrostatic, hydrophobic, and van der Waals forces. Consequently, for a significant interaction, the antibody combining site and the epitope require a close steric fit like a lock and key.

2. Only the reaction between a multivalent antigen and at least a bivalent antibody can bring about secondary antigen—antibody reactions that depend on crosslinking of antigen molecules by antibodies. These secondary reactions do not take place with haptens or monovalent Fab.

3. The interaction between a soluble antibody and an insoluble particulate antigen results in agglutination. The extent of agglutination depends on the proportions of the interacting antibody and antigen. At high antibody levels, excess agglutination may not occur. This is referred to as a prozone. The term titer refers to the highest serum dilution at which agglutination still takes place and beyond which, at higher dilution, no agglutination occurs.

4. Precipitation reactions occur on mixing, at the right proportions, of soluble multivalent antigen and (at least) divalent antibodies. The precipitation reaction may take place in aqueous media or in gels.

5. The reaction in gels, between soluble antigen and antibodies, may be used for the qualitative and quantitative analysis of antigen or antibody. Examples are gel diffusion tests, radial diffusion tests, and immunoelectrophoresis.

6. Radioimmunoassay (RIA) is a very sensitive test used to quantitate antibody or antigen. It employs the use of radiolabeled antigen or antibody and is based on competitive inhibition of nonlabeled and labeled antigen. Antibody-bound antigen must be separated from nonbound labeled antigen. Separation is usually achieved by precipitation with anti-immunoglobulins.

7. Solid-phase immunoassay is a test that employs the property of many proteins to adhere to plastic and form a monomolecular layer. Antigen is applied to plastic wells, antibodies are added, the well is washed, and any antibodies bound to antigen are measured by the use of radiolabeled or enzyme-linked anti-immunoglobulins.

8. The enzyme-linked immunosorbent assay (ELISA) is essentially a solid-phase immunoassay in which an enzyme is linked to the anti-immunoglobulin. Quantitation of enzyme-linked, anti-immunoglobulins is achieved by colorimetric evaluation, after the addition of a substrate, which changes color on the action of the enzyme.

9. Immunofluorescence is a method in which an antigen is detected by the use of fluorescence-labeled immunoglobulins. In direct immunofluorescence, the antibody to the antigen in question carries a fluorescent label. In indirect immunofluorescence, the antigen-specific antibody is not labeled; it is detected by the addition of fluorescently labeled anti-immunoglobulin. Fluorescence-activated cell sorters (FACS) are instruments that can be used to quantitate and sort fluorescently-labeled cells.

10. Assays used to assess lymphocyte function typically measure their proliferative responses or effector functions. For example, B cells can be functionally assessed by measuring their ability to produce antibodies in response to LPS. T cells are often assessed by measuring their ability to provide help for other cells (in the case of CD4[+]cells) or to kill antigen-bearing targets (in the case of CD8[+] cells). In addition, T cells can be assessed by measuring their ability to produce certain cytokines.

11. Monoclonal antibodies are highly specific reagents consisting of homogeneous populations of antibodies, all of precisely the same specificity toward an epitope.

REFERENCES

Camper SA (1987): Research applications of transgenic mice. *Biotechniques* 5:638.

Channing-Rodgers RP (1994): Clinical laboratory methods for detection of antigens and antibodies. In Stites DP, Terr AI, Parslow TG (eds): Basic and Clinical Immunology, 8th ed. E Norwalk, CT: Appleton & Lange.

Harlow E, Lane D (1988): Antibodies: A Laboratory Manual. Cold Spring Harbor, NY: Cold Spring Harbor Laboratory Press.

Hudson L, Hay FC (1989): Practical Immunology, 3rd ed. Oxford, UK: Blackwell.

Johnstone A, Thorpe R (1987): Immunochemistry in Practice. Oxford, UK: Blackwell.

Koller BH, Smithies O (1992): Altering genes in animals by gene targeting. *Annu Rev Immunol* 10:705.

Mayforth RD (1993): Designing Antibodies. San Diego, CA: Academic Press.

Mishell BB, Shiigi SM (1980): Selected Methods in Cellular Immunology. New York: Freeman.

Rose NR, Friedman H, Fahey J (1986): Manual of Clinical Immunology, 3rd ed. Washington, DC: American Society for Microbiology.

Thompson KM (1988): Human monoclonal antibodies. *Immunol Today* 9:113.

Weir DM (1986): Handbook of Experimental Immunology, Vol 12, 4th ed. Oxford, UK: Blackwell.

Winter G, Griffith AD, Hawkins RE, et al. (1994): Making antibodies by phage display technology. *Annu Rev Immunol* 12:433.

● REVIEW QUESTIONS

For each question, choose the ONE BEST answer or completion.

1. Primary interactions between antigens and antibodies involve all of the following except
   A) covalent bonds.
   B) van der Waals forces.
   C) hydrophobic forces.
   D) electrostatic forces.
   E) a very close fit between an epitope and the antibody.

2. If an IgG antibody preparation specific for hen egg lysosome (HEL) is treated with papain to generate Fab fragments, which of the following statements concerning the avidity of such fragments is true?

A) They will have a lower avidity for HEL as compared with the intact IgG.
B) They will have a higher avidity for HEL as compared with the intact IgG.
C) There will have the same avidity for HEL as the intact IgG.
D) They will have lost their avidity to bind to HEL.
E) They will have the same avidity but will have a lower affinity for HEL.

3. Western assays used to test serum samples for the presence of antibodies to infectious agents, such as HIV, are particularly useful as diagnostic assays because

A) they are more sensitive than ELISA.
B) antibodies specific for multiple antigenic epitopes can be detected.
C) they provide quantitative data for sample analysis.
D) they allow multiple samples to be tested simultaneously.
E) they are less expensive and take less time to perform as compared with ELISA.

4. The major difference between transgenic mice and knockout mice is that

A) transgenic mice always employ the use of cloned genes derived from other species.
B) transgenic mice have foreign genes that integrate at targeted loci through homologous recombination.
C) transgenic mice have a functional foreign gene added to their genome.
D) knockout mice always have a unique phenotype.

5. SCID mice have a genetic defect that prevents development of functional

A) hematopoietic cells.
B) B cells and T cells.
C) T cells and NK cells.
D) pluripotential stem cells.
E) myeloid cells.

6. Which of the following statements regarding B cell hybridomas is false?

A) They are immortal cell lines that produce antibodies of a single specificity.
B) They are derived from B cells that are first cloned and grown in cell culture for short periods.
C) They contain a large nucleus formed by the fusion of two nuclei.
D) They can be used to manufacture diagnostic or therapeutic monoclonal antibodies.
E) They are derived by fusing B cells with malignant plasma cells that are unable to secrete immunoglobulin.

7. An ELISA designed to test for the presence of serum antibody for a new strain of pathogenic bacteria is under development. Initially, a monoclonal antibody specific for a single epitope of the organism was used both to sensitize the wells of the ELISA plate and as the enzyme-labeled detecting antibody in a conventional sandwich ELISA. The ELISA failed to detect the antigen despite the use of a wide range of antibody concentrations. What is the most probable cause of this problem?

A) The antigen is too large.
B) The antibody has a low affinity for the antigen.
C) The monoclonal antibody used to sensitize the wells is blocking access of the epitope, thus when the same antibody is enzyme-labeled, it cannot bind to the antigen.
D) The enzyme-labeled antibody used should have been a different isotype than the sensitizing antibody.
E) The monoclonal antibody used is probably unstable.

Answers To Review Questions

1. *A* No covalent bonds are involved in the interaction between antibody and antigen. The binding forces are relatively weak and include van der Waals forces, hydrophobic forces, and electrostatic forces. A very close fit between an epitope and the antibody is required.

2. *A* Avidity denotes the overall binding energy between antigens and multivalent antigens. Since the valency of the Fab fragments is one as compared with the HEL-specific IgG molecule, which has a valence of 2 (due to the presence of two Fab regions), the avidity of the fragments will be lower. Choice E is incorrect since the affinity of the Fab fragments will be the same as each of the Fab regions of the intact IgG molecule.

3. *B* In Western assays, electrophoretic separation techniques are used to resolve the molecular mass of a given antigen or mixtures of antigens. Since antibody responses to infectious agents generate polyclonal responses by virtue of the complex antigenic determinants expressed by such agents, Western assays can confirm the presence of these antibodies, which react with the electrophoretically separated antigens of known molecular weights.

4. *C* Cloned foreign genes from either the same or other species are introduced into mice to generate a transgenic strain. Integration is random and occurs in both somatic and germ line cells. Choice D is incorrect because sometimes knockout mice do not have a phenotype unique caused by the replacement of a functional gene with one that is nonfunctional, probably due to the activity of redundant or compensatory mechanisms.

5. *B* SCID mice possess an autosomal recessive mutation that causes a disorder in which B and T cells fail to develop. Like their human counterparts, SCID mice are compromised with respect to lymphoid defense mechanisms. Pluripotential stem cells present in SCID mice can give rise to other hematopoietic lineages, including cells in the myeloid lineage and NK cells.

6. *B* The method used to generate B cell hybridomas employs the fusion of B cells (e.g., from the spleen and lymph nodes) harvested from immunized mice with a selected population of malignant plasma cells unable to secrete immunoglobulin. Antigen-specific B cells are not cloned first and then fused with such plasma cells.

7. *C* In a sandwich ELISA, an antibody (often monoclonal) is used to coat ELISA wells followed by blocking with a nonspecific protein to saturate any unbound sites. The antigen is then added, followed by the addition of a second antigen-specific antibody that is enzyme-labeled. A polyclonal, antigen-specific antibody is often used as the enzyme-labeled reagent. This is done because the epitope detected by the coating antibody (a monoclonal antibody in this case) may be blocked by that antibody, thus preventing its access if the same monoclonal were used as the enzyme-labeled detecting antibody.

6

THE GENETIC BASIS OF ANTIBODY STRUCTURE

 INTRODUCTION

One characteristic of the immune response is its enormous diversity. Estimates of the number of B and T cells with different antigenic specificities that can be generated in a given individual range from 10^{15} to 10^{18}. If every immunoglobulin (Ig) or T-cell receptor (TCR) were coded for by one gene, then an individual would have to have this same number of genes—10^{15} to 10^{18}—devoted exclusively to coding for these structures. Since such a large number of genes would occupy a significant percentage of the individual's *genome* (inherited DNA), it seemed hard to understand how all these genes could be fitted in. As a result of the work of several investigators over the last 25 years, however, we now know Ig and TCR genes use a unique strategy to achieve the degree of diversity required. This strategy, which we discuss below, uses a much more limited set of genes, numbering in the hundreds rather than millions.

The first key finding was that the variable and constant regions of an immunoglobulin molecule are coded by different genes. In fact, many different variable (V) region genes can be linked up to a single constant (C) region gene. The combining of V and C region genes (rather than having a single gene coding for every individual antibody molecule) considerably reduces the amount of genetic information required to encode different antibody molecules.

A subsequent crucial finding by Susumu Tonegawa (who was awarded the Nobel Prize) was that antibody genes could move and *rearrange* themselves within the genome of a differentiating cell. A V region gene can be located in one position in the DNA of an inherited chromosome (the *germ line*), and can then move to another position on the chromosome during lymphocyte differentiation. This process of rearrangement during differentiation brings together an appropriate set of genes for the

V and C regions. The set of rearranged genes is then transcribed and translated into a complete H or L chain.

Subsequent studies of Mark Davis and others have shown that the organization of genes that code for the TCR and the mechanisms used to generate TCR diversity obey many of the same principles (this is discussed in more detail in Chapter 9). Thus, the generation of diversity of antigen-specific receptors on both B and T lymphocytes has many common features.

The mechanisms used to generate antigen-specific receptors on T and B cells seem to be unique in the entire body: to date, no other genes behave in the same way because they do not use these rearrangement strategies.

A BRIEF REVIEW OF NONIMMUNOGLOBULIN GENE STRUCTURE AND GENE EXPRESSION

Before discussing the molecular arrangement and rearrangement of the genes involved in immunoglobulin synthesis, we will review the organization and expression of nonimmunoglobulin genes. We will focus on the components of genes that code for a typical protein expressed at the cell surface, which is illustrated diagrammatically in Figure 6.1.

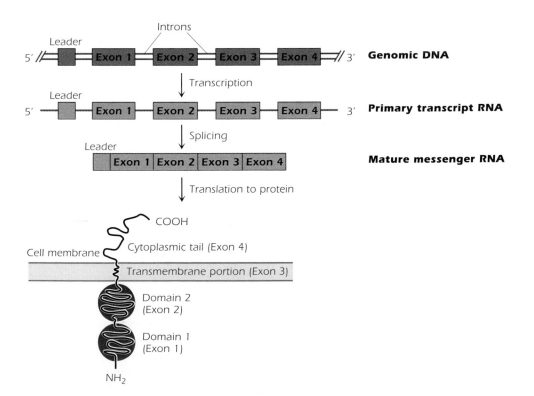

Figure 6.1. A prototypical gene coding for a membrane protein.

1. The genome (total inherited DNA) of an individual consists of linear arrays of genes in the DNA strands of the various chromosomes. Genes are transcribed into RNA, and RNA is translated into protein.

2. Every diploid cell in the human body contains the same set of genes as every other cell. The only exceptions are lymphocytes, which, as we shall discuss shortly, differ from other cells and each other in the actual content of genes coding for their antigen-specific receptor. Cells within an individual differ from each other because they transcribe and translate different genes. We say that these cells *express* different patterns of genes.

3. The expression of a specific pattern of genes determines the cell's function. Thus, for example, while every cell contains an insulin gene, only pancreatic β cells express that gene, enabling them to make insulin. Similarly, all cells contain immunoglobulin genes; however, only B lymphocytes (and their differentiated form, plasma cells) express immunoglobulin genes and therefore synthesize immunoglobulin molecules. Like all other cells except B cells, T cells contain immunoglobulin genes but do not express them.

   Control of gene expression exists at multiple levels, including the activity of transcription factors, the rate of transcription, and the half-life of messenger RNA (mRNA). Understanding the mechanisms that regulate gene expression and, in particular, how genes are turned on and off in different cell types is an area of intense research interest. Aberrant gene expression can lead to disease, so studying how genes are turned on or off in lymphocytes will help researchers design therapies for treating diseases at the molecular level.

4. Most genes coding for a protein have a characteristic structure comprising *exons* and *introns*. Exons are sequences of base pairs, which are later transcribed into mature mRNA. Exons are separated from each other by introns —noncoding regions of base pairs.

5. When a gene is transcribed into RNA, the entire stretch of DNA (exons plus introns) is transcribed into a primary RNA transcript. Enzymes modify this primary RNA transcript by *splicing* out the noncoding introns, bringing together all the coding exons needed to encode the final protein. This yields a processed mature mRNA segment that is much shorter than the original transcript because noncoding introns have been deleted. This mRNA is translated into protein on ribosomes. Notice in Figure 6.1 that exons generally code for a discrete region of the protein, such as an extracellular *domain*, a transmembrane piece, or a cytoplasmic tail. Thus, proteins are assembled by putting together multiple functional regions, and each region is coded by a separate gene segment.

6. Preceding each gene that codes for a protein expressed at the cell surface is a *leader sequence* (L exon) at the $5'$ end coding for a signal peptide that is about 20 amino acids in length. This provides a hydrophobic amino-terminus that is used to transport the nascent polypeptide chain through the membrane of the endoplasmic reticulum and into the Golgi apparatus, where the signal peptide is cleaved off and the protein is inserted into the cell membrane.

There are many ways in which membrane immunoglobulin structure differs from the structure of the surface molecule depicted in Figure 6.1. Most obviously, an immunoglobulin molecule is a multichain glycoprotein. To make a complete immunoglobulin, the newly synthesized individual heavy and light chains must be assembled and glycosylated inside the cell before the four-chain multimer reaches the cell surface. Another important difference is that each Ig chain has a very short cytoplasmic tail.

The surface molecule depicted in Figure 6.1 is shown with its amino terminus outside the cell, a single transmembrane region and the carboxy-terminus inside the cell. For the surface molecule in the figure, its large cytoplasmic tail would also allow it to interact with other molecules inside the cell. However, other molecules involved in the immune response are expressed at the cell surface with different configurations, for example, with their C-terminus extracellular and their N-terminus intracellular. Other membrane molecules, such as LFA-1 (CD58), are completely extracellular but are linked to the surface of the cell via a covalent bond to an oligosaccharide, which in turn is bound to a phospholipid in the membrane, phosphatidylinositol. These molecules are thus referred to as glycosylphosphatidylinositol (GPI)-linked membrane molecules. (The function of LFA-1 as an adhesion molecule is discussed in Chapter 10.) Some molecules, such as CD16, the low-affinity Fc receptor, may be expressed at the surface in both GPI-linked as well as classical transmembrane versions.

GENETIC EVENTS IN THE SYNTHESIS OF IMMUNOGLOBULIN CHAINS

Organization and Rearrangement of Light-Chain Genes

As we saw in Chapter 4, the light-chain polypeptides κ and λ each consists of two major domains, a variable region and a constant region (V_L and C_L). The variable region of the light chain, V_L, the amino-terminal portion of approximately 108 residues (see Chapter 4), is coded for by *two separate gene segments*: a *V (variable) segment* that codes for the amino-terminal 95 residues and a small *J (joining) segment* coding for about 13 residues (96–108) at the carboxy-terminal end of the variable region. One V gene and one J gene are brought together in the genome to create a gene unit that, together with the C region gene, codes for an entire immunoglobulin light chain. This unique *gene rearrangement* mechanism is referred to as *V(D)J recombination* (D gene segments are discussed below in the heavy-chain gene section.) This mechanism is used only by genes coding for immunoglobulin light and heavy chains and, as we shall see in Chapter 9, by genes coding for T cell receptors.

The molecular events involved in rearrangement are only just beginning to be understood. Many of the steps in rearrangement appear to be common to both B cells and T cells. An enzyme complex, known as *V(D)J recombinase*, mediates the rearrangement of receptor genes in B and T cells. V(D)J recombinase is found in all cells and is involved in the repair of DNA strands. The products of two genes expressed exclusively in lymphocytes, however, are required in the first stages of cutting Ig (and TCR) DNA. These two genes, *RAG-1 and RAG-2* (recombination-activating genes) are critical for the development of both T and B cells. RAG-1 and RAG-2 need to be expressed together in the precursor cells: mice lacking one of these genes (called "RAG knockout mice") are deficient in both B and T cells.

κ-Chain Synthesis. We will first examine the synthesis of κ light chains. In humans, the set of genes coding for κ chains and referred to as the *κ locus*, is found on chromosome 2. Genetic analysis has shown that the arrangement of κ genes in the germ line, that is, in *any* cell in the body is as follows: there are approximately 40 different V_κ genes, each of which can code for the N-terminal 95 amino acids of a κ variable region. These V_κ genes are arranged linearly, each with its own L (leader) sequence, all separated by introns, as shown in Figure 6.2 (for simplicity, the leader sequences have been omitted in the figure). A series of 5 J_κ gene segments is found downstream (that is, 3′) of this region. Each J_κ gene segment can encode the remaining 13 amino acid residues (96–108) of the κ variable region. Separated by another long intron is the single gene segment coding for the single constant region of the κ-chain (C_κ).

To make a κ-chain, an early cell in the B-lymphocyte lineage selects one of the V_κ genes from its DNA and physically joins it to one of the J_κ segments (in Figure 6.2, V_2 rearranges to J_4). How this selection of V and J genes is made is not known but is probably a random process. Joining involves the linking of **recognition sequences**, which are found at the ends of all genes (both Ig and TCR) which use rearranging gene segments to generate polypeptides. Figure 6.3 illustrates this V_2 to J_4 rearrangement in more detail; note that the DNA in this cell still contains the unrearranged gene segments V_1 and J_5. When joining occurs during rearrangement, in most cases the intervening DNA is looped, cut out, and ultimately broken down.

From this rearranged DNA a primary RNA transcript is made (Figure 6.2), which is then spliced to remove all intervening noncoding sequences to bring the Vκ, Jκ, and C_κ exons together. This results in a mature mRNA. This mRNA is then translated into the κ polypeptide chain on the cell's rough endoplasmic reticulum, and, after transport, the leader sequence is cleaved off and the κ chain is free to join with an H chain to form an immunoglobulin molecule.

λ Chain Synthesis. The λ genes are found on chromosome 22 in the human; that is, on a chromosome distinct from κ and from heavy-chain genes. The synthesis

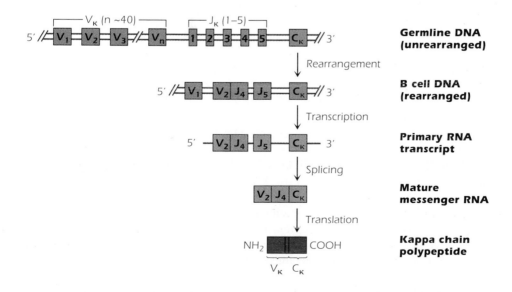

Figure 6.2. The genetic events leading to the synthesis of a kappa light chain.

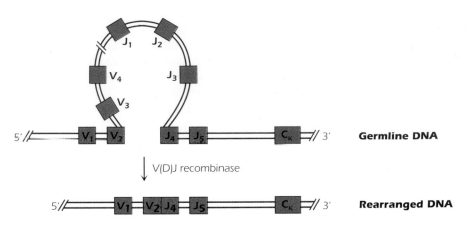

Figure 6.3. Rearrangement of DNA coding for a kappa light chain.

of λ chains is similar in principle to the synthesis of κ chains, in that it involves rearrangement of DNA, which joins a V_λ gene, coding for the N-terminal region of a λ variable region, with a J_λ segment, coding for the remaining 13 amino acids of the λ variable region. The human λ locus comprises about 40 V_λ and 4 J_λ genes, which are known to be functional. (The J_λ region contains sequences known as "pseudogenes," long stretches of DNA that have some defect that prevents them from being transcribed or translated.) The organization of the λ gene locus is slightly different from the organization of the κ gene locus which contains only one C_κ gene: by contrast, each J_λ is associated with a different C_λ gene. Thus, there are four different types of C_λ polypeptides in the human.

Organization and Rearrangement of Heavy-Chain Genes

Heavy-chain genes are found on a chromosome distinct from either light chain (chromosome 14 in humans). The organization of genes encoding the heavy chain is different from those encoding light chains (see Figure 6.4). In contrast to the variable region of a light chain that is constructed from two gene segments, the variable region of a heavy chain is constructed from three gene segments (V_H, D_H, and J_H). Thus, in addition to V and J segments, genes coding for the varible region of a heavy chain also use a D ("diversity") segment. The D and J segments code for amino acid sequences in the third hypervariable or *complementarity determining region* (CDR3) of the heavy chain (see Chapter 4). The human heavy-chain locus includes approximately 50 V_H genes, about 20 D_H gene segments, and 6 J_H gene segments (see Figure 6.4).

The second key feature of the H-chain genes is the presence in the germ line of multiple genes coding for the C region of the immunoglobulin. The C region determines the class and hence biological function of the particular antibody (see Chapter 4 on the function of antibody molecules). The C genes, each flanked by introns, are separated from the V_H genes by a large intron. The order of C genes in the human is shown in Figure 6.4. The C genes closest to the V region genes are μ and δ, which are transcribed first during B-cell development.

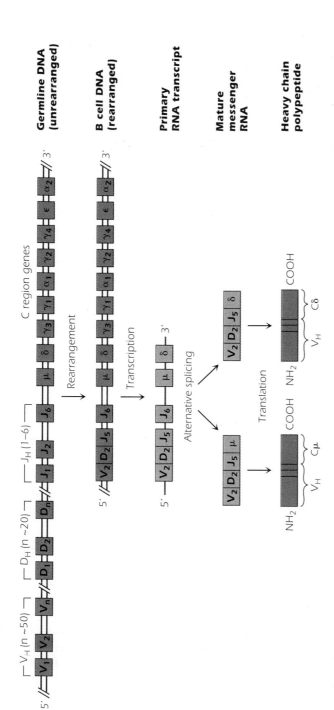

Figure 6.4. The genetic events leading to the synthesis of a human heavy chain.

123

Heavy chain synthesis uses the same mechanisms of rearrangement described for light chains; namely, the use of the V(D)J recombinase to mediate the joining of different gene segments. In the early stages of the life of a particular B cell, two rearrangements of germ line DNA must occur. The first brings one D segment alongside one J segment. The second brings one V segment next to the DJ unit ($V_2 D_2 J_5$ in Figure 6.4), fixing the antigen specificity of the heavy chain. The rearranged DNA is then transcribed along with the closest C region genes μ and δ. This primary transcript can be spliced in two different ways (*alternative splicing*) to yield a VDJ-μ or a VDJ-δ mRNA. These two messages may then be translated in rough endoplasmic reticulum to yield either a μ or δ polypeptide. In this way an individual resting B cell may express both μ and δ with identical antigenic specificity.

Regulation of Immunoglobulin Gene Expression

Theoretically, any one B cell has many genes from which to choose to synthesize an immunoglobulin molecule: multiple V, D, and J genes to form the variable regions, and different genes for the light chains, κ and λ. In reality, each B cell uses only one set of VDJ genes and one type of light chain. As a result, *a single B cell produces an immunoglobulin of only one antigenic specificity.*

Furthermore, a given B cell has two sets of chromosomes, one set from each parent, so theoretically, Ig genes located on both chromosomes could synthesize Ig molecules. This does not occur. In contrast to all other gene products, which are derived from genes from *both* parental chromosomes, Ig (and T-cell receptor) chains are coded for by *only* one set of genes, either from the maternal or paternal chromosome. For example, the H chain may be coded for by genes on the paternal chromosome and the L chain (either κ or λ) by genes on the maternal chromosome. This phenomenon of using genes of only one parental chromosome is known as *allelic exclusion*.

We now know that the steps in rearrangement, allelic exclusion, and hence the synthesis of a complete immunoglobulin (and, as we shall see later, T-cell receptor) molecule are very tightly controlled, although all the controlling mechanisms are not yet completely clear. It seems that in the differentiating cell the clusters of H-chain genes on both chromosomes begin to rearrange. If a successful rearrangement of V-, D-, and J-gene DNA occurs on one of the parental chromosomes, and an H-chain polypeptide is produced, the other parental H-chain DNA stops rearranging as a result of some kind of suppressive mechanism. If the first attempt to rearrange the V, D, and J genes is unsuccessful (i.e., if it fails to produce a polypeptide chain), then the second parental chromosome continues rearrangement. Thus, even though there are two chromosomal copies of the H chain in each cell, only one is functionally expressed. The same process then occurs with the light chain, first with the κ- and then with the λ-chain genes. Successful rearrangement by V to J fusion of any one of these genes causes the others to remain in germ line form. In this way, the cell progresses through some or all of its chromosomal copies until it has successfully completed the productive rearrangement of genes for one H and one L chain. These chains then become the basis of the antibody specificity of that particular cell. (A cell that fails to make functional H and L chain rearrangements makes no immunoglobulin receptors, and it dies by *apoptosis*, also known as *programmed cell death*. The death of precursor and mature lymphocytes by this pathway is a critical regulatory feature of the immune response and is discussed in more detail in Chapter

11.) This mechanism of gene exclusion ensures that every B cell and the antibody it synthesizes is monospecific; that is, specific for only one epitope. In this way, an individual B cell is prevented from forming and expressing immunoglobulin molecules with different antigenic specificities on its cell surface.

CLASS OR ISOTYPE SWITCHING

As we have described above, one B cell makes antibody of just one single specificity that is fixed by the nature of VJ (light chain) and VDJ (heavy-chain) rearrangements. These rearrangements occur *in the absence of antigen* in the early stages of B-cell differentiation. During the lifetime of an individual cell, however, *it can switch to make a different class of antibody, such as IgG, IgE, or IgA, while retaining the same antigenic specificity*. This phenomenon is known as *class* or *isotype switch* (see Chapter 4 for more on the function of antibody isotypes). It involves further DNA rearrangement, juxtaposing the rearranged VDJ genes with a different heavy-chain C region gene (Figure 6.5).

Class switching occurs in mature B cells and is dependent on antigenic stimulation of the cell and the presence of factors released by T cells. These factors are known as *cytokines* (see below and further discussion in Chapters 10 and 12). In the absence of such T cell-derived cytokines there is little or no class switching by B cells.

The cytokines that affect class switch induce further rearrangement of B cell DNA and produce switching to other immunoglobulin classes in a downstream progression (e.g., to IgG_4 or IgE). Thus, a single B cell with a unique specificity is capable of making an antibody of all possible classes depending on the switches occurring in the DNA coding for its heavy chain.

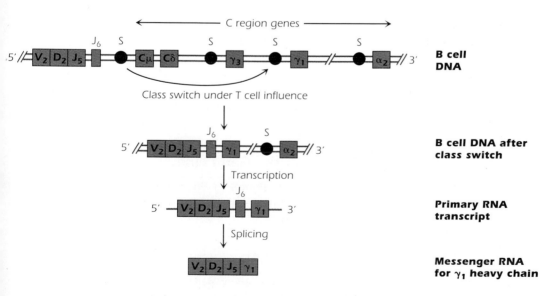

Figure 6.5. Mechanism of class switching in immunoglobulin synthesis. S = switch region, upstream of each heavy-chain constant region.

The mechanism by which mature B cells undergo class switch is as follows: each C region gene of the H chain (C_H) has at its 5′ end a stretch of repeating base sequences called a **switch (S) region** (Figure 6.5). This S region permits any of the C_H regions to associate with the VDJ unit. (The only exception is the δ gene, which has no switch region.) Under the stimulating influence of antigen and T-cell-derived cytokines, a B cell with a VDJ unit linked to Cμ and Cδ further rearranges its DNA to link the VDJ to an S region in front of another C region gene (γ_1 in Figure 6.5). In so doing, the intervening C region DNA is removed. Thus, at this stage the cell loses its ability to revert to making a class of antibody whose C-region gene has been deleted (e.g., IgM, IgD, or IgG_3). Again, a primary RNA transcript is made from this rearranged DNA. The transcript has all the introns spliced out to give a mRNA coding for the IgG_1 heavy chain.

The phenomenon of class switching is unique to immunoglobulin H chains. Whereas gene rearrangement mechanisms are used for synthesizing individual H and L Ig and TCR chains, only genes coding for Ig H chains undergo DNA rearrangement using switch (S) regions 5′ of their C_H genes. Class switching is a unique mechanism which allows an antibody with a single antigenic specificity to associate with a variety of different effector functions.

It is also noteworthy that the C_H gene selected in isotype switching is critically dependent on the cytokine present at the time of antigen activation of the B cell. Thus, in the mouse, in the presence of the cytokine interferon-γ, the B cell can rearrange its VDJ to the $C\gamma_2$ heavy chain and the cell will switch to IgG_2 synthesis. By contrast, in the presence of the cytokine interleukin 4 (IL-4) a human or mouse B cell can rearrange its VDJ to $C\gamma_4$ or Cε, and the cell will switch to IgG_4 or IgE synthesis, respectively. Each cytokine is thought to loosen the structure of the DNA double helix at only certain points along the immunoglobulin locus, allowing an enzyme known as a "switch recombinase" to recognize DNA coding for specific C regions.

GENERATION OF ANTIBODY DIVERSITY

Thus far we have described the unique genetic mechanisms involved in generating an enormously varied set of antibodies to cope with the universe of antigens without using a great deal of DNA. Still more mechanisms for generating diversity exist, some of which are discussed briefly below.

Presence of Multiple V Genes in the Germ Line

The number of different genes for the V region in the germ line constitutes the baseline from which antibody is derived and represents the minimum number of different antibodies that could be produced.

VJ and VDJ Combinatorial Association

As we have already seen, the association of any V gene segment with any J gene segment can occur to form a light-chain variable region, and similarly, any V can associate with any J or D gene segments in heavy-chain gene rearrangement. All these distinct segments contribute to the structure of the variable region. As there are about 40 V_κ and 5 J_κ genes coding for the κ-chain variable region, assuming random association, then 40×5 or 200 κ chains can be formed; with $40V_\lambda$ and $4J_\lambda$ genes 160λ chains can be formed. Similarly, if there are about 50 V genes, 20 D genes, and 6 J genes that can code for an H-chain variable region, and these may also associate in any combination, $50 \times 20 \times 6$ or 6000 different heavy chains can be formed.

Random Assortment of H and L Chains

In addition to VJ and VDJ combinatorial association, any H chain may associate with any L chain. Thus, if any H chain can associate with any κ or λ chain, a total of 1.2×10^6 different κ-containing immunoglobulin molecules (200×6000), and 0.96×10^6 (160×6000) λ-containing molecules can be generated from just 165 different genes (adding up all the H, κ and λ segments)! This illustrates very effectively how a limited set of genes can generate a large number of different antibodies.

Junctional and Insertional Diversity

The precise positions at which the genes for the V and J, or the V, D, and J, segments are fused together are not constant, and imprecise DNA recombination can lead to changes in the amino acids at these junction sites. The absence of precision in joining during DNA rearrangement leads to deletions or changes of amino acids (*junctional diversity*) that affect the antigen-binding site, since they occur in parts of the hypervariable region, where complementarity to antigen is determined. In addition, small sets of nucleotides may be inserted (*insertional diversity*) at the V–D, and D–J junctions. The major mechanism for inserting nucleotides into the DNA sequence is mediated by the enzyme *terminal deoxynucleotidyltransferase (TdT)*. The additional diversity generated is termed *N region diversity*.

Somatic Hypermutation

Mutations that occur in V genes of heavy and/or light chains during the lifetime of a B cell also increase the variety of antibodies produced by the B cell population. Generally, an antibody of low affinity is produced in the primary response to antigen. DNA and polypeptide sequencing of antibodies formed in the primary response indicate that they follow very closely the sequence of the protein that would be encoded by germ line DNA. As the response matures, however, especially after secondary stimulation by the antigen, an increase in affinity of the antibody for the antigen occurs, and a divergence is found from the amino acid sequence that is encoded in germ line DNA.

This divergence results predominantly from point mutations in the V(D)J recombined unit of antibody V genes, which result in changes in individual amino acids. This phenomenon is referred to as *somatic hypermutation* because it occurs at a rate at least ten thousand-fold higher than the normal rate of mutation. Somatic hypermutation results in the observed increased affinity of antibodies for antigen in the secondary response. As a consequence of this ''fine-tuning'' of the immune response, somatic hypermutation increases the variety of antibodies produced by the B cell population. The evidence suggests that there is a narrow window for somatic hypermutation to occur; that is, after antigenic stimulation in the germinal centers of spleen and lymph node (see Chapter 7).

Somatic Gene Conversion

The paradigm that Ig diversity is generated by V(D)J recombination and somatic hypermutation evolved from studies of mouse and human B cells. Subsequent studies in other species, most notably in birds and rabbits, however, revealed that these animals use a mechanism known as ***somatic gene conversion*** to generate a repertoire of diverse B cell specificities. Somatic gene conversion involves the nonreciprocal exchange of sequences between genes: part of the donor gene or genes is "copied" into an acceptor gene, but only the acceptor gene is altered. The precise mechanism by which this occurs is currently not clear. This process is illustrated in the outline in Figure 6.6. It shows the chicken Ig heavy-chain locus, which comprises a single functional V_H gene that rearranges in all B cells, and approximately 20 defective V_H genes (pseudogenes) that cannot rearrange. The bottom line of the Figure 6.6 shows that in this particular B cell a diversified variable gene unit is generated by incorporating two short sequences from pseudogene 3 and one from pseudogene 8 into the rearranged VDJ gene. Somatic gene conversion can also generate light-chain diversity.

It is now clear that, in contrast to mouse and humans, many species rely on somatic gene conversion and somatic hypermutation to generate diversity within the *primary* Ig repertoire, that is, before antigen stimulation. For example, chickens use somatic gene conversion as a major mechanism to generate the primary repertoire, whereas sheep use somatic hypermutation. Other species, such as rabbit, cattle, and swine, use very limited V(D)J recombination plus somatic gene conversion and somatic hypermutation to generate their primary Ig diversity.

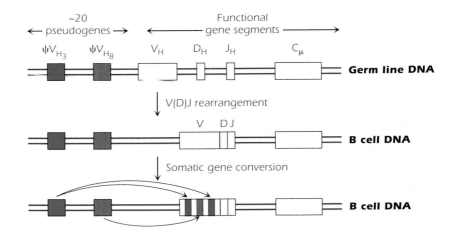

Figure 6.6. Somatic gene conversion generates diversity in Ig genes of several species. The figure illustrates the phenomenon in the chicken Ig heavy-chain locus: short sequences of DNA from one or more pseudogenes (3 and 8 in the figure) are copied into the rearranged B-cell VDJ unit.

Receptor Editing

Under some circumstances, a cell in the B cell lineage can undergo a second rearrangement of its heavy- or light-chain variable gene segments, after it has formed a recombined V(D)J unit. This process is known as *receptor editing*. The mechanism of receptor editing can be understood by looking at Figure 6.3. The rearranged DNA of this particular B cell contains the unrearranged elements, V_1 and J_5, which can be used in a second rearrangement. As described in Chapter 7, receptor editing can occur when a B cell interacts with a self-antigen; the second rearrangement may generate a V(D)J recognition unit for a foreign, rather than a self-, antigen. Thus, receptor editing may increase the diversity of the overall response to foreign antigens.

All these mechanisms contribute to the formation of a huge *library* or *repertoire* of B lymphocytes that contain all the specificities required to deal with the universe of diverse epitopes. Estimates of the number of total Ig specificities that can be generated in an individual are of the order of 10^{15}, which is increased even higher by somatic hypermutation.

SUMMARY

1. Every individual synthesizes an enormous number of different immunoglobulin (Ig) molecules, each of which can act as a receptor on the B-cell surface, specific for a particular epitope.

2. The variable region of a heavy-chain Ig molecule is coded for by three separate genes, referred to as V_H (variable), D_H (diversity), and J_H (joining) gene segments. A distinct gene segment codes for the constant region of the heavy chain, C_H. The variable region of a light-chain Ig molecule is coded for by two gene segments, V_L and J_L, distinct from the gene segments used for heavy-chain synthesis. DNA from every cell in the body (the germ line) contains multiple V, D, and J gene segments for immunoglobulin H- and L-chain synthesis.

3. In the course of differentiation, a B cell rearranges its heavy-chain DNA so as to join one V_H gene segment to one D_H gene segment and one J_H gene segment. The joined VDJ unit codes for the entire variable region of the heavy chain. These gene rearrangements put the VDJ unit next to the heavy-chain constant region genes, $C\mu$ and $C\delta$.

4. The same type of rearrangement occurs to produce a gene unit coding for the entire V region of an Ig L chain; one V_L gene segment is joined to one J_L segment, putting the VJ unit next to a light-chain constant region gene. In a B cell committed to making a κ chain, the $V_\kappa J_\kappa$ unit is juxtaposed to the C_κ gene. In a B cell committed to making a λ chain, $V_\lambda J_\lambda$ is put next to a C_λ gene.

5. Primary RNA transcripts are made from the rearranged DNA. Noncoding RNA is spliced out of the primary transcripts, resulting in mRNA for light and heavy chains, which are then translated into the L and H chains of IgM and IgD.

6. After antigenic stimulation, a B cell can further rearrange its DNA. The VDJ unit, which has joined to the $C\mu$ and $C\delta$ genes, can rearrange to join another

C region gene, such as $C\gamma$, $C\alpha$, or $C\varepsilon$. This phenomenon is known as class switching. As a result, the B cell that was synthesizing IgM and IgD can now synthesize antibody of a different isotype (IgG, IgA, or IgE) but with the same antigenic specificity.

7. Diversity in antibody specificity is achieved by
   a. multiple inherited genes for the V regions of both L and H chains;
   b. rearrangement of V, D, and J segments in different combinations, and random assortment of H and L chains;
   c. junctional and insertional diversity when V, D, and J genes are joined;
   d. somatic hypermutation, which primarily occurs after stimulation by antigen, leading to selection for mutations that endow the antibody with higher affinity for the antigen;
   e. somatic gene conversion in species other than the human or mouse: Short DNA sequences from nonrearranging genes are copied into a rearranged V(D)J gene unit.

Thus, these mechanisms allow a small number of genes to generate a vast number of antibody molecules with different antigenic specificities.

REFERENCES

Agrawal A, Eastman QM, Schatz DG (1998): Transposition mediated by RAG1 and RAG2 and its implications for the evolution of the immune system. *Nature* 394:744–751.

Gellert M (1997): Recent advances in understanding V(D)J recombination. *Adv Immunol* 64: 39–64.

Gorman JR, Alt FW (1998): Regulation of immunoglobulin light chain isotype expression. *Adv Immunol* 69:113–181.

Grawunder U, West RB, Lieber MR (1998): Antigen receptor gene rearrangement. *Curr Opin Immunol* 10:172–180.

Nussenzweig MC (1998): Immune receptor editing: revise and select. *Cell* 95:875–878.

Rajewsky K (1998): Burnet's unhappy hybrid. *Nature* 394:624–625.

Wabl M, Steinberg C (1996): Affinity maturation and class switching. *Curr Opin Immunol* 8: 89–92.

Wagner SD, Neuberger MS (1996): Somatic hypermutation of immunoglobulin genes. *Annu Rev Immunol* 14:441–457.

Weill JC, Reynaud CA (1996): Rearrangement/hypermutation/gene conversion: when, where, and why. *Immunol Today* 17:92–97.

REVIEW QUESTIONS

For each question, choose the ONE BEST answer or completion.

1. The DNA for an H chain in a B cell making IgG$_2$ antibody for diphtheria toxoid has the following structure: $5'-V_{17}D_5J_2\ C\gamma_2-C\gamma_4-C\varepsilon-C\alpha_2-3'$ How many individual rearrangements were required to go from the embryonic DNA to this B-cell DNA?

A) 1
B) 2
C) 3
D) 4
E) none

2. If you had 50 V, 20 D, and 6 J regions able to code for a heavy chain, and 40 V and 5 J region genes able to code for a light chain, you could have a maximum repertoire of
    A) 76 + 45 = 121 antibody specificities
    B) 76 × 45 = 3420 specificities
    C) (40 × 5) + (50 × 20 × 6) = 6200 specificities
    D) (40 × 5) × (50 × 20 × 6) = 1,200,000 specificities
    E) more than 1,200,000 specificities

3. The antigen specificity of a particular B cell
    A) is induced by interaction with antigen.
    B) is determined only by the L-chain sequence.
    C) is determined by H + L-chain variable region sequences.
    D) changes after isotype switching.
    E) is determined by the heavy-chain constant region.

4. If you could analyze, at the molecular level, a plasma cell making IgA antibody, you would find all of the following *except*
    A) a DNA sequence for V, D, and J genes translocated near the $C\alpha$ DNA exon.
    B) mRNA specific for either κ or λ light chains.
    C) mRNA specific for J chains.
    D) mRNA specific for μ chains.
    E) a DNA sequence coding for the T-cell receptor for antigen.

5. The ability of a single B cell to express both IgM and IgD molecules on its surface at the same time is made possible by
    A) allelic exclusion.
    B) isotype switching.
    C) simultaneous recognition of two distinct antigens.
    D) selective RNA splicing.
    E) use of genes from both parental chromosomes.

6. Which of the following statements concerning the organization of immunoglobulin genes is correct?
    A) V and J regions of embryonic DNA have already undergone a rearrangement.
    B) Light-chain genes undergo further rearrangement after surface IgM is expressed.
    C) V_H gene segments can rearrange with $J\kappa$ or $J\lambda$ gene segments.
    D) The VDJ segments coding for an immunoglobulin V_H region may associate with different heavy-chain constant region genes.
    E) After VDJ joining has occurred, a further rearrangement is required to bring the VDJ unit next to the $C\mu$ gene.

7. Which of the following does not contribute to the generation of diversity of B-cell antigen receptors?
    A) multiple V genes in the germ line
    B) random assortment of L and H chains
    C) imprecise recombination of V and J or V, D, and J segments
    D) inheritance of multiple C-region genes
    E) somatic hypermutation

8. Which of the following concerning Ig expression on a B cell is *incorrect*:

A) The light chains of the IgM and IgD have identical amino acid sequences.
B) The constant parts of the heavy chains of the IgM and IgD have different amino acid sequences.
C) The IgM and IgD have different antigenic specificities.
D) If the B cell is triggered by antigen and T-cell signals to proliferate and differentiate into antibody secreting plasma cells, the cell can potentially secrete IgG, IgE, or IgA antibody.
E) The IgM on the surface will have either κ light chains or λ light chains, but not both.

9. Which of the following plays a role in changing the antigen binding site of a B cell *after* antigenic stimulation?:

A) junctional diversity
B) combinatorial diversity
C) germ-line diversity
D) somatic hypermutation
E) differential splicing of primary RNA transcripts

Case Study

As a member of a research team studying a tribe found in a remote region of New Guinea, you make the astonishing discovery that they have only two V genes for the L chain and three V genes for the H chain of immunoglobulins. Nevertheless, they seem healthy and able to resist the diversity of pathogenic organisms endemic to the area. Suggest how this might be accomplished.

Answers to Review Questions

1. *C* Three DNA rearrangements are required. First, $D_5 \rightarrow J_2$ rearrangement occurs, followed by $V_{17} \rightarrow D_5J_2$. This permits synthesis of IgM and IgD molecules using $V_{17}D_5J_2$. The third rearrangement is the class switch of $V_{17}D_5J_2C\mu C\delta$ to $V_{17}D_5J_2C\gamma2$, leading to the synthesis of IgG_2 molecules.

2. *E* While 1,200,000 would be the product of all possible combinations of genes, the generation of many more antibody specificities is likely as a result of imprecise recombinations of VJ or VDJ segments, insertional diversity, and somatic hypermutation.

3. *C* The antigenic specificity is determined by the sequences and hence the structure formed by the combination of heavy- and light-chain variable regions.

4. *D* As a consequence of the rearrangement of the VDJ to $C\alpha$ in the IgA producing cell, the $C\mu$ gene will have been deleted. The other DNA sequences and mRNA species will be found in the cell.

5. *D* The simultaneous synthesis of IgM and IgD is made possible by the alternate splicing of the primary RNA transcript $5'$–VDJ—$C\mu$—$C\delta$–$3'$; to give either $VDJC\mu$ or $VDJC\delta$ messages.

6. *D* This is the basis of isotype or class switching.

7. **D** The presence of multiple C_H region genes, although the basis for functional diversity, does not contribute to the diversity of antigen-specific receptors.

8. **C** The IgM and IgD expressed on a single B cell use the same heavy- and light-chain V(D)J gene units and therefore have the same antigenic specificity.

9. **D** Of the mechanisms described for generating diversity of Ig molecules, only somatic hypermutation affects the antigen binding site *after* antigen stimulation.

Answer to Case Study

Despite the paucity of V-region genes, these individuals presumably retain other mechanisms for generating diversity. These include the presence of multiple J and D gene segments in the germ line, junctional diversity due to deletion or insertion of bases at joining sites, random assortment of H and L chains, and somatic hypermutation. It is therefore conceivable that, even with their limited V-gene repertoire, they can generate sufficient diversity of antibody specificity to survive.

7

BIOLOGY OF THE B LYMPHOCYTE

 INTRODUCTION

In Chapter 6 we described how B lymphocytes can develop a vast repertoire of antigenic specificities. This explained one of the key features of the immune response: *diversity*, the ability to respond to many different antigenic determinants, or epitopes, even if they had not been previously encountered. In this chapter and Chapter 9, we consider the development of lymphocytes, the cells responsible for other major characteristics of the immune response. These characteristics are as follows:

Specificity: the ability to discriminate among different antigenic epitopes, and to respond only to those that necessitate a response rather than making a random response.

Memory: The ability to recall previous contact with a particular antigen, such that subsequent exposure leads to a more rapid and more effective immune response.

Discrimination between "self" and "nonself": The ability to respond to those antigens that are "foreign" or "nonself" and to prevent responses to those antigens that are part of "self."

This chapter focuses on the differentiation of B lymphocytes, the cells that synthesize antibody in response to antigen. In Chapter 9, we will discuss the differentiation of T lymphocytes.

Sites of Early B-Cell Differentiation

Our understanding of B-cell differentiation has been facilitated by studying different animals in which the early embryonic stages can be manipulated. For this reason,

B-cell differentiation in chickens, as well as in mammals, is particularly well characterized. Many of the differentiation steps are common to humans, chickens, and mice.

B lymphocytes acquired their name from early experiments in birds: the synthesis of antibody was shown to require the presence of an organ called the **bursa of Fabricius** (an outpouching of the cloacal epithelium). Surgically removing the bursa prevented antibody synthesis. Thus, *the cells that developed into mature, antibody-forming cells were called bursa-derived* or B cells. In contrast to birds, mammals do not appear to have a bursa; rather, B-cell differentiation occurs in a restricted number of critical sites. B-cell differentiation is first noted in the liver of the early fetus. Later in fetal development and throughout the rest of life, the bone marrow is the predominant site of B-cell differentiation. The bone marrow is therefore considered *the primary lymphoid organ for B-cell differentiation* in the human and other mammals (see Chapter 2).

ONTOGENY OF THE B LYMPHOCYTE

Figure 7.1 illustrates the key stages in the B-cell differentiation pathway. Many of the gene rearrangement steps described in the text and figures of Chapter 6 define important stages in this pathway.

Early Phases of B-Cell Differentiation: Pro-B and Pre-B Cells

B lymphocytes arise from **hematopoietic stem cells** that commit to the B-cell lineage in response to signals from a variety of soluble factors (cytokines), and as a result

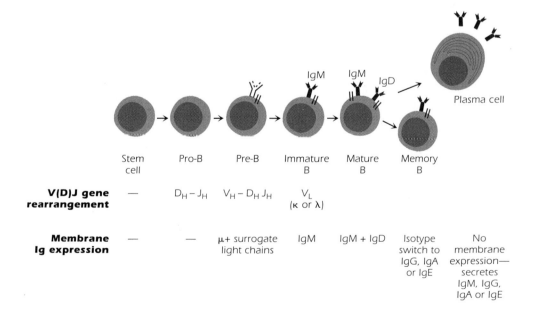

Figure 7.1. Differentiation pathway of B lymphocytes. Dashed lines on the pre-B cell indicate surrogate light chains. The two lines associated with the cell surface heavy chain represent the molecules Igα and Igβ.

of interactions with cells in their environment. The earliest distinguishable cell in the B lineage is known as a ***pro-B cell***, in which a heavy-chain D_H gene segment rearranges to a J_H gene segment (described in Chapter 6), but no immunoglobulin product is made. In the next cell in the B-cell pathway, the ***pre-B cell***, a heavy-chain V_H gene segment rearranges to join the rearranged DJ segments, forming a VDJ unit. This rearranged VDJ is thus put next to $C\mu$ (see Figure 6.3), and the pre-B cell synthesizes a μ chain. A key characteristic of the pre-B cell is that it expresses the μ chain as a transmembrane molecule at the cell surface in conjunction with the products of two nonrearranging genes, called $\lambda 5$ and VpreB. $\lambda 5$ and VpreB together function as ***surrogate light chains*** (see Figure 7.2A).

As shown in Figure 7.2A, the μ chain and surrogate light chains of the pre-B cell are also expressed at the cell surface with two closely associated transmembrane molecules known as ***Igα (CD79a) and Igβ (CD79b)*** which are disulfide-linked to each other. The complex of μ and surrogate light chains in conjunction with Igα and Igβ is referred to as the ***pre-B-cell receptor or pre-BCR***. Igα and Igβ are associated with immunoglobulin molecules on all cells of the B cell lineage, from the pre-B cell to the memory B cell (Figure 7.1). The complex of Igα and Igβ associated with immunoglobulin molecules on cells in the B cell lineage more mature than the pre-B cell is known as the ***B-cell receptor, or BCR***, and is depicted in Figure 7.2B.

Igα and Igβ do not bind antigen. Their function is to transmit a signal into the cell after antigen binds to the V regions of the immunoglobulin heavy and light chains. Igα and Igβ are thus referred to as ***signal transduction molecules*** associated with the BCR and pre-BCR. As we shall discuss in Chapter 9, similar signal transduction molecules are associated with the antigen-specific receptor expressed at different stages of T-lymphocyte development.

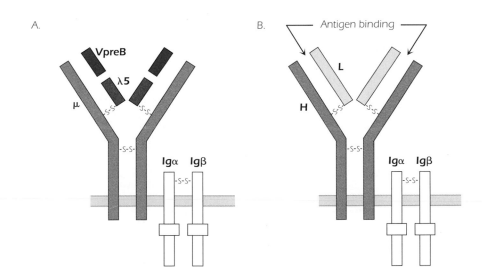

Figure 7.2. **A:** The pre-B-cell receptor (pre-BCR). **B:** The B-cell receptor (BCR). The heavy chain of the pre-BCR is a μ chain; the heavy chain of the BCR may be a μ, δ, γ, α, or ε chain. The immunoreceptor tyrosine-based activation motif (ITAM, discussed later in this chapter) is depicted as a rectangle in the Igα and Igβ polypeptides.

During the early stages of B cell differentiation, cells that do not express the pre-BCR (because they fail to productively rearrange their heavy chain loci or for any other reason) die by apoptosis. Cells expressing a pre-BCR undergo further differentiation, referred to as ***positive selection***, mediated by signals transmitted via the pre-BCR. It is not currently clear if unknown ligands bind to the pre-BCR or whether just the expression of the pre-BCR on the membrane triggers these signals and results in further differentiation of the pre-B cell. As a result of these signals, the cell is induced to proliferate, surrogate light-chain synthesis is shut down, light-chain gene rearrangement starts, and further heavy-chain gene rearrangement is stopped.

Immature B Cells

At the next stage of B-cell differentiation, light chains now pair with μ chains to form monomeric IgM, which is inserted in the membrane. The cell bearing only monomeric surface IgM as its antigen-specific receptor is referred to as an ***immature B cell***. Early experiments showed that immature B cells can recognize and respond to foreign antigen, but this interaction resulted in long-lasting ***inactivation***, rather than expansion and differentiation. More recent studies indicate that immature B cells can interact with self-molecules in the bone marrow, which can also result in inactivation. The interaction of self-molecules and immature B cells is important in the development of ***self-tolerance in the B-cell lineage: cells with potential reactivity to self are prevented from responding.*** This can occur in two ways, depicted in Figure 7.3. If the immature B cell is exposed to a self-molecule expressed on the surface of bone marrow cells, it dies by apoptosis (***deletion***). In contrast, if the immature B cell is exposed to a non-cell surface molecule (***soluble antigen***) in the

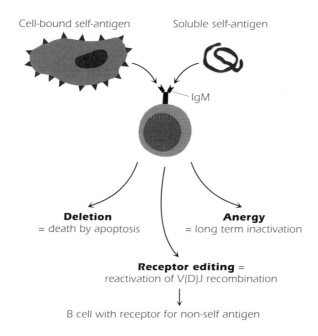

Figure 7.3. Interaction of the immature B cell with self-antigens.

bone marrow, the cell is inactivated, but not deleted; it is said to be **anergized**. (Deletion and anergy are described further in Chapter 11.) The inactivation of immature B cells with potential reactivity to self through interaction with self-molecules is known as **negative selection**. As described in Chapter 9, developing T lymphocytes also undergo positive and negative selection steps during differentiation in the thymus.

Figure 7.3 also depicts a third possible outcome for the interaction of an immature B cell and a self-molecule, namely reactivation of the cell's V(D)J recombinase. As a consequence, the cell's immunoglobulin-heavy or -light chain genes undergo secondary rearrangement, using unrearranged V, D, or J elements. This may generate a specificity for a non-self (foreign) antigen, and the immature B cell is "rescued" from inactivation. This phenomenon is known as **receptor editing** (see Chapter 6).

Mature B Cells

The next step in the B cell differentiation pathway is the development of the **IgM^+IgD^+ mature B cell**, which occurs predominantly in the bone marrow but can also take place in secondary lymphoid organs. The signals which drive the differentiation of the IgM^+ B cell to the IgM^+IgD^+ stage are not known. The antigenic specificities of the IgM and IgD expressed on the mature B cell are identical; this results from the alternative splicing of a single RNA species transcribed from VDJ plus μ and δ genes which was discussed in Chapter 6.

Antibody Synthesis and Class Switching.

By contrast with the response of immature B cells to antigen, the interaction of antigen with the mature B cell generally results in **activation**, rather than inactivation. The response of mature B cells to foreign antigen occurs primarily in the secondary lymphoid organs, the lymph node and spleen, and, more specifically, in specialized regions of these organs, known as **germinal centers**. Interaction with antigen triggers IgM^+IgD^+ B cells with the appropriate surface Ig receptor to enlarge (to become B-cell **blasts**) and to proliferate. Several different events may occur after the initial stages of activation by antigen. Activated IgM^+IgD^+ B cells may differentiate further into **plasma cells**, which are the specialized end stage of B-cell development (depicted on the far right of Figure 7.1). Plasma cells synthesize and secrete antibody of the same antigenic specificity as that of the immunoglobulin on the surface of the B cell that was initially triggered by antigen.

In the early stages of an immune response, plasma cells secrete antibody of the IgM class. If, however, antigen-activated IgM^+IgD^+ B cells receive appropriate signals from T cells, the B cells may differentiate along different pathways. **Class (isotype) switching** may occur. Under the influence of different T-cell-derived cytokines and T–B-cell-surface interaction, progeny of the IgM^+IgD^+ B cell that was involved in the initial response to antigen may switch to synthesize IgG, IgA, or IgE molecules. Whatever the isotype of the Ig produced, all the daughter cells have the same antigenic specificity.

Memory Cell Formation.

The second major pathway after antigen activation is to become a **memory B cell** (see Figure 7.1). These are B cells capable of being activated for a subsequent (secondary) and more rapid response to antigen. Memory

B cells are nonproliferating, generally long-lived B cells that can be distinguished from other mature B cells by the differential expression of a number of cell-surface molecules. Most importantly, memory cells express isotypes other than IgM and IgD on their surface. Although the precise stage at which memory cells develop is not clear, it is apparent that plasma cells do not become memory cells.

The generation of memory B cells is associated with class switch and somatic hypermutation (see Chapter 6). These processes also occur in the germinal centers of spleen and lymph node (shown in Figure 2.9). Each germinal center consists predominantly of activated B cells, a few helper T cells and a small number of specialized cells known as follicular dendritic cells, which retain antigen on their surface and present it to B cells. The germinal center provides an environment where B cells with mutations for high affinity to the antigen are clonally selected and expanded (see discussion of somatic hypermutation in Chapter 6). There is some evidence that B cells with low affinity for antigen are selected against in the germinal center, and that these unselected cells die there. These events in the germinal center result in an increase in the production of high-affinity antibodies, a process known as *affinity maturation*. B cells which are thus selected in the germinal center exit the lymphoid organ and make antibody of the appropriate class, or serve as memory cells for subsequent responses.

The overall result of the differentiation steps described above is that the individual builds up a continuously replenished library of diverse B-cell antigen specificities (*a repertoire*) directed against a wide array of antigens. The development of a response to antigen therefore depends on the interaction of antigen with an existing B-cell clone contained in this library. It should be noted, however, that most B cells in the vast B-cell repertoire do not interact with antigen during their lifetime, but remain as resting unstimulated IgM^+IgD^+ cells.

Anatomical Distribution of B-Cell Populations

As described above, the early phases of B-cell differentiation take place in bone marrow. Mature B cells circulate through blood to secondary lymphoid organs, primarily lymph nodes, spleen, and Peyer's patches of the intestine. If the B cell does not interact with antigen it either leaves the lymphoid and continues to circulate in blood or it dies in the organ. If it does interact with antigen and helper T cells in the lymphoid organ a germinal center is formed, which is a site of proliferation and further differentiation. The final stage of B-cell development is differentiation into plasma cells, found in the region of the lymph node known as the "medullary cords." Plasma cells secreting IgG migrate to the bone marrow and continue to synthesize immunoglobulin; plasma cells secreting IgA are found in mucosal tissue. The migration of naive B cells into secondary lymphoid organs, and of antigen-activated and memory B cells into other tissues, is governed by the same types of "homing" interactions which are described in Chapter 9 for T cells.

B-1 or CD5$^+$ B Cells

A second subset of B cells has been described in humans, mice, and other animals. They are referred to as B-1 cells as they arise earlier in ontogeny than conventional or B-2 type B cells. B-1 cells are also characterized by the surface expression of the molecule CD5. In the adult, B-1 cells are minor populations in spleen and lymph

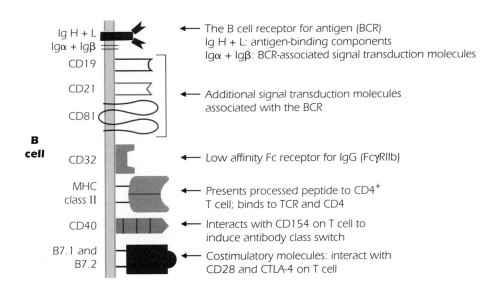

Figure 7.4. Important molecules expressed on the surface membrane of the mature B cell.

node but predominate in the peritoneal and pleural cavities. They synthesize predominantly low-affinity IgM antibodies in response to bacterial polysaccharide antigens.

B-CELL MEMBRANE PROTEINS

The key characteristic of B cells is their ability to synthesize antibody after antigenic stimulation. As we shall describe in more detail in subsequent chapters, production of antibody by B cells is a multistep process that generally requires the mutual interaction of B cells with T cells. In the following paragraphs we describe briefly some of the B-cell membrane proteins that play a role in antibody synthesis and some that have other important functions (see Figure 7.4).

Antigen-Binding Molecules: Membrane Immunoglobulin

The quintessential property of the B lymphocyte lineage is its expression of immunoglobulin molecules at the surface of the cell as membrane-bound proteins, with the concomitant ability to bind antigen. (It is noteworthy, however, that the pro-B cell, the most immature B cell, and the plasma cell, the end-stage cell of B-cell differentiation that secretes Ig, do not express Ig on their surface.) The expression of surface Ig can thus be used to identify B cells, and to separate them from other lymphocytes and mononuclear cells. In addition, antibodies specific for different portions of the immunoglobulin molecule (i.e., anti-immunoglobulin antibodies) can be used experimentally to distinguish distinct subsets of B cells (e.g., B cells expressing only IgM or only IgG).

Signal Transduction Molecules Associated With Membrane Immunoglobulin

Immunoglobulin-heavy and light-chains have very short intracellular domains and do not directly transmit a signal into the B cell after antigen binding. It is the role of the previously described Igα (CD79a) and Igβ (CD79b) molecules, which are noncovalently associated in the membrane of B cells with Ig-heavy and light-chains (see Figure 7.2) to transmit the activation signal into the interior of the B cell. As discussed in Chapter 10, one of the earliest events in B cell activation following antigen binding to the BCR is the phosphorylation of tyrosine residues — the addition of a phosphate group — in the cytoplasmic regions of Igα + Igβ by enzymes known as protein kinases. These Igα + Igβ tyrosine residues are contained in a sequence of amino acids referred to as an *immunoreceptor tyrosine-based activation motif (ITAM)*. The amino acid sequence is referred to as a "motif" because it is found in a number of other signal transduction molecules on cells of the immune system (for example, those associated with the T cell receptor, which are discussed in Chapter 9).

Other molecules on the B-cell membrane (CD19, CD21, and CD81[TAPA-1]) have been shown to increase the activatory signal after antigen binds to Ig. Thus, these molecules function as another set of signal transduction molecules associated with the BCR. Intracellular events in B cell activation are described in more detail in Chapter 10.

Molecules Involved in Antigen Presentation

As we shall see in Chapters 8–10 in detail, to activate T cells, antigen must be presented by cells referred to as *antigen-presenting cells (APC)*. B cells, like other cells in the body, act as APC for T cells, and B cells share several important characteristics with other APC. In common with other presenting cells, B cells express on their surface proteins referred to as *MHC class II molecules*, coded for by genes of the major histocompatibility complex (MHC). These proteins are essential for presenting antigen to a major set of T cells known as CD4$^+$ T cells. Unlike the expression pattern of many other cell types, B-cell expression of MHC class II molecules is *constitutive*; that is, the molecules are always expressed. Interestingly, MHC class II molecule expression on B cells can be further increased by exposure to certain cytokines such as IL-4. MHC class II is expressed on all cells in the B-cell lineage apart from the pro-B cell.

Another crucial requirement for APC function is the expression of *costimulatory molecules*. These are molecules expressed on B cells and other APCs that interact with T-cell membrane molecules and enhance the activation of T cells (see Chapter 10). Several costimulatory molecules have been defined on the APC surface, the most prominent of which are *B7* and *CD40*. Resting mature B cells express low levels of B7 and are poor APC, whereas activated B cells express high levels of B7 and are very efficient APCs. CD40 on the B cell plays a critical role in isotype switching, via interaction with CD154 (CD40 Ligand or CD40L) on the T cell. The importance of this interaction is underscored by a condition known as human X-linked hyper-IgM syndrome. Boys who have a mutation in their CD40 ligand gene and whose T cells either do not express or have a non-functional CD40 ligand make only IgM antibodies; their B cells cannot switch to any other isotype.

Fc Receptor, CD32

Virtually all mature B cells express a low affinity receptor for the Fc portion of IgG, FcγRII or CD32. CD32 binds IgG when it aggregates in the absence of antigen (see Chapter 4), and when the IgG is in the form of an antigen–antibody complex. CD32 plays an important role in *"antibody feedback,"* the inactivation of B cells by antibody, by delivering a negative signal to the B cell. The mechanism of this CD32-mediated inhibition is discussed further in Chapter 11.

CD21

As described above, CD21 is a B-cell surface molecule involved in B-cell activation. CD21 is also a receptor for a complement component, C3d (see Chapter 13). In addition, CD21 acts as a receptor for Epstein–Barr virus (EBV), which is responsible for the conditions mononucleosis and in Africa, Burkitt's lymphoma. This is one important example of a pathogen using a normally expressed cell-surface molecule to gain access to the cell. Other examples include human immunodeficiency virus (HIV) binding to CD4 on T cells and rhinovirus binding to ICAM-1 (CD54) on epithelial cells.

SUMMARY

1. The differentiation of B cells occurs in the bone marrow throughout the life of an individual. The earliest recognizable cell in the B-cell lineage is the pro-B cell, in which the first stage of immunoglobulin heavy chain gene rearrangement takes place: a D_H gene segment rearranges to a J_H gene segment

2. The next stage is the pre-B cell, in which a V_H gene segment rearranges to the joined DJ segments to form a VDJ unit, which is thus put next to the $C\mu$ gene. The pre-B cell transcribes and translates the VDJCμ gene unit and thereby synthesizes a μ chain. This μ chain can reach the surface of the pre-B cell in association with molecules referred to as surrogate light chains.

3. On the surface of the pre-B cell, the μ chain and surrogate light chains are expressed with two closely associated transmembrane molecules Igα (CD79a) and Igβ (CD79b). The complex of μ and surrogate light chains in conjunction with Igα and Igβ is referred to as the pre-B-cell receptor (pre-BCR). Cells expressing a pre-BCR undergo further differentiation, referred to as positive selection.

4. In the next stage of differentiation, light-chain genes start to rearrange, surrogate light-chain synthesis is shut down and a κ or λ chain is formed that associates with the cell's μ chain. This results in the formation of an IgM molecule, which is expressed on the surface of the cell in the absence of IgD. This cell is referred to as an immature B cell.

5. If the immature B cell interacts with antigen it is generally inactivated. The interaction of immature cells with self-molecules which results in inactivation or deletion of cells with potential reactivity to self is one of the important ways of maintaining self-tolerance (negative selection).

6. The next step in B-cell differentiation is the expression of IgD together with IgM on the cell surface. The IgM and IgD expressed on a single cell have identical antigenic specificity. The cell expressing IgM and IgD is referred to as a mature B cell.

7. Further development of the mature B cell occurs predominantly outside the bone marrow and as a result of exposure to antigen.

8. Activation of the B cell leads to proliferation and differentiation into a plasma cell, the end stage of B-cell differentiation. Plasma cells are B cells that synthesize and secrete antibody. In the primary response, predominantly IgM is synthesized.

9. In secondary responses, in which both B and T cells have been primed by antigen, B cells can differentiate further. They may (a) undergo class or isotype switch, that is, produce antibody of different isotypes, or (b) develop into memory B cells. These differentiation events occur in specialized regions of secondary lymphoid organs, the germinal centers. In these areas, somatic hypermutation of antibody molecules also takes place, leading to the selection of mutations that code for higher affinity antibodies.

10. Isotype switching involves a rearrangement mechanism unique to B cells. In the presence of antigen and cytokines secreted by T cells, the VDJ heavy-chain unit that was joined to the Cμ and Cδ genes rearranges to join another C-region gene, such as Cγ, Cα, or Cε. The B cell that was synthesizing IgM and IgD can now synthesize antibody of a different isotype (IgG, IgA, or IgE) but with the same antigenic specificity.

11. Expression of membrane immunoglobulin is unique to B cells. The molecules Igα and Igβ, and other molecules associated with membrane Ig, transduce signals into the B cell following antigen binding to Ig. The B cell also expresses an array of molecules on its cell surface, which play a vital role in interactions with other cells, particularly T cells. These include MHC class II molecules, B7, and CD40.

REFERENCES

Cornall RJ, Goodnow CC, Cyster JG (1995): The regulation of self-reactive B cells. *Curr Opin Immunol* 7:804–811.

Fearon DT, Carter RH (1995): The CD19, CR2/TAPA-1 complex of B lymphocytes: linking natural to acquired immunity. *Annu Rev Immunol* 13:127–19

Karasuyama H, Rolink A, Melchers F (1996): Surrogate light chain in B cell development. *Adv Immunol* 63:1–41.

LeBien TW (1998): B-cell lymphopoiesis in mouse and man. *Curr Opin Immunol* 10:188–195.

Möller G (1993): The B-cell antigen receptor complex. *Immunol Rev* 132:5.

Nossal GJV (1994): Negative selection of lymphocytes. *Cell* 76:229.

Pfeffer K, Mak T (1994): Lymphocyte ontogeny and activation in gene targeted mice. *Annu Rev Immunol* 12:367.

Reth M (1994): B cell antigen receptors. *Curr Opin Immunol* 6:3.

REVIEW QUESTIONS

For each question, choose the ONE BEST answer or completion.

1. The earliest stages of B-cell differentiation
   A) occur in the embryonic thymus.
   B) require the presence of antigen.
   C) involve rearrangement of κ-chain gene segments.
   D) involve rearrangement of surrogate light-chain gene segments.
   E) involve rearrangement of heavy-chain gene segments.

2. Which of the following is expressed on the surface of the mature B lymphocyte?
   A) CD40
   B) MHC class II molecules
   C) CD32
   D) IgM and IgD
   E) All of the above.

3. Which of the following statements is *incorrect*?
   A) Antibodies in a secondary immune response generally have a higher affinity for antigen than antibodies formed in a primary response.
   B) Somatic hypermutation of V region genes may contribute to changes in antibody affinity observed during secondary responses.
   C) Synthesis of antibody in a secondary response occurs predominantly in the blood.
   D) Isotype switching occurs in the presence of antigen.
   E) Predominantly IgM antibody is produced in the primary response.

4. Immature B lymphocytes
   A) produce only μ chains.
   B) are progenitors of T as well as B lymphocytes.
   C) express both IgM and IgD on their surface.
   D) are at a stage of development where contact with antigen may lead to unresponsiveness.
   E) must go through the thymus to mature.

5. Antigen binding to the B-cell receptor
   A) transduces a signal through the antigen-binding chains.
   B) invariably leads to B-cell activation.
   C) transduces a signal through the Igα and Igβ molecules.
   D) results in macrophage activation.
   E) leads to cytokine synthesis, which activates T cells.

6. Which of the following would *not* be found on a memory B cell:
   A) Igα and Igβ
   B) γ heavy chains
   C) ε heavy chains
   D) surrogate light chains
   E) κ light chains

Answers to Review Questions

1. *E* The earliest events in B-cell differentiation take place in fetal liver and bone marrow in the adult and involve rearrangement of heavy-chain V, D, and J gene segments.

2. *E* All the molecules are expressed on the surface of the mature B cell.

3. *C* Antibody synthesis in secondary responses occurs predominantly in lymph nodes, not blood.

4. *D* In immature B cells, which express only IgM, contact with antigen leads to unresponsiveness rather than activation.

5. *C* The molecules Igα and Igβ, which are associated with the surface Ig molecule, transduce a signal following antigen binding to surface Ig.

6. *D* Surrogate light chains are expressed only at the pre-B cell stage of B-cell differentiation.

8

THE ROLE OF THE MAJOR HISTOCOMPATIBILITY COMPLEX IN THE IMMUNE RESPONSE

● INTRODUCTION

Thus far, we have focused on one set of lymphocytes, the B lymphocytes, and their receptor for antigen, immunoglobulin. The products of B cells, antibodies, play a critical role in interacting with antigens when they are found *outside* cells, such as occurs when viruses are encountered in blood or at mucosal surfaces. Once an antigen gets into a cell, however, antibodies do not generally have access to it, and so antibodies are ineffective in dealing with antigens *inside* cells. It is generally believed that T cells evolved to deal with the crucial phase of the response to pathogens such as viruses, bacteria, and parasites that invade cells and live inside them. T cells respond predominantly to the protein component of antigens. Since nearly all antigens contain protein, T cells play a critical role in the intracellular phase of the response to nearly all the agents to which an individual is exposed.

As T cells interact with antigens that come from inside cells, they use an antigen recognition system which is distinct from the antigen recognition system of B cells. As we shall describe in this and subsequent chapters, the *T-cell receptor (TCR)* for antigen interacts with antigen almost exclusively only when a fragment of the antigen is on the surface of the cell, and bound to a molecule known as a *major histocompatibility complex (MHC)* gene product. Thus, the role of molecules coded for by the MHC is to bind to peptide fragments derived from protein antigens. Since this binding of MHC molecules to peptide is *selective*, that is, MHC molecules bind to only certain peptides, *MHC molecules may be viewed as a third set of recognition molecules for antigen in the immune response, in addition to the antigen-specific T-cell and B-cell receptors.*

Before describing the characteristics and functions of T lymphocytes, we will focus in this chapter on the MHC genes and products that play such a central role in the recognition of antigen by T cells.

The importance of MHC molecules was originally recognized from studies, particularly in mice, of the rejection of tissues between different members of the same species (see Chapter 19). Later studies indicated that *every vertebrate species has MHC genes and products*, and that transplantation rejection responses were dominated by T cells. As individuals are not normally the subjects of transplantation responses, the function of the MHC in "everyday" responses became the focus of intense investigation. Only within the last 25 years has the relevance of MHC molecules to T cell responses within individuals been understood. We now recognize that molecules coded for by MHC genes are critical both for the development of immature T cells in the thymus and for the responses of mature T cells to antigen. The centrality of MHC molecules to T cell interactions is referred to as the *MHC restriction of T-cell responses*.

We shall focus first on the characteristics of MHC genes, then describe the structure of MHC gene products, and finally discuss their role in processing and presenting antigen to T cells.

VARIABILITY OF MHC GENES AND PRODUCTS

Two major sets of MHC genes and products are involved in T-cell responses: *MHC class I* and *MHC class II*. Figure 8.1A illustrates a simplified view of the region of the chromosome that contains the human MHC region, known as *HLA (human leukocyte antigen)*, and which is located on chromosome 6. (The names of the MHC regions of species other than the mouse generally follow the human designation; for example, BoLA for bovine and SLA for swine leukocyte antigen.) The MHC is referred to as a "complex" because the genes are closely linked and inherited as a unit. The set of genes inherited by an individual from one parent is known as a *haplotype*.

Figure 8.1A depicts the three independent human MHC class I genes and their cell surface products, HLA-A, HLA-B, and HLA-C. MHC class I molecules are always expressed at the surface in association with a molecule known as *β2-microglobulin (β2m)* described in more detail below. The products of human MHC class II genes are the three cell surface molecules HLA-DP, HLA-DQ, and HLA-DR, each comprising an α and a β chain. The DPα chain always pairs with DPβ, and not with DQβ or DRβ, and the other pairs of chains behave similarly. The α and β chain of each molecule are coded for by an A and a B gene, respectively. The genes coding for DP α and β are known as DPA1 and DPB1, and for DQ α and β DQA1 and DQB1, respectively. The DR region comprises approximately seven known DRB genes (not shown in the figure) and one A gene: the product of the A gene DRA1 combines with the product of one of the DRB genes to generate a DR $\alpha\beta$ molecule.

Figure 8.1B shows the murine MHC, *H-2*, located on chromosome 17, which has also been intensely studied. There is a high degree of *homology* (similarity in sequence and structure) between the human and mouse MHC class I genes and molecules, indicating a common ancestral origin. MHC class I molecules are members of the immunoglobulin superfamily, and contain Ig-like domains. Figure 8.1B shows the three mouse MHC class I genes and products, H-2K, H-2D, and H-2L, which like their human MHC class I counterparts, are expressed at the cell surface

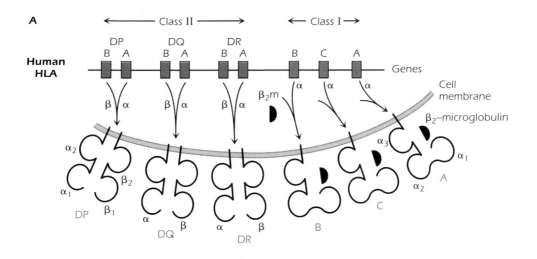

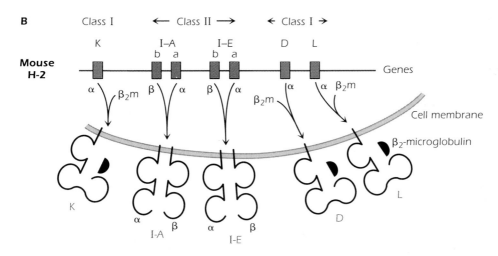

Figure 8.1. Simplified depiction of the human (A) and mouse (B) MHC, showing regions and genes coding for polymorphic MHC class I and II molecules. β2m = β2- microglobulin, encoded outside the MHC.

with β2m. In contrast to humans, who express three different types of MHC class II cell surface heterodimers — DP$\alpha\beta$, DQ$\alpha\beta$, and DR$\alpha\beta$ — the mouse expresses just two, I-A$\alpha\beta$ and I-E$\alpha\beta$. (Some mouse strains are unable to synthesize I-E molecules, and cells from these mice express only MHC class II I-A molecules at their cell surface.) The mouse MHC class II genes are referred to as H-2I-Aa and Ab and H-2I-Ea and Eb. The mouse I-A genes and product are homologous to the human MHC class II DP, and the mouse I-E genes and product are homologous to the human MHC class II DR.

Genetic Polymorphism

A key point to note is that different individuals within a species can have slightly different forms, *alleles*, of each MHC class I or II gene; that is, at a single MHC locus, different individuals can have different types of a prototypical gene. (In humans, different alleles are given numbers, such as HLA-B15 or B27, whereas in mice alleles are given superscripted small letters such as H-2K^b or K^d.) The phenomenon of having multiple stable forms of one gene in the population is known as *genetic polymorphism*. Genetic polymorphism generates diversity of MHC molecules within the population; that is, MHC-distinct individuals express different MHC molecules. Every cell in one individual, however, expresses the products of the same set of MHC genes. (This contrasts with the strategy of gene rearrangement for generating diversity of antigen-specific T- and B-cell receptors, discussed in Chapters 6 and 9: each lymphocyte has a unique set of genes coding for an antigen-specific receptor. As a result, every clone of lymphocytes within an individual expresses a different antigen-specific receptor.)

The MHC is the most highly polymorphic gene system in the body, and hence in the population (see box below). This extensive polymorphism of MHC genes therefore makes it very unlikely that two random individuals will express identical sets of MHC molecules. As we shall describe in Chapter 19, this polymorphism is the basis for rapid graft rejection between genetically different individuals.

Pattern of Expression

MHC class I molecules are expressed on almost every nucleated cell in the body. MHC class II molecules have a somewhat more limited distribution than class I molecules: they are expressed *constitutively* (i.e., under all conditions) only on B lymphocytes, dendritic cells, and thymic epithelial cells. Nonetheless, many other cells, such as macrophages and endothelial cells, may be *induced* to express MHC class II molecules by activating factors such as IFN-γ. (Interestingly, human but not mouse T cells can be induced to express MHC class II molecules following antigen stimulation.)

It is also worth noting that the expression of MHC class I molecules is *coordinate*, in that all three MHC class I molecules are expressed on the cell surface at the same time. Similarly, MHC class II molecules are also coordinately expressed, but under distinct regulation. Thus, MHC class I molecules can be expressed in the absence of any MHC class II molecule. The level of MHC class I and II expression at the cell surface can be coordinately up- or downregulated by a number of stimuli;

The advent of PCR technology has shown the extent of HLA polymorphism; individuals formerly designated identical at a particular HLA locus by the use of serologic techniques (reaction with antibodies specific for HLA molecules) have been shown to differ in their HLA gene sequences. To better define HLA gene variability in the population, a new nomenclature employs a more extensive definition of an HLA allele. For example, in place of the serologically defined DR7, the newer definition of an allele comprises the locus (e.g., DRB1), followed by an asterisk, then two digits to define the allele group, usually the same as the serologically defined specificity (e.g., DRB1*07), and two digits that identify the subtype, e.g., DRB1*0701 or DRB1*0704. This more extensive and precise characterization of HLA alleles has been invaluable in trying to match transplant donors and recipients, and for identifying individuals who may be at risk for different autoimmune diseases.

for example, in the mouse the cytokine interferon-γ (IFN-γ) enhances expression of all MHC class I and class II molecules.

In summary, in the absence of inducing factors, most cells express MHC class I molecules without expressing MHC class II molecules. Certain cells, such as B cells, constitutively express both MHC class I and class II molecules. By contrast, very few, if any, cells express MHC class II in the absence of MHC class I.

Codominant Expression

One further point worth noting is that MHC molecules (both classes I and II) are **codominantly expressed**; that is, each cell expresses MHC proteins, which are transcribed from both maternal and paternal chromosomes. (This again contrasts with the formation of Ig and TCR molecules, described in Chapters 6 and 9, in which only one chromosome is used, the unique phenomenon of allelic exclusion.) As a consequence of codominant expression of MHC molecules, each cell within an individual therefore expresses six different MHC class I molecules: in the human, HLA-A, -B, and -C proteins encoded by the paternal chromosome, and HLA-A, -B, and -C proteins encoded by the maternal chromosome. Thus, for example, all the cells in one individual may express the molecules HLA-A2 and -A5, HLA-B7 and -B13, and HLA-C6 and -C8 on their surface. Cells in another individual may express six completely different HLA class I molecules.

MHC class II molecules also exhibit codominant expression. Mouse cells may express four different MHC class II molecules (I-A and I-E from each chromosome). For the human MHC class II, there is more than one functional DRB gene and the α chain can pair with the products of each of the different DRB genes. This results in the expression of between 10 and 20 different DP, DQ, and DR molecules on its surface.

STRUCTURE OF MHC MOLECULES

MHC molecules have two critical functions: (1) to bind to peptides derived from protein antigens, and (2) once peptide has bound, to interact with a TCR. Over the last 10 years, investigators have provided important genetic, molecular, and crystallographic evidence about how peptide, MHC, and TCR interact. The crystallographic studies in particular have provided important structural information. They have shown three-dimensional structures of human and mouse MHC class I and class II molecules, and more recently of MHC molecules complexed with peptide and the external domains of a TCR (see Chapter 9). We will consider first the structure of MHC class I molecules, and then discuss the structure of MHC class II molecules.

Structure of MHC Class I Molecules

Each MHC class I gene codes for a transmembrane glycoprotein of approximate molecular weight 43 kDa, which is referred to as the α or "heavy" chain. It comprises three extracellular domains α_1, α_2, and α_3. As shown in Figure 8.2, every MHC class I molecule is expressed at the surface of a cell in noncovalent association with an invariant small polypeptide called **β2-microglobulin (β2m**, molecular weight 12 kDa), which is coded for on another chromosome. β2m has a structure homol-

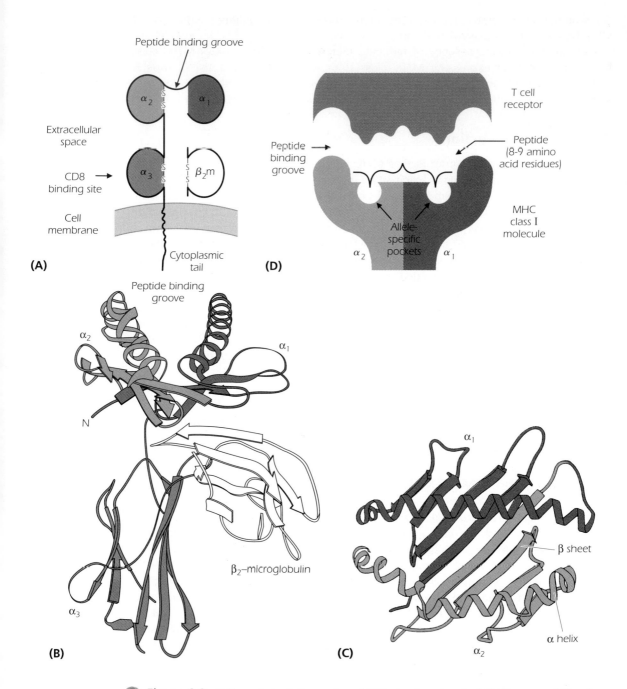

Figure 8.2. Different depictions of an MHC class I molecule. **(A)** Diagram of the structures of an MHC class I molecule associated at the cell surface with β2m. **(B)** Side view of the MHC class I molecule with β2m, showing the peptide-binding groove. **(C)** Top view of the peptide-binding groove. **(D)** Diagram of the interaction of a T-cell receptor with an MHC class I molecule and peptide bound in the peptide-binding groove. [Figures B and C from Bjorkman et al., 1987, with permission; Figure D adapted from Rammensee et al., 1993.]

ogous to a single Ig domain, and indeed, β2m is also a member of the Ig superfamily. Thus, the cell surface complex of MHC class I and β2m appears like a four-domain molecule, with the α_3 domain of the class I molecule and β2m juxtaposed closest to the membrane.

From sequencing different MHC class I molecules it became apparent that different allelic forms of the molecule have very similar sequences. Sequence differences are confined to a limited region, found in their extracellular α_1 and α_2 domains. Thus, an individual class I molecule can be divided into a ***nonpolymorphic or invariant region*** (similar in all class I allelic forms) and a ***polymorphic or variable region*** (sequence unique to that allele). The T cell molecule CD8 binds to the invariant region of all MHC class I molecules (see Figure 8.2A).

All MHC class I molecules from the human and mouse have the same general structure, depicted in Figures 8.2B and C. The most striking feature is that the part of the molecule furthest from the membrane contains a deep groove or cleft. This cleft is made up of parts of the α_1 and α_2 domains. ***This groove in the MHC class I molecule is the binding site for peptides.*** As shown in Figure 8.2D, peptide bound in this cleft and parts of the MHC class I molecule interact with the variable regions, Vα and Vβ, of a T-cell receptor. The cleft resembles a basket with an irregular floor made up of 8 β-pleated sheets and each surrounding wall forming an α-helix. The cleft can fit peptides 8–9 amino acids long in a linear array because it is closed at both ends. When the structure of different MHC class I molecules is compared, it is found that amino acid differences between the alleles are confined primarily to the region of this cleft, while the rest of the molecule is relatively constant. Comparing clefts between different MHC class I molecules, the floor of each is different, consisting of a number of ***allele-specific pockets*** (see Figure 8.2D). The shape and charge of these pockets at the bottom of the cleft help to determine which peptides bind to a particular MHC molecule. The pockets also help to secure peptides in a position in which they can be recognized by specific T-cell receptors.

A single MHC class I molecule can bind to a variety of peptides but binds preferentially to peptides with certain ***motifs***; that is, peptides with either invariant or closely related amino acids at certain positions (***anchor residues***) in the 8 or 9 amino acid sequence, but variability at the other positions. Thus, for example, the peptides that bind to mouse MHC class I molecule K^b have as their anchor residues the amino acids phenylalanine or tyrosine at position 5, and leucine at position 8, whereas the human class I molecule HLA-A2 binds peptides with leucine at position 2 and valine at position 9. The other positions on the bound peptides can be occupied by a variety of different amino acids. This indicates that any one MHC molecule can bind to a large number of peptides with different sequences. This helps to explain why T-cell responses are made, with very few exceptions, to at least one epitope from almost all protein antigens, and why failing to respond to a protein antigen is so rare. It also indicates that the binding of peptides to MHC molecules has a degree of flexibility that is not seen with the binding of antigens to B- or T-cell receptors for antigen.

Structure of MHC Class II Molecules

MHC class II α and β genes code for chains of approximate molecular weight 35,000 and 28,000 Da, respectively. MHC class II molecules, like MHC class I molecules, are transmembrane glycoprotein molecules with cytoplasmic tails and extracellular

Ig-like domains (see Figure 8.3A); the domains are referred to as α_1 and α_2, and β_1 and β_2. MHC class II molecules are also members of the immunoglobulin superfamily. As was described with MHC class I molecules, MHC class II molecules also comprise variable or polymorphic regions (differing between alleles) and invariant or nonpolymorphic regions (common to all alleles). The T-cell molecule CD4 binds to the invariant portion of all MHC class II molecules.

One of the key features of the MHC class II molecule crystal structure is a peptide-binding groove or cleft at the top of the molecule, structurally analogous to the MHC class I groove (see Figures 8.3B and C). In the MHC class II molecule, however, the cleft is formed by interactions between domains of different chains, the α_1 and β_1 domains. As shown in Figure 8.3C, the floor of the MHC class II groove comprises 8 β-pleated sheets, with the α_1 and β_1 domains each contributing four; helical sections of the α_1 and β_1 domains each comprise one wall of the cleft. In contrast to the class I groove, however, the class II groove is open at both ends, allowing larger peptides to bind. Thus, the MHC class II groove binds peptides varying in length from 12 to approximately 20 amino acids in a linear array, with the ends of the peptide outside the groove. Peptide bound in the groove of the MHC class II molecule, and parts of the MHC class II molecule, interact with the variable regions, $V\alpha$ and $V\beta$, of a T-cell receptor (Figure 8.3D). Peptides that bind to different MHC class II molecules also exhibit motifs — as the lengths of the peptides are more variable than those that bind to MHC class I molecules the motif is generally seen in the central region of the peptide, the region that fits inside the MHC class II binding groove.

FUNCTION OF MHC MOLECULES

As we have mentioned previously, pathogens such as bacteria and viruses can penetrate and infect the cells of the body. To deal with these infections, T cells are required to mount an immune response against the cell harboring the invading organism. T cells must therefore be able to distinguish between infected and noninfected cells. The ability of T cells to discriminate between infected and noninfected cell is achieved by displaying peptides derived from the foreign antigen on the surface of the host cell in which they were generated. *Only those cells displaying "foreign" peptides in association with an MHC molecule trigger a T-cell response.* In a sense, the foreign peptides that reach the cell surface are a representative sampling of all the peptides derived from the pathogen inside the infected cell. In this way, T cells are able to recognize the difference between an infected and a noninfected cell.

The events involved in the generation of peptides from proteins inside cells, the binding of peptides to MHC molecules, and the display of such peptides at the cell surface is known collectively as *antigen processing and presentation*. MHC molecules play a central role in these phenomena because they bind to selected peptide fragments inside the cell and transport them to the cell surface. At the surface of the cell, the complex of peptide and MHC molecule can now be recognized by a T cell with the appropriate receptor. As we mentioned in the Introduction, because of the critical role that MHC molecules play in these interactions, T-cell responses are said to be MHC-restricted. In every vertebrate species studied, *the function of MHC class I molecules is to present peptides derived from protein antigens to the set of*

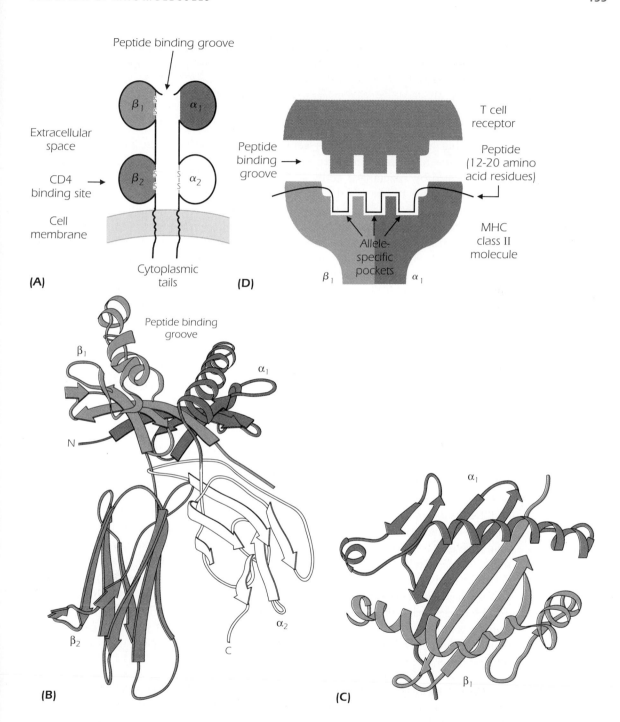

Peptide binding groove

Figure 8.3. Different depictions of an MHC class II molecule. **(A)** Diagram of the structure of an MHC class II molecule at the cell surface. **(B)** Side view of the MHC class II molecule showing the peptide-binding groove. [Adapted from Stern and Wiley, 1994, with permission.] **(C)** Top view of the peptide-binding groove. [Adapted from Stern et al., 1994, with permission.] (D) Diagram of the interaction of a T-cell receptor with an MHC class II molecule and peptide bound in the peptide-binding groove. [From Rammensee et al., 1993.]

T cells known as CD8$^+$, and the *function of MHC class II molecules is to present peptides to CD4$^+$ T cells.* In the sections that follow we will describe these phenomena in more detail.

Antigen Processing and Presentation

Determining how protein antigens activate T cells has been the subject of intense study for several years. Early experiments in the field suggested that antigens had to be ingested by specialized cells, such as macrophages, and then broken down to peptide fragments before T cells would respond. In which part of the cell and how this occurred were not understood. Tracing the fate of antigen inside the cell was difficult because it became apparent that only a tiny fraction of the input antigen generated an immune response; almost all of the antigen was broken down to very small fragments that were not immunogenic. It was thus not possible to follow the intracellular fate of that crucial portion of the antigen that generated a T-cell response. Furthermore, although the immunogenic antigenic moieties were suspected to be on the surface of the macrophage, they could not be detected by antibodies specific for the protein.

The involvement of MHC molecules in processing and presentation was suggested by a key early finding: antibody specific for MHC molecules was able to block macrophage presentation of antigen to T cells. Since the antibody directed at MHC molecules presumably sterically blocked the interaction of MHC on the APC with the T-cell receptor, this finding strongly suggested that MHC molecules and antigen were closely associated on the surface of the APC.

Several findings over the last twenty years have revolutionized our understanding of the nature of antigen processing and presentation, as well as the role of MHC molecules in these phenomena. One of the most important advances came from studying the immune response to small protein antigens whose complete sequence was known (rather than complex multimeric proteins), for example, cytochrome c and lysozyme molecules obtained from a variety of animals. In conjunction with advances in the in vitro culture of T cells using growth factors, it was determined that a single T cell was able to respond to a specific linear peptide region of the molecule. Generally, these peptides are 10–20 amino acids long. Another key finding was that many different cells — such as dendritic cells, B cells, and epithelial cells, and not macrophages alone — have the machinery to process and present antigen to T cells, and so have the ability to act as antigen-presenting cells for T cells. A further finding with crucial impact was that MHC molecules purified from the cell surface could bind selectively to peptides in vitro. This finding established the role of MHC molecules as selective peptide binders.

Cell Biology of Antigen Processing and Presentation: What Determines Whether an Antigen Elicits an MHC Class I or Class II Restricted Response? Over the last few years, we have begun to understand the processes that occur inside a cell to determine how a particular protein antigen is processed and presented by either MHC class I or class II molecules. In addition, we have come to realize that the phenomena of antigen processing and presentation are aspects of normal cell physiologic pathways. Thus, a great deal of recent attention has focused on understanding basic cellular physiology, including how normal (and abnormal) cellular proteins move through the cell to its surface, how long they remain on the cell surface, and what happens to them after they leave the cell surface; in short, to gain an understanding of the dynamic aspects of intracellular traffic and turnover.

We now understand that to activate the T-cell response to any foreign protein, the protein must be broken down into peptides, at least one of which must bind to an MHC molecule. Protein catabolism to peptides takes place in two cellular compartments: (1) within acid vesicles and (2) within the cytoplasm. *Peptides generated in acid vesicles bind to newly synthesized MHC class II molecules, whereas peptides generated in the cytoplasm bind to newly synthesized MHC class I molecules.* The interaction of peptide with MHC molecules and the movement of peptide−MHC complexes through the cell to the cell surface is facilitated by a series of molecular *chaperones*. The following paragraphs summarize our current knowledge of these areas.

Generation of MHC Class II−Peptide Complexes.

We will deal first with the set of antigens known as *exogenous antigens*. Exogenous antigens are taken into cells by endocytosis if the antigen is soluble or by phagocytosis, in specialized cells such as macrophages, if the antigen is particulate (see Figure 8.4). These exogenous antigens include bacteria, viruses taken up by macrophages, and potentially harmless foreign proteins, such as ovalbumin or sheep red blood cells.

Once internalized, the antigen is contained in an intracellular vesicle that then fuses with existing endosomal or lysosomal vesicles. The endosomal and lysosomal vesicles are highly acidic (pH ~ 4.0) and contain an array of degradative enzymes, including proteases and peptidases. Recent studies indicate that a protease that clips protein at asparagine residues may make the first cut in a protein antigen; other proteases, known as cathepsins, which function at low pH, are also thought to be involved in selective cutting of proteins in these vesicles. Some regions of the antigenic protein are thus catabolized to single amino acids, but at least some portions of the protein seem less sensitive to degradation and remain as peptides for a finite period.

As shown in Figure 8.4, acid vesicles containing the immunogenic peptides derived from protein antigens intersect with vesicles containing newly synthesized MHC class II molecules. MHC class II α and β chains are synthesized on ribosomes of the rough endoplasmic reticulum (ER). The chains associate in the ER with a molecule known as *invariant chain (Ii, CD74)*; a region of the Ii interacts with the groove of the newly formed MHC class II molecule, preventing the binding of endogenous peptides found in the ER (see Figure 8.4). Ii also acts as a "chaperone" for the newly synthesized MHC class II chains: interaction with Ii allows the MHC class II α plus β chains to leave the ER and enter the endocytic pathway. Removal of Ii from the complex occurs in stages in acid vesicles; initially, Ii is degraded proteolytically, leaving a fragment known as CLIP bound to the MHC class II groove. In acid vesicles containing peptides derived from exogenous antigens, a molecule known as *HLA-DM* facilitates peptide exchange between the MHC class II−CLIP complex and peptides derived from exogenous protein antigens. (Exactly where this occurs in the cell is not completely understood, although it is believed to occur in a specialized compartment.) In this way, a peptide-MHC class II complex is generated, which then moves to the cell surface where it can interact with a $CD4^+$ T cell expressing the appropriate receptor.

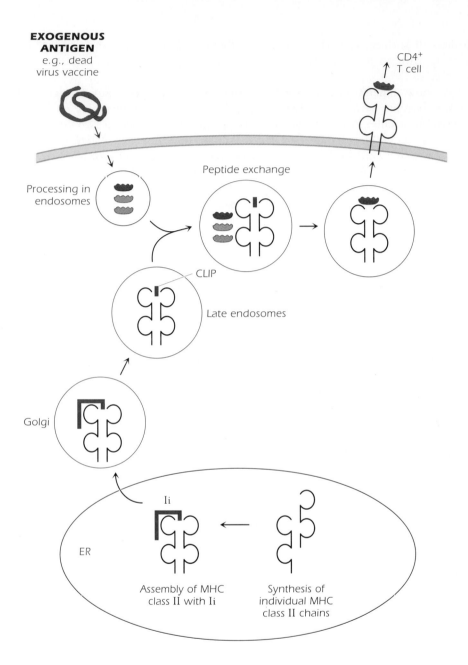

Figure 8.4. Processing of an exogenous antigen in the MHC class II pathway. Ii = invariant chain, CLIP = fragment of Ii bound to MHC class II groove.

As shown in Figure 8.5, the association of MHC class II molecules and processed peptides is *selective* for peptides between approximately 12 and 20 amino acids in length, and a single peptide binds with high affinity to some but not other allelic forms of the molecule. The sequence and charge of the amino acids forming the peptide-binding groove of the MHC molecule determine which processed peptides

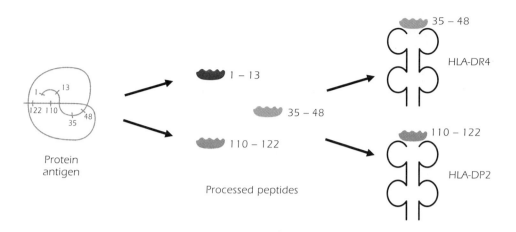

Figure 8.5. Selective binding of processed peptides by different MHC alleles. The numbers refer to positions of amino acids in the sequence of the protein antigen.

are accommodated. Figure 8.5 illustrates that catabolism of a typical protein antigen yields a number of peptides. In a person who expresses the HLA molecules DR4 and DP2, peptide 35-48 binds to HLA-DR4, and peptide 110-122 to HLA-DP2, and likely trigger CD4$^+$ T cell responses. These peptides are said to be the ***immunodominant T cell epitopes*** of the antigen in this individual. Peptide 1-13 does not bind to the HLA molecules of the individual shown, and therefore does not trigger a T cell response. Peptide 1-13 may, however, be the immunodominant epitope of the antigen in an individual expressing a different set of HLA molecules.

Generation of MHC Class I–Peptide Complexes. Proteins that generate peptides able to bind MHC class I molecules follow a different pathway of processing (see Figure 8.6). These antigens (generally viral or parasitic in origin) are ***endogenous, in that they are generally synthesized within the cell***; processing of these antigens occurs in the cytosolic compartment rather than in acid vesicles. The major mechanism for generating peptide fragments in the cytoplasm is via a giant protein complex known as the ***proteasome***. The proteasome cuts the protein into peptide fragments eight or nine residues long, and these peptides are selectively transported into the ER by the products of two transporter genes, known as TAP-1 and TAP-2. Binding of peptides with newly synthesized MHC class I molecules takes place in the ER. Binding of peptide to MHC class I molecules is also selective, based on the structure of the binding groove of the MHC class I molecule and the peptide. Because the groove in the MHC class I binding site is closed at both ends, MHC class I molecules preferentially bind peptides of 8–9 amino acids in length, the length which results from cutting by the cytosolic proteasome.

Before peptide loading, the MHC class I and β2-microglobulin chains synthesized in the ER associate with ***chaperones***, which assist in the correct folding of the MHC class I plus β2-microglobulin and directing the molecule through the ER. Peptide that binds to an MHC class I molecule in the ER moves via the Golgi

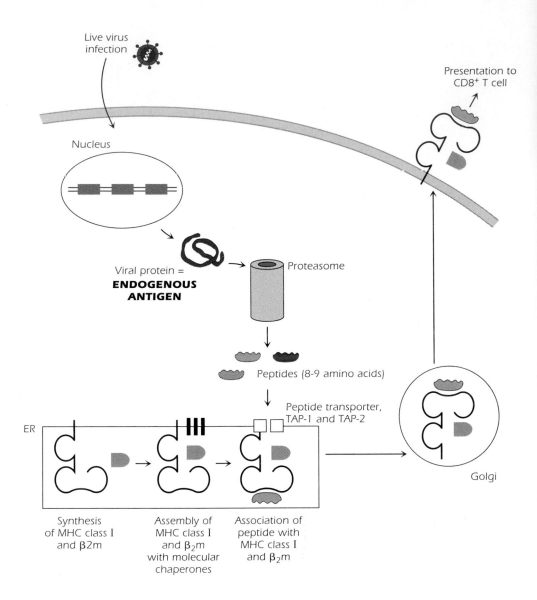

Figure 8.6. Processing of an endogenous antigen in the MHC class I pathway. β2m = β2-microglobulin.

apparatus to the cell surface where it may interact with a CD8$^+$ T cell expressing the appropriate receptor.

Current research favors the view that peptide binds to newly synthesized MHC class I and II molecules on their way to the cell surface, but cannot exclude that some peptide binding may take place with MHC molecules that are recycling from the membrane of the cell. It is also possible that peptide may bind to some MHC molecules at the cell surface, either to MHC molecules not containing peptide or by displacing previously bound peptide.

MHC Molecules Bind Peptides Derived From Self-Molecules

As a consequence of the normal pathways of intracellular turnover and metabolism of cellular constituents, peptides derived from self-components such as ribosomal and mitochondrial proteins can also bind to MHC molecules. These self-components do not, however, generally result in T-cell activation. Either these components are present at a number too low to activate T cells, or the T cells have been made tolerant to this combination of MHC and peptide (see Chapter 11). (As discussed in Chapter 9, most T cells reactive to self-molecules are removed during differentiation in the thymus, so that the mature T cells are depleted of reactivity to self.)

This binding of peptides derived from self-molecules raises an interesting issue because it indicates that MHC molecules do not discriminate self- from nonself-peptides. Since an individual's cells are bathed in an ocean of self-proteins, which they are continually processing and binding to their MHC molecules, how can the individual respond to a tiny amount of foreign protein? The answer appears to be that only a very small number of MHC–foreign peptide complexes is required at the surface of the APC to generate an immune response. It is believed that as few as 80–100 MHC–foreign peptide complexes on the surface of a cell (which may express about 10^5 total MHC molecules on its surface) is sufficient to trigger a T-cell response.

Inability to Respond to an Antigen

As we have described in the preceding sections, a limited number of different MHC class I molecules (6) and MHC class II molecules (10–20 in the human, 6 in the mouse) is expressed on the cells of any one individual. For an antigen to generate a T-cell response, at least one peptide derived during processing must bind to one of these MHC molecules. A peptide that does not bind to an MHC molecule does not activate a T-cell response. Thus, it is possible that some individuals may respond to a small peptide, but other MHC-distinct individuals may not. If an entire antigen fails to generate a single peptide able to bind to an MHC molecule, the individual will not mount a T-cell response to that particular antigen. This kind of unrespon-siveness to an entire antigen can occur, for example, in the response of certain strains of mice to synthetic polymers of amino acids that contain a very limited number of epitopes. An inability to respond to naturally occurring pathogens is very rare, as pathogens generally contain multiple epitopes.

One Antigen Can Trigger MHC Class I- or Class II-Restricted Responses

It is important to note that a single antigen can induce MHC class I *or* class II-restricted responses; the outcome is dependent on the processing pathway the antigen takes through the cell. Thus, if a viral antigen is taken up by macrophages, for example, as may occur when a noninfectious viral particle is presented in a vaccine, processing occurs in acid vesicles and peptides bind to MHC class II molecules. If, however, the same viral antigen is synthesized following the infection of a cell, processing occurs in the cytoplasm of the cell and peptides associate with MHC class I molecules. The peptides that associate with MHC class I may be different from those that bind to MHC class II. Thus, as a consequence of the selective binding of peptides to MHC molecules, CD4$^+$ and CD8$^+$ T cells in one individual may respond to different epitopes on the same antigen.

 ## DIVERSITY OF MHC MOLECULES: MHC ASSOCIATION WITH RESISTANCE AND SUSCEPTIBILITY TO DISEASE

In this chapter we have described the extensive polymorphism of MHC genes and molecules. We have indicated that such polymorphism is a great impediment to the acceptance of tissue between individuals, because it is highly unlikely that two random individuals are genetically identical (discussed more fully in Chapter 19). Since nearly every vertebrate species has developed a similarly diverse array of MHC genes and molecules, it suggests that the maintenance of MHC diversity must have some major benefit to be so widespread.

It is believed that the maintenance of diversity of MHC molecules is an important mechanism that the species uses to protect itself from the surrounding array of pathogenic organisms. To illustrate this point, imagine the situation if there were only one MHC molecule in the population and a new pathogen emerged that did not produce an epitope able to bind to the single MHC molecule. In this extreme case, no T-cell response would be mounted, and the entire species could be wiped out. Thus, maintaining a large number of MHC genes and molecules in the species would greatly reduce the risk of one pathogen having such a negative effect.

A recent example of how diversity among HLA alleles may affect the progress of a disease was reported in a study of HIV-1-infected patients. Individuals who were HLA heterozygotes (expressing *different* paternal and maternal chromosome products) at one or more HLA class I loci progressed more slowly to AIDS than individuals who were homozygotes (expressing the *same* gene product). One possible explanation of these findings is that HLA heterozygotes are able to present a wider range of pathogen-derived peptides to their T cells than homozygotes, and thus may be more likely to induce some type of protective response.

Over the last few years it has also become apparent that the expression of a specific MHC allele is one of the important factors associated with *susceptibility* and with resistance to different infectious agents. In humans, expression of specific HLA alleles has been associated with either susceptibility or resistance to a number of different infectious diseases, such as human T-lymphotropic virus (HTLV-1), hepatitis B, leprosy, malaria, tuberculosis, and rapid progression to AIDS. Similar MHC associations with susceptibility or resistance have also been shown in infectious diseases of other species. These include Marek's disease (a viral disease in chickens) and bovine leukemia virus infection in cows. For almost all known cases of association of a disease with a particular MHC allele, definitive mechanisms connecting possession of the gene with the onset or progress of the disease have not been established. Some theories to account for these associations are described at the end of this chapter.

It has also been recognized for many years that *individuals with certain HLA alleles have a higher risk of contracting certain autoimmune or inflammatory diseases*. Some of these diseases and associations with HLA molecules are illustrated in Table 8.1. A recent focus of research in this area has been to show that the disease association is with a particular HLA allele, rather than the serologically defined specificity; for example, not all individuals designated HLA-DR4$^+$ are equally at risk

TABLE 8.1. Association of Diseases and HLA Types

Disease	HLA molecule
Rheumatoid arthritis	DR4
Multiple sclerosis	DR2
Myasthenia gravis	DR3
Celiac disease	DR3, DR7
Insulin-dependent diabetes mellitus	DR3 and DR4
Ankylosing spondylitis	B27
Reiter's disease	B27
Narcolepsy	DR2

for rheumatoid arthritis: those with the DR4 alleles DRB1*0405 and *0402 have the highest risk (see Chapter 17 for further discussion.)

One of the most dramatic examples of all HLA-associated diseases is **ankylosing spondylitis** (an inflammatory disease that leads to stiffening of the vertebral joints of the spine) in which almost 90% of people with the disease carry one particular HLA allele (the B27 allele). Only a very small fraction of B27$^+$ individuals develop ankylosing spondylitis, however, indicating the role of other factors, such as environment or infection, in the induction of the disease process. Narcolepsy (a sleep disorder) is also very strongly associated with HLA-DR2, but the etiology of the disease is unknown and it has no known immunologic component.

In the case of many autoimmune diseases, the autoantigen believed responsible for the condition has not yet been identified, complicating explanations of possible mechanism. Many of these diseases are suspected of being initiated by viruses or bacteria (see Chapter 17). The following are among the hypotheses that have been proposed to account for the associations of MHC type and disease:

TABLE 8.2. Comparison of the Properties and Function of MHC Class I and Class II Molecules

	MHC class I	MHC class II
Structure	α chain + β2m	α and β
Domains	α_1, α_2 and α_3 + β2m	α_1 + α_2 and β_1 + β_2
Constitutive cellular expression	Nearly all nucleated cells	Antigen presenting cells (B cells, dendritic cells, thymic epithelial cells)
Peptide binding groove	Closed, binds 8–9 amino acid peptides formed by α_1 and α_2 domains	Open, binds 12–20 amino acid peptides formed by α_1 and β_1 domains
Peptides derived from	Endogenous antigens, catabolized in the cytoplasm	Exogenous antigens, catabolized in acid compartments
Peptide presented to	CD8$^+$ T cells	CD4$^+$ T cells

1. MHC molecules serve as *receptors* for the attachment and entry of pathogens into the cell. Thus, individuals with a certain MHC type could be more susceptible to an infection by a particular virus that uses that MHC molecule as a receptor.

2. Serendipitous *resemblance* between the antigenic determinants of the pathogen and the MHC or other molecules of the host (molecular mimicry). One result of this mimicry may be the failure to induce an immune response to the pathogen because it is seen as self; alternatively, if the pathogen does activate T and/or B cells, these activated cells may initiate a response to the self-antigens expressed in the host and lead to an autoimmune reaction.

3. As described earlier in the chapter, distinct regions of a single protein may be bound by different MHC molecules (Figure 8.5). Thus, it is possible that the peptides binding to the MHC molecules of disease-susceptible individuals may be different from the peptides binding to the MHC molecules of nonsusceptible individuals. It is also possible that as a result of these differences in peptide–MHC binding in susceptible vs nonsusceptible individuals, different patterns of cytokines are synthesized by subsets of T cells and different effector cells activated. (This is discussed further in Chapters 10, 11, and 17.)

     As an alternative possibility, the complex of peptide derived from a certain pathogen with a particular MHC molecule may not be recognized by an individual's T cells. Such a combination would thus be ignored by the host and slip through a "hole" in the host's T-cell repertoire.

4. It is possible that an allele in the MHC itself is not responsible for the disease, but rather that some other genetic locus closely linked to the MHC causes the disease.

Whatever the explanation of the association between MHC and disease, it is of great practical value in trying to identify individuals at risk, in making more precise diagnoses, and in projecting the course of treatment.

● OTHER GENES WITHIN THE MHC REGION

Over the last fifteen years, the MHC regions of the human and of the mouse have been mapped by molecular biologic approaches, and an understanding of the true complexity of the regions is still emerging. Each MHC complex contains about 40 genes and pseudogenes. The function of many of these genes awaits clarification. Why all these genes are linked in a complex with genes coding for crucial cell interaction molecules is currently not known.

The MHC region contains genes coding for serum complement components C2, C4, and factor B (see Chapter 13). These genes were formerly referred to as "MHC class III genes." The region between class I and class II genes in the human also contains several different genes: two cytokines [tumor necrosis factor (TNF) α and β], two heat-shock proteins (hsp 70-1 and 70-2), and an enzyme involved in the hydroxylation of steroids. Additional human (HLA-E, -F, -G, and -H) and murine MHC class I genes (Qa and TLa) have been identified which are not variable like other class I genes. The function of the products of most of these class I genes is not well understood, but they may also be involved in the presentation of antigens to T cells. The expression of HLA-G by placental trophoblast cells has been suggested as a potential mechanism by which rejection of the fetus by the maternal host is prevented.

The MHC class II region includes genes other than those coding for the cell-surface molecules described earlier in the chapter. These include genes known as DM, DN, and DO in the human class II region, and the homologous genes M and O in the mouse. As described earlier in the chapter, DM catalyzes peptide exchange between foreign peptides and the invariant chain-derived CLIP protein. DO is expressed only in B cells and thymic epithelial cells and acts as a negative regulator of DM-mediated peptide exchange. Genes coding for molecules involved in the MHC class I pathway of antigen presentation, the peptide transporter molecules TAP-1 and TAP-2, and the major subunits of the proteasome, LMP-2 and LMP-7, are also found in the MHC class II region.

SUMMARY

1. MHC molecules play a crucial role in the response of T cells to antigens that penetrate or live inside cells of the body. MHC molecules bind peptides derived from protein antigens and present them to T cells with the appropriate receptor. Thus, T-cell responses are said to be MHC-restricted.

2. The MHC codes for two major categories of cell surface transmembrane molecules, MHC class I and class II molecules. The outer region of every MHC class I and class II molecule contains a deep groove that binds peptides derived from the catabolism (processing) of protein antigens. The binding of peptides to MHC molecules is selective. Each MHC molecule binds peptides with a particular motif.

3. Within one individual, the MHC class I and II molecules expressed are the same on all cells of the body. An individual expresses only a limited number of different MHC class I molecules (6) and class II molecules (10–20 in the human) per cell.

4. Different individuals express a distinct array of MHC class I and class II molecules. This diversity comes about because different individuals within a species have a range of slightly different forms, alleles, of MHC class I and class II genes ("genetic polymorphism"). Because of the extensive polymorphism of MHC genes, every individual has an almost unique array of inherited MHC genes.

5. MHC molecules are codominantly expressed at the cell surface (products of both maternal and paternal chromosomes). The expression of MHC molecules is inducible on many cell types, particularly in response to cytokines.

6. Peptide + MHC class II at the cell surface interacts with T-cell receptors on $CD4^+$ T cells, whereas peptide + MHC class I complexes interact with T-cell receptors on $CD8^+$ T cells. Thus, the response of $CD4^+$ T cells is referred to as restricted by MHC class II, and $CD8^+$ T cells by MHC class I.

7. Since proteins are generally structurally complex they usually generate at least one peptide able to bind to an MHC molecule, ensuring that a T-cell response is made to at least some part of a foreign antigen.

8. Susceptibility and resistance to many diseases in humans and other species are associated with the expression of a particular MHC allele.

REFERENCES

Bjorkman PJ, Saper MA, Samraoui B, Bennet WS, Strominger JI, Wiley DC (1987): Structure of the human class I histocompatibility antigen HLA-A2. *Nature* 329:506–512.

Bogyo M, Ploegh HL (1998): A protease draws first blood. *Nature* 396:625–626.

Carrington M, Nelson GW, Martin MP, Kissner T, Vlahov D, Goedert JJ, Kaslow R, Buchbinder S, Hoots K, O'Brien SJ (1999): HLA and HIV-1: heterozygote advantage and B*35-Cw*04 disadvantage. *Science* 283:1748–1753.

Garboczi DN, Biddison WE (1999): Shapes of MHC restriction. *Immunity* 10:1–7.

Germain RN (1994): MHC-dependent antigen processing and peptide presentation providing ligands for T lymphocyte activation. *Cell* 76:287–299.

Geuze HJ (1998): The role of endosomes and lysosomes in MHC class II functioning. *Immunol Today* 19:282–287.

Hill AV (1998): The immunogenetics of human infectious diseases. *Annu Rev Immunol* 16: 593–617.

Monaco JJ (1993): Structure and function of genes in the MHC class II region. *Curr Opin Immunol* 5:17.

Rammensee H-G, Falk K, Rötzschke O (1993): MHC molecules as peptide receptors. *Curr Opin Immunol* 5:35–44.

Stern LJ, Brown JH, Jardetzky TS, Gorga JC, Urban RG, Strominger JL, Wiley DC (1994): Crystal structure of the human class II MHC protein HLA-DR1 complexed with an influenza virus peptide. *Nature* 368:215–21.

Stern LJ, Wiley DC (1994): Antigenic peptide binding by class I and class II histocompatibility proteins. *Structure* 2:245–251.

Watts C (1997): Capture and processing of exogenous antigens for presentation on MHC molecules. *Annu Rev Immunol* 15:821–850.

● REVIEW QUESTIONS

For each question, choose the ONE BEST answer or completion.

1. All the following are characteristics of both MHC class I and class II molecules *except:*

   A) They are expressed codominantly.
   B) They are expressed constitutively on all nucleated cells.
   C) They are glycosylated polypeptides with domain structure.
   D) They are involved in presentation of antigen fragments to T cells.
   E) They are expressed on the surface membrane of B cells.

2. MHC class I molecules are important for which of the following?

    A) binding to CD8 molecules on T cells

    B) presenting exogenous antigen (e.g., bacterial protein) to B cells

    C) presenting viral protein to antigen-presenting cells such as macrophages

    D) binding to CD4 molecules on T cells

    E) binding to Ig on B cells

3. Which of the following is *incorrect* concerning MHC class II molecules?

    A) B cells may express different MHC class II molecules on their surface.

    B) MHC class II molecules are synthesized in the endoplasmic reticulum of many cell types.

    C) Genetically different individuals express different MHC class II alleles.

    D) MHC class II molecules are associated with β2-microglobulin on the cell surface.

    E) A peptide that does not bind to an MHC class II molecule will not trigger a CD4$^+$ T cell response.

4. Products of TAP-1 and -2 genes

    A) bind β2-microglobulin.

    B) prevent peptide binding to MHC molecules.

    C) are part of the proteasome.

    D) transport peptides into the endoplasmic reticulum for binding to MHC class I.

    E) transport peptides into the endoplasmic reticulum for binding to MHC class II.

5. Which of the following is *incorrect* concerning the processing of an antigen, such as a bacterial protein, in the acid compartments of the cell?

    A) It results in production of potentially immunogenic peptides that associate with MHC class II molecules.

    B) Predominantly exogenous antigens are processed by this pathway.

    C) It may lead to activation of CD4$^+$ T cells.

    D) It may lead to the activation of CD8$^+$ T cells.

    E) Bacterially derived peptides displace a fragment of the invariant chain from the MHC class II binding groove.

6. Which of the following statements about the MHC is *incorrect*?

    A) It codes for complement components.

    B) It codes for both chains of the MHC class I molecule.

    C) It codes for both chains of the MHC class II molecule.

    D) It is associated with susceptibility and resistance to different diseases.

    E) The total set of MHC alleles on the chromosome is known as the MHC haplotype.

Answers to Review Questions

1. **B** MHC class I molecules are expressed on nearly all nucleated cells, but the constitutive expression of MHC class II molecules is more limited (B cells, dendritic cells, and thymic epithelial cells). MHC class II expression can be induced on other cell types (such as macrophages, endothelial cells, and human T cells) by cytokines.

2. **A** As described further in Chapters 9 and 10, the interaction of CD8 on the T cell and an invariant region of MHC class I molecule is crucial in the triggering of CD8$^+$ T cells.

3. **D** The MHC class I molecule, not the MHC class II molecule, associates with β2-microglobulin.

4. *D* The products of the TAP-1 and -2 genes selectively transport peptides 8–9 amino acids in length from the cytoplasm into the ER where they bind to MHC class I molecules.

5. *D* CD8$^+$ T cells are generally not activated by processing in acid compartments; exogenous antigen processing in acid compartments results in the generation of peptides, some of which can displace the CLIP fragment of the invariant chain from the MHC class II binding groove. The peptide–MHC class II complexes move to the cell surface and can interact with a CD4$^+$ T cell with the appropriate receptor.

6. *B* The β2-microglobulin gene is located outside the MHC, on a different chromosome.

9

BIOLOGY OF THE T LYMPHOCYTE

INTRODUCTION

In this chapter we will focus on the ***T-cell receptor for antigen (TCR)***—the structure on the T cell that interacts with the complex of MHC and peptide molecules. We will compare and contrast its characteristics with those of the B-cell receptor for antigen. We will also describe how T cells differentiate.

NATURE OF THE ANTIGEN-SPECIFIC T-CELL RECEPTOR

Molecules That Interact With Antigen

Each T cell bears on its surface a disulfide-linked two-chain molecule (***heterodimer***) that interacts with antigen. The disulfide bond links the two chains to form a structure similar to the hinge region of an antibody molecule. The predominant form of the TCR, depicted on the left side of Figure 9.1, comprises the glycoprotein chains α and β (molecular weights between 40 and 60 kDa). The TCR, like the previously discussed B-cell receptor for antigen, is clonally distributed; that is, every clone of cells expresses a different receptor.

There are striking similarities in the structure of the TCR and immunoglobulin (Ig) molecules and in the organization of the genes that code for these structures (discussed later in this chapter). These similarities or homologies between the TCR and Ig (and, indeed, many other molecules expressed at the cell surface) suggest that they have evolved from a common ancestral gene. These genes are said to belong to the ***immunoglobulin gene superfamily***, and the molecules are referred to as members of the ***immunoglobulin superfamily***.

Like Ig, the TCR is a transmembrane molecule with a short cytoplasmic tail. ***The extracellular portion of the TCR resembles the Fab fragment of an antibody***. It comprises both variable (V) and constant (C) regions, which form domains. The

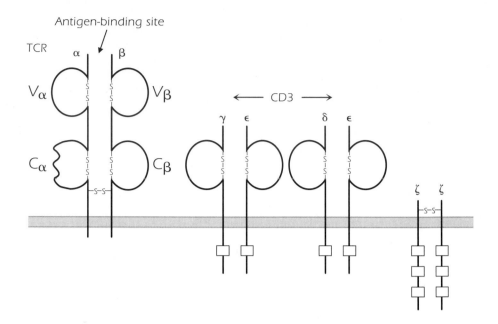

Figure 9.1. The structure of the T-cell receptor (TCR) complex showing the predominant form of the antigen-binding chains, α and β, and the associated signal transduction complex, CD3 (γ, δ, and ε chains) plus ζ or η. ITAMs are indicated by the rectangular boxes.

β chain of the TCR has V and C domains homologous to an Ig domain, but only the V region of the α chain is Ig-like. The interaction of the V regions creates three hypervariable or **complementarity determining regions (CDRs 1, 2, and 3)**, which form the antigen binding site for a peptide + MHC complex. As we will describe below, the CDR3 region of the TCR exhibits the most variability from molecule to molecule.

One difference between the TCR and an Ig molecule is that, as described, the C_{α} region of the TCR does not fold into an Ig-like domain. In addition, the conformation of the TCR appears more rigid than that of Ig because of extensive interactions between the domains of each TCR chain. This may reflect differences in the nature of the epitopes bound by Ig and the TCR: Ig with the flexibility to bind to antigens of different shapes, contrasting with the TCR's interaction only with an MHC + peptide complex.

The T-Cell Receptor Complex

The TCR is expressed on the surface of T cells in noncovalent association with a complex of transmembrane polypeptides (see right side of Figure 9.1). The entire set of molecules is referred to as the **T-cell receptor complex**, analogous to the B-cell receptor complex described in Chapter 7.

One of the molecules associated with the antigen-recognizing α + β chains is **CD3**, comprising three distinct polypeptides known as $\boldsymbol{\gamma}$, $\boldsymbol{\delta}$, and $\boldsymbol{\varepsilon}$ (molecular weights 25, 20, and 20 kDa, respectively). All the CD3 polypeptide chains are members of the Ig superfamily. It is currently believed that ε associates with both γ and δ chains in the complex, as shown in Figure 9.1. Because CD3 plays a "chaperone" role in transporting the newly synthesized TCR molecule through the cell to the cell surface, it is always found associated with the TCR and is expressed exclusively on T cells.

On most human T cells, CD3 and TCR polypeptides are also tightly associated at the cell surface with another molecule comprising two identical ζ *(zeta)* chains, molecular weight 16 kDa (see Figure 9.1). Unlike CD3 and the TCR, ζ is not T-cell specific, but is also found on macrophages and NK cells. (Some mouse T cells also express an alternatively spliced form of ζ known as η [eta], molecular weight 22 kDa, and thus an individual mouse T cell may express $\eta\eta$, $\zeta\eta$, and $\zeta\zeta$ molecules. The ζ and η chains appear to function similarly.)

CD3 and ζ polypeptides do not bind antigen. When antigen binds to the $\alpha + \beta$ chains of the TCR some change occurs in the closely linked CD3 and ζ molecules that transfers a signal into the T cell ultimately leading to a change in gene expression in the nucleus. Thus, CD3 and ζ play a crucial role as transducer molecules after antigen binding to the TCR, analogous to the role played by the Igα and Igβ molecules associated with the BCR, described in Chapter 7. Each chain of the CD3 complex contains one tyrosine-containing sequence referred to as an ***immunoreceptor tyrosine-based activation motif*** (ITAM) (Chapter 7), and the ζ chain contains three. As discussed in Chapter 10, following antigen binding to the α and β chains of the TCR, the ITAMs of the associated CD3 and ζ chains also act as docking sites for protein kinases that activate intracellular T-cell proteins and result in T-cell activation.

CD4 and CD8

The TCR is expressed on the cell surface in association with another transmembrane molecule referred to as a ***coreceptor or accessory molecule***. This coreceptor, a member of the Ig superfamily, can be one of two molecules on the mature T cell, either ***CD4*** or the two-chain molecule, ***CD8*** (see Figure 9.2), thus, T cells are either CD4$^+$ CD8$^-$ or CD4$^-$ CD8$^+$. (A cell expressing the gene of interest is referred to as "+", and a cell not expressing this gene is "−".) Coreceptor molecule expression splits the T-cell population into one of two major subsets, either CD4$^+$ CD8$^-$ or CD4$^-$ CD8$^+$. (Only immature T cells at a specific stage of differentiation in the thymus are CD4$^+$CD8$^+$.) In blood and most tissues, the ratio of CD4$^+$ to CD8$^+$ T cells is normally a little greater than 2 to 1; for example, CD4$^+$ T cells constitute 50–60% and CD8$^+$ T cells about 20–25% of total blood lymphocytes.

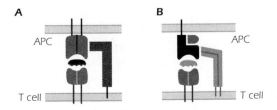

Figure 9.2. The TCR coreceptors and their interaction with MHC molecules. **(A)** CD4 and **(B)** CD8.

The functions of CD4 and CD8 are at least twofold. First, the extracellular portions of these molecules bind to the invariant portion of MHC molecules on the surface of cells that present antigen to T cells (see Chapter 8). Thus, CD4 and CD8 act as **adhesion molecules** that help to tighten the binding of T cells to antigen-presenting cells. Because CD4 binds selectively to MHC class II molecules and CD8 binds selectively to MHC class I molecules, $CD4^+$ cells interact with cells expressing antigen + MHC class II, and $CD8^+$ T cells with cells expressing antigen + MHC class I. This forms the basis of MHC restriction of the T-cell response, described in Chapter 8.

The second major function of CD4 and CD8 is to act as **signal transducers** in T cells; the intracellular portions of CD4 and CD8 are linked to specific kinases, which are activated after binding of peptide + MHC to the TCR. As discussed in Chapter 10, these CD4- and CD8-associated kinases play an important role in T-cell activation.

A unique characteristic of the CD4 molecule, which we shall describe later in more detail (see Chapter 18), is that it binds to the human immunodeficiency virus (HIV), allowing the virus to enter T cells expressing CD4, eventually leading to the disease AIDS.

INTERACTION OF THE TCR WITH MHC MOLECULES

Recent crystallographic studies have provided a striking view of how the external regions of the TCR bind to peptide + MHC complexes. Figure 9.3 depicts some of the major features of the interaction. The CDR3 regions of the TCR α and β, the regions of most variability in the TCR, interact with the center of the peptide bound in the groove of the MHC molecule. This central area of the peptide sticks out of

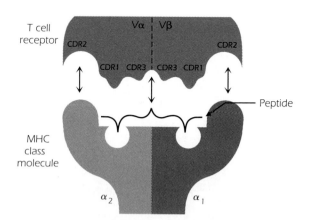

Figure 9.3. The interaction of TCR, MHC, and peptide. The complementarity determining regions (CDRs) of the TCR V regions and peptide bound in the peptide-binding groove of an MHC class I molecule are depicted. [Based on the crystal structure described by K. C. Garcia et al. (1998): Science 279: 1166.]

the MHC groove and is the only part of the peptide not buried in the MHC molecule. This suggests that limited contacts with amino acids in the center of the peptide are critical for recognition by the TCR. In contrast, the majority of the TCR-MHC interactions are with conserved MHC amino acids for that allele. In particular, the CDR2 regions of the TCR α and β make a number of contacts with the helical walls of the MHC molecule, "anchoring" the interaction of MHC and TCR. Thus, the TCR appears to make different types of contacts with the peptide on the one hand and the MHC molecule on the other. Another feature, which is not depicted in the figure, is that the TCR binds diagonally across the groove in the MHC molecule; this orientation is thought to maximize the interactions among the TCR, peptide, and MHC molecules. To date, all the crystallized structures have been TCRs complexed with MHC class I molecules, but it is believed that the interaction of TCRs with MHC class II molecules is similar.

$\gamma\delta$ T CELLS

Some T cells express a TCR distinct from $\alpha\beta$. This alternative TCR is known as $\gamma\delta$, and thus the cells expressing this receptor are referred to as $\gamma\delta$ T cells. $\gamma\delta$ is expressed in association with CD3 and ζ. (Note that the $\gamma\delta$ chains of the TCR are different from the γ and δ chains of CD3.) Generally, $\gamma\delta$ cells lack the CD4 coreceptor molecule found on $\alpha\beta$-expressing T cells, but some $\gamma\delta$ cells do express CD8.

In normal adult humans $\gamma\delta$ T cells are found at much lower numbers than $\alpha\beta$ cells, but their numbers are increased by infectious agents. $\gamma\delta$ T cells are present in all mammals at some level; the peripheral blood of ruminant species, which include the cow and deer, can have higher circulating levels of $\gamma\delta$ T cells than $\alpha\beta$ T cells.

The $\alpha\beta$ and $\gamma\delta$ lineages diverge early in intrathymic development, but less is known about the steps in $\gamma\delta$ T-cell differentiation than $\alpha\beta$ differentiation. During development of the individual $\gamma\delta$ cells appear in the thymus before $\alpha\beta$-bearing cells. There are at least two subpopulations of $\gamma\delta$ cells, defined by different Vγ-gene usage. The subpopulations migrate to different sites: skin or, alternatively, epithelial areas, such as lung and intestine.

The functions of $\gamma\delta$ T cells are not well understood; in general, $\gamma\delta$ T cells do not respond to a wide range of protein antigens. Some have been found to be activated by mycobacterial antigens and some to heat-shock proteins (proteins that form in cells when they are heated or stressed in different ways). $\gamma\delta$ T cells can produce many of the cytokines synthesized by $\alpha\beta$ TCR cells in response to antigen, and may exhibit other functions associated with $\alpha\beta$ T cells, such as cytotoxicity. From this sparse information, it has been suggested that $\gamma\delta$ TCR cells may provide a first line of defense against invading pathogens.

Unlike $\alpha\beta$ T cells, some $\gamma\delta$ T cells do not respond to complexes of peptide and MHC molecules. Some $\gamma\delta$ can recognize native antigen (such as viral proteins) and some interact with other cell surface structures, such as nonpolymorphic MHC class I and CD1(discussed in Chapters 8 and 10, respectively), that can present antigen. Recent crystallographic evidence indicates that the framework structure of a Vδ domain more closely resembles the V region of an immunoglobulin heavy chain than the corresponding regions of an $\alpha\beta$ TCR. This suggests that antigen binding to the $\gamma\delta$ TCR may have more in common with antigen binding to antibody than to $\alpha\beta$ TCRs.

GENES CODING FOR T-CELL RECEPTORS

The organization of the human gene loci coding for the α, β and δ T-cell receptor chains is shown in Figure 9.4. (Because of its complexity, the organization of γ genes is not shown.) Several other features are noteworthy. First, α and γ chains are constructed from V and J gene segments, like Ig light chains, whereas β and δ chains are constructed from V, D, and J gene segments, like Ig heavy chains. Second, the β and γ loci are each found on different chromosomes, while gene segments of the α and δ loci are interspersed on the same chromosome. Genes coding for the δ chain are flanked on both the 5′ and 3′ sides by genes coding for the α chain. Third, there are many more Vα and Vβ genes than Vγ and Vδ genes (5–10) in the germ line.

Individual TCR V regions have been given numbers, for example, $V_\alpha 2$ or $V_\beta 7$. Interestingly, the use of certain TCR V regions is associated with the response to particular antigens. This has been shown to be particularly important in the response to **superantigens**, discussed in Chapters 3 and 10.

 GENERATION OF T-CELL RECEPTOR DIVERSITY

The mechanisms for generating diversity in T-cell receptors are very similar to the mechanisms of generating diversity in B-cell receptors. The same fundamental principles of gene rearrangement, as described in Chapter 6 for Ig, apply in synthesizing the V and C regions of each chain of the T-cell receptor α, β, γ, and δ. **Recombinases and joining sequences** are used to link up a VJ or a VDJ unit, generating the variable region specificity of a particular TCR polypeptide chain. The same enzymes are probably involved in the recombination events in both B and T cells. As described in Chapter 6, two genes known as **recombination activation genes** (RAG-1 and RAG-2) have been shown to play a crucial role in activating the recombinase genes in both early B and T cells. T-cell receptor genes also show **allelic exclusion**, just like Ig, ensuring that a single T cell makes a receptor with only a single antigenic specificity.

The generation of diversity in T-cell receptors is thus very similar to the generation of diversity in the B-cell receptor, immunoglobulin, described in Chapter 6. As in the generation of Ig diversity, TCR diversity is generated by (1) multiple V

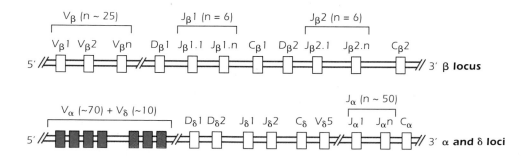

Figure 9.4. Organization of the α, β, and δ genes coding for the human T-cell receptor. The organization of the γ-gene locus is not shown because of its complexity.

genes in the germ line, (2) random combination of chains, and (3) junctional and insertional variability. Unlike immunoglobulin molecules, however, T-cell receptors do not undergo somatic hypermutation following antigenic stimulation.

The repertoire of different TCRs is believed to be as large or larger than the repertoire of Ig molecules (estimated in the range of 10^{15} different potential specificities for $\alpha\beta$ and 10^{18} for $\gamma\delta$ TCRs). TCRs have enormous junctional and insertional variability, which results in tremendous diversity of the CDR3 regions. As described earlier in this chapter, only the CDR3 regions of the $\alpha\beta$ TCR interact with peptide residues bound in the cleft of the MHC molecule. It is likely that the large number of possible sequences for the CDR3 regions ensures that TCR binding to the peptide portion of the peptide-MHC complex is highly specific.

T-CELL DIFFERENTIATION IN THE THYMUS

Introduction

The thymus is absolutely required for the differentiation of immature precursor cells into cells with the characteristics of T cells: children born without a thymus (Di-George syndrome, discussed in Chapter 18) or mice genetically lacking a thymus (known as nude mice because they also lack hair) do not have mature T cells. T-cell differentiation in the thymus occurs throughout the life of the individual but diminishes significantly after puberty. The size of the thymus itself decreases with the onset of puberty in mammals (thymic involution), presumably because of the synthesis of steroid hormones at this time. In some species, particularly the mouse, if the thymus is removed shortly after birth, the mature T-cell population is drastically depleted. Indeed, these were the pioneering observations of Jacques Miller in the 1950s, who established the crucial role of the thymus in T-cell responses. Removing the thymus later in the development of the animal has much less impact on the mature T-cell population.

In the thymus the rearrangement events occur that determine whether a T cell expresses $\alpha\beta$ or $\gamma\delta$ as its receptor, and determine the specificity of the particular TCR for an antigenic epitope. Thus, as described in Chapter 2, the thymus is the *primary lymphoid organ* for the development of T cells, analogous to the bone marrow as the primary organ for mammalian B-cell differentiation.

As we shall discuss later in this chapter, there are two other major consequences of differentiation in the thymus. First, mature T cells emerge that recognize antigen only when it is associated with MHC molecules; that is, *T cells are MHC-restricted*. Second, mature T cells emerge that do not respond to self components, that is, *T cells are self-tolerant*.

Thymocytes Interact With Thymic Nonlymphoid Cells

T-cell differentiation in the thymus is a complex multistep process (see Figure 9.5). It has been easiest to study in the mammalian embryo and in vitro where the sequence of events can be determined from the very earliest stages. We shall focus on a number of key steps in T-cell differentiation in the thymus.

At every stage of thymic maturation, from precursor to mature T cell, the developing T lymphocytes (*thymocytes*) are in contact with, and interact with, a mesh

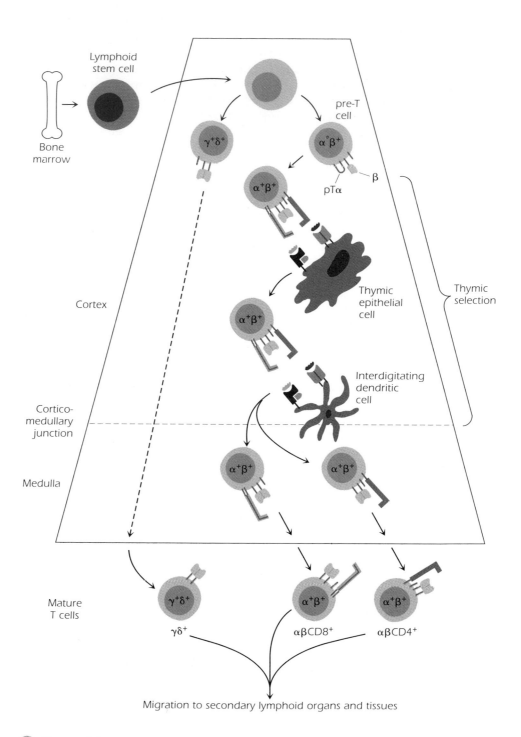

Figure 9.5. The developmental pathways of T cells in the thymus. Genes coding for the α, β, γ, and δ chains of the T-cell receptor are designated as α^0 etc. if unrearranged and α^+ if rearranged.

formed by the nonlymphoid (*stromal*) cells of the thymus. The thymocytes trickle through this network of nonlymphoid cells, starting at the top of the thymus (*the thymic cortex*) and continuing into the lower area (*the thymic medulla*). As we shall describe in more detail below, the nonlymphoid cells provide critical cell surface interactions required for the development of maturing T cells. They also produce cytokines such as IL-7, which are important for the early stages of T (and B) lymphocyte development. The most important thymic nonlymphoid cells are (1) *cortical epithelial cells*, and (2) *interdigitating dendritic cells (IDC)*, found predominantly at the junction of the cortex and medulla. IDC are closely related to the bone-marrow-derived, antigen-presenting dendritic cells described at the end of this chapter and in Chapter 10.

 ## T-CELL RECEPTOR GENE REARRANGEMENT

The earliest cell in the T-lymphocyte lineage enters the thymus with its TCR genes in an unrearranged or germ line configuration. In the thymus, the thymocytes which differentiate from this precursor undergo an ordered sequence of TCR gene rearrangements (see Figure 9.5) analogous to the ordered rearrangement of Ig genes during B-cell development. As in the B-cell lineage, if a developing T cell fails to generate both chains of the antigen-specific receptor, it dies via apoptosis.

In the early stages of differentiation in the thymic cortex, TCR β- and γ-chain genes start to rearrange, more or less simultaneously. If the γ-chain genes rearrange successfully, then δ-chain genes also start to rearrange. If both γ and δ genes rearrange "productively," that is, if they can be transcribed and translated into polypeptides, no further rearrangement occurs and the cell remains a $\gamma\delta$ T cell. Thus, cells that express $\gamma\delta$ as their TCR separate from the lineage of cells expressing $\alpha\beta$ at an early stage in intrathymic differentiation.

If, however, γ and/or δ rearrangements are not functional, β-gene rearrangement continues. If this results in a productive rearrangement, the β polypeptide is expressed on the surface with an invariant molecule known as *pTα* or *gp33*, together with CD3. These molecules constitute the *pre-T-cell receptor*, analogous to the pre-B-cell receptor, discussed in Chapter 7. The cell which expresses them is the *pre-T cell*. It is currently not clear if the signal for further differentiation of the cell is the interaction of the pre-TCR with currently unknown ligands, or whether the expression of the pre-TCR in the membrane is itself sufficient. (If the cell does not receive these signals it dies by apoptosis.) As a consequence of signaling through the pre-TCR, further rearrangement of β genes stops. This ensures that the cell expresses only one type of β chain (*allelic exclusion*), expression of pTα is downregulated, α genes start to rearrange, and the cell proliferates.

The next important cell in the $\alpha\beta$ lineage expresses *both* coreceptor molecules CD4 and CD8 on its surface. This $\alpha\beta^+CD3^+CD4^+CD8^+$ *thymocyte*, referred to as a CD4$^+$CD8$^+$ T cell, is found in the thymic cortex, and forms the majority of thymocytes in the young mammalian thymus. It is important to note that as a consequence of the more or less random nature of the recombination events involved in receptor generation, T cells expressing TCRs with specificities for all antigens, including self antigens, can arise in the thymus. Allowing T cells reactive to self antigens to leave the thymus and interact with these antigens in tissues could result in undesirable autoimmune responses. To prevent these responses, CD4$^+$CD8$^+$ T cells differentiate further before leaving the thymus, as described in the following section.

 THYMIC SELECTION

The CD4$^+$CD8$^+$ thymocyte expressing $\alpha\beta$ as its TCR undergoes a multi-step process known as ***thymic selection*** (see Figure 9.6). (Whether $\gamma\delta$+ T cells undergo a similar selection process before they leave the thymus is currently not clear.) In the first stage, ***positive selection***, the TCR of the CD4$^+$CD8$^+$ T cell interacts with MHC molecules expressed on epithelial cells in the thymic cortex. A CD4$^+$CD8$^+$ T cell which does not make this critical interaction with the thymic epithelial cell dies by apoptosis. Positive selection results in the proliferation and expansion of the CD4$^+$CD8$^+$ T cell, and the termination of RAG-1 and RAG-2 gene expression, so no further gene rearrangement occurs.

As a consequence of this positive selection step, the $\alpha\beta$ T cell becomes ***"educated"*** to the MHC molecules expressed by the thymic cortical epithelial cells. This means that for the rest of the life of the T cell, even as a mature cell when it leaves the thymus, it will respond to antigen only when the antigen is bound to the type of MHC molecules that the developing T cell encountered in the thymus. This is the origin of the phenomenon known as ***MHC restriction of T-cell responses***, and emphasizes again the critical importance of the MHC in T-cell responses.

Thymocytes expressing TCRs specific for self *and* nonself antigens are expanded by positive selection. To prevent T cells with potential reactivity to self-antigens from leaving the thymus, the CD4$^+$CD8$^+$ cell undergoes a second selection step, known as ***negative selection***. This occurs by interaction with interdigitating dendritic cells (IDC) at the corticomedullary junction. The TCR, CD4, and CD8 on the CD4$^+$CD8$^+$ T cell interact with MHC class I and II molecules plus peptides derived from self-antigens which are expressed on the IDC (see Figure 9.6). A T cell expressing a TCR which reacts with too high an affinity to the combination of MHC and peptide is deleted by apoptosis. Thus, negative selection removes T cells expressing T cell receptors with reactivity to self components. The thymocytes which survive the negative selection step because they have a lower affinity for MHC + peptides constitute the body of T cells which the individual uses to mount responses to non-self (foreign) antigens.

A number of questions remain about the mechanisms involved in selection. One is the role and nature of ***peptides*** expressed by the thymic non-lymphoid cells at different stages of the selection processes. Current evidence indicates that peptides expressed by cortical epithelial cells play a critical role in the positive selection step. These peptides are derived from self antigens either expressed in the thymus or which are brought into the thymus. It is not currently clear, however, how these peptides derived from self antigens select T cells with TCR specificities for non-self as well as self antigens. In addition, it is not clear whether the peptides expressed by the cortical epithelial cells in positive selection differ from those expressed by the IDC in negative selection. A further unresolved issue is how the interaction of the TCR expressed on a CD4$^+$CD8$^+$ T cell with peptides and MHC molecules of the cortical epithelial cell induces a positive signal (proliferation and expansion) whereas a similar interaction with a thymic dendritic cell induces a negative signal (cell death). These topics are the subject of intense research activity.

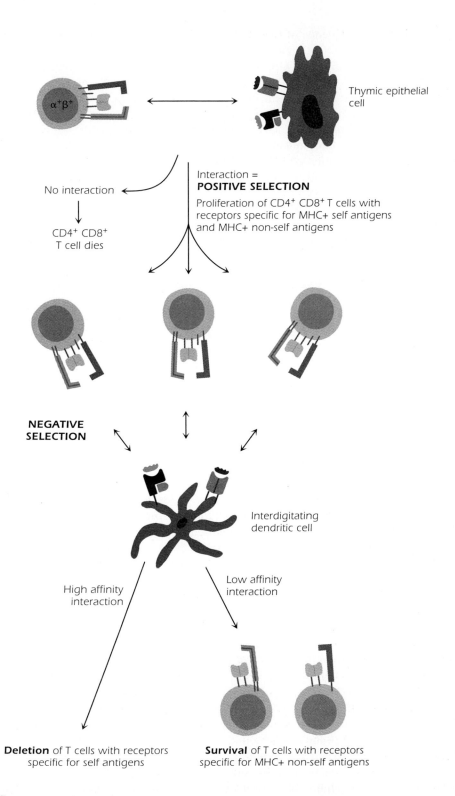

Thymic epithelial cell

No interaction

CD4⁺ CD8⁺ T cell dies

Interaction =
POSITIVE SELECTION

Proliferation of CD4⁺ CD8⁺ T cells with receptors specific for MHC+ self antigens and MHC+ non-self antigens

NEGATIVE SELECTION

Interdigitating dendritic cell

High affinity interaction

Low affinity interaction

Deletion of T cells with receptors specific for self antigens

Survival of T cells with receptors specific for MHC+ non-self antigens

Figure 9.6. Positive and negative selection of $\alpha\beta^+$ CD4⁺CD8⁺ T cells in the thymus.

As a further consequence of their interaction with the MHC molecules and peptides expressed on the IDC, thymocytes which survive negative selection also downregulate expression of either CD4 or CD8 by a mechanism that is currently not well understood. This results in the development of either *CD4⁺CD8⁻ or CD4⁻CD8⁺ T cells*. These two sets of cells are the end point of the complex pathway of $\alpha\beta$ TCR cell differentiation in the thymus. They leave the thymus and comprise the *peripheral (i.e., outside the thymus)* mature CD4⁺ and CD8⁺ T-cell lineages.

In summary, as a consequence of the steps in intrathymic differentiation of $\alpha\beta$TCR⁺ T cells, a repertoire of CD4⁺ T cells and CD8⁺ T cells is constructed which is able to respond to the universe of non-self antigens. These T cells have two other important characteristics: (1) *they are MHC-restricted*; they react to peptides derived from non-self antigens only when these peptides are associated with MHC molecules that were expressed in the thymus in which the T cells developed and (2) *they are self-tolerant*; T cells expressing receptors for self antigens are eliminated or functionally inactivated.

 ## LYMPHOCYTE TRAFFICKING TO TISSUES

Mature T cells leave the thymus and circulate via the blood to secondary lymphoid organs, in which most responses to antigen subsequently occur. In addition, lymphocytes may leave the circulation and enter tissues. This is a critical feature of the immune system, allowing lymphocytes to reach the site of exposure to antigen, no matter where it occurs. This rapid redistribution of lymphocytes from blood to tissues is particularly vital when the effects of the antigen result in damage to the tissue: lymphocytes, as well as other leukocytes, play a key role in the inflammatory response in the damaged tissue. As we shall describe more fully in Chapter 12, all leukocytes use fundamentally similar processes to leave the circulation and move into tissues; *these involve multiple paired adhesive interactions between surface molecules on the circulating leukocytes and those on endothelial cells at the boundary of the tissue*. In addition to these paired cell surface interactions, cytokines and chemokines released by inflamed tissues play a role in attracting leukocytes into tissues by binding to specific receptors on the cells' surface.

One of the most interesting aspects to emerge from studies of lymphocyte traffic is the understanding that *different lymphocytes preferentially enter different tissues*, a phenomenon known as *homing*. Differences between the homing patterns of naive and activated lymphocytes are well documented: *naive lymphocytes home to peripheral and mucosal lymph nodes, whereas activated and memory T cells move out of the nodes and to sites in the skin and other tissues*.

Homing of naive T cells to nodes is mediated by the binding of *CD62L (L-Selectin or MEL-14)* expressed on the T cell surface to glycoprotein molecules known as *addressins*, which are expressed specifically on cells in a specialized region of the vascular endothelium at the boundary of the nodes. The CD62L-addressin binding triggers further paired interactions which tighten the binding between the lymphocyte and endothelial surfaces, notably between LFA-1 on the T cell and ICAM-1 on the endothelium, and ultimately result in the naive lymphocyte leaving the circulation and entering the node by squeezing through adjacent endothelial cells.

It is worth noting that these adhesive interactions occur in the absence of antigen and do not involve the TCR.

If naive T cells are stimulated by antigen in the node, however, most down-regulate expression of CD62L, and upregulate expression of other cell-surface molecules, such as CD49d (VLA-4) and CD44. These molecules mediate lymphocyte homing to tissues outside the node. Thus, as a consequence of this change in pattern of expression of homing molecules, activated and memory cells exit from the node and home to tissues such as the skin or sites of inflammation, where ligands for these molecules are expressed. Recent evidence indicates that naive and memory T cells differ not only in their expression of homing molecules but also in their expression of chemokine receptors. Thus, differences in expression of both homing molecules and of chemokine receptors result in different subsets of T cells selectively migrating to distinct sites in the body.

 ## SPECIALIZED CELLS PRESENT ANTIGEN TO T CELLS

In general, the interaction of mature T cells takes place in secondary lymphoid organs, especially lymph nodes. As described in the preceding section, however, this interaction can also occur in any tissue which has been exposed to or damaged by antigen. Because antigen can enter the body via several different routes (via the airways or gastrointestinal tract, through the skin, or by injection), specialized *antigen-presenting cells (APC)* are found at all these distinct antigen entry sites as well as in lymphoid organs. The function of these APC is to take up antigen, process it, and present it to T cells; in particular, to present antigen to CD4$^+$ T cells that play a central role in responses to protein antigens. This frequently involves the APC transporting processed antigen from the site at which it interacts with antigen via lymph vessels to the T cell area of the closest (draining) lymph node.

Bone marrow-derived cells of the myeloid type, and *dendritic cells* in particular, are extremely efficient APC at initiating *primary T cell responses* because they express high levels of MHC class II molecules, costimulatory molecules such as CD40 and B7, and other adhesion molecules. (These dendritic cells, depicted in Figure 2.1, are in the same family of cells as the interdigitating dendritic cells of the thymus which play such a crucial role in thymic selection, described earlier in the chapter.) For example, antigen that enters via the skin is taken up by specialized skin APC known as *Langerhans cells*, which belong to the macrophage/dendritic cell family of cells. These antigen-bearing Langerhans cells migrate via the lymph to the draining node. Antigen uptake and migration result in the differentiation of the APC to a cell known as the *mature dendritic cell* in the lymph node. In the T-cell area of the node, the antigen-bearing mature dendritic cells interact with a T cell which expresses the appropriate antigen receptor specificity, and initiates the cascade of events involved in T cell activation described further in Chapter 10.

As described in Chapter 7, B cells can also act as very efficient APC, especially in responses in which both CD4$^+$ T cells and B cells have already been primed by antigen. The interaction of primed T cells and B cells takes place in specialized areas of the node, the follicles, and the production of antibody in distinct areas known as germinal centers, as discussed in Chapter 7. The role of the B cell in T-B cell interactions is discussed further in Chapter 10.

SUMMARY

1. As with B cells, the individual has an enormous number of different T cells. Each T cell bears a unique, clonally distributed receptor for antigen, known as the T-cell receptor (TCR). The same rearrangement strategies and recombinase machinery are used to generate a repertoire of T cells with different TCRs as are used by B cells to generate immunoglobulin diversity.

2. On the majority of human and mouse T cells, the TCR is a two chain transmembrane molecule, $\alpha\beta$. The extracellular portion of the TCR resembles the Fab fragment of an antibody.

3. The $\alpha\beta$ TCR interacts with both an MHC molecule and peptide bound in the peptide-binding cleft of the MHC molecule. The TCR makes a limited number of critical contacts with amino acids in the center of the peptide, and interacts more extensively with conserved amino acids in the helical walls of the MHC binding cleft.

4. The antigen-binding $\alpha\beta$ chains of the TCR are expressed on the surface of the T cell in a multimolecular complex (the TCR complex) in association with CD3 and ζ polypeptides, which act as a signal transduction unit after antigen binding to $\alpha\beta$.

5. Coreceptor (accessory) molecules are associated with the $\alpha\beta$ TCR. On mature T cells the coreceptor is either CD4 or CD8, dividing T cells into two subsets, either $\alpha\beta^+CD4^+$ or $\alpha\beta^+CD8^+$. The function of these coreceptor molecules is to (a) bind MHC molecules on an antigen-presenting cell and (b) act as signal transduction molecules after antigenic stimulation.

6. A different two-chain structure, $\gamma\delta$, is the TCR on a minor population of human and mouse T cells. $\gamma\delta$ is also expressed on the surface of the cell in association with CD3 and ζ. Most $\gamma\delta$ do not express CD4, but some express CD8. The functions of $\gamma\delta^+$ T cells are not as well understood as those of $\alpha\beta^+$ T cells.

7. The TCR is initially expressed on the surface of developing T cells during differentiation in the thymus. The divergent development of T cells using $\alpha\beta$ as their receptor from those using $\gamma\delta$ as their receptor occurs early in the differentiation pathway in the thymus.

8. A key feature of $\alpha\beta^+$ T-cell differentiation is thymic selection. This is mediated by interactions of the $\alpha\beta$ TCR and coreceptor molecules on the developing T cell with MHC molecules and peptides expressed by the thymic non-lymphoid cells. Positive selection on thymic cortical epithelial cells "educates" the developing T cell: as a mature cell, it responds to antigen only when presented by a cell that expresses the same MHC molecules that the T cell interacted with during differentiation in the thymus (MHC restriction of the T-cell response). Negative selection on thymic interdigitating dendritic cells removes T cells with potential reactivity to self-molecules, ensuring self-tolerance.

9. Mature T cells leave the thymus and constitute the peripheral population of T cells able to respond to nonself (foreign) antigen. They circulate, migrate to secondary lymphoid organs, and move into tissues in response to antigen. In general, T cells are activated by specialized antigen-presenting cells.

REFERENCES

Anderson G, Moore NC, Owen JJT, Jenkinson EJ (1996): Cellular interactions in thymocyte development. *Annu Rev Immunol* 14:73–99.

Ashton-Rickardt PG, Tonegawa S (1994): A differential avidity model for T cell selection. *Immunol Today* 15:362.

Banchereau J, Steinman RM (1998): Dendritic cells and the control of immunity. *Nature* 392: 245–252.

Butcher EC, Picker LJ (1996): Lymphocyte homing and homeostasis. *Science* 272:60–66.

Cresswell P (1998): Proteases, processing, and thymic selection. *Science* 280:394–395.

Davis MM, Boniface JJ, Reich Z, Lyons D, Hampl J, Arden B, Chien Y-h (1998): Ligand recognition by $\alpha\beta$ T-cell receptors. *Annu Rev Immunol* 16:523–544.

Garcia KC, Degano M, Pease LR, Huang M, Peterson PA, Teyton L, Wilson IA (1998): Structural basis of plasticity in a T cell receptor recognition of a self peptide-MHC antigen. *Science* 279:1166–1177.

Haas W, Pereira P, Tonegawa S (1993): Gamma/delta cells. *Annu Rev Immunol* 11:637.

Robey E, Fowlkes BJ (1998): The $\alpha\beta$ versus $\gamma\delta$ T-cell lineage choice. *Curr Opin Immunol* 10:81–187.

von Boehmer H, Fehling HJ (1997): Structure and function of the pre-TCR. *Annu Rev Immunol* 15:432–452.

von Boehmer H, Aifantis I, Azogui O, Feinberg J, Saint-Ruf C, Zober C, Garcia C, Buer J (1998): Crucial function of the pre-T-cell receptor (TCR) in TCRβ selection, TCRβ allelic exclusion and $\alpha\beta$ versus $\gamma\delta$ lineage commitment. *Immunol Rev* 165:111–119.

 REVIEW QUESTIONS

For each question, choose the ONE BEST answer or completion.

1. Which of the following statements concerning T-cell development is correct?

A) Progenitor T cells that enter the thymus from the bone marrow have already rearranged their T cell receptor genes.

B) Interaction with thymic non-lymphoid cells is critical.

C) Maturation in the thymus requires the presence of foreign antigen.

D) MHC class II molecules are not involved in positive selection

E) Mature, fully differentiated T cells are found in the cortex of the thymus.

2. The development of self-tolerance in the T-cell compartment is important for the prevention of autoimmunity. Which of the following results in T-cell self-tolerance?

A) allelic exclusion

B) somatic hypermutation

C) thymocyte proliferation

D) positive selection

E) negative selection

3. Which of the following statements is correct?

A) The TCR $\alpha\beta$ chains transduce a signal into a T cell.

B) A cell depleted of its CD4 molecule would be unable to recognize antigen.

C) T cells with fully rearranged $\alpha\beta$ chains are not found in the thymus.

D) T cells expressing the $\gamma\delta$ receptor are found only in the thymus.

E) Immature $CD4^+CD8^+$ T cells form the majority of T cells in the thymus.

4. Which of the following is *incorrect* regarding mature T cells that use $\alpha\beta$ as their antigen-specific receptor?

   A) They coexpress CD3 on the cell surface.

   B) They may be either $CD4^+$ or $CD8^+$.

   C) They interact with peptides derived from nonself antigens.

   D) They can further rearrange their TCR genes to express $\gamma\delta$ as their receptor.

   E) They circulate through blood and lymph and migrate to secondary lymphoid organs.

5. CD4

   A) binds directly to peptide antigen.

   B) binds to an invariant portion of MHC class I molecules.

   C) binds to an invariant portion of MHC class II molecules.

   D) binds to CD8 on the T cell surface.

   E) binds to the peptide-binding site of MHC class II.

6. Which of the following statements is *incorrect* concerning TCR and Ig genes?

   A) In both B- and T-cell precursors, multiple V-, D-, J-, and C-region genes exist in an un-rearranged configuration.

   B) Rearrangement of both TCR and Ig genes involves specific recombinase enzymes that bind to specific regions of the genome.

   C) Both Ig and TCR are able to switch C-region usage.

   D) Both Ig and TCR exhibit allelic exclusion.

   E) Both Ig and the TCR use combinatorial association of V, D, and J genes and junctional imprecision to generate diversity.

7. Which of the following statements is *incorrect* concerning antigen-specific receptors on both B and T cells?

   A) They are clonally distributed transmembrane molecules.

   B) They have extensive cytoplasmic domains that interact with intracellular molecules.

   C) They consist of polypeptides with variable and constant regions.

   D) They are associated with signal transduction molecules at the cell surface.

   E) They can interact with peptides derived from nonself antigens.

Answers to Review Questions

1. *B* Interaction of thymocytes with thymic stromal cells—cortical epithelial cells and inter-digitating dendritic cells at the corticomedullary junction—is critical in T cell development.

2. *E* Negative selection removes developing T cells with potential reactivity to self-molecules.

3. *E* $CD4^+CD8^+$ T cells form the majority of cells in the thymus.

4. *D* The genes of T cells that use $\alpha\beta$ as their receptor cannot further rearrange to use $\gamma\delta$ as their receptor; TCR δ gene segments are interspersed with the α locus and are deleted when the α locus rearranges.

5. *C* CD4 expressed on T cells binds to an invariant or nonpolymorphic region of all MHC class II molecules.

6. *C* The ability to change the heavy-chain constant region while retaining the same antigen specificity is a property unique to Ig. The other features are common to both the TCR and Ig.

7. *B* Both the TCR and Ig have short cytoplasmic tails. The signal transduction molecules associated with the antigen-binding chains interact with intracellular molecules.

10

ACTIVATION AND FUNCTION OF
T AND B CELLS

 INTRODUCTION

The interaction of antigen with antigen-specific receptors on either T or B cells initiates a cascade of events that results in the cells' proliferation and further differentiation. As a result of antigenic stimulation, both B and T cells differentiate into *effector cells*, and a small fraction of both populations becomes *memory cells*.

The consequences of B- and T-cell activation (i.e., their effector functions), however, are completely different. In the case of B cells, antigen-driven differentiation results in antibody production, and to the generation of antibody of distinct isotypes. By contrast, antigen-driven differentiation of T cells leads to the synthesis and secretion of an array of cytokines that affect many different cell types or, alternatively, to the development of cells that are directly cytotoxic.

In this chapter we will describe in more detail how T and B cells are activated, and how they exert their effector functions.

 ACTIVATION OF CD4$^+$ T CELLS

In previous chapters we have described how protein antigens are broken down to peptide fragments, some of which associate with MHC class II molecules. We have also described how specialized *antigen-presenting cells* (APC), such as the dendritic cell, are important in presenting complexes of peptide and MHC class II molecules to CD4$^+$ T cells in primary responses, and that B cells are likely to be the major APC in the responses of primed (memory) T cells. In this section we shall describe in more detail the interactions between the T cell and APCs, which are critical in CD4$^+$ T-cell activation (see Figure 10.1).

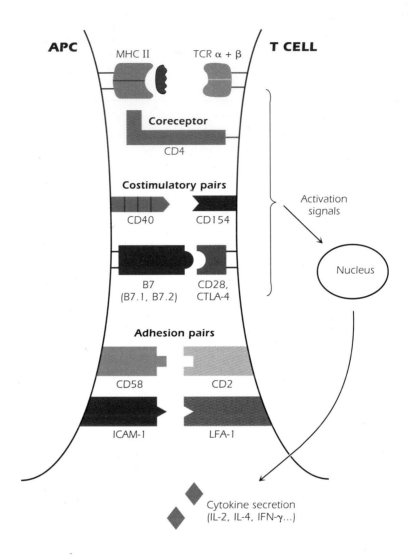

Figure 10.1. Key cell surface interactions leading to T-cell activation and cytokine secretion.

Paired Interactions Between the APC and the CD4⁺ T Cell

The variable regions, $V_\alpha + V_\beta$, of the antigen-specific receptor (TCR) on a CD4⁺ T cell expressing the appropriate receptor interact with a peptide bound to the groove of an MHC class II molecule. Contact between the TCR and MHC molecules of the APC is necessary but generally not sufficient for T-cell activation. This is likely due to the low affinity of the interaction between the TCR and peptide–MHC complex, and to the small number of complexes of MHC and foreign peptide at the surface of an individual APC (as few as 100 per cell, as described in Chapter 8). Sets of paired interactions between the APC and T-cell surfaces are required for full T-cell activation. The most important involve the *coreceptor, CD4, binding to MHC class II*, interactions of molecules known as *costimulatory pairs* and the effects of *other pairs of adhesion molecules* (Figure 10.1). In our current view, these paired interactions contribute to the formation of what is known as the ***immunological synapse***, the area of contact between the APC and the T cell containing the MHC class II plus peptide and the TCR. The formation of the synapse brings larger areas of the cell surfaces into contact, increases the time that the two cells are in contact, and leads to sustained intracellular signaling. These interactions are discussed briefly in the following subsections, and more extensively in the sections "Intracellular Events in CD4⁺ T-cell Activation," and "Functions of Costimulatory Pairs."

CD4–MHC Class II. The interaction of CD4 on the T cell with the invariant or nonpolymorphic region of an MHC class II molecule enhances the binding of a CD4⁺ T cell to an MHC class II⁺ APC. In addition, as described below, CD4 acts as an important component of T-cell activation pathways; after the peptide–MHC complex binds to the TCR, CD4 is believed to move closer to the TCR. The cytoplasmic tail of CD4 is associated with an enzyme involved in T-cell activation; "clustering" of CD4 with the TCR brings this enzyme into a signal transduction complex.

Costimulatory Molecules. The interaction of the MHC and TCR is referred to as the first signal. Additional signals, known as ***costimulatory*** or ***second signals***, are required for full T-cell activation. Costimulatory interactions are believed to be vital in activating unprimed, resting T cells but are probably less important for the activation of primed or memory T cells. The most important interactions are between ***CD40 and CD154 (CD40 Ligand*** or ***CD40L)***, and ***B7 and its ligands CD28 and CTLA-4***.

Based on recent studies, costimulatory interactions are thought to help bring molecules involved in T-cell activation inside the T cell, such as the enzymes described later in this chapter, to the area where the TCR is in contact with the APC. This redistribution also pushes molecules not involved in the APC–T-cell interaction out of the contact area. As a result, costimulatory interactions enhance and sustain signals delivered by MHC⁺ peptide to the TCR.

Other Adhesive Interactions. ***CD2***, a T-cell-specific molecule and one of the first to be expressed during T-cell development, binds to ***CD58 (leukocyte function-associated antigen-3 [LFA-3])***, which is expressed on many cells. This interaction enhances the binding (adhesion) of T cells to the other cells. In addition, ***LFA-1*** (a heterodimer of ***CD11a*** and ***CD18***) an adhesion molecule on the T-cell surface but whose expression is not confined to T cells, binds to CD54 (***intercellular adhesion molecule-1 [ICAM-1]***) on the APC. As a result of the interaction between the adhesion molecules on T cells and other cells, the binding of T cells to these other cells is considerably enhanced. These antigen nonspecific adhesive interactions slow down the movement apart from the APC and T cell and allow time for the TCR to "sample" the MHC class II + peptide expressed by the APC. In this way, these adhesive interactions stabilize what would be a transient interaction between the cells.

In summary, a combination of antigen-specific and nonspecific interactions are generally required to initiate T-cell activation. As a result of these activation processes the CD4⁺ T-cell proliferates, secretes cytokines, and differentiates into a memory cell. The activated CD4⁺ T cell also up- and downregulates cell surface molecules, which allow it to migrate from the site at which it was activated (generally the secondary lymphoid organs) to infected tissues (also see Chapter 9).

Intracellular Events in CD4⁺ T-cell Activation

In this section we discuss the roles of the interacting pairs of molecules on the APC and CD4$^+$ T cell. A great deal of recent research has focused on identifying the sequence of events inside the CD4$^+$ T cell, which is initiated by interaction with an APC (such as a dendritic cell or B cell) expressing peptide associated with an MHC class II molecule. A complex and as yet incomplete picture has emerged. Ordered cascades of activation take place inside the cell, some events occurring within seconds, others within minutes, and yet others within hours of the initial interaction. These activatory pathways spread from the surface of the membrane, through the cytoplasm to the nucleus. The critical events in T-cell activation are described in the following paragraphs and in Figure 10.2.

The binding of peptide-MHC to the extracellular variable regions ($V_\alpha + V_\beta$) of

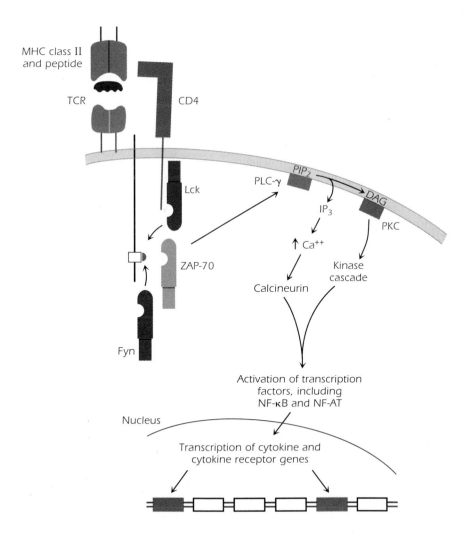

Figure 10.2. Intracellular events in T-cell activation. For simplicity, only one chain of CD3 and ζ (zeta) and one phosphorylated ITAM are shown.

the TCR transmits a signal via the tightly associated CD3 and ζ molecules into the interior of the T cell. The nature of the signal across the membrane is not currently clear. It may involve a conformational change in the transmembrane region of the TCR chains or a signal that induces the aggregation of multiple TCRs in the cell membrane. Such aggregation of the TCR upon activation would be similar to the initial steps in activation through the BCR that are described later in the chapter.

One of the earliest detectable events inside the T cell after binding to the TCR is the activation within seconds of *tyrosine kinases* — enzymes which activate proteins by adding phosphate groups to tyrosine residues — which are associated with the cytoplasmic regions of the TCR complex and CD4 molecules. The tyrosine kinases associated with CD3 + ζ and with CD4 are known as *Fyn* and *Lck*, respectively, and they belong to a family of tyrosine kinases known as Src (pronounced "sark"). It is believed that the membrane protein CD45 activates Fyn and Lck by removing inhibitory phosphate groups. As a result of the activation of Fyn and Lck, they cluster in proximity to the regions of the CD3 and ζ chains which contain the previously described *immunoreceptor tyrosine based activation motifs (ITAMs)*, and phosphorylate them. (Clustering also pulls CD4 in to closer association with the TCR complex.) These phosphorylated ITAMs then act as docking sites for another tyrosine kinase, *ZAP-70* (belonging to a second tyrosine kinase family known as Syk). In this way, *a multi-protein complex of signal transduction molecules is assembled in sequence and activated.*

Subsequent activation of complexed ZAP-70 by Lck and Fyn appears critical for T-cell activation; T cells from the rare individuals who lack ZAP-70 are unresponsive to antigen. Activation of ZAP-70 leads to the activation of phospholipase C-gamma (PLC-γ), a membrane enzyme that catalyzes the breakdown of membrane phospholipids. PLC-γ splits phosphatidylinositol bisphosphate (PIP$_2$) into diacylglycerol (DAG) and inositol triphosphate (IP$_3$) leading to the activation of two major signaling pathways. DAG activates protein kinase C, which in turn activates a cascade of kinases, ultimately leading to the activation of a transcription factor, NF-κB. IP$_3$ increases intracellular free calcium levels, which activates the cytoplasmic molecule calcineurin, and leads to the activation of the transcription factor NF-AT. Activated NF-κB, NF-AT and other transcription factors enter the nucleus, selectively binding to the chromosomes. This results in the transcription of genes involved in the subsequent stages of T-cell activation, such as those coding for cytokines and for cytokine receptors.

At later times, genes for cytokine receptors are transcribed into mRNA and translated into protein. In particular, T-cell activation results in the transcription of one chain of the IL-2 receptor, IL-2Rα (CD25). Within 24 hours, the cell enlarges and IL-2 protein is secreted from the cell. The IL-2 can then bind to its receptor on the same or on a different T cell. After about 48 hours, DNA is synthesized and after approximately 72 hours the cells undergo division. Thus, the end result of the activation pathways is T-cell proliferation and differentiation.

In addition to the events described, most activated T cells stop expressing the homing receptor, CD62L (L-Selectin), which allows naive T cells to enter the node (see Chapter 9). Consequently, activated T cells leave the node and move to sites of infection in the body where antigen is present. Trafficking of the activated T cell is also enhanced by induction of expression of the cell surface molecules, CD49d (VLA-4) and CD44, which bind to molecules on the surface of endothelial cells in an infected tissue. In this way, the activated T cell changes its pattern of circulation so that it can migrate to and be effective in an area away from the node in which it was activated (also see Chapter 9).

Functions of Costimulatory Pairs

At the beginning of this chapter we mentioned briefly the contribution of two pairs of costimulatory molecules to T-cell activation. The first is **CD40** on the APC with **CD154**. The interaction of MHC + peptide with the TCR upregulates the expression of CD154 on the CD4$^+$T cell, which interacts with CD40 expressed on the surface of the APC (dendritic cell, B cell, or macrophages). This interaction is critical in T-cell activation: inhibition of the binding of CD40 to CD154 severely impairs T-cell responses to many protein antigens. In addition, recent evidence indicates that a pair of costimulatory molecules known as RANK and TRANCE (expressed on the dendritic cell and T cell surfaces, respectively), related to but distinct from CD40 and CD154, are involved in the response to viral proteins.

As a consequence of this initial interaction, interaction is induced between another set of molecules: B7 on the APC and CD28 on the T cell, which is the best-characterized costimulatory pair. CD28 is a transmembrane molecule, and a member of the Ig supergene family, expressed on a large percentage of human peripheral T cells (and some activated B cells). B7 is now known to comprise at least two molecules, **B7.1 and B7.2 (CD80 and CD86**, respectively), which are expressed on APC such as activated B cells, dendritic cells, and activated macrophages. It is currently not clear if CD80 and CD86 have different functions.

The interaction of the CD28–B7 costimulatory pair induces the phosphorylation and activation of T-cell proteins including CD28 itself. The recruitment and activation of a kinase, phosphatidylinositol-3 kinase, is important in this pathway. One of the major consequences of activation of CD28 is that the lifetime of specific mRNAs, in particular IL-2 mRNA, is increased. As a result, the activated T cell can synthesize IL-2. Thus, *the costimulatory B7–CD28 interaction enhances and sustains the T-cell activation signals transmitted by the peptide–MHC–TCR interaction*. The importance of the B7–CD28 interaction is underscored by studies which show that the CD4$^+$ T cell may be tolerized or turned off rather than activated in the absence of the B7–CD28 interaction (see Chapter 11 for further details.)

A T-cell surface molecule very closely related to CD28, known as **CTLA-4 (CD152)**, is induced later in the sequence of T-cell activation events. CTLA-4 interacts with the same B7 ligands on the APC as CD28, namely, B7.1 and B7.2. The B7–CTLA-4 interaction, however, transmits a negative signal to the activated T cell, which is thought to occur by inhibiting the signal transduction function of the TCR complex. This turns off the production of IL-2, limits the extent of the immune response, and leads to differentiation of T cells into memory cells.

● SUBSETS OF CD4$^+$ CELLS DEFINED BY CYTOKINE PRODUCTION

The synthesis of antigen-nonspecific soluble factors known as *cytokines* is a key effector function of the activated CD4$^+$ cell (bottom of Figure 10.1). The cytokines produced by CD4$^+$ T cells affect the function of multiple cell types, including CD4$^+$ and CD8$^+$ T cells, B cells, myeloid cells, such as macrophages and eosinophils, and the differentiation of bone marrow precursors. For this reason, the loss of the CD4$^+$

T cell in AIDS is devastating. The properties of cytokines produced by T cells and other cells, and the nature of their receptors, is discussed in detail in Chapter 12.

In the preceding sections we have described how the naive CD4+ T cell initially synthesizes IL-2 following stimulation by peptide + MHC molecules. This cell can differentiate further to synthesize a large number of cytokines. It is now apparent that not every activated CD4+ T cell synthesizes the same array of cytokines following antigenic stimulation. Studies of mouse and, more recently, of human T cells indicate that antigen-primed CD4+ T cells can be divided into at least three subsets based on the different cytokines they produce; these subsets are known as T_H0, T_H1, *and T_H2*. As shown in Figure 10.3, T_H1 and T_H2 are generated from the antigen-driven differentiation of T_H0 cells, which synthesize IL-2, interferon γ-(IFN-γ), and IL-4.

T_H1 cells, which synthesize IL-2, IFN-γ, and tumor necrosis factor beta (TNF-β), and T_H2 cells, which synthesize IL-4, IL-5, IL-10, and IL-13, play important but distinct roles in the immune response. Since different cytokines interact with different target cells, a major consequence of the production of unique sets of cytokines by T_H1 and T_H2 cells is that *each subset has different effector functions*. Thus, the cytokines synthesized by T_H1 cells activate cells involved in cell-mediated immunity: CD8+ T cells, NK cells, and macrophages. By contrast, the cytokines synthesized by T_H2 cells trigger B cells to class-switch to IgE production, and activate eosinophils. To date, the results of studies attempting to characterize cell surface molecules whose expression would distinguish T_H1 from T_H2 subsets have been controversial, and are an area of intense research interest. Some recent studies have suggested that T_H1 and T_H2 cells may express different molecules expressed in homing interactions,

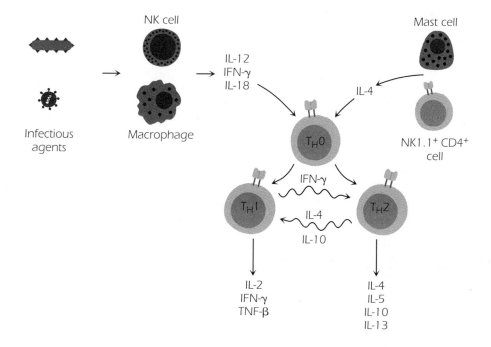

Figure 10.3. Cytokine control of T_H1 and T_H2 CD4+ T cell subset generation.

including different chemokine receptors (discussed in Chapters 9 and 12), but further research is needed either to confirm or modify these conclusions.

Many antigens give rise to all three subsets of CD4$^+$ T cells, but some antigens produce more of one subset than the others. In particular, *viruses and bacteria favor the production of T_H1 cells, whereas allergens and parasites favor T_H2 cell induction.* One of the major factors driving the differentiation to either T_H1 or T_H2 cells by different antigens is the presence of cytokines at the time of T cell stimulation (Figure 10.3). (Other factors, such as the concentration and route of exposure to antigen, the affinity of interaction between peptide + MHC and the TCR, and the nature of the APC in the response, have also been suggested to play a role in determining which subset of CD4$^+$ T cell develops.) T_H1 cells develop when IL-12, IFN-γ, and the recently described IL-18 are present during antigen stimulation of T cells. These cytokines are synthesized by cells of the innate immune system (particularly natural killer [NK] cells and macrophages) early in the response to pathogens such as viruses or bacteria. By contrast, the presence of IL-4 early in the response results in differentiation to T_H2 cells. This IL-4 is thought to be produced by either mast cells or the NK1.1 CD4$^+$ T cell (so named because it expresses a surface molecule found on NK cells).

Figure 10.3 also illustrates that cytokines produced by T_H1 can inhibit the function of T_H2 and vice versa. For example, IFN-γ produced by T_H1 cells inhibits the generation of T_H2 cells, and IL-4 and IL-10 produced by T_H2 cells inhibit the generation of T_H1 cells. Table 10.1 illustrates two other important points about the T_H1 and T_H2 subsets of CD4$^+$ T cells. First, the subsets synthesize a number of cytokines in common, including IL-3 and granulocyte-macrophage colony stimulating factor (GM-CSF). Second, mouse T_H1 and T_H2 CD4$^+$ T subsets show more clearcut differences in cytokine production than human subsets.

The functional differences between the CD4$^+$ T cell subsets may have some clinical significance in humans. In particular, a preponderance of T_H1 cells and T_H1-produced cytokines has been found in the response to many viruses and bacteria,

● TABLE 10.1. The Synthesis of Cytokines by the T_H1 and T_H2 Subsets of CD4$^+$

Cytokine	T_H1	T_H2
IL-2	+	−
IFN-γ	+	−
TNF-β (lymphotoxin)	+	−
IL-4	−	+
IL-5	−	+
IL-6	− (+)	+ (++)
IL-10	− (+)	+ (++)
IL-13	− (+)	+ (++)
IL-3	+	+
GM-CSF	+	+

The pluses in parentheses indicate that in humans IL-6, IL-10, and IL-13 are also made by T_H1 cells, but at lower levels than by T_H2 cells.

delayed-type hypersensitivity (described in Chapter 16), and in diseases such as the tuberculoid form of leprosy. By contrast, the presence of T_H2 cells and increases in levels of cytokines synthesized by T_H2 cells have been linked to allergic and parasitic responses (see Chapter 14). These observations suggest that regulating the balance of T_H1 and T_H2 subsets may be a way to treat different diseases.

 ## CD4⁺ T Memory Cells

Following antigen stimulation, CD4⁺ T cell numbers increase substantially. During the course of response to antigen, most of the activated cells die off by apoptotic mechanisms described in the next chapter. The surviving cells form the long-lived antigen-specific *CD4⁺ memory cells*. The clonal size of this memory population is still larger than the size of the unprimed population, which contributes to the greater effectiveness of a secondary or memory T-cell response than a primary response. The memory cell also expresses some molecules that are different from those expressed on unprimed cells; for example, an increase in CD44 and decrease in CD62L as described in Chapter 9. Changes in the membrane phosphatase CD45 have also been described; activation is thought to change CD45 from a form known as CD45RA to CD45RO. It is also thought that the memory cell does not need B7– CD28 costimulatory interactions to induce full T-cell activation. It is not clear whether the persistence of memory cells requires the presence of antigen, even at some very low level; some studies indicate that in the absence of the priming antigen, memory cells die.

 ## FUNCTION OF CD8⁺ T CELLS

In the sections above we have described the function of one of the major sets of T cells, CD4⁺ T cells, which produce a plethora of cytokines and thus interact with a vast array of cells. We now turn our attention to the other major population of T cells, CD8⁺ T cells. The major function of CD8⁺ T cells is to kill cells that have been infected by pathogens, such as bacteria and viruses. CD8⁺ T cells are also involved in killing transplanted foreign cells during graft rejection, and tumor cells (see Chapters 19 and 20). For this reason, CD8⁺ T cells are frequently referred to as *T killer* or *cytotoxic T lymphocytes* (CTL). The cell killed by a CTL is known as a *target*, which can be a specialized antigen presenting cell such as a dendritic cell, or any other cell in the body. In contrast to the TCR of CD4⁺ T cells, the TCR of a CD8⁺ T cell recognizes a combination of peptide in association with an MHC class I molecule on the surface of a cell. Recognition of a peptide–MHC class I complex by the TCR of a CD8⁺ T cell results in the death of the cell presenting the foreign peptide.

CD8⁺ T cells also synthesize cytokines: many produce cytokines associated with the T_H1 CD4⁺ phenotype. These include IFN-γ, which regulates certain viral and bacterial infections, as well as TNF-β, which plays a role in target cell killing. Other CD8⁺ T cells, however, synthesize cytokines such as IL-4, which are associated with the T_H2 CD4⁺ T-cell pattern.

CTLs must be activated before they kill their targets. One major pathway of activation involved in the response to many viruses is *via the activation of virus-*

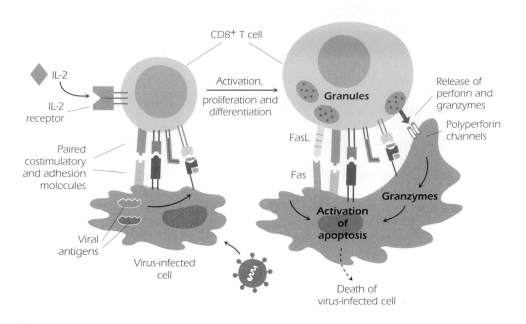

Figure 10.4. Activation and target cell killing by a CD8$^+$ CTL.

specific CD4$^+$ T cells. These CD4$^+$ T cells are activated by viral antigens presented by the MHC class II molecules of an APC such as a macrophage. As shown on the left side of Figure 10.4, the combination of virus-infected cell and IL-2 produced by activation of the CD4$^+$ T cells induces CD8$^+$ T cell proliferation and differentiation. In this pathway, the viral epitope which activates CD4$^+$ T cells may be distinct from the viral epitope which interacts with CD8$^+$ T cells.

Other CD8$^+$ T-cell activation mechanisms have been described that do not require activated CD4$^+$ T cells or IL-2. For example, some viruses do not appear to need CD4$^+$ T cells for the induction of CD8$^+$ T cells. These alternative pathways of CTL activation likely involve the presentation of virus antigens to CD8$^+$ T cells by potent antigen presenting cells such as dendritic cells, which express high levels of costimulatory and MHC class I (as well as MHC class II) molecules.

Whatever the cellular interactions involved in activating the CD8$^+$ cell, it is likely that similar early intracellular activation events are involved as were described above in the activation of CD4$^+$T cells. Like CD4, CD8 is associated with the tyrosine kinase Lck, and the same pairs of costimulatory and adhesion molecules described in the activation of CD4$^+$ T cells — CD28-B7, LFA-1–ICAM-1 and CD2–CD58 — are also involved. Once activated, the CD8$^+$ T cell can kill infected target cells expressing viral peptides associated with MHC class I molecules.

KILLING OF TARGET CELLS BY CYTOTOXIC T CELLS

As shown in Figure 10.4, the activated CTL initiates killing by attaching to the target cell via its TCR. Contact between the CTL and target is enhanced by interactions between the paired adhesion molecules described earlier in this chapter.

Killing by cytotoxic T cells appears to occur by two pathways, shown on the right of Figure 10.4. The first involves the action of cytotoxic substances contained in granules inside the T cell which produce lesions in the membranes of target cells. After attaching to the target cell, the killer cell mobilizes its granules directionally toward the target and, by a process known as exocytosis, releases the contents of these granules onto the target cell. The major constituents of the granules involved in target-cell killing are *perforin* and *granzymes*. Perforin is a molecule that polymerizes to form ringlike transmembrane channels or pores in the target-cell membrane. The resulting increase in permeability of the cell membrane contributes to the eventual death of the cell. The action of perforin on cell membranes is similar to that of the complement membrane attack complex, described in Chapter 13. CTL killing via this pathway also involves granzymes, a set of serine proteases. Granzymes pass into the target cell through the pores created by polyporphyrin molecules and interact with intracellular components of the target cell to induce apoptosis. Since death by apoptosis does not result in the release of the cell's contents, killing infected cells by apoptotic mechanisms may prevent the spread of infectious virus into other cells.

A second pathway of target cell killing occurs via the interaction of the molecule *Fas ligand* on the activated CTL with *Fas* on the target cell. This interaction activates the apoptosis of the target cell via a sequential activation of proteolytic enzymes known as *caspases* inside the target cell. As a result, the cell dies within hours. Recent studies indicate that the Fas−FasL pathway is not as important as the perforin−granzyme pathway for CD8$^+$T cell killing of targets.

Once the CTL has initiated the killing mechanisms, it detaches from the target cell to attack and kill additional target cells. When the target cells expressing the foreign antigen have been eliminated, the overwhelming majority of the activated CTL die by the process known as *activation-induced cell death*, which is described in the subsequent chapter. A small minority of the activated CD8$^+$ T cells survive to constitute the memory CD8$^+$ T-cell population.

As the foregoing paragraphs illustrate, activation of CTL and killing of the target cell are separable events. This can be demonstrated by preparing CTL from an individual who has been infected with a virus. These virus-specific cytotoxic cells (shown on the top right-hand side of Figure 10.4) are able to kill virus-infected targets outside the body. In vitro killing of the infected target does not require the addition of any further factors. The assay for CTL killing of targets is described in Chapter 5.

It is worth repeating that the killing of a target cell by a virus-specific CD8$^+$ CTL occurs via the recognition of a specific combination of viral peptide associated with a particular MHC class I molecule. This means that a CD8$^+$ CTL specific for a flu virus peptide and isolated from an individual expressing HLA-A2 will kill a target cell that expresses HLA-A2 that has bound the flu-derived peptide. However, uninfected or normal cells from the same individual expressing HLA-A2 in the absence of the flu peptide are not killed. Furthermore, this virus-specific CD8$^+$ T cell will not kill targets expressing different combinations of peptides plus MHC molecules, such as a measles virus-derived peptide bound to HLA-A2 or even the same flu peptide bound to HLA-B3. These findings, by Rolf Zinkernagel and Peter Doherty (both awarded the 1996 Nobel Prize), established the concept of *MHC restriction of T-cell responses*, indicating that T cells recognize the combination of antigen plus MHC molecule rather than antigen alone.

It is also worth noting that the recognition of peptide–MHC class I by a CD8$^+$ T cell occurs irrespective of the expression of any MHC class II molecule by the target cell. The ability of CD8$^+$ T cells to kill cells expressing peptides derived from nonself antigens in association with MHC class I is of enormous biological importance. In Chapter 8 we described how MHC class I molecules are expressed on almost every cell in the body, and the relevance of this ubiquitous MHC class I expression is now apparent: since an infectious pathogen (such as a virus, parasite or bacterium) may infect any nucleated cell in the body, the pathogen will generate foreign peptides in its cytoplasmic or endoplasmic reticulum compartment able to associate with MHC class I molecules. Expression of these foreign peptide–MHC class I complexes at the cell surface leads to recognition by CD8$^+$ T cells, followed by the killing of the infected cell. Thus, killing by CD8$^+$ T cells provides a mechanism to eliminate any cell in the body that becomes infected with a pathogen. Clearly, elimination of the pathogen does result in the destruction of host cells, but this is the bearable price the individual pays to remove the source of infection.

It is also worth repeating that only pathogens such as viruses, parasites, and some bacteria that infect cells and generate peptides that reach the cell's cytoplasmic or ER compartments and associate with MHC class I molecules evoke CD8$^+$ T cell responses. These pathogens generally activate antigen-specific CD4$^+$ T cells and antibody synthesis as well as CD8$^+$ T cells, all of which may be involved in the host's protective immune response against the pathogen (discussed further in Chapter 21). In contrast, harmless or noninfectious antigens (such as a killed virus protein in a vaccine) do not generally trigger CD8$^+$ T cell responses, but can trigger CD4$^+$ T cell and antibody responses because they are brought into an APC's acidic compartments and interact with MHC class II molecules.

CD8$^+$ T cells almost invariably function as cytotoxic T cells in both the human and mouse. A considerable proportion of human CD4$^+$ T cells and some mouse CD4$^+$ T cells, however, also display cytotoxic function. As might be expected from our foregoing discussion of MHC restriction, these cytotoxic CD4$^+$ T cells are activated to kill by the recognition of peptide–MHC class II complexes on the APC or target cell. The mechanisms used by CD4$^+$ and CD8$^+$ to kill targets appear to be very similar; the evidence suggests that for mouse CD4$^+$ T cells with cytotoxic function the Fas–FasL pathway may be more important than the perforin–granzyme pathway for target cell killing.

 ## T-CELL RECOGNITION OF LIPIDS

In the last ten years, it has become apparent that T cells can recognize lipids and glycolipids in addition to protein-derived antigens. The T-cell response to the lipid and glycolipid cell wall products derived from mycobacteria has been well documented. The genes and products of a family known as *CD1* play a role in the presentation of these lipids and glycolipids in a number of species. CD1 molecules are distantly related to MHC class I and II molecules, and it is believed that they constitute a third family of antigen-presenting molecules that have evolved to present lipid and glycolipid antigens derived from microbial pathogens to T cells.

CD1 molecules are cell surface glycoproteins which are non-MHC and non-polymorphic; that is, not varying from cell to cell. They are expressed in association with β2-microglobulin on APC such as dendritic cells and B cells. Binding of lipid antigens to CD1 is believed to take place in acidic cellular compartments, similar to the loading of exogenous peptides to MHC class II molecules. The structure of a recently crystallized CD1 molecule shows overall similarities to an MHC class I molecule but containing a larger binding groove with a deep cavity (see Figure 10.5A). The cavity probably binds the hydrophobic backbone of a lipid antigen, with the polar region of the lipid or glycolipid exposed in the groove for binding to the T-cell receptor.

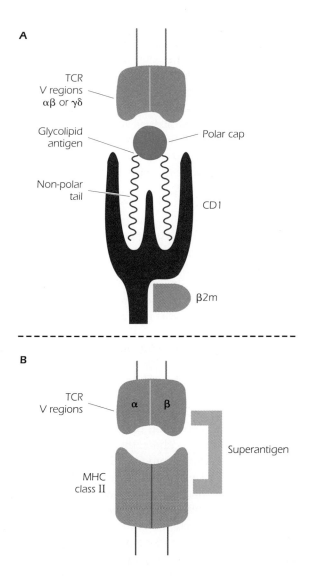

Figure 10.5. Recognition of different antigens by TCR. **(A)** Glycolipid presentation by CD1; **(B)** Superantigen binding to V$_\beta$.

Different members of the CD1 family have been shown to present antigens to $\gamma\delta^+$ T cells, to $\alpha\beta^+$ CD8$^+$ T cells, and to a subset of $\alpha\beta^+$ T cells known as NK1.1 CD4 T cells (cells which express both natural killer and T-cell surface molecules.) Activation of NK1.1 CD4 T cells by CD1$^+$ cells in response to antigens derived from infectious agents results in the synthesis of high levels of IL-4. Consequently, it has been suggested that NK1.1 CD4 T cells may be one of the sources of IL-4 which drives the differentiation of the T_H2 subset of CD4$^+$ T cells.

 ## OTHER WAYS TO ACTIVATE UNPRIMED T CELLS

In the preceding sections, we focused on how peptide–MHC complexes on APC activate T cells by means of the latter's antigen-specific receptor, the TCR. Since T cells expressing any one particular peptide specificity are rare, approximately 1 in 10^4 T cells, only a small fraction of the total T-cell pool is activated by any one peptide–MHC complex. Detecting the response to antigen of those rare antigen-specific cells in the total T cell population has thus proved difficult. Naive or un-primed T cells can be activated in a number of different ways, however, allowing us to measure the function of more than just a rare subpopulation of antigen-specific T cells. In general, the consequences of activation via these alternative pathways result in similar consequences, most notably cytokine production and cell prolifer-ation. A few of these alternative ways of activating the population of unprimed T cells are described below.

Superantigens

Superantigens (SAg) are a class of antigen that activate T cells expressing a specific V_β segment, such as $V_\beta3$ or $V_\beta11$, as a component of their TCR, irrespective of the V_α molecule used by the TCR. Since individual V_β segments may be expressed in up to 10% of the T-cell population, a high percentage of T cells of various antigenic specificities may become activated by the interaction of superantigens with the T-cell population.

There are several unique aspects of SAg interactions with T cells (see Figure 10.5B). SAg bind more or less exclusively to the V_β region of the TCR and not to the V_α region. SAg are presented by class II MHC molecules of APC, but are not bound in the peptide groove. They are not believed to be processed by APC. The intracellular pathways following SAg activation may also be different from those following peptide–MHC complex activation of the TCR.

More importantly, there are several clinically relevant features of SAg. The first is that several disease-causing organisms produce SAg. These include staphylococci, some of which are responsible for food poisoning and toxic shock, and viruses such as rabies. In the case of *Staphylococcus aureus*, the bacterial toxin acts as a super-antigen, and activates a large percentage of T cells. It is believed that the massive release of cytokines following SAg action results in injury to the host.

Plant Proteins and Antibodies to T-Cell Surface Molecules

Several naturally occurring materials have the ability to trigger the proliferation and differentiation of many if not all clones of T lymphocytes. These substances are referred to as ***polyclonal activators or mitogens*** because of their ability to induce mitosis of the cell population. The plant glycoproteins ***concanavalin A*** (Con A) and ***phytohemagglutinin*** (PHA) are particularly potent mitogens for T cells. These molecules are lectins, molecules that bind to carbohydrate moieties on proteins. Both Con A and PHA are thought to act through the TCR. Another plant lectin, ***pokeweed mitogen***, activates both T and B cells. As we shall also describe later in the chapter, certain substances such as bacterially derived lipopolysaccharide are specifically mitogenic for mouse B cells. Some antibodies specific for CD3 have the ability to activate T cells. Since CD3 is expressed on all T cells in association with the T-cell receptor, these anti-CD3 antibodies thereby induce all T cells to proliferate.

 ## B-CELL ACTIVATION AND FUNCTION

T–B Cooperation

Antigens that have multiple repeating epitopes have the ability to crosslink the BCR and directly activate the B cell. Most protein antigens, however, do not contain multiple repeating units. They contain small discrete single epitopes that cannot crosslink the BCR by itself. For this reason, B-cell responses to nearly all protein antigens require additional signals provided by CD4$^+$ T cells. The major class of antigens that requires CD4$^+$T cells is referred to as ***thymus-dependent (TD) antigens***, and the set of CD4$^+$ T cells that participates in TD-antigen responses is referred to as ***helper T cells (T$_H$)***.

The production of antibody in response to a TD antigen requires that both B and T cells be activated and interact. In addition, for T–B cooperation to occur, the B and T cells must respond to epitopes that are physically linked in the same antigen. The B and T cells may respond to different epitopes on that antigen, but these epitopes must be physically linked in order to produce antibody. Thus, the phenomenon of T–B cell cooperativity is also known as ***linked recognition***.

As a consequence of antigen binding and the effects of T cell-secreted cytokines, the B cell is activated to proliferate and to differentiate to an antibody-producing cell. The nature of the cytokine secreted by the T cell determines to which immunoglobulin isotype the B cell switches. The importance of T-cell involvement in B-cell antibody production can be gauged from findings with antigens that do not use T-cell help, so-called T-independent (TI) antigens, discussed later in the chapter. These TI antigens do not induce memory B cells, and B cells do not undergo Ig class switching from IgM to other Ig isotypes.

As we described earlier in the chapter, in the primary response T cells are most effectively activated by antigen processed and presented by dendritic cells. Activated T cells are then likely to interact with and activate B cells, using the mechanisms described below. In secondary responses, both the relevant B and T cells have been previously activated and expanded by antigen, and in contrast to primary responses, very efficient T–B cooperation is thought to be achieved between B and T cells only, with no requirement for a dendritic cell. This is depicted in Figure 10.6. In this response, the B cell captures antigen by binding it to its specific immunoglobulin receptor. Following antigen binding at the B-cell surface, the complex of antigen and immunoglobulin is taken into the cell (internalized) and degraded in acid compartments, which also contain MHC class II molecules. As described in Chapter 8, some

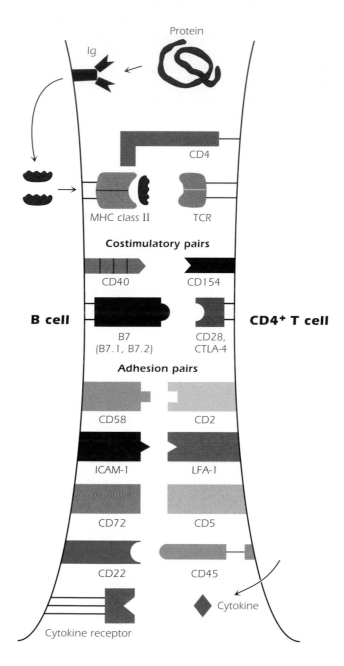

🔵 Figure 10.6. Key cell surface interactions involved in T–B cooperation.

of the peptides formed by the degradation of antigen selectively bind to MHC class II molecules. Peptide–MHC class II complexes traffic through the cell to the B-cell surface, where the complexes can interact with a CD4$^+$ T cell with the appropriate TCR.

As described earlier in the chapter, interaction between peptide + MHC on the B cell and the TCR of the CD4$^+$ T cell is accompanied by paired interactions at the surface of the B and T cells, which result in mutual activation: T cells are activated to synthesize cytokines and B cells to synthesize antibody. The most important of these paired interactions are shown in Figure 10.6. Adhesion pairs, such as **LFA-1–ICAM-1, CD5–CD72, and CD45–CD22** strengthen the T–B interaction and enhance activation. A key interaction is between **CD40** on the B cell and its ligand **CD154** on the activated T cell. As described earlier in the chapter, this interaction promotes the upregulation of the costimulatory **B7** molecules on the B cell. Induction of B7 expression enhances the ability of a B cell to act as an effective antigen-presenting cell to a T cell via its interaction with **CD28** on the activated T cell.

The interaction of CD40 and CD154 promotes proliferation and is also required for the B cell to switch the class of antibody that it can synthesize. In the absence of this CD40-CD154 interaction, only IgM is made. This is demonstrated in humans with nonfunctional CD154, a clinical condition known as hyper-IgM syndrome (see Chapter 18), and in so-called CD154 knockout mice. IgM antibody, but no other isotype, is made at normal levels in these two situations.

In addition to the CD40–CD154 interaction, class switching by the B cell in the secondary response also requires T cell-derived cytokines. The nature of the cytokine produced by the primed T cell determines which class of antibody is produced by the B cell. Thus, if the T cell makes IL-4, B cells will switch to producing predominantly IgE, whereas if the T cell produces IFN-γ, B cells will switch to producing IgG subtypes.

The Carrier Effect

One further point should be made about B- and T-cell epitope recognition in primary and secondary responses. To achieve linked recognition, it is important that the B-cell epitope and the T-cell epitope be the same in both primary and secondary responses. If primary immunization is given with a B-cell epitope linked to one T-cell epitope, but the secondary immunization is given with the same B-cell epitope linked to a different T-cell epitope, no secondary response is generated. This is because the second immunization does not prime a sufficient number of T cells specific for the new T-cell epitope to allow effective cooperation with B cells specific for the B-cell epitope. This phenomenon was originally observed in the secondary response to **haptens**, a set of small molecules, which, by themselves, cannot induce immune responses (described in Chapter 3). Secondary antibody responses to a hapten could be generated only if the hapten were linked to the same large protein or carrier in both primary and secondary immunizations. For this reason, the phenomenon is known as **the carrier effect**. The carrier effect has present application in the immunization of individuals with peptide vaccines. In such vaccinations, it is crucial to use the peptide linked to the same carrier in both primary and secondary immunizations.

T-INDEPENDENT RESPONSES

B-Cell Activation in the Absence of T-Cell Help

Although most of the antigens involved in immune responses are proteins that require help by T cells to evoke a response (i.e., they are T-dependent antigens), some antigens are capable of activating B cells to produce antibody in the absence of T cells or cytokines produced by T cells. These antigens, referred to as ***thymus-independent (TI) antigens***, are ***generally large polymeric molecules*** with multiple, repeating, antigenic determinants; for example, the components of bacterial cell walls such as lipolysaccharides, and the capsule polysaccharide component of *Haemophilus influenzae*. It appears that the multivalent TI antigens activate the B cell through extensive crosslinking of its surface receptors (see below) (Figure 10.7).

A subset of TI antigens referred to as TI-1 are ***mitogenic*** at high concentrations; that is, they are able to activate multiple B-cell clones to proliferate and to produce antibody. Because of this antigen-nonspecific activation property, such antigens are

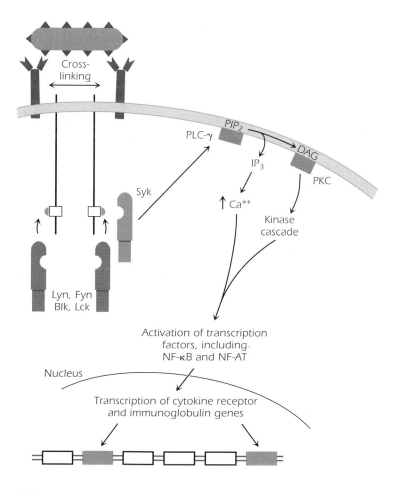

Figure 10.7. Intracellullar events in B-cell activation. For simplicity, only one chain of Igα and Igβ associated with each Ig molecule is shown.

called *polyclonal B-cell activators*. In mice, lipopolysaccharide derived from a number of gram negative bacteria such as *E. coli* are TI-1 antigens; in humans, however, such lipopolysaccharides do not activate human B cells to proliferate. A second subset of TI antigens known as TI-2, which includes bacterial and fungal polysaccharides, such as pneumococcal polysaccharide, dextrans, and ficoll, are not mitogenic at high concentrations.

There are two biologically relevant features of TI responses. First, unlike responses involving T-dependent antigens, responses to *TI antigens generate primarily IgM and they do not give rise to memory*. In other words, a second injection of a TI antigen leads to the same level of production of IgM as the first, with no increase in level, speed of onset, or class switch. This finding reinforces the importance of T cell-derived cytokines in the development of memory cells and B-cell isotype switch. Second, a protective immune response can still be made against TI antigens even if an individual lacks T cells. Thus, patients with T-cell immune deficiencies can still make protective IgM responses against extracellular bacteria, even if they cannot make significant responses to viruses that are T cell-dependent.

Intracellular Pathways in B-Cell Activation

Multivalent antigens with repeating epitopes, and some antibodies reactive with immunoglobulin chains, directly activate the B cell. Activation is initiated by *receptor crosslinking*; that is, by bringing together more than one BCR complex in the cell membrane (see Figure 10.7). Immunoglobulin heavy and light chains have very short intracellular domains and are not directly involved in signal transduction. Crosslinking induces an activation cascade inside the B-cell similar to the events that were described earlier in the chapter during the activation of CD4$^+$ T cells. One of the earliest events is the activation of the src-family tyrosine kinases Lyn, Blk, Lck, and Fyn which are associated with the BCR. (These kinases are believed to be activated by CD45.) Activation of these kinases results in the phosphorylation of tyrosine residues in ITAMs of the Igα and Igβ molecules associated with Ig chains in the membrane. Phosphorylation of these ITAMs recruits another kinase, Syk, to the cluster of molecules and Syk is phosphorylated and activated.

Activation of Syk leads to the activation of PLC-γ, which splits PIP$_2$ into DAG and IP$_3$, leading to the activation of two major signaling pathways. DAG activates protein kinase C, which in turn activates a cascade of kinases; IP$_3$ increases intracellular free calcium levels and leads to the activation of calcium-dependent enzymes. As a result of this sequence of early activation events, transcription factors such as NF-AT and NF-κB enter the nucleus of the B cell and promote the transcription of specific genes, the most important of which are immunoglobulin and cytokine receptor genes. Approximately 12 hours after antigenic stimulation, the B cell increases in size (becoming a B-cell blast) and if it receives the appropriate signals, generally from T-helper cells, the B-cell blast proliferates and differentiates into a cell that synthesizes and secretes immunoglobulin (a plasma cell).

The B-cell surface molecules CD19, CD21, and CD81 (TAPA-1), discussed in Chapter 8, are noncovalently associated with the BCR, and function as a coreceptor complex. These molecules enhance the signal transmitted through the BCR after antigen binding. CD21 binds to a product of the complement pathway (C3d) which attaches to antigens, but the ligands for the other molecules of the coreceptor complex are not known.

SUMMARY

1. Binding of MHC class II plus peptide to the TCR of the CD4$^+$ T cell, in conjunction with the interaction of costimulatory and adhesion pairs of molecules on the surface of the APC and the T cell, leads to T-cell activation. In primary CD4$^+$ T-cell responses, dendritic cells are the major APC.

2. T-cell activation involves a cascade of events inside the cell after initiation at the cell surface. The earliest activation events include the phosphorylation of intracellular proteins by tyrosine kinases, phospholipid breakdown, and increases in intracellular calcium. As a consequence of these early intracellular changes, changes occur in the nucleus of the T cell. This results in the transcription of specific genes in the nucleus. Among the important genes transcribed as a consequence of T-cell activation are genes coding for cytokines, such as IL-2, and cytokine receptors. Ultimately, the activation of these genes results in the proliferation and differentiation of the T cell.

3. As a consequence of activation by antigen, CD4$^+$ T cells secrete cytokines, soluble factors that affect T cells, B cells, and many other cell types. Subsets of CD4$^+$ T cells have been defined by the range of cytokines they produce. T$_H$1 cells secrete IL-2, IFN-γ, and TNF-β, but not IL-4, IL-5, IL-10, and IL-13. Cytokines produced by T$_H$1 cells activate other T cells, NK cells, and macrophages. By contrast, a second subset of CD4$^+$ T cells, T$_H$2 secretes IL-4, IL-5, IL-10 and IL-13, but not IL-2, IFN-γ, or TNF-β. The cytokines synthesized by T$_H$2 cells result in B cell class switch to IgE synthesis and in eosinophil activation.

4. CTL kill cells infected by microorganisms, such as bacteria or viruses. The two main pathways of CTL killing of targets involve: a) secretion of perforin + granzymes, and b) cell surface Fas–FasLigand interaction. In mice, CTL are almost exclusively CD8$^+$, but in humans CD4$^+$T cells are also cytotoxic. The TCR of a CD8$^+$ T cell interacts with peptide derived from the pathogen bound to an MHC class I molecule on the surface of an infected cell, and the TCR of a cytotoxic CD4$^+$ T cell interacts with peptide + MHC class II.

5. Some T cells recognize lipids and glycolipids. These antigens are presented by CD1 rather than MHC molecules to the TCR.

6. Certain substances stimulate multiple clones of T and B cells to proliferate. These substances are referred to as mitogens. Superantigens activate all T cells that use a specific V$_\beta$ segment to form its TCR. Plant lectins such as Concanavalin A and phytohemagglutinin activate all T cells by binding to cell-surface glycoproteins. Similarly, lipopolysaccharide from bacterial cell walls activates all mouse B cells. Some antibodies specific for molecules on the T- and B-cell surface are also mitogenic.

7. The generation of antibody in the response to T-dependent antigens (the vast majority of responses to proteins) requires antigen, CD4$^+$ T cells, and B cells. This T–B cell cooperation involves (a) interaction between pairs of molecules on the surface of the CD4$^+$ T cell and the B cell, resulting in mutual activation and (b) cytokine secretion by T cells. A further requirement for antibody to be generated by T–B cooperation is linked recognition: the antigenic epitope that

the T cell responds to and the epitope that the B cell responds to must both be on the same molecule. T and B cells may, however, respond to different epitopes on the same antigen.

8. Class or isotype switching to IgG, IgA, or IgE requires the interaction of CD40 on the B cell with its ligand CD40L on the T cell. The cytokine produced by the T cell determines the isotype of antibody synthesized by the switched B cell.

9. Some antigens, such as polysaccharides that have many repeating, identical epitopes on each molecule, are capable of triggering B cells without significant help from T cells. These so-called T-independent responses involve predominantly the production of IgM and do not include the development of immunologic memory.

REFERENCES

Chu DH, Morita CT, Weiss A (1998): The Syk family of protein tyrosine kinases in T-cell activation and development. *Immunol Rev* 165:167–180.

Clark EA, Ledbetter JA (1994): How B and T cells talk to each other. *Nature* 367:425.

Coffman RL, von der Weid T (1997): Multiple pathways for the initiation of T_H2 responses. *J Exp Med* 185:373–375.

Dustin ML, Shaw AS (1999): Costimulation: building an immunologic synapse. *Science* 283: 649–650.

Grewal I, Flavell RA (1998): CD40 and CD154 in cell-mediated immunity. *Annu Rev Imunol* 111–135.

Isakov N (1998): Role of immunoreceptor tyrosine-based activation motif in signal transduction from antigen and Fc receptors. *Adv Immunol* 69:183–247.

Paul WE, Seder RA (1994): Lymphocyte responses and cytokines. *Cell* 76:241.

Powell JD, Ragheb JA, Kitagawa-Sakakida S, Schwartz RH (1998): Molecular regulation of interleukin-2 expression by CD28 co-stimulation and anergy. *Immunol Rev* 165:287–300.

Reth M, Wienands J (1997): Initiation and processing of signals from the B cell antigen receptor. *Annu Rev Immunol* 15:453–479.

Viola A, Schroeder S, Sakakibara Y, Lanzavecchia A (1999): T lymphocyte costimulation mediated by reorganization of membrane microdomains. *Science* 283:680–682.

Zeng Z-H, Castano AR, Sengelke BW, Stura EA, Peterson PA, Wilson IA (1997): Crystal structure of mouse CD1: an MHC-like fold with a large hydrophobic binding groove. *Science* 277:339–345.

 ## REVIEW QUESTIONS

For each question, choose the ONE BEST answer or completion.

1. The role of the antigen-presenting cell in the immune response is all of the following *except*

   A) the limited catabolism of polypeptide antigens.

   B) to allow selective association of MHC gene products and peptides.

C) to supply second signals required to fully activate T cells.

D) to present non-self peptides associated with MHC class II molecules to B cells.

E) to present peptide-MHC complexes to T cells with the appropriate receptor.

2. Which of the following statements about interleukin 2 (IL-2) is *incorrect*?

A) It is produced primarily by activated macrophages.

B) It is produced by CD4$^+$ T cells.

C) It can induce the proliferation of CD4$^+$ T cells.

D) It binds to a specific receptor on CD4$^+$ T cells.

E) It can activate CD8$^+$ T cells in the presence of antigen.

3. CD40 Ligand (CD154) is expressed by which of the following?

A) B cells

B) dendritic cells

C) resting T cells

D) activated T cells

E) all leukocytes

4. Which of the following statements about the activation of CD4$^+$ cells is *incorrect*?

A) Binding of peptide + MHC to the TCR results in rapid phosphorylation of tyrosine residues in proteins associated with the TCR.

B) Intracellular calcium levels rise rapidly following activation.

C) Only peptide bound in the groove of MHC class II activates the CD4$^+$ T cell.

D) Interaction of B7 and CD28 stabilizes IL-2 mRNA so effective IL-2 translation occurs.

E) The activated cell synthesizes IL-2 and a receptor for IL-2.

5. Which of the following statements about cytokines synthesized by CD4$^+$ T$_H$1 and T$_H$2 subsets is *incorrect*?

A) Cytokines produced by T$_H$1 cells include IFN-γ and TNF-β.

B) Cytokines produced by T$_H$2 cells are important in allergic responses.

C) T$_H$1 cells secrete cytokines that induce macrophage and NK cell activation.

D) T$_H$2 cells secrete cytokines that activate CD8$^+$ T cells.

E) T$_H$2 cell cytokines may inhibit the action of T$_H$1 cells.

6. Which of the following statements about CD8$^+$ CTL is *incorrect*?

A) They lyse targets by synthesizing perforin and granzymes.

B) They cause target cell apoptosis.

C) They cannot kill CD4$^+$ T cells.

D) They interact with their target through paired cell surface molecules.

E) They must be activated before exerting their cytotoxic function.

7. Infection with vaccinia virus results in the priming of virus-specific CD8$^+$ T cells. If these vaccinia virus-specific CD8$^+$ T cells are subsequently removed from the individual, which of the following cells will they kill in vitro?

A) vaccinia-infected cells expressing MHC class II molecules from any individual

B) influenza-infected cells expressing the same MHC class I molecules as the individual

C) uninfected cells expressing the same MHC class I molecules as the individual

D) vaccinia-infected cells expressing the same MHC class I molecules as the individual

E) vaccinia-infected cells expressing the same MHC class II molecules as the individual

8. Bacterial lipopolysaccharide (LPS), a T-independent antigen, stimulates antibody production in mice. Which of the following is *incorrect*?

A) The antibody produced will be predominantly IgM.

B) Memory B cells will not be induced.

C) IL-4 and IL-5 are required for the production of antibody during the response.

D) The polymeric nature of the antigen crosslinks B-cell surface receptors.

E) B cell activation involves phosphorylation of intracellular molecules.

Case Study

Great effort is now being directed at developing vaccines for a variety of diseases. In one study, it was found that antibody to a particular epitope on a protein of the pathogens surface membrane was protective. The structure of this epitope was determined to be a peptide 10 amino acids in length. This peptide was synthesized and used to immunize individuals exposed to the pathogen. Disappointingly, no protection was seen. Can you suggest any reasons for this failure?

Answers to Review Questions

1. *D* The antigen-presenting cell does not present peptide + MHC class II to B cells. The other statements are all features of the antigen-presenting cell.

2. *A* IL-2 is produced almost exclusively by activated T cells.

3. *D* CD40 ligand (CD154) is expressed on the surface of the CD4$^+$ T cell as a consequence of the activation that follows the binding of peptide + MHC class II to the TCR.

4. *C* Agents other than peptides bound to MHC class II can activate CD4$^+$ T cells; these include superantigens, antigens presented by CD1, and polyclonal activators.

5. *D* T$_H$1 rather than T$_H$2 cells secrete cytokines that activate CD8$^+$ T cells.

6. *C* A CD8$^+$ CTL can kill any cell expressing an MHC class I molecule in association with a non-self peptide, including, for example, a CD4$^+$ T cell infected with HIV.

7. *D* The principle of MHC restriction indicates that the TCR of CD8$^+$ T cells interacts with target cells that express specific peptide bound to self-MHC class I molecules. Thus, vaccinia-primed CD8$^+$ T cells recognize and hence kill only vaccinia-infected targets that express self MHC class I.

8. *C* T-independent antigens, because they do not generate T cell-derived cytokines, do not produce IL-4 or IL-5. Thus, no isotype switching or memory cell induction occurs in the response to T-independent antigens.

Answer to Case Study

Several possibilities may be considered, such as size and complexity of the peptide, which are required for immunogenicity. The more likely failure, however, was that the response to the pathogens membrane protein was almost certainly a thymus-dependent response. Therefore, immunization with the epitope seen by the B cells would not work unless epitopes seen by helper T cells were also present.

Attempts at producing synthetic vaccines are now directed toward incorporating the B cell-specific epitopes in carriers containing adequate helper T epitopes that will induce both help and memory responses. This would provide a better possibility for protection following exposure to the pathogen.

11

CONTROL MECHANISMS IN THE IMMUNE RESPONSE

 INTRODUCTION

An understanding of the immune response as a complete physiologic system requires some understanding of the "off" signals, in addition to an understanding of the "on" signals described in previous chapters. Only with such a complete understanding of the system is it possible to approach such questions as why the development of a response against antigens of our own tissues is exceptional rather than commonplace, and why the response to any particular antigen does not continue to increase in magnitude until it takes over the whole immune apparatus.

In this chapter we will discuss the multiple levels of control of the immune response, and indicate how breakdown of these control mechanisms may lead to autoimmunity and autoimmune disease, subjects that are discussed more fully in Chapter 17.

 TOLERANCE

One of the key mechanisms for controlling the lymphocyte response to antigen is by the induction of *tolerance* rather than activation. Tolerance is the *state of unresponsiveness to a particular antigenic epitope*. In general, it occurs when the interaction of antigen with an antigen-specific lymphocyte results in signals that inactivate, rather than activate the cell. As a consequence of this *tolerizing* interaction, the cell, or the individual exposed to the antigen, is said to be *tolerant*.

Only cells with antigen-specific receptors, that is, lymphocytes, can be tolerized. Tolerance can be achieved any time in the ontogeny of the cell, provided it expresses a receptor for the antigen. We refer to tolerance induced during the early stages of lymphocyte development as *central tolerance*, and to tolerance induced in mature lymphocytes as *peripheral tolerance*.

There are two major consequences of lymphocyte inactivation: *deletion*, in which exposure to antigen results in the elimination of cells by apoptosis, or, alternatively, *anergy*, in which exposure to antigen results in an unresponsive or inactivated state. These mechanisms are not mutually exclusive, as cells that are initially anergized by exposure to antigen may be deleted at a later time.

In the following sections we will discuss how both immature and mature lymphocytes can be made tolerant to antigen. We will also describe how tolerance is a dynamic state which can be modified by a number of factors.

Induction of Tolerance in Immature T and B Lymphocytes

Negative Selection and the Prevention of Autoimmunity. As we have already discussed in Chapters 6 and 9, the enormous numbers of T- and B-cell receptors for antigen are generated by the process of V(D)J rearrangement. Since the assortment of chains (H and L for Ig and α and β for the TCR) is more or less random, the process inevitably generates some receptors that can interact with self-molecules present in the individual. To prevent potential reactivity to self, both immature T and B cells undergo a process of *negative selection* throughout the life of an individual; cells with potential reactivity to self-molecules are *functionally inactivated in the primary lymphoid organs (central tolerance)*. For the developing T cell, this occurs in the thymus when an $\alpha\beta^+$ $CD4^+$ $CD8^+$ cell (see Chapter 9) binds with too-high affinity to MHC and peptide expressed on the interdigitating cells at the corticomedullary junction. The cell is deleted by apoptosis. As described in Chapter 8, negative selection of potentially self-reactive developing B cell occurs in the bone marrow when the immature B cell binds to antigens expressed on other cells in the bone marrow (resulting in deletion by apoptosis), or if it encounters soluble antigen (resulting in anergy).

Negative selection, however, does not remove every lymphocyte potentially able to react with self. If this were the case, autoimmune responses should never occur. Why do such autoimmune reactions happen at all? Some T lymphocytes with reactivity for self-components, especially those that express a TCR with an affinity for MHC plus antigen just below a critical threshold required for deletion in the thymus, may escape the negative selection process and migrate to the periphery. In addition, T cells specific for self-molecules absent from the thymus or present in low levels may avoid deletion or anergic induction in the thymus, and enter the peripheral T-cell pool. Nonetheless, these cells do not normally cause autoimmune responses. Many mechanisms have been proposed to explain this lack of reactivity, including:

1. Self-reactive cells are removed in the periphery by the process of activation induced cell death (AICD), involving Fas and Fas Ligand (FasL). This mechanism is described later in this chapter.

2. The tissue cells expressing the self-antigen to which the T cells may respond do not express costimulatory molecules (also described later in this chapter).

3. There is evidence that negative selection of self-reactive B cells may not be as stringent as negative selection of T cells, and thus the presence of B cells with potential reactivity to self-components can be found in the periphery. As

responses to self-antigens generally require both T-helper cells and B cells, however, the mere presence of autoreactive B cells does not necessarily mean that they will be activated to participate in harmful immunologic responses. In fact, stringent conditions are imposed on lymphocytes before they become activated to function. As was discussed in Chapter 10 and will be discussed later in this chapter, activation requires stimulation by costimulatory molecules and cytokine signals.

Tolerance Induction by Foreign Antigen in Immature Animals. If immature B and T cells are exposed to foreign antigens the result is generally tolerance induction (inactivation) rather than activation. One of the earliest experiments that demonstrated this phenomenon came from the observations of Ray Owen in 1945. He showed that dizygotic cattle twins, which shared a common vascular system in utero, were mutually tolerant of skin grafts from one another as adults. Thus, exposure of one twin's developing lymphoid system to the "foreign" antigens expressed by cells of the other twin had produced long-lasting tolerance.

These observations provided the basis for experiments by Peter Medawar and his colleagues in the 1950s, resulting in a Nobel Prize. These studies led to an understanding of the mechanisms underlying both transplantation rejection and the induction of ***neonatal tolerance***. As depicted in Figure 11.1, line 1, Medawar and his colleagues showed that adult mice of one strain, A, rejected skin grafts from mice of a strain B which differed in expression of MHC molecules, that is, from a ***histoincompatible*** strain. We now know that rejection occurred because MHC molecules expressed by cells in the donor-grafted skin activated T cells in the recipient; this is discussed further in Chapter 19. By contrast, the second line of Figure 11.1

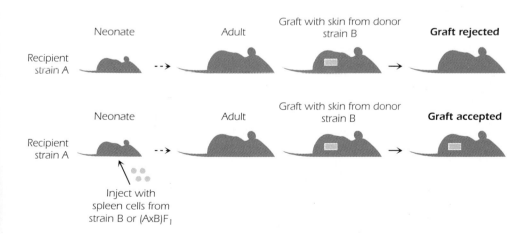

Figure 11.1. Rejection or acceptance of a skin graft from an MHC-distinct mouse. **Line 1:** Adult recipient of strain A mouse rejects skin graft from MHC-distinct strain B donor. **Line 2:** Adult strain A mouse which was injected within 24 hours after birth with spleen cells from strain B or from an (A × B)F$_1$ accepts a strain B skin graft. The neonatally-injected mouse is tolerant to B-strain MHC molecules.

indicates that strain A mice injected within 24 hours after birth with spleen cells from strain B did not reject skin grafts from the donor B strain when they grew to adulthood. In most of these and subsequent studies of neonatal tolerance, Medawar and colleagues injected the neonatal mice of strain A with cells derived from a cross of A with B, referred to as an (A × B) F$_1$ hybrid. Injecting spleen cells of strain B into the neonatal histoincompatible A mouse generally results in a severe, frequently fatal graft versus host disease [discussed in Chapter 19]. This part of the study indicated that the developing immune system (and we now know the T-cell component in particular) of the neonatal mouse was tolerized, rather than activated, by the foreign MHC antigens expressed on the strain B donor cells.

These studies also showed that tolerance to cells expressing the foreign MHC was long lasting. The mechanism by which tolerance is induced in the neonatal tolerance system is still not completely understood, but is likely to be through deletion of T cells specific for the histoincompatible MHC molecules. Persistence of cells of the donor type in very small numbers (*microchimerism*) appears to be crucial for the maintenance of the tolerant state.

Regulation of Cell Death in Immature and Mature Lymphocytes

The maintenance of lymphocyte homeostasis, that is, the mechanisms that regulate the production and the removal of cell populations, is a critical component of the immune response. As we describe below, humans and animals that have defects in regulating these pathways show faulty immune regulation.

The numbers of developing lymphocytes are carefully regulated in the primary lymphoid organs. For example, the thymus is the site of enormous cellular proliferation, particularly early in life. Many more cells are produced in the thymus, however, than actually leave it or can be accounted for in the circulation. In fact, it is estimated that as many as 90% of the developing T cells produced in the thymus die there. This can occur at several stages of thymic differentiation; the most prominent are (1) when a precursor fails to rearrange successfully the genes needed to code for either an $\alpha\beta$ or a $\gamma\delta$TCR, (2) when a precursor is not positively selected on the MHC molecules of thymic epithelial cells, and (3) as discussed earlier in this chapter and in Chapters 7 and 9, when a cell is eliminated at the negative selection stage because it expresses a receptor specific for a self-antigen. In all these cases death is believed to occur via apoptotic pathways.

The number of mature lymphocytes is also under tight regulation. Antigen stimulation increases the number of lymphocytes specific for the antigen, as well as the numbers of lymphocytes and other effector cells that are recruited during the course of the response. Once the antigen has been eliminated, however, it is critical to decrease the size of this pool of activated cells, otherwise the body would fill quickly with expanded populations of cells.

It is now clear that the end result of the response to most antigens is the survival of a minor population of long-lived antigen-specific cells that constitute the *memory T or B cells* for that antigen, and the *death by apoptosis* of the majority of the activated cells (for example, the death of mature B cells in the germinal center that do not produce high-affinity mutations [see Chapter 7]). The mechanism of T-cell death following activation (*activation-induced cell death* [AICD]) is the subject of intensive current research interest. These studies show that after the T cell has been activated, and particularly after repeated antigenic stimulation, it is susceptible to

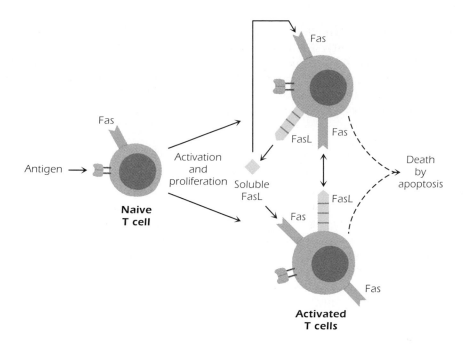

Figure 11.2. Activation-induced cell death. Following antigen stimulation, the T cell can kill itself by secreting a soluble form of FasL that interacts with Fas on the same cell **(top cell)**, or a different T cell via either soluble or membrane FasL interaction with Fas **(bottom cell)**.

apoptosis as a result of the Fas−FasL interaction described in Chapter 10: "Killing of Target Cells by Cytotoxic T Cells." This occurs as a consequence of the expression of both FasL *and* Fas by activated T cells (see Figure 11.2). Once the activated CTL cells have killed their targets, they interact with each other via Fas−FasL. As FasL can also be secreted by activated cells, the cells may be induced to commit suicide. The Fas−FasL interaction is believed to play a critical role in the elimination of the majority of activated CD4+ and CD8+ T cells following antigen stimulation.

INDUCTION OF TOLERANCE IN MATURE T AND B LYMPHOCYTES

Fas−FasL Interactions

In addition to its role in clonal downsizing, the Fas−FasL pathway described in the previous section is currently thought to play a crucial role in the removal of T and B cells with potential reactivity to self, which escape negative selection in the primary lymphoid organs and escape to the periphery. The importance of the Fas−FasL pathway was initially shown by studying mouse strains with autoimmune conditions, which accumulated enormous numbers of T cell subpopulations in the spleen and lymph nodes. The defects in these mice, strains known as *lpr* for lymphoproliferative, and *gld* for generalized lymphoproliferative disease, were shown to be mutations in Fas and FasL, respectively. These mutations prevented the mice from deleting autoreactive T cells and from reducing the size of their T-cell populations. Children with a mutated Fas have also been described; they have an autoimmune condition known as autoimmune lymphoproliferative syndrome (ALPS), with characteristics similar to those described for the mutant mice.

Mechanisms That Inhibit T- and B-Cell Activation

As we described in Chapter 10, antigen-specific activation of mature lymphocytes is a complex multistep process. The end result of this process is proliferation and differentiation. Much recent work has shown that interfering with one of the many steps in cellular activation can result in the cell being able to complete some but not all of its program. As a result, the cell may be rendered tolerant. A complete picture, however, of what intracellular changes determine whether a cell is activated or tolerized has not emerged; possible mechanisms include a change in the balance of positive and negative signals received in the nucleus, or in the production of qualitatively or quantitatively different signals at different steps in the activation cascade. The following sections describe some of the mechanisms thought to be involved in the induction of tolerance in T and B cells by preventing their activation.

Inhibition of T-Cell Activation. As we described in Chapter 10, stimulation of naive CD4$^+$ T cells to active proliferation and secretion of T-cell products such as IL-2 requires ***costimulatory*** interactions with the antigen-presenting cell (APC) in addition to MHC–TCR interactions. ***APC–T interactions in which the costimulatory or second signals are blocked or absent tolerize rather than activate the T cell***. It is rendered anergic, unable to make IL-2, and unresponsive to subsequent antigen challenge.

The results of blocking the interaction between the costimulatory pair B7 on the APC and CD28 on the T cell have been extensively studied. Delivery of the first signal (MHC + peptide) to the TCR leads to the induction of several transcription factors, one of which binds to the promoter region of the IL-2 gene allowing for its transcription in the T cell. As a result of the B7–CD28 interaction, the half-life of mRNA specific for IL-2 is increased, and IL-2 protein is synthesized. If the first signal is not followed by the costimulatory B7–CD28 signal, however, the IL-2 mRNA is rapidly degraded, and IL-2 protein is not made. Thus, the activation process is aborted and the T cell is anergized. The anergized T cell may still be able to produce certain other cytokines, such as IL-3. In some situations, anergy can result when cells produce IL-2 but do not express an IL-2 receptor and thus are unable to respond to IL-2.

The induction of T-cell anergy in the absence of costimulatory interactions was originally described in in vitro studies of T-cell unresponsiveness to foreign antigens. It is now believed to be a major mechanism for inducing unresponsiveness to self-molecules in the periphery which do not reach the thymus, and so do not induce clonal deletion in developing T cells. For example, cells from tissues such as pancreas, kidney, liver, and other organs do not normally express costimulatory molecules. Thus, antigens presented by these cells under normal circumstances are likely to induce anergy rather than activation. Following infection or other activation processes, however, the cells may express MHC class II molecules by exposure to IFN-γ

and costimulatory molecules and become capable of triggering T cells. Thus, the tissue cells become susceptible to immunologic attack with resultant damage and disease. Alternatively, it is even more likely that an antigen-presenting cell with costimulatory activity may acquire a tissue-specific antigen and trigger T cells leading to autoreactivity (see Chapter 17).

Attempting to block steps in APC–T and T–B interactions to induce tolerance is currently being tested as a therapeutic tool in a number of clinical situations. These include the prevention of transplantation rejection and the treatment of autoimmune diseases. Almost every stage in the T-cell activation pathway represents a potential target for disruption that may lead to tolerance induction. Blocking the function of critical cell surface molecules has attracted a great deal of interest. Strategies have included trying to block the function of CD3 and CD4 on the T cell with specific antibodies (used in transplantation), and the blocking of CD40–CD154 or B7–CD28 interactions with specific antibodies or similar molecules (autoimmune diseases and transplantation models). T-cell tolerance can also be induced by interfering with the intracellular steps in T-cell activation: the mode of action of cyclosporine and other molecules used to prevent graft rejection is discussed in Chapter 19.

Inhibition of B-Cell Activation. As we saw in Chapter 10, B cells require multiple sequential signals to proliferate and differentiate into antibody-secreting cells. Most of this signaling after the Ig receptors are engaged comes from T-cell help in the form of cytokines. In the absence of such T-cell help, B cells can also undergo negative signaling associated with a calcium flux, resulting in anergy. Thus, administration of antigen in ways that avoid the engagement of T cells (such as large doses, and soluble antigen, as we describe later in this chapter) leads to the partial activation of B cells by engagement of its specific Ig receptors and the development of unresponsiveness when the costimulatory signals are absent.

 ## OTHER POTENTIAL MECHANISMS OF REGULATING THE FUNCTION OF LYMPHOCYTES

Active Suppression via T Cells

Certain T cells appear to be capable of specifically suppressing the functional response of other lymphocytes to antigen. T cells with these inhibitory properties are referred to as ***suppressor*** or ***regulatory*** T cells. These cells may play a role in inhibiting or limiting responses to foreign antigens; they have been described as being involved in the downregulation of responses to antigens that enter through the mucosa, and in the prevention of graft rejection. In addition, suppressor or regulatory cells may provide a fail-safe mechanism for preventing the activation of cells with receptors for self-molecules that escape the protective screen of clonal deletion and clonal anergy.

Suppressive function has generally been shown by ***transferring*** T cells from one individual into another. Characterization of cells with suppressive function, however, has proved difficult, as the cells do not have a unique phenotype that distinguishes them from other $\alpha\beta^+$ CD4$^+$ or CD8$^+$ T cells. There may not be a unique population of T cells whose sole function is to suppress immune responses. It is possible that a population of T cells may temporarily function as a suppressor cell if it produces an appropriate cytokine; for example, by synthesizing TGF-β, a potent suppressor of the proliferation of many subsets of T and B cells. (For example, regulatory T cells have been described to induce tolerance after oral administration of antigen in some animal models by synthesizing TGF-β.) In addition, as described in Chapter 10 and later in this chapter, cytokines produced by one subset of CD4$^+$ T cells can inhibit the development or function of another CD4$^+$ subset.

One further mechanism of control by one lymphocyte type on another is that CD8$^+$ cells may be cytotoxic to other T cells or B cells that express foreign peptides in association with MHC molecules. They may recognize and lyse activated cells using mechanisms common to all cytotoxic CD8$^+$ T cells.

Idiotype Network

An alternative view of immune regulation was put forward by Niels Jerne (a Nobel Prize winner), who postulated that the immune system was controlled by a network, in which the products of V-region genes (idiotypes), present on antibody and on the antigen-specific receptors of T and B cells, would be recognized as immunogenic in the host. Adherents of this view proposed complex control loops involving multiple sets of B and T cells. Although some of these phenomena have been demonstrated in experimental situations, the relevance of these observations is still unclear.

REGULATION OF THE RESPONSE IN THE INDIVIDUAL

In the previous sections we discussed the tolerization of T and B cells as a key regulator of the immune response. In this section, we discuss a number of factors that can regulate or influence the level or type of response produced in the individual.

Age

Age extremes have an effect on the immune responsiveness to almost all antigens. Very young individuals do not respond to many antigens. While the fetus may respond with IgM antibodies to some antigens, IgG responses in the fetus are rare because of its still undeveloped immunocompetence. As described in Chapter 21, generalized immunocompetence develops only a few months after birth, accompanied by the waning of protective immunity derived from maternal antibody which circulates in the young child. Thus, vaccination against several diseases can be ineffective if given too early in life.

As described earlier in this chapter, injection of neonatal mice with cells from a different strain can lead to long-term tolerance to the tolerizing antigen. These results had suggested that the presentation of foreign antigen to the lymphocytes of very young mice generally resulted in the induction of tolerance rather than activation. Recent studies, however, have indicated that lymphocytes from neonatal mice are able to respond to a number of antigens, indicating that they can be activated under a number of conditions. For example, injecting dendritic cells with the tolerizing dose resulted in activation rather than tolerance induction. This suggests that diminished or absent populations of antigen-presenting cells, which are noted in neonatal mice, may contribute to the induction of tolerance in response to antigen.

In addition, diminution of immunocompetence has also been documented in aging individuals. The mechanisms accounting for decreased immune function in the elderly are currently the subject of intense research activity. It should be noted that immunizations to several organisms are recommended for older people (Chapter 21).

Neurologic and Endocrine Factors

Interactions between the immune system and other physiologic systems are complex and difficult to study, and the results of studies investigating these connections have frequently been controversial. *Steroid hormones* are thought to play a role in the immune system. Stress, presumably mediated through the production of endogenous *corticosteroids*, can increase susceptibility to infectious diseases, such as shingles in adults (reemergence of the virus that causes chicken pox). Corticosteroids are used to treat a number of conditions because they are potent inhibitors of the function of a wide range of cell types, including lymphocytes. *Sex hormones* are also believed to play a role in immune responsiveness. One important manifestation is that women are more prone to autoimmune diseases such as multiple sclerosis and systemic lupus erythematosus than men (see Chapter 17). Studies have also shown that hormones such as estradiol, progesterone, and androgens may influence the pattern of cytokines secreted in in vitro human and animal immune responses. In addition, androgens have been shown to reduce disease severity in an animal model of multiple sclerosis. Peptides such as somatostatin and substance P, which are involved in the interaction of cells in the nervous system, have also been shown to affect T-cell responses.

Nutritional status is a key regulator of the immune response. *Dietary deficiencies* in vitamins or trace metals such as zinc can induce profound immunodeficiency. Moreover, *malnutrition* is probably the leading cause of immunodeficiency in the world (see Chapter 18). The most dramatic effects are seen in *protein-energy malnutrition* cases, which can result from the combined effects of infection and poor nutrition. One of the human body's responses to an infectious agent is to produce the cytokines, TNF-α and IL-1. As a further illustration of the connections between the immune and nervous system described above, these cytokines act on the hypothalamus in the brain to induce fever (*pyrogens*). Fever leads to appetite reduction and increased requirement of energy to drive intracellular reactions. These factors combine to break down the individual's protein and fat stores, leading to weight loss and problems with several physiologic systems including the immune system. Reduced circulating T-lymphocyte count and poor delayed skin reactions are early indicators of protein-energy malnutrition. The complement system and phagocytic killing mechanisms are also impaired.

Recent studies have indicated additional connections between the immune system and nutritional status. *Leptin*, a recently discovered protein associated with obesity, reverses the immunosuppression that results from starvation, and enhances some T-cell responses in vitro. Mice defective in leptin also have impaired T-cell immunity.

Expression of MHC Molecules

The key role of MHC molecules in antigen presentation to T cells has been discussed in detail in Chapters 8 and 10. (Lack of expression of these molecules results in a rare immunodeficiency known as "bare lymphocyte syndrome," which results in severe depletion of T-cell responses [see Chapter 18 for more detail.]) The individual's expression of a unique set of MHC molecules determines which peptides are recognized by the immune system. As we discussed previously, peptide recognition is dependent binding to the antigen-binding groove of either an MHC class I or MHC class II molecule. Thus, it is highly likely that in the response to a single protein an individual expressing a particular pattern of MHC molecules presents peptides to his or her T cells, which are distinct from the peptides presented in another individual. Differences in the levels as well as the nature of the peptides bound by MHC molecules are also believed to influence the pattern of T-cell response. As a result, one individual may make one pattern of cytokines and thus activate one set of effector cells, and another individual may make a completely different response (see the next section.) As discussed in Chapter 8, this selective interaction of MHC and peptide is a plausible explanation for the association of certain diseases with specific MHC haplotypes.

When the antigen has a limited number of epitopes, MHC-dependent T-cell responses may also be very different in different individuals. This may be relevant in the response to certain peptide vaccines. In addition, responses to antigens with a limited number of epitopes (such as the response to small proteins or synthetic polypeptides) can vary widely in humans and other species, depending on the MHC molecules they express. Some may make weak or no response to the antigen, while others may generate a strong response.

Effects of Cytokines

As we described in Chapter 10, one of the major consequences of $CD4^+$ T-cell activation is the synthesis of a plethora of cytokines that affect the function of many different cell types. We now know that different subsets of $CD4^+$ T cells synthesize distinct patterns of cytokines. Because these distinct cytokines activate different effector cells, the result of synthesizing one set of cytokines rather than another may have important ramifications. For example, T_H1 cells produce IFN-γ and TNF-β, which are important in activating cells, such as macrophages, which play a key role in cell-mediated immunity. By contrast, T_H2 cells secrete IL-4, IL-5, and IL-13. These cytokines play a role in B-cell switching to IgE production and the activation of eosinophils, which are involved in responses to allergens and parasites. Furthermore, cytokines secreted by one set of T cells can inhibit the function of the other subset. Thus, IL-4 (as well as IL-10 and IL-13) inhibits IFN-γ activation of macrophages and conversely, IFN-γ may prevent IL-4-mediated switching of B cells.

The pattern of cytokines synthesized by subsets of $CD4^+$ cells exerts a powerful level of control on the immune response. What governs the synthesis of the subsets, however, is less clear, and is an area of intense research interest. As described in Chapter 10, one key factor is the presence of different cytokines during the priming of $CD4^+$. Priming of $CD4^+$ cells in the presence of IL-12 or IL-18, and IFN-γ favors the development of the T_H1 subset, and the presence of IL-4 and possibly IL-6 the formation of T_H2 cells. Other factors such as the concentration and route of exposure to antigen, the affinity of interaction between peptide–MHC complexes and the TCR, and the nature of the antigen-presenting cell in the response, have been suggested to play a role in determining which type of $CD4^+$ T cell develops and thus what pattern of cytokines is synthesized.

Regulation of the cytokine pattern generated may have therapeutic application. For example, individuals who demonstrate allergic responses to a particular allergen synthesize predominantly T_H2 cytokines and activate IgE- and eosinophil-mediated responses, whereas individuals who do not have allergic symptoms do not have this reactivity (also see Chapter 12). One treatment of allergic individuals has been to inject multiple low levels of the allergen over several months (***immunotherapy*** or hyposensitization, discussed in more detail in Chapter 14). Some studies indicate that effective immunotherapy is associated with decreased IL-4 production, and with decreased IgE and increased IgG levels by the end of the treatment. These results suggest that immunotherapy may shift the cytokine response away from a T_H2 pattern and toward a T_H1 or T_H0 pattern.

Effects of Antigen

Not every injection of an antigen results in an immune response. Generation of a response is a highly empirical process, depending on ***dose, route of exposure, the nature and form of the antigen, and timing***.

Dose. Early experiments investigated the ability of adult animals such as mice to respond to different concentrations of antigen. Avrion Mitchison showed in 1964 that immunologic tolerance could be induced by opposite extremes of dosage: tolerance could be induced by the use of relatively large doses of antigen, given repeatedly over long periods of time. Very small doses given similarly were also found to induce tolerance. Intermediate doses resulted in immunity.

Jacques Chiller and William Weigle expanded on these results to show that both mouse T and B cells could be tolerized by injecting the antigen human gamma globulin, but the cells behaved differently with respect to dose, timing, and duration of tolerance. They found that low (around 10 μg) and high (1 to 10 mg) doses induced tolerance in T cells, whereas only concentrations in the high range tolerized

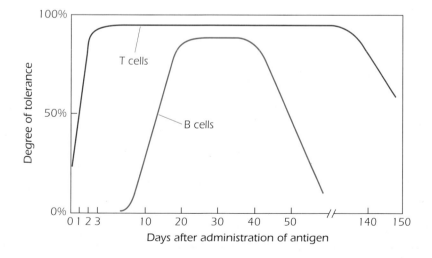

Figure 11.3. The kinetics of induction, maintenance, and loss of tolerance in T and B cell populations following antigen injection into mice.

B cells. As shown in Figure 11.3, they also demonstrated that the kinetics of tolerance induction were different in T- and B-cell populations. Tolerance was more rapidly induced in T cells and lasted longer; by contrast, B cells were tolerized for shorter periods. This difference in duration of T- and B-cell tolerance is attributable to the fact that the T-cell population is long-lived, whereas the B-cell population is replenished with nontolerized cells derived from bone marrow precursors. In addition, they noted that the animals remained tolerant to the injected antigen for the period that the T cells were tolerant. Thus, even though B cells were potentially able to respond to antigen, the animal was tolerant because the T-cell compartment was still tolerant. These findings also help to explain the observation made earlier that responses to self-molecules (which normally involve T and B cells) occur infrequently: even though B cells with self-reactivity may be present, tolerance of the T-cell compartment prevents reactivity.

Route of exposure. The individual is exposed to antigen through multiple sites. The predominant routes of exposure are through the air and in food, and also via injection, which prime mucosal and systemic immunity, respectively. Results from animal studies in particular indicate that the *route of exposure* to antigen and the type of *adjuvant* (see Chapter 3) used to boost immunity to the administered antigen, may play a role in determining the outcome of the response. Immunity induced by injection into the muscle, into the peritoneal cavity or subcutaneously, is enhanced by the use of adjuvants, and different adjuvants may skew the outcome of the response by activating different antigen-presenting cells (APC). For example, Freund's complete adjuvant, an emulsion that contains mycobacterial antigens, activates monocytic cells and favors the synthesis of T_H1 cytokines by $CD4^+$ T cells, whereas antigens injected with alum are thought to activate B cells, enhancing their effectiveness as APC, and favor the induction of T_H2 cytokines.

Exposure by different routes, however, may induce tolerance rather than activation; for example, by the *intravenous* injection of proteins into unprimed animals such as mice. (Previously primed animals, i.e., containing memory cells, are not tolerized by intravenous injection.) Antigen injected into the blood rapidly reaches the spleen, where it is presented to T cells by resting B cells. As resting B cells lack costimulatory molecules, their presentation of antigen induces T-cell tolerance rather than activation (described earlier in this chapter). It is not clear whether intravenous injection in humans also results in tolerance induction.

In addition, *oral* exposure to antigens has been shown to lead to tolerance in animal models. The mechanisms invoked to explain the induction of oral tolerance are complex; one involves the generation of regulatory cells that secrete cytokines, including TGF-β, which inhibits the response of other antigen-reactive cells. Oral exposure has been tested in humans as a means to downregulate autoimmune responses, by feeding the putative autoantigen. To date, however, feeding collagen to rheumatoid arthritis patients and myelin to multiple sclerosis sufferers has shown little or no clinical benefit.

Nature and Form of Antigen. The inherent *immunogenicity* of the substance being used to induce tolerance is critically related to the ease of induction of tolerance. For example, a very weak immunogen in mice, such as bovine γ-globulin (BGG), requires a less stringent regimen for induction of tolerance than a very strong immunogen, such as hen egg albumin or diphtheria toxoid. In general, the more chemically complex the antigen is, the more immunogenic it is. This is because complexity increases the number of epitopes and the chances for cell interaction necessary to trigger a response.

The *form* of the antigen is also important. BGG in soluble form is not immunogenic, and it also readily induces tolerance in mice; however, if it is given in an adjuvant or in an aggregated form, BGG is immunogenic. If a normally antigenic material is injected in solution in its monomeric form, tolerance rather than immunity frequently results. This effect is exemplified by the following: if a suspension of BGG in saline, which is normally immunogenic in rabbits, is subjected to ultracentrifugation, then the supernatant that contains the monomeric BGG is no longer immunogenic, but is, in fact, tolerogenic, while the sediment, which consists of aggregated BGG, is highly immunogenic. *Nonmetabolizable substances*, such as synthetic D-polypeptides (made with the unnatural D- rather than L-isomers of amino acids) also readily induce tolerance.

Regulation by Antibody. *Antibody feedback* is the process by which antibody produced in response to antigen can inhibit further response to that particular antigen. This can occur as a consequence of the normal immune response; the antibody produced in response to the antigen binds to it and removes it via the activation of phagocytic cells or the complement pathway. It can also occur if antibodies are injected into an individual shortly before or during an immune response. This has been used clinically to treat Rh disease of the newborn (see Chapter 15). Injection of antibody specific for Rh (an erythrocyte antigen) at the time of delivery of an Rh^+ baby into an Rh^- mother prevents the potentially damaging anti-Rh immune response of the mother to subsequent Rh^+ fetuses.

One important way in which the presence of antibody may inhibit further antibody production is through the formation of an *antigen-antibody complex* which can interact with a B cell as shown in Figure 11.4. The figure shows the Fc end of the antigen-antibody complex binding to the low affinity Fc receptor for IgG, CD32 (FcRγIIb) on the B cell, while the antigen end of the complex simultaneously binds to the Ig on the same cell. This simultaneous binding to Ig and to the FcR results in a negative signal to the B cell. Binding to the extracellular portion of CD32 recruits a *phosphatase* to an intracellular portion of CD32 which contains a tyrosine-containing sequence of amino acids. By analogy to the previously described ITAMs, the sequence in CD32 and other molecules is known as an *immunoreceptor tyrosine-based inhibitory motif (ITIM).* The phosphatase which binds to the CD32 ITIM removes phosphate groups from tyrosine residues in the signal transduction polypeptides associated with the BCR. As a result, the activatory signal through the BCR is inhibited.

IMMUNOLOGICALLY PRIVILEGED SITES

Grafts placed in certain sites in the body, such as the anterior chamber of the eye, and the cheek pouch of the hamster are not rejected. These sites are referred to as *immunologically privileged* (see Chapter 19). It was originally thought that these and other sites (such as the brain and the testes) provided an anatomic barrier: potential self-antigens, which were expressed by the cells of the organ or deliberately introduced antigens, were "sequestered," so that they were not in contact with lym-

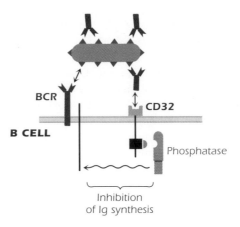

Figure 11.4. Antibody feedback inhibits B-cell activation. Simultaneous binding of the antigen and antibody components of an antigen–antibody complex to receptors on a B cell (antigen to the Ig, and the Fc portion of the antibody component to the FcR, CD32) results in a negative signal to the cell. The rectangle in the cytoplasmic region of CD32 represents the immunoreceptor tyrosine-based inhibitory motif (ITIM).

phoid cells or tissues. More recent studies have indicated, however, that antigens from these sites can interact with lymphoid cells, and that the mechanisms which underlie immunological privilege are more complicated than simple sequestration. It is currently believed that both local and systemic factors prevent inflammatory responses that might damage the organ. These include the secretion of cytokines, notably TGF-β and IL-10. TGF-β inhibits the function of many lymphoid populations, and as described in Chapters 10 and 12, IL-10 suppresses the induction of an inflammatory T_H1-type T-cell response and favors the induction of a T_H2 cytokine pattern. In addition, unlike cells of other organs, the testis and eye constitutively express FasL, and it is possible that Fas–FasL interactions inducing apoptosis play a role in preventing inflammatory responses at these sites.

The fetus may also be considered to develop in a privileged site. The fetus is in contact with elements of the maternal circulation, which include cells and IgG, but is generally not rejected. Several mechanisms exist for preventing fetal rejection; for example, fetal cells do not appear to express the standard MHC class I (or class II molecules), and thus may not be destroyed by CTL. In addition, trophoblast cells express a nonpolymorphic MHC class I molecule, HLA-G, which may inhibit killing by natural killer cells. The fetus is also believed to synthesize cytokines that may be suppressive to the maternal host.

Immunosuppression by Drugs or Radiation

Finally, we will briefly mention *nonspecific* methods for inhibiting responses by using *immunosuppressive agents* and *irradiation*. Some of these are also described in Chapter 19 dealing with transplantation immunology.

The most commonly used immunosuppressive drugs include *cytotoxic agents* (such as methotrexate and cyclophosphamide) that kill rapidly dividing cells and thus target lymphocytes (as well as hematopoietic cells of the bone marrow, gastrointestinal lining cells, and hair follicles). As discussed earlier in this chapter, corticosteroids are potent inhibitors of inflammatory responses. A major class of immunosuppressive agents acts specifically on T cells to prevent activation. These include *cyclosporine and FK506*, which block the action of nuclear transcription factors and inhibit the synthesis of IL-2 and other cytokines, and *rapamycin*, which interferes with protein kinases used in the signaling pathway of the IL-2–IL-2 receptor complex.

The hematopoietic and lymphoid systems are extremely sensitive to *radiation*. The dose rate of exposure is important, however, as whole-body irradiation may be lethal. This susceptibility can be exploited as a treatment therapy for lymphocyte disorders, such as leukemias and lymphomas.

SUMMARY

1. Tolerance is the state of lymphocyte unresponsiveness to antigen. Tolerance generally results from an interaction with antigen that functionally inactivates the antigen-specific cell. As a result, the tolerized cell may be deleted or alternatively anergized.

2. Self-tolerance is a critical feature of the immune system. One of the major mechanisms of inducing and maintaining self-tolerance is through the functional inactivation of developing T and B cells with potential reactivity to self (negative selection).

3. Tolerance can be induced in both immature and mature lymphocytes. To be tolerized, a cell must express an antigen-specific receptor (BCR or TCR).

4. Inhibiting one or more of the multiple steps required for T and/or B cell activation can result in tolerance. This may be manipulated to prevent the activation of lymphocytes in different conditions, such as autoimmune disease or graft rejection.

5. Multiple levels of control regulate the correct functioning of the immune response. Regulating the number of cells through "death pathways" is critical. Other potential mechanisms of regulating the function of lymphocytes include the action of suppressor (regulator) cells, and the idiotype network.

6. A number of factors control whether or not an individual makes a response to an antigen and determine what type of response is made. These include age, neurologic and endocrine factors, the expression of MHC molecules, the pattern of cytokines synthesized, the nature and level of antigen introduced, the site of antigen exposure, the presence of antibody, and exposure to drugs or radiation.

REFERENCES

Alberola-Ila J, Takaki S, Kerner JD, Perlmutter RM (1997): Differential signaling by lymphocyte antigen receptors. *Annu Rev Immunol* 15:125–154.

Goodnow CC, Adelstein S, Basten A (1990): The need for central and peripheral tolerance in the B cell repertoire. *Science* 248:1373.

Healy JI, Goodnow CC (1998): Positive versus negative signaling by lymphocyte antigen receptors. *Annu Rev Immunol* 16:645–670.

Nossal GJV (1994): Negative selection of lymphocytes. *Cell* 76:229.

Peter ME, Krammer PH (1998): Mechanisms of CD95(Apo-1/Fas)-mediated apoptosis. *Curr Opin Immunol* 10:545–551.

Powrie F, Coffman RL (1993): Cytokine regulation of T cell function: potential for therapeutic intervention. *Immunol Today* 14:270.

Raff M (1998): Cell suicide for beginners. *Nature* 396:119–122.

Starzl TE, Zinkernagel RM (1998): Antigen localization and migration in immunity and tolerance. *N Engl J Med* 339:1905–1913.

Stockinger B (1999): T lymphocyte tolerance: from thymic deletion to peripheral control mechanisms. *Adv Immunol* 71:229–265.

REVIEW QUESTIONS

For each question, choose the ONE BEST answer or completion.

1. An individual does not make an immune response to a self-protein because
   A) self-proteins cannot be processed into peptides.
   B) peptides from self-proteins cannot bind to MHC class I.
   C) peptides from self-proteins cannot bind to MHC class II.
   D) lymphocytes that express a receptor reactive to a self-protein are inactivated by deletion or anergy.
   E) developing lymphocytes cannot rearrange V genes required to produce a receptor for self-proteins.

2. Which of the following statements is *incorrect*?
   A) Interaction of Fas and FasL can lead to apoptosis.
   B) Both Fas and Fas L can be expressed on activated T cells.
   C) Both Fas and Fas L can be expressed on B cells.
   D) Cells in immunologically privileged sites can express FasL.
   E) Fas–FasL-mediated apoptosis prevents uncontrolled T-cell clone growth.

3. Which of the following is *incorrect* concerning immune tolerance?
   A) Tolerance induction is antigen-specific.
   B) Tolerance results from inactivation and/or elimination of B and/or T cells.
   C) Tolerance can be induced in both young and old individuals.
   D) Immature neutrophils are more susceptible to tolerance than mature neutrophils.
   E) The breakdown of tolerance can result in autoimmunity.

4. Which of the following statements is *incorrect* concerning the immune response to antigens?
   A) Reactivity is influenced by extremes of age.

B) Greater immune responses are produced when antigen is given with adjuvant.

C) Impaired nutrition depresses immunity.

D) The presence of preexisting antibody does not affect the subsequent response to antigen.

E) Different protein antigens stimulate different levels of antibody production.

5. All of the following procedures would be likely to induce tolerance to a protein antigen *except*

A) intramuscular injection of the antigen in adjuvant.

B) intravenous injection of deaggregated protein.

C) injection of cyclosporine with the antigen.

D) injection of antigen at a stage in development before mature lymphocytes appear.

E) intravenous injection of small amounts of antigen.

6. When a tolerogenic injection of a protein antigen is given experimentally, it can be shown that

A) B-cell tolerance is more rapidly induced than T-cell tolerance.

B) B-cell tolerance is lost as new B cells come from the bone marrow.

C) B-cell tolerance can be induced only when low doses are used.

D) T-cell tolerance can be induced only when high doses are used.

E) T-cell tolerance is shorter lasting than B-cell tolerance.

7. Blocking any of the following processes can result in peripheral tolerance in mature T cells *except*

A) the interaction of costimulatory molecules on T cells with their ligands on APC.

B) intracellular signal transduction mechanisms.

C) negative selection of thymocytes.

D) activation of the IL-2 gene.

E) the binding of antigen with MHC molecules.

Answers to Review Questions

1. *D* Negative selection generally ensures that a lymphocyte expressing a receptor reactive to a self-protein is inactivated by deletion or anergy.

2. *C* B cells express Fas but not FasL.

3. *D* Tolerance can be induced only in lymphocytes that express an antigen-specific receptor.

4. *D* Preexisting antibody may exert a negative feedback on the subsequent response to antigen.

5. *A* Injection into muscle and in the presence of adjuvant are likely ways to induce activate rather than tolerize the immune response. The remaining procedures generally induce tolerance. The use of cyclosporine in blocking transplantation rejection is discussed further in Chapter 19.

6. *B* T-cell tolerance is more rapidly achieved, occurs with lower doses, and lasts longer than B-cell tolerance. As new B cells are produced by the bone marrow, tolerance in this compartment wanes. T-cell tolerance, by contrast, persists because the thymus of an adult no longer actively produces new T cells.

7. *C* Interfering with negative selection of thymocytes disrupts central rather than peripheral T cell tolerance.

12

CYTOKINES

 INTRODUCTION

As we have already discussed in several of the preceding chapters, the immune system is regulated by soluble mediators collectively called *cytokines*. These low-molecular-weight proteins are produced by virtually all cells of the innate and adaptive immune systems and, in particular, by T_H cells, which orchestrate many effector mechanisms. Their major functional activities are concerned with the *regulation of the development and behavior of immune effector cells*. Some cytokines possess direct effector functions of their own. A simple way to understand how cytokines work is to compare them with hormones—the chemical messengers of the endocrine system. *Cytokines serve as chemical messengers within the immune system*, although they also communicate with certain cells in other systems, including those of the nervous system. Thus, they can function in an integrated fashion to facilitate homeostasis. By contrast, they also play a significant role in driving hypersensitivity and inflammatory responses and in some cases they can promote acute or chronic distress in tissues and organ systems.

As we will discuss later in this chapter, cells regulated by a particular cytokine must express a receptor for that factor. Thus, cells are regulated by the quantity and type of cytokines to which they are exposed and by the expression or downregulation of cytokine receptors. Normal regulation of innate and adaptive immune responses is largely controlled by a combination of these methods.

 THE HISTORY OF CYTOKINES

In the late 1960s when the activities of cytokines were first discovered, it was believed that they served as amplification factors that acted in an antigen-dependent fashion to elevate proliferative responses of T cells. Gery and colleagues were the

229

first to demonstrate that macrophages released a thymocyte mitogenic factor termed *lymphocyte activating factor* (LAF). This view changed radically when it was found that supernatants of mitogen-stimulated peripheral blood mononuclear cells promoted the long-term proliferation of T cells in the absence of antigens and mitogens. Soon afterward, it was found that this factor was produced by T cells and could be used to isolate and clonally expand functional T-cell lines. This T-cell-derived factor was given several names by different investigators, including thymocyte mitogenic factor (TMF), T cell growth factor (TCGF), and killer-cell helper factor (KHF). In 1979, an international workshop was convened to address the need to develop a consensus regarding the definition of these macrophage- and T-cell-derived factors. Since they mediated signals between leukocytes, the term *interleukin* was coined. The macrophage-derived LAF and T-cell-derived factors were given the names *interleukin-1* (IL-1) and *interleukin-2* (IL-2), respectively. Currently, numbers have been assigned to 18 interleukins, and this will undoubtedly continue to grow as research efforts continue to identify new members of this cytokine family. Cytokines produced by lymphocytes were collectively called *lymphokines*, whereas those produced by monocytes and macrophages were called monokines. To complicate matters, studies of the cellular sources of lymphokines and *monokines* ultimately revealed that these factors were not the exclusive products of lymphocytes and monocytes/macrophages. Thus, the more appropriate term cytokine was coined as a generic name for these glycoprotein mediators. To further illustrate the degree to which the cytokine field has outgrown the terminology established in 1979, knowledge of the functional properties of various cytokines has engendered a more liberal meaning of terms originally designed to define what a given factor does. It is well known that many interleukins have important biologic effects on cell types outside of the immune system. For example, *IL-2* not only acts to *promote T cell proliferation* in an autocrine fashion, it also stimulates osteoclasts, the bone-forming cells. TGF-β similarly acts on many cells, including connective tissue fibroblasts, as well as T cells and B cells. Thus, cytokines commonly have *pleiotropic properties*, since they can affect the activity of many different cell types. In addition, there is a great deal of *functional redundancy* among cytokines as evidenced, for example, by the ability of more than one cytokine to promote the growth, survival, and differentiation of B or T cells (e.g., IL-2 and IL-4 both function as T cell growth factors). As we shall see later in this chapter, this redundancy is explained, in part, by the common use of cytokine receptor signaling subunits by certain groups of cytokines. Finally, cytokines rarely, if ever, act alone in vivo. Thus target cells are exposed to a milieu containing cytokines, which often exhibit *additive*, *synergistic* or *antagonistic* properties. In the case of synergism, the combined effects of two cytokines is sometimes greater that the additive effects of the individual cytokines. Conversely, antagonism occurs when one cytokine inhibits the biologic activity of another.

The cytokine field has evolved rapidly over the past three decades due to the identification, functional characterization, and molecular cloning of a growing list of cytokines. The convenient nomenclature previously developed to define the sources of origin or the functional activities of certain cytokines has, in general, not held up. Nevertheless, occasionally, the field recognizes that common functional features of several glycoproteins merits the creation of yet another collective term to help define a family of cytokines. For example, the term *chemokines* was adopted in 1992 to describe a family of closely related chemotactic cytokines with conserved sequences, known to be potent attractors for various leukocyte subsets, such as lymphocytes, neutrophils, and monocytes. As students of immunology, learning about the rapidly expanding list of cytokines with diverse functional characteristics may appear to be a formidable task. However, by focusing on some that deserve special mention, the assignment can become an interesting and manageable exercise.

GENERAL PROPERTIES OF CYTOKINES

As noted above, cytokines are similar to polypeptide hormones, since they facilitate communication between cells and do so at very low concentrations (typically 10^{-10} to 10^{-15} M). Cytokines are short-lived and may act locally either on the same cell that secreted it (*autocrine*), on other cells (*paracrine*), or, like hormones, they may act systemically (*endocrine*) (Figure 12.1). In common with other polypeptide hormones, cytokines exert their functional effects by binding to specific receptors on target cells. Thus, cells regulated by specific cytokines must have the capacity to express a receptor for that factor. In turn, the activity of a responder cell may be regulated by the quantity and type of cytokines to which they are exposed or by the up- or downregulation of cytokine receptors, which, themselves, may be regulated by other cytokines. A good example of the latter is the ability of IL-1 to upregulate IL-2 receptors on T cells. This illustrates another common feature of cytokines, namely, their ability to act in concert with one another to create synergistic effects that reinforce the other's action on a single cell. Alternatively, some cytokines behave antagonistically toward one or more other cytokines and thus inhibit each other's action on a given cell. Finally, when certain cytokines (chemokines) are produced by cells in response to various stimuli (e.g., infectious agents), they establish a concentration gradient that serves to control or direct cell migration patterns, also known as **chemotaxis**. As discussed later in this chapter, cell migration (e.g., neutrophil

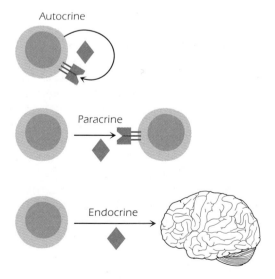

Figure 12.1. Autocrine, paracrine, and endocrine properties of cytokines. The brain is illustrated as an example of an organ that responds to cytokines in an endocrine fashion.

chemotaxis) is essential to the development of inflammatory responses resulting from localized injury or other trauma.

Interactions of the multiple cytokines generated during a typical immune response are often referred to as the ***cytokine cascade***. This cascade largely determines whether a response to an antigen will be primarily antibody-mediated (and, if so, which classes of antibodies will be made) or cell-mediated (and, if so, whether cells engaged in delayed hypersensitivity or cytotoxicity will be activated). Later in this chapter, we will discuss the cytokine-mediated control mechanisms that help determine the pattern of cytokines that develop following T_H cell activation. The antigenic stimulus appears to play a key role in the initiation of cytokine responses by effector T_H cells. Thus, depending on the nature of the antigenic signal, and the cytokine milieu associated with T cell activation, naive effector T_H cells will generate a particular cytokine profile—one that ultimately controls the type of immune response generated (antibody versus cellular). The cytokine cascade associated with immune responses also determines what other systems are activated or suppressed, as well as the level and duration of the response.

Cytokines have several functional features in common. They are nonantigen-specific glycoproteins that are generally synthesized and rapidly secreted in response to a stimulus; thus, they are usually not stored within the cell that makes them. Most cytokines have very short half-lives; consequently, cytokine synthesis and function occur in a burst.

Cytokines can act over both short and long range, with consequent systemic effects. Cytokines thus play a crucial role in the amplification of the immune response because the release of cytokines from just a few antigen-activated cells results in the activation of multiple different cell types, which are not necessarily located

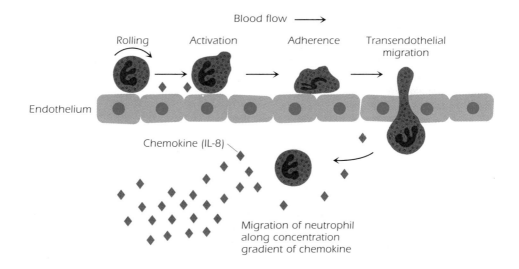

Figure 12.2. Steps involved in neutrophil transendothelial migration showing reversible binding followed by activation, adherence, and movement between the endothelial cells forming the wall of the blood vessel (extravasation).

in the immediate area. This is apparent in a response such as delayed-type hyper-sensitivity, discussed in detail in Chapter 16, in which the activation of rare antigen-specific T cells is accompanied by the release of cytokines. As a consequence of cytokine effects, monocytes are recruited into the area in great numbers, dwarfing the originally antigen-activated T cell population. It is also worth noting that the production of high levels of cytokines by a powerful stimulus can trigger deleterious systemic effects, such as toxic-shock syndrome as discussed later in this chapter.

A given cell may make many different cytokines. Moreover, one cell may be the target of many cytokines, each binding to its own cell-surface receptor. Consequently, one cytokine may affect the action of another, which may lead to an additive, synergistic, or antagonistic effect on the target cell.

As noted earlier in this chapter, it is common for cytokines to have overlapping (redundant) functions; for example, both IL-1 and IL-6 induce fever and several other common biologic phenomena. Nonetheless, these cytokines also have properties that are unique. One reason for this functional overlap is now understood: several cytokines share at least one chain of a common multichain receptor. For example, the cytokines IL-3, IL-5, and granulocyte-macrophage colony-stimulating factor (GM–CSF) use a shared chain of the cell-surface receptor as a signal transduction molecule. This is discussed in more detail later in this chapter. Finally, cytokines are a crucial link between cells of the immune system and other systems in the body. Thus, therapeutic manipulation of the immune system that target specific cytokines (e.g., cytokine replacement therapy; use of cytokine antagonists) can affect multiple physiologic systems depending on the range of biologic activity associated with a particular cytokine.

FUNCTIONAL CATEGORIES OF CYTOKINES

We will not attempt to list all of the currently well-characterized and molecularly cloned cytokines in this chapter. The major cytokines that play a role in the immune response and a brief description of their functions are listed in Table 12.1. A convenient way to begin this exercise is to classify cytokines into five categories on the basis of their general properties. It is important to state that this subdivision, although convenient, is somewhat arbitrary, given the pleiotropic effects of many cytokines.

Cytokines That Regulate Specific Immune Responses

As discussed in Chapter 10, many cytokines regulate B and T lymphocytes following their stimulation with antigen. Depending on the cytokines involved, regulation can be positive or negative and can impact cell proliferation, activation, and differentiation. Ultimately, cytokines regulate the intensity and duration of immune responses. A major feature of all immune responses is their antigen specificity. In the face of these potent immunoregulatory cytokines, how does the immune system ensure that antigen-nonspecific B and T cells are not activated during an immune response? One mechanism to ensure the specificity of the immune response is through the selective expression of functional cytokine receptors only on lymphocytes that have been stimulated by antigen. As a consequence, cytokines tend to act only on antigen-

● T A B L E 12.1. Selected Cytokines and Their Functions

Cytokine	Produced by	Major functions
Interleukin-1 (IL-1)	Monocytes, many other cell types	Produces fever, stimulates acute-phase protein synthesis, promotes proliferation of T_H2 cells
Interleukin-2 (IL-2)	T_H0 and T_H1 cells	T cell growth factor
Interleukin-3 (IL-3)	T_H cells, NK cells, mast cells	Growth factor for hematopoietic cells
Interleukin-4 (IL-4)	T_H2, CD4$^+$ T cells, mast cells	Growth factor for B cells and T_H2 CD4$^+$ T cells, promotes IgE and IgG, synthesis; inhibits T_H1 CD4$^+$ T cells
Interleukin-5 (IL-5)	T_H2 cells, mast cells	Stimulates B-cell growth and Ig secretion; growth and differentiation factor for eosinophils
Interleukin-6 (IL-6)	T cells and many others	Induces acute-phase protein synthesis, T-cell activation, and IL-2 production; stimulates B-cell Ig production and hematopoietic progenitor cell growth
Interleukin-7 (IL-7)	Bone marrow and thymic stromal cells, some T cells	Growth factor for pre-T and pre-B cells
Interleukin-9 (IL-9)	T cells	Mast-cell activation
Interleukin-10 (IL-10)	T_H2 cells and macrophages	Inhibits production of T_H1 cells and macrophage function
Interleukin-11 (IL-11)	Fibroblasts	Stimulates megakaryocyte (platelet precursor) growth
Interleukin-12 (IL-12)	B cells and macrophages	Activates NK cells and promotes generation of T_H1 CD4$^+$ T cells
Interleukin-13 (IL-13)	T cells	Shares characteristics with IL-4 such as Ig switch to IgE synthesis, but does not affect T cells; growth factor for human B cells
Interleukin-14 (IL-14)	T cells	Involved in the development of memory B cells
Interleukin-15 (IL-15)	T cells and epithelial cells	T-cell growth factor, similar to IL-2
Interferon-gamma (IFN-γ)	T_H1 cells	Activates NK cells, macrophages, and NK cells; inhibits T_H2 CD4$^+$ T cells; induces expression of MHC class II on many cell types
Transforming growth factor β (TGF-β)	Lymphocytes, macrophages, platelets, mast cells	Enhances production of IgA; inhibits activation of monocyte and T-cell subsets; active in fibroblast growth and wound healing
TNF-α	Macrophages, mast cells	Involved in inflammatory responses; activates endothelial cells and other cells of immune and nonimmune systems; induces fever and septic shock
TNF-β (lymphotoxin)	T cells	Involved in inflammatory responses; also plays a role in killing target cells by cytotoxic CD8$^+$ T cells
Granulocyte-monocyte-stimulating factor (GM-CSF)	T cells and monocytes	Promotes growth of granulocytes and macrophages; growth of dendritic cells in vitro
Macrophage-stimulating factor (M-CSF)	T cells and monocytes	Promotes macrophage growth
Granulocyte-stimulating factor (G-CSF)	T cells and monocytes	Promotes granulocyte growth

activated lymphocytes. A second mechanism that protects antigen-nonspecific lymphocytes from being regulated by cytokines involves the need for cells to interact with each other in a cognate fashion through cell-to-cell contact. Such interactions that might occur, say, between T_H cells and APCs (e.g., dendritic cells, macrophages, B cells), generate high concentrations of cytokines at the juncture between the interacting cells. In this way, only the target cell(s) participating in the interaction are affected by the cytokines produced. Finally, since the half-life of cytokines is very short, particularly in the bloodstream and extracellular spaces, they have a very limited period to act on other target cells.

Cytokines Produced by T_H1 and T_H2 Cells

T_H cells are a major source of cytokines that regulate immune responses. We have already discussed some of the diverse functional properties of several T cell-derived cytokines including IL-2 and IL-4 (see Chapter 10). Naive $CD4^+$ T cells differentiate into subpopulations of T_H1 or T_H2 cells, each of which possesses characteristic cytokine profiles (see Figure 10.3). During an initial immune response, antigens play a key role in determining which direction naive T_H0 cells will take in this differentiation pathway. While the mechanism controlling these events is not yet fully defined, it is known that the cytokines produced by other cells as a result of their exposure to antigen (e.g., antigen-presenting cells, NK cells, mast cells) profoundly influence the initial proliferative phase of T-cell activation when T_H0 cells differentiate into T_H1 or T_H2 cells. For example, many intracellular bacteria (e.g., *Listeria*) and viruses activate dendritic cells, macrophages, and NK cells to produce IL-12 and IFN-γ. In the presence of these cytokines, T_H0 cells tend to develop into T_H1 cells. By contrast, other pathogens (e.g., parasitic worms) do not induce IL-12 production by these cells but instead cause release of IL-4 by other cells (e.g., mast cells). IL-4 promotes the development of T_H0 cells into T_H2 cells.

Another way in which antigen plays a role in determining which direction naive T_H0 cells will take in developing into T_H1 or T_H2 subsets concerns the amount and nature of antigenic peptide presented to these cells during primary stimulation. Low levels of antigenic peptide bind poorly to the T cell receptor of T_H0 cells. Under these conditions, the naive T cells differentiate preferentially into T_H2 cells to produce IL-4 and IL-5. By contrast, when naive $CD4^+$ T cells are presented with a high density of ligand that binds strongly to the T cell receptor, they tend to differentiate into T_H1 cells to produce IL-2, IFN-γ and TNF-β. Ultimately, the cytokines generated determine whether the response will be dominated by macrophage activation or antibody production. *The T_H1 pathway facilitates cell-mediated immunity* with the activation of macrophages, NK cells, and CTL responses, whereas *the T_H2 pathway is essential for humoral immunity*.

The two subsets of $CD4^+$ T cells can also regulate the growth and effector functions of each other. This phenomenon occurs as a result of the activity of cytokines produced by the subset that is being activated and its apparent purpose is to make it difficult to shift the response to the other subset. For example, production of IL-10 and TGF-β by T_H2 cells inhibits activation and growth of T_H1 cells. Similarly, production of IFN-γ by T_H1 cells inhibits proliferation of T_H2 cells. These effects permit either subset to dominate a particular immune response by inhibiting the outgrowth of the other subset.

Cytokines That Facilitate Innate Immune Responses and Activate Inflammatory Responses

Innate Immune Responses. Several cytokines facilitate innate immune responses stimulated by viruses and microbial pathogens. Included in this group are *IL-1, IL-6, TNF-α, interferon-α and interferon-β.* IL-1, IL-6, and TNF-α initiate a wide spectrum of biologic activities that help coordinate the host's responses to infection. They are produced largely by phagocytes (e.g., macrophages and neutrophils) and are termed *"endogenous pyrogens"* because they cause fever. Elevated body temperature is beneficial to host defenses because adaptive immune responses are more intense and most pathogens grow less efficiently at raised temperatures. Another important effect of IL-1, IL-6 and TNF-α is their initiation of a response known as the *acute-phase response* following production of *acute-phase proteins* produced by hepatocytes. As discussed below, acute inflammation (e.g., in response to infections) is generally accompanied by a systemic acute-phase responses. Typically, changes in acute-phase protein plasma levels occur within 2 days following infection. One of these proteins, *C-reactive protein* (CRP), binds to phosphorylcholine on bacterial surfaces and act like an opsonin and also activate the classical complement pathway. Another acute-phase protein with opsonin and complement-activating activity is *mannan-binding lectin* (MBL) that binds mannose residues accessible on many bacteria. Given these functional properties, they mimic the actions of antibodies, which opsonize bacteria and activate the complement cascade. In concert with the other members of the acute-phase protein family, CRP and MBL lead to bacterial clearance.

Another effect of the endogenous pyrogens (IL-1, IL-6, and TNF-α) is to induce an increase in circulating neutrophils that are summoned from the bone marrow and the blood vessels where leukocytes attach loosely to endothelial cells. Finally, dendritic cells from peripheral tissues migrate to the lymph nodes in response to these cytokines. There, they serve as potent antigen-presenting cells to facilitate adaptive immune responses needed to control infections.

The term interferon was coined because they interfere with viral replication thus blocking the spread of viruses to uninfected cells. *Interferon-α* (IFN-α) and *interferon-β* (IFN-β) are synthesized by many cell types following viral infection. They are distinguished from another glycoprotein called interferon-γ, which is produced by activated NK cells and effector T cells and thus appears after the induction of adaptive immune responses.

In addition to their antiviral activities, IFN-α and IFN-β induce increased MHC class I expression on most uninfected cells, thus enhancing their resistance to NK cells as well as making newly infected cells more susceptible to killing by CD8$^+$ cytotoxic T cells. Finally, they activate NK cells, which contribute to early host responses to viral infections.

Inflammatory Responses. Many cytokines, including IL-1, IL-6, and TNF-α, activate functions of inflammatory cells. During localized acute inflammatory responses, all three cytokines cause increased vascular permeability, which ultimately leads to the swelling and redness associated with inflammation. As *inflammatory mediators*, they act in concert with the chemokines to ensure the development of physiologic responses to a variety of stimuli such as infections and tissue injury. Acute inflammatory responses develop rapidly and are of short duration. This short time course is probably related to the short half-lives of the inflammatory mediators involved as well as the regulatory influence of cytokines such as TGF-β which limits the inflammatory response (see below). Typically, systemic responses accompany these short-lived responses and are characterized by a rapid alteration in levels of acute-phase proteins (see above). Sometimes, persistent immune activation can occur (e.g., in chronic infections) leading to chronic inflammation, which subverts the physiologic value of inflammatory responses and causes pathologic consequences.

The neutrophil plays a key role in the early stages of inflammatory responses. Neutrophils infiltrate within a few hours into the tissue area where the inflammatory response is occurring. Their migration from the blood to the tissue site is controlled by the expression of adhesion molecules by vascular endothelial cells—a mechanism regulated by mediators of acute inflammation including IL-1 and TNF-α. Following exposure to these cytokines, vascular endothelial cells increase their expression of adhesion molecules (e.g., E- and P-selectin, ICAM-1; see Chapter 9), which, in turn, bind to selectin ligands (e.g., sialyl Lewis moiety) expressed on the surface of neutrophils. The neutrophils attach securely to the endothelial cells and undergo a process of end-over-end rolling. Chemokines also activate the neutrophil causing a conformational change in their membrane integrin molecules. Figure 12.3 shows a schematic illustration of the conformational change in the heterodimeric (α and β chain) integrin molecule, LFA-1, which allows it to ligate ICAM-1. This change increases the affinity of neutrophils for the adhesion molecules on the endothelium. Finally, the neutrophil undergoes transendothelial migration resulting in extravasation of the neutrophil, which continues its journey to the damaged or infected tissue site under the directional influence of chemokines, a process known as chemotaxis. It should be noted that lymphocytes and monocytes also undergo extravasation using the same basic steps as the neutrophil, although different combinations of adhesion molecules are involved. Other cytokines that play a significant role in inflammatory responses include IFN-γ and TGF-β. In addition to its role in activating macrophages to increase their phagocytic activity, *IFN-γ* has been shown to chemotactically attract macrophages to the site where antigen is localized. The migration of all of these cell types, including neutrophils, lymphocytes, monocytes, macrophages, as well as eo-

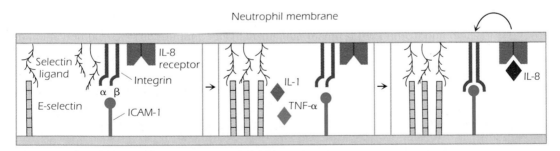

Figure 12.3. Cell membrane adhesion molecules and cytokine activation events associated with neutrophil transendothelial migration. **Left:** Weak binding of selectin ligands on the neutrophil to E-selectin on the endothelial cells. **Middle:** IL-1 and TNF-α upregulation of E-selectin, which facilitates stronger binding. **Right:** The activation effects of IL-8 on neutrophils which causes a conformational change in the integrins (e.g., LFA-1) to allow them to bind ICAM-1.

sinophils and basophils, which are attracted to the site of tissue damage by complement activation, leads to clearance of the antigen and healing of the tissue. TGF-β plays a role in terminating the inflammatory response by promoting the accumulation and proliferation of fibroblasts and the deposition of extracellular matrix proteins required for tissue repair.

Chemokines: Cytokines That Affect Leukocyte Movement

The term *chemokine* was adopted in 1992 to describe a family of closely related, low-molecular-weight *chemotactic cytokines* containing 70–80 residues with conserved sequences, and known to be potent attractors for various leukocyte subsets, such as neutrophils, monocytes, and lymphocytes. Table 12.2 lists some of the important chemokines among the 40 that have been identified. Structurally, this large superfamily consists of four subfamilies that display one of four highly conserved NH$_2$-terminal cysteine amino acid residues as follows: CXC, CC, C, or CX3C, where X represents a nonconserved amino acid residue. Most chemokines fall into the CXC and CC groups. As discussed above, they function in concert with inflammatory mediators to regulate the expression and conformation of cell adhesion molecules in leukocyte membranes. Some cytokines have also been shown to induce respiratory burst, enzyme release, intracellular Ca^{2+} mobilization, and angiogenesis. The latter functional property of some chemokines is a biologic feature consistent with the important role they play in wound healing and tissue repair. Production of chemokines may either be induced or constitutive. Those whose production is inducible or strongly upregulatable in peripheral tissues by inflammation are primarily involved in wound healing/tissue repair mechanisms. By contrast, constitutively produced chemokines fulfill housekeeping functions and may be involved in normal leukocyte traffic.

Among the more than 40 chemokines that have been identified to date, *IL-8*, a member of the CXC subfamily, is the most well-characterized. It is produced by many different cell types such as monocytes, macrophages, endothelial cells, fibroblasts and neutrophils and plays a major role in inflammatory responses and wound healing mainly due to its ability to attract neutrophils to sites of tissue damage. Another important function of IL-8 is its ability to activate neutrophils following their attachment to vascular endothelium (Figure 12.3).

An exciting and important finding emerging from the field of chemokine research in 1995 concerned the ability of certain CC chemokines (e.g., RANTES, MIP-1α, and MIP-1β) to suppress infection of T cells with the macrophage-tropic (M-tropic) HIV strains (see Chapter 18). Subsequently, it was found that the chemokine receptor CCR5, which binds to certain CC chemokines, including the ones listed above, is the coreceptor for M-tropic HIV-1. By contrast, the chemokine receptor that binds to certain members of the CXC subfamily (CCR4) is the coreceptor responsible for entry of T-trophic strains of HIV-1 into target cells. The establishment of a heterotrimeric complex between the viral envelope protein gp120, CD4, and one of these chemokine receptors facilitates viral entry into cells although the molecular mechanisms associated with this phenomenon are only beginning to be understood.

Cytokines That Stimulate Hematopoiesis

As discussed in Chapter 2, myeloid and lymphoid cells are derived from pluripotential stem cells (see Figure 2.1). Cytokines capable of inducing growth of hemato-

● T A B L E 12.2. Selected Chemokines and Their Functions

Chemokine	Produced by	Chemoattracted cells	Major functions
Interleukin-8 (IL-8)	Monocytes, macrophages, fibroblasts, keratinocytes, endothelial cells	Attracts neutrophils, naive T cells	Mobilizes and activates neutrophils; promotes angiogenesis
Regulated on activation normal T cell expressed and secreted (RANTES)	T cells, endothelial cells, platelets	Attracts monocytes, NK and T cells, basophils, eosinophils	Degranulates basophils, activates T cells
Monocyte chemotactic protein-1 (MCP-1)	Monocytes, macrophages, fibroblasts, keratinocytes	Attracts monocytes, NK and T cells, basophils, and dendritic cells	Activates macrophages, stimulates basophil histamine release, promotes T_H2 immunity
Macrophage inflammatory protein-1α (MIP-1α)	Monocytes, macrophages, T cells, mast cells, fibroblasts	Attracts monocytes, NK and T cells, basophils, and dendritic cells	Promotes T_H1 immunity, competes with HIV-1
Macrophage inflammatory protein-1β. (MIP-1β)	Monocytes, macrophages, neutrophils, endothelium	Attracts monocytes, NK and T cells, and dendritic cells	Competes with HIV-1 for chemokine receptor binding

poietic cells in vitro were initially characterized using cultures of bone marrow cells grown in soft agar and thus are referred to as *colony-stimulating factors (CSF)*. Several biochemically distinct CSFs were identified by the particular lineage of hematopoietic cells that were stimulated to form colonies. These include macrophage–CSF (M–CSF), which supports the clonal growth of macrophages, granulocyte–CSF (G–CSF), which supports the clonal growth of granulocytes, and GM–CSF, which supports the clonal growth of both macrophages and macrophages. IL-3 is another cytokine capable of stimulating clonal growth of hematopoietic cells but unlike the CSFs is capable of promoting proliferation of a large number of cell populations, including granulocytes, macrophages, megakaryocytes, eosinophils, basophils, and mast calls. Moreover, in the presence of erythropoietin, a kidney-derived growth factor that has the ability to support the growth and terminal differentiation of cells of the erythroid lineage, IL-3 is also capable of stimulating development of normoblasts and red cells. IL-7, a cytokine produced largely by bone marrow and thymic stromal cells, induces differentiation of lymphoid stem cells into progenitor B and T cells. Like other functional categories of cytokines, the list of factors that are involved in hematopoiesis has grown significantly in recent years. Perhaps more than any other category of cytokines, CSFs have emerged as important therapeutic agents. For example, G-CSF is used to treat patients undergoing high-dose chemotherapy to reverse the neutropenia casued by such therapies. GM–CSF is used to treat patients undergoing bone marrow transplantation to boost clonal expansion of the granulocyte and macrophage populations.

 ## CYTOKINE RECEPTORS

Cytokines can only act on target cells that express receptors for that cytokine. Often, cytokine receptor expression, like cytokine production itself, is highly regulated, such that resting cells either do not express a given receptor or express a low- or intermediate-affinity version of that receptor. An example of the latter is seen in the case of the IL-2 receptor, which can be expressed on the membranes of cells in one of three forms: (1) a low-affinity monomer (α chain); (2) an intermediate-affinity dimer (β and γ chains); and (3) a high-affinity trimer containing three subunit chains α, β, and γ. IL-2 is capable of activating cells expressing the high-affinity form of the IL-2 receptor— a property unique to T cells undergoing antigen stimulation. The relative importance of these receptor subunits in binding to IL-2, and signaling the target cell is discussed later in this chapter. Suffice to say, the regulation of the receptor level expressed on the target cell membrane and/or the receptor form expressed helps to ensure that only an activated target population will respond to the cytokine(s) within its local microenvironment.

Understanding how cytokines affect their target cells has been the subject of many recent studies. Clinically, knowledge about cytokine–cytokine receptor interactions may be useful in devising strategies to prevent the action of cytokines involved in inflammatory responses, such as rheumatoid arthritis, or in responses such as transplantation rejection.

Receptors for cytokines can be divided into five families of receptor proteins (Figure 12.4):

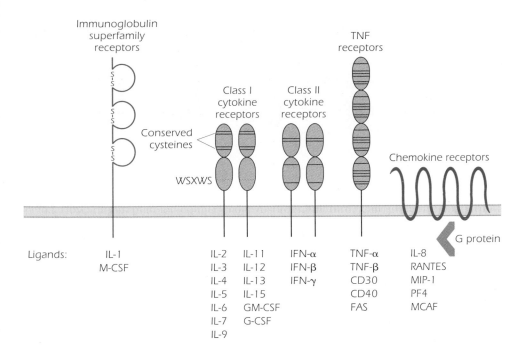

Figure 12.4. Schematic diagram showing the structural features of the five types of cytokine receptors. Many contain highly conserved cysteine residues.

- Immunoglobulin superfamily receptors
- Class I cytokine receptor family
- Class II cytokine receptor family
- TNF receptor family
- Chemokine receptor family

   The immunoglobulin superfamily receptors contain the domain structure of the typical member of a member of the immunoglobulin superfamily. Class I cytokine receptors (also known as the hematopoietin receptor family) are usually composed of two types of polypeptide chains: a cytokine-specific subunit (α chain) and a signal-transducing subunit (β or γ chain). Most cytokines identified to date utilize the class I family of cytokine receptors. Exceptions for the two subunit structural feature of these cytokine receptors are seen in the case of the high-affinity receptors for IL-2 and the IL-15 receptor, which are trimers (see below). An interesting feature of class I cytokine receptors is that they often share common signal transducing subunits with other members of the same family. For example, the high-affinity IL-2 receptor (IL-2R) consists of an IL-2-specific α chain and two additional chains (β and γ) responsible for signal transduction (discussed below). ***The γ subunit is utilized by several other cytokine receptors as the signal transducing subunit***—a structural feature that helps to explain the redundancy and antagonism often exhibited by some cytokines (Figure 12.5). As mentioned above, the IL-2 receptor can be expressed on the membranes of cells in one of three forms: (1) a low-affinity monomer (α-chain); (2) an intermediate-affinity dimer (β and γ chains); and, (3) a high-affinity trimer

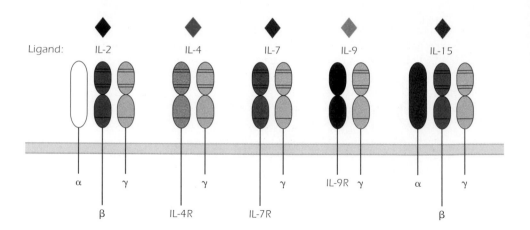

Figure 12.5. Schematic diagram showing structural features of members of the class I cytokine receptor family which share the common γ chain (green) that mediates intracellular signaling.

containing three subunit chains α, β, and γ (Figure 12.6). IL-2 is capable of activating cells expressing the high-affinity form of the IL-2 receptor—a property reserved for T cells undergoing antigen stimulation. A defect in the common IL-2Rγ chain has been shown to cause a profound immune deficiency in males suffering from X-linked severe combined immunodeficiency disease (X-linked SCID; Chapter 18). This defect abolishes the functional activity of multiple cytokines owing to their shared use of the IL-2Rγ chain for normal ligation of their receptors.

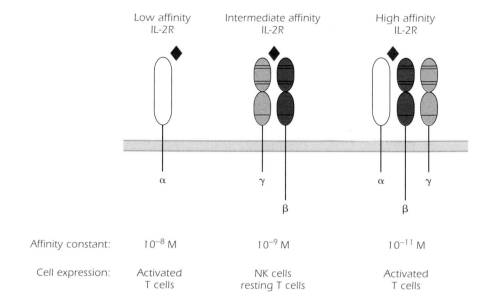

⬤ **Figure 12.6.** Comparison of the three forms of IL-2 receptors expressed on cells.

Class II cytokine receptors are also known as the interferon receptor family because their ligands include interferons α, β, and γ. Ligands for the TNF cytokine receptor family can be membrane-associated or secreted proteins. For example, most effector T cells express membrane forms of members of the TNF protein family including TNF-α and TNF-β—both of which can also be released as secreted proteins. Other ligands for the TNF receptor family include CD40 and Fas, both of which play crucial roles in cell–cell interactions. Finally, the ***chemokine receptors*** belong to a superfamily of serpentine G-protein-coupled receptors—so-called because of their unique snakelike extracellular–cytoplasmic structural configuration and their association with G proteins, which mediate signal transduction (Figure 12.4). To date, eight CC and five CXC chemokine receptors have been cloned, and some have been found to be promiscuous, since they can bind not only to chemokines but also to a diverse set of pathogens, including bacteria (e.g., *Streptococcus pneumonia*, which binds to the platelet activating-factor receptor [PAFR]), parasites (e.g., *Plasmodium vivax*, which binds to the chemokine receptor known as Duffy blood-group antigen), and certain viruses (e.g., T-tropic HIV-1 strains that use the CXCR4 chemokine receptor and M-tropic HIV-1 strains that use the CCR5 chemokine receptor for viral entry into T cells and macrophages, respectively).

 ## CYTOKINE RECEPTOR-MEDIATED SIGNAL TRANSDUCTION

In order for cytokines to mediate their biologic effects on target cells, they must generate intracellular signals that result in the production of active transcription factors and, ultimately, gene expression. A simple model for cytokine activation of cells is shown in Figure 12.7. Binding of a cytokine to its cellular receptor induces ***dimerization or polymerization of receptor*** polypeptides at the cell surface. The mechanism illustrated applies to most, if not all, class I and class II cytokines receptor families. It should be noted that it is not known how signal specificity is maintained when different cytokine receptors use the same cytoplasmic signaling pathways. In the case of these two receptor families, the dimerization/polymerization of receptor subunits juxtaposes their cytoplasmic tails thus allowing the dimeric receptor to engage the intracytoplasmic signaling machinery. Signaling is initiated by the ***activation of JAK kinases***, a family of cytosolic protein tyrosine kinases that interact with the cytoplasmic domains of the receptor. This results in the ***phosphorylation of tyrosine residues*** present on the cytoplasmic domain of the receptor and on a family of transcription factors known as ***STATs*** (signal transducers and activators of transcription). Once phosphorylated, the STAT transcription factors dimerize and subsequently translocate from the cytoplasm to the nucleus where they bind to enhancer regions of genes induced by the cytokine. This culminates in the biologic properties of the cytokine at the cellular level.

 ## ROLE OF CYTOKINES AND CYTOKINE RECEPTORS IN DISEASE

Given the complex regulatory properties of cytokines, it is not surprising that overexpression or underexpression of cytokines or cytokine receptors have been implicated in several diseases. Here we discuss some examples of diseases with cytokine-associated pathophysiology.

Toxic Shock Syndrome

Toxic shock syndrome is initiated by the release of ***superantigen*** (enterotoxin) from certain microorganisms. For example, the toxins derived from *Staphylococcus aureus* or *Streptococcus pyogenes* cause a burst of cytokine production by T cells. As discussed in Chapter 10, the toxin does this by activating large numbers of CD4$^+$ T cells which use certain Vβ segments as part of their TCR. The toxin crosslinks the Vβ segment of the TCR with a class II MHC molecule expressed on antigen-presenting cells (see Figure 10.5). It has been estimated that one in every five T cells can be activated by superantigens. Superantigen-activated T cells results in excessive production of cytokines that ultimately cause dysregulation of the cytokine network leading to extremely high levels of IL-1 and TNF-α. These cytokines induce systemic reactions including fever, blood clotting, diarrhea, a drop in blood pressure, and shock. Sometimes these reactions are fatal.

Bacterial Septic Shock

Overproduction of cytokines is also associated with infections caused by certain gram-negative bacteria, including *Escherichia coli, Klebsiella pneumonia, Entero-*

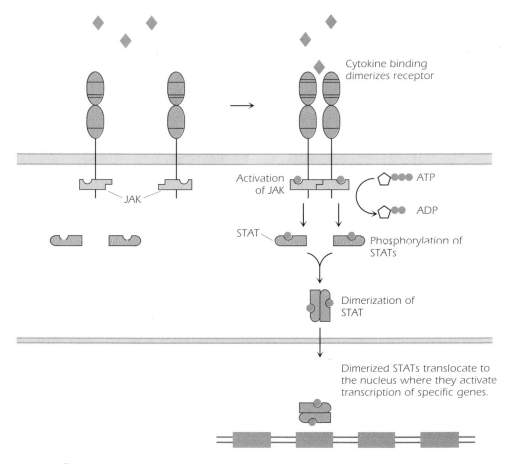

Figure 12.7. Model of cytokine receptor signaling using receptor-associated kinases to activate specific transcription factors.

bacter aerogenes, Pseudomonas aeruginosa, and *Neisseria meningitidis.* Endotoxins produced by these bacteria stimulate macrophages to overproduce IL-1 and TNF-α that cause an often fatal form of bacterial septic shock.

Cancers

Several lymphoid and myeloid cancers have been shown to be associated with abnormally high levels of cytokines and/or cytokine receptor expression. Perhaps the best example of an association between malignancy and overproduction of both a cytokine and its receptor is seen in patients with adult T cell leukemia—a disease that is strongly associated with the human T cell lymphoma (HTLV-1) retrovirus. T cells infected with HTLV-1 constitutively produce IL-2 and express the high-affinity IL-2 receptor in the absence of activation by antigen. This results in autocrine stimulation of infected T cells, leading to their uncontrolled growth. Other examples of malignancies associated with overproduction of cytokines include myelomas (neoplastic B cells), which produce large amounts of the autocrine IL-6, and Hodgkin's disease, a lymphoma in which the reactive milieu is the result of abundant cytokine production, particularly IL-5 (also see Chapter 18).

Autoimmunity

Much evidence suggests that T cells exert a controlling influence on the generation of autoantibodies and on the regulation of autoimmunity (see Chapter 17). It is likely that some of the observed phenomena are manifestations of the actions of T_H subset-derived cytokines, including IL-10, IFN-γ, and IL-4. Several cytokine and cytokine receptor abnormalities have been shown to be associated with systemic autoimmune diseases. Some occur late in illness and are probably not causal, while others may be involved in dysregulation of immune responses and may help promote autoreactivity. The autoimmune disease systemic lupus erythematosus (SLE) has been shown to be associated with elevated levels of IL-10. Recent studies of cytokines involved in autoimmune diseases have examined whether skewing of the T_H cell subset phenotype contributes to disease initiation or disease progression. While most of this work has been performed using experimental animal models of autoimmune disease, the importance of T_H2 cells in promoting systemic autoimmunity has been reported. Future studies will be needed to clearly elucidate the disease-related roles played by cytokines and T_H subsets in autoimmunity.

CYTOKINE ANTAGONISTS AND INHIBITORS

Several proteins that are capable of antagonizing the effects of cytokines have been identified. Among these, the best characterized is the naturally occurring ***IL-1 receptor antagonist*** (IL-1Ra). This protein appears to play a role in regulating the intensity of inflammatory responses by binding to the IL-1 receptor on T_H cells thus preventing their activation. Binding of IL-1Ra to the IL-1 receptor does not mediate cell signaling through this receptor. IL-1Ra has been cloned and is currently under clinical investigation to determine whether it can be used as a therapeutic agent for chronic inflammatory diseases.

Several cytokine inhibitors have been identified in the bloodstream and extra-cellular fluids. In contrast to cytokine antagonists, which are secreted by cells, these inhibitors are **soluble cytokine receptors**, which are released from the cell surface as a result of enzymatic cleavage of the extracellular domain of the cytokine receptor. Circulating soluble cytokine receptors maintain their ability to bind to the cytokine for which the receptor is specific thus neutralizing their activity. Examples of such inhibitors include those that bind to IL-2, IL-4, IL-6, IL-7, IFN-γ, and TNF-β. Among these, the soluble IL-2 receptor (IL-2R) has been studied extensively. It is formed by the proteolytic release of a 45-kDa portion of the IL-2 α chain of the IL-2R. Chronic T-cell activation is associated with very high bloodstream levels of soluble IL-2R. Thus, it has been used as a clinical marker for chronic T-cell activation in patients with certain autoimmune diseases and those undergoing transplant rejection.

THERAPEUTIC USES OF CYTOKINES AND CYTOKINE RECEPTORS

Knowledge of the cellular and molecular components of immune responses to in-fectious microbes and, specifically, the roles played by cytokines in regulation and homeostasis of hematopoietic cells has opened opportunities for new forms of ther-apeutics. Throughout this chapter, and elsewhere in this book (for example, see Figure 20.3), we have noted several examples of cytokines that have been exploited as therapeutic agents to modulate the immune response or selectively promote he-matopoiesis. The many opportunities for clinical uses of cytokines, cytokine recep-tors, cytokine analogs, and anti-cytokine or anti-cytokine receptor antibody therapies have sparked a great deal of commercial interest in cytokines. These biologic ther-apeutics have shown promise in several ways.

Reversing Cellular Deficiencies

Cytokines have been used to treat acute events such as cellular deficiencies arising from chemotherapy or radiotherapy by administration of growth factors (e.g., G– or GM–CSF). As discussed earlier in this chapter, treatment with these hematopoietic growth factors escalates the rate of natural reconstitution of desired hematopoietic cell lineages.

Treatment of Immunodeficiencies

Cytokines have also been used in immunodeficiency diseases to enhance T-cell ac-tivation. Several cytokines have been used with varying degrees of clinical success in this area, including IL-2, IFN-γ and TNF-α.

Treatment of Cancer

Patients with cancer have also benefited from the use of cytokines in tumor therapies that utilize **lymphokine-activated killer** (LAK) cells as discussed in Chapter 20. Culturing populations of NK cells or cytotoxic T cells in the presence of high con-centrations of IL-2 generates effector cells with potent anti-tumor activities. The use of antibodies to neutralize the activity of cytokines has also proven useful in the treatment of certain cancers. The relative accessibility of leukemic cells has encouraged numerous trials with native as well as toxin-conjugated antibodies. In one subset of leukemia, the adult T-cell leukemia, antibodies to the IL-2R α chain (anti-CD25, also known as anti-Tac) has been shown to induce therapeutic responses in a third of the patients treated.

Treatment of Chronic Inflammatory Diseases

There is evidence that many signs and symptoms of rheumatoid arthritis can be controlled by biologics (antibodies and receptor analogs) that neutralize the activities of proinflammatory cytokines such as TNF-α. As noted above, the cytokine antagonist IL-1Ra may also be useful in treating chronic inflammatory responses by preventing T_H cell activation. Similarly, a cloned soluble form of the IL-1 receptor has also been shown to act as a cytokine inhibitor to block activation of T_H cells.

Treatment of Transplant Patients

Antibodies have been widely investigated in organ transplantation, both as prophylactics and as therapeutics to reverse rejection (see Chapter 19). In the cytokine arena, *anti-IL-2R (CD25) therapy* has been used as part of a regimen of immunosuppressive therapy to treat patients with renal transplants. Experiments in animals are also examining the possible uses of soluble IL-1R and IL-1Ra to block activation of T_H cells in response to alloantigens.

Treatment of Allergies

Our current understanding of the functional properties of T_H2 cells, and, more specifically, the roles played by specific cytokines they produce (e.g., IL-4, IL-13) in IgE production suggests that therapies that target these cytokines or their receptors may prove to be effective in the treatment of allergies. Given the cross-antagonistic effects of T_H1 cells and T_H2 cells, it may be possible to skew the production of IgE in response to a given allergen using strategies that selectively silence the undesired T_H2 subset. At present, this remains an experimental goal, which is being aggressively investigated in animal models. Progress has emerged using a related strategy that specifically targets IL-4, the major cytokine responsible for promoting B-cell isotype class switching to IgE. Antibodies against IL-4 have been shown to dramatically decrease IL-4 production in mice. The clinical applications of such research cannot be underestimated given the enormous number of individuals who suffer from allergies worldwide.

SUMMARY

1. Cytokines are nonantigen-specific low-molecular-weight proteins that mediate cellular interactions involving immune, inflammatory, and hematopoietic systems.

2. Cytokines exhibit properties of pleiotropy and redundancy and often display synergism or antagonism with other cytokines.

3. Cytokines are short-lived and may act locally either on the same cell that secreted it (autocrine), on other cells (paracrine), or, like hormones, they may act systemically (endocrine).

4. Cytokines have a wide variety of functional activities as illustrated by their ability to (1) regulate specific immune responses; (2) facilitate innate immune responses; (3) activate inflammatory responses; (4) affect leukocyte movement; and, (5) stimulate hematopoiesis.

5. Subsets of CD4$^+$ T$_H$ cells have been defined by the range of cytokines they produce. T$_H$1 cells secrete IL-2 and IFN-γ (as well as several other cytokines), but not IL-4 or IL-5. Cytokines produced by T$_H$1 cells activate other T cells, NK cells, and macrophages (cell-mediated immune responses). By contrast, T$_H$2 cells secrete IL-4 and IL-5 (as well as other cytokines), but not IL-2 or IFN-γ. Cytokines produced by T$_H$2 cells predominantly affect antibody responses.

6. Cytokines can only act on target cells that express receptors for that cytokine. Cytokine receptor expression is highly regulated such that resting cells either do not express a given receptor or express a low- or intermediate-affinity version of that receptor. Increased levels of cytokine receptor expression or expression of high-affinity forms of a given receptor predispose target cells to respond to a cytokine.

7. Class I cytokine receptors (also known as the hematopoietin receptor family) are usually composed of two types of polypeptide chains: a cytokine-specific subunit (α chain) and a signal-transducing subunit (β or γ chain). Most cytokines, identified to date, including IL-2, IL-4, G-CSF and GM-CSF, utilize the class I family of cytokine receptors.

8. The cytokine receptor γ subunit is utilized by several cytokine receptors as the signal transducing subunit—a structural feature that helps to explain the redundancy and antagonism often exhibited by some cytokines.

9. Ligation of class I and class II cytokine receptors by cytokines generates intracellular signals that result in the production of active transcription factors and, ultimately, gene expression. Binding of a cytokine to its cellular receptor induces dimerization or polymerization of receptor polypeptides at the cell surface and permits association of JAK kinases with the receptor cytoplasmic domain. This association activates the kinases and causes phosphorylation of tyrosine residues in STATs (signal transducers and activators of transcription). Once phosphorylated, the STAT transcription factors dimerize and subsequently translocate from the cytoplasm to the nucleus where they bind to enhancer regions of genes induced by the cytokine.

10. Overexpression or underexpression of cytokines or cytokine receptors have been implicated in several diseases including bacterial toxic shock, bacterial sepsis, certain lymphoid and myeloid cancers, and autoimmunity.

11. Cytokine-related therapies offer promise for the treatment of certain immunodeficiencies, in preventing graft rejection, and in treating cetrain cancers. The utility of cytokine-related therapies is best seen in the use of: (a) hematopoietic growth factors (G–CSF, GM–CSF) to reverse certain cellular deficiencies associated with chemo- or radiotherapy; (b) the use of anti-IL-2 receptor therapy to help reduce graft rejection; and (c) the use of IL-2 to generate lymphokine-activated killer cells (NK and cytotoxic T cells) employed in the treatment of patients with certain cancers.

REFERENCES

Cocchi RI, DeVico AL, Garzino-Demo A, Arya SK, Gallo RC, Lusso P (1995): Identification of RANTES,MIP-1α and MIP-1β as the major HIV-suppressive factors produced by CD8[+] T cells. *Science* 270:1811.

Hogg N, Landis RC (1993): Adhesion molecules in cell membranes. *Curr Opin Immunol* 5: 383.

Ihle JN (1995): Cytokine receptor signaling. *Nature* 377:591.

Jain J, Loh C, Rao A. (1995): Transcriptional regulation of the IL-2 gene. *Curr Opin Immunol* 7:333.

Lindley IJD, Westwick J, Kunkel SL (1993): Nomenclature announcement: the chemokines. *Immunol Today* 14:24.

Minami Y, Kono T, Miyazaki T, Taniguchi T. (1993): The IL-2 receptor complex: its structure, function, and target genes. *Ann Rev Immunol* 11:245.

Picker LC (1994): Control of lymphocyte homing. *Curr Opin Immunol* 6:394.

Powrie F, Coffman RL (1993): Cytokine regulation of T cell function: potential for therapeutic intervention. *Immunol Today* 14:270.

Rubinstein M, Dinarello CA, Oppenheim JJ, Hertzhog P (1999): Recent advances in cytokines, cytokine receptors, and signal transduction. *Cytokine Growth Factor Rev* 9:175.

Springer TA (1994): Traffic signals for lymphocyte recirculation and leukocyte emigration: the multistep paradigm. *Cell* 76:301.

Taga T, Kishimoto T (1994): Signaling mechanisms through cytokine receptors that share signal transducing receptor components. *Curr Opin Immunol* 7:17.

Waldman H, Gililand LK, Cobbold SP, Lane G (1999): Immunotherapy. In Paul WE (ed): Fundamental Immunology, 4th ed. New York: Lipincott-Raven. Ward SG, Bacon K, Westwick J (1998): Chemokines and T lymphocytes: more than an attraction. *Immunity* 9:1.

REVIEW QUESTIONS

For each question, choose the ONE BEST answer or completion.

1. Which of the following statements regarding the functional properties of cytokines is *false*?

A) They typically have pleiotropic properties.

B) They often exhibit functional redundancy.

C) They often display antigen specificity.

D) They exhibit synergistic or antagonistic properties.

E) They assist in the regulation and development of immune effector cells.

2. When IL-2 is secreted by antigen-specific T cells activated due to presentation of antigen by APCs, what happens to naive antigen-nonspecific T cells in the vicinity?

    A) They proliferate due to their exposure to IL-2.
    B) They often undergo apoptosis.
    C) They begin to express IL-2 receptors.
    D) They secrete cytokines associated with their T_H phenotype.
    E) Nothing happens.

3. Which of the following cytokines have receptors that exhibit structural similarity that helps to account for their functional redundancy?

    A) IL-3, IL-15, and GM–CSF
    B) IL-1, IL-2, and M–CSF
    C) IL-2, IL-3, and IL-8
    D) IL-3, TNF-β, and RANTES
    E) IL-3, IL-4, and IFN-γ

4. What type of immune response is *not* mediated by the T_H1 subset?

    A) responses to viral infections
    B) delayed-type hypersensitivity
    C) activation of cytotoxic T cells
    D) activation of IgE synthesis
    E) responses to intracellular pathogens

5. IL-1, IL-6, and TNF-α are proinflammatory cytokines that are known to

    A) cause increased vascular permeability.
    B) act in concert with chemokines to promote migration of inflammatory cells to sites of infection.
    C) initiate acute-phase responses.
    D) have endogenous pyrogen properties.
    E) All of the above.

6. Which of the following cytokines plays a role in terminating inflammatory responses?

    A) IL-2
    B) IL-4
    C) TGF-β
    D) IFN-α
    E) IL-3

7. All of the following are induced by the chemokine IL-8 *except*

    A) activation of neutrophils.
    B) attraction of neutrophils to sites of tissue damage.
    C) wound healing.
    D) extravasation of neutrophils.
    E) reduction of cytokine production by T_H1 cells.

8. Superantigens cause a burst of cytokine production by T cells due to their ability to

    A) crosslink the Vβ segments of T cell receptors with class II MHC molecules on APCs.
    B) crosslink the Vα segments of T cell receptors with class II MHC molecules on APCs.
    C) crosslink T cell receptors and CD3.
    D) crosslink multiple cytokine receptors on a large population of T cells.
    E) crosslink CD3.

Case Study

A 7-year-old boy with an infected wound on his leg is admitted to the emergency department. His mother states that a high fever with diarrhea occurred during the last 12 hours. Within the last 2 hours he had become very lethargic, was unable to stand, and was very disoriented. The attending physician observes that his blood pressure is dangerously low and suspects that the boy is suffering from bacterial septic shock caused by the wound infection. Discuss the etiology of bacterial septic shock as well as the role of cytokines in the pathogenesis of this disease. Speculate on future therapeutic strategies that might be employed by using monoclonal antibodies or other biologic agents to treat this disease.

Answers to Review Questions

1. *C* Cytokines secreted by a single lymphocyte following antigen-specific activation do not exhibit antigen specificity. Instead, they regulate the activities of other cells involved in an immune response by binding to cytokine receptors expressed by these cells.

2. *E* Since these cells have not been activated by antigen, they do not express the high affinity IL-2 receptor. Hence they remain quiescent.

3. *A* The receptors for IL-3, IL-5, and GM-CSF contain the common γ chain, which is responsible for signal transduction. Therefore, cytokine binding to each of these receptors probably induces a similar activation signal.

4. *D* The T_H1 subset is responsible for classical cell-mediated functions (answers A, B, C, and E). Synthesis of IgE is mediated by cytokines produced by T_H2 cells.

5. *E* The answer is self-explanatory.

6. *C* Among the cytokines listed, TGF-β plays a role in terminating inflammatory responses by promoting the accumulation and proliferation of fibroblasts and the deposition of extracellular matrix proteins required for tissue repair.

7. *E* IL-8 chemotactically attracts and activates neutrophils and induces their adherence to vascular endothelium. Thus, IL-8 also plays an important role in wound healing. It also promotes their extravasation into tissues. It plays no role in regulation of cytokine production by T_H1 cells—a biologic property ascribed to IL-10 produced by T_H2 cells.

8. *A* Superantigens bind simultaneously to class II MHC molecules and to the Vβ domain of the T cell receptor activating all T cells bearing a particular Vβ domain. Thus, they activate large numbers of T cells (between 5% and 25%), regardless of their antigen specificity causing them to release harmful quantities of cytokines.

Answer to Case Study

Bacterial septic shock is a condition that can develop within a few hours following infection by certain gram-negative bacteria, including *Escherichia coli, Klebsiella pneumonia, Pseudomonas aeruginosa, Enterobacter aerogenes,* and *Neisseria meningitidis.* The symptoms are often fatal and include a drop in blood pressure, fever, diarrhea, and widespread blood clotting in various organs. It develops when bacterial cell wall endotoxins stimulate macrophages to overproduce IL-1 and TNF-α. Therapeutic strategies using monoclonal antibodies capable of neutralizing the effects of IL-1 and TNF-α or antagonists such as IL-1 receptor antagonist (IL-1Ra) may offer hope for the treatment of bacterial septic shock in humans.

13

COMPLEMENT*

 INTRODUCTION

The complement system serves as an important effector arm of both innate and acquired immunity. ***Comprising over 30 circulating and membrane-fixed proteins, complement acts in a wide variety of host defense, inflammatory, homeostatic, and immune reactions.*** It was the ability of complement to kill certain bacteria that led to its discovery, and the ensuing years have been spent elucidating these mechanisms, purifying and characterizing the proteins and genes responsible, and learning more about the other roles that complement plays in an ever-increasing number of normal as well as abnormal physiologic processes.

 HISTORICAL BACKGROUND

In the late 1800s, scientists studying the reaction of the body to infection by bacteria noticed that if bacteria were injected into the circulation and blood was drawn at later time points, the bacteria disappeared rapidly. In an effort to sort out the process of clearance, in 1888 Nuttall placed bacteria into freshly drawn defibrinated guinea pig blood and showed that the bactericidal activity was still present. Separation of the blood components defined the activity as a humoral rather than cellular process, and, in 1889, led Buchner to propose a theory of immunity based on serum borne components he called ***alexin*** derived from the Greek for "to ward off."

At the same time, current studies suggested that immunized and "normal" animals differed in their responses to bacterial challenge. In 1894, Pfeiffer and Issaeff injected *Vibrio cholera* intraperitoneally into guinea pigs and observed that animals that had survived a previous infection rapidly killed the bacteria, whereas normal

*Contributed by Patricia C. Giclas, National Jewish Medical & Research Center, Denver, CO.

animals were overcome by the same number of bacteria. Heating the serum from the immunized animals destroyed its antibacterial activity in vitro, but the heated serum still conferred immunity when given to normal animals. The heat-stable immune factors were shown to be antibodies, but the heat-labile alexin activity present in normal serum was required to kill the bacteria. Paul Ehrlich suggested that antibodies could bind both antigen and alexin, allowing the combination to kill the cell bearing the antigen. He proposed that the name ***complement*** replace the previous designation, alexin, to denote that the activity described "complemented" the action of the antibodies.

During the first half of the twentieth century, several laboratories devoted their efforts to purifying complement components. As they were purified, the components were designated by the symbol C', for complement, with a digit denoting the order of their discovery.[1] The early proteins were defined in terms of their activities rather than their biochemical purity, and many of the first to be described were crude mixtures.

The first nine components of complement were perceived as individual proteins with the designations C1, C4, C2, C3, C5, C6, C7, C8, and C9. As we now know, these proteins comprise the ***classical pathway*** of complement activation, so called because it was the first to be worked out.

By the early 1980s the proteins of the ***alternative pathway*** had been purified, and it was possible to reconstruct a functional pathway using only the purified components. The known sequence of activation for the alternative pathway was C3b, also known as $C3 \cdot H_2O$, factor B, factor D, properdin, and the same late components shared by the classical pathway: C3, C5, C6, C7, C8, and C9. There are still unresolved questions as to the exact requirements for alternative pathway initiation and propagation of the amplification loop that allows for the efficient cleavage of C3 characteristic of alternative pathway activation.

In the last ten years, a new pathway has been added to the classical and the alternative. It has been known for some time that ***under certain conditions the C1 activation step can be bypassed and yet activation of C2, C4, and the late components can still occur***. A protein with structure very similar to C1q was known by its ability to bind to mannan–Sepharose, but little was known of its function. Kawasaki and his coworkers showed that this ***mannose-binding lectin (MBL) can activate the classical pathway of complement in the absence of C1q***, and since that time two other proteins have been found that have been named ***MASPs***, for ***MBL-associated serine proteases***. Much is still to be discovered about this new pathway and its role in the complement system. Table 13.1 lists the known complement proteins that can be found in the circulation.

 ## THE ACTIVATION PATHWAYS AND THEIR PROTEINS

Complement activation can be thought of as a three-step process: 1) recognition, 2) enzyme activation, and 3) expression of biologic activities. Each pathway (Figure 13.1) has unique proteins and enzymes for the first two steps, but the activities that result are the same for all three. It is important to remember that complement acti-

---

[1]The prime symbol (') was dropped by a World Health Organization committee on nomenclature in 1976.

TABLE 13.1. Components of the Human Complement System

Component symbol	Concentration in plasma (μg/ml)	Molecular weight (dalton)	Number of chains in native form	Associated pathway*	Enzymatic activity
C1q	180	462,000	18 (6 ea A, B, C)	CP	No
C1r	100	92,000	1	CP	Yes
C1s	110	86,000	1	CP	Yes
C2	25	117,000	1	CP, MBL	Yes
C4	640	206,000	3	CP, MBL	Cofactor
C3	1200	185,000	2	CP, MBL, AP	Cofactor
C5	80	180,000	2	Terminal	Cofactor
C6	75	120,000	1	Terminal	Yes?
C7	55	110,000	1	Terminal	No
C8	80	163,000	3	Terminal	No
C9	50	71,000	1	Terminal	No
MBL (mannan-binding lectin)	0.1–5	540,000	18	MBL	No
MASP$_1$	ND	94,000	1	MBL	Yes
MASP$_2$	ND	90,000	1	MBL	Yes
C3b or C3·H$_2$O	Trace	170,000	2	AP	Cofactor
D (factor D)	2	25,000	1	AP	Yes
B (factor B)	200	93,000	1	AP	Yes
P (properdin)	25	220,000		AP	No
C1-inhibitor	25	110,000	1	CP control	No
Factor I (I, C3b-Ina, KAF)	35	88,000	1	Control, all pathways	Yes
H (factor H, β1H)	500	150,000	1	AP control	Cofactor
C4-binding protein	250	550,000	7	CP control	Cofactor
CFI (CPB-N)	35	310,000	1	Control	Yes
SP40,40	50	80,000	1	Terminal control	No
S (vitronectin)	500	83,000	1	Terminal control	No
C4a	1.6	12,000		CP split prod.	No
C4d	8.9	30,000		CP split prod.	No
C3a	0.6	11,000		TP split prod.	No
iC3b	8.5	170,000		TP split prod.	No
C5a	0.01	11,000		TP split prod.	No
Bb	0.4	60,000		AP split prod.	No
SC5b-9 TCC	0.3	>1,000,000		Terminal C complex	No

*CP, classical pathway; MBL, mannose-binding lectin pathway; AP, alternate pathway; TP, terminal pathway.

vation is a dynamic process with many interactive steps between the components of the different pathways and with other plasma or cell-derived enzyme systems, as well. Although some compounds activate predominantly one pathway, others may involve several different routes, including mechanisms outside the complement system. A list of some of the complement activators is given in Table 13.2.

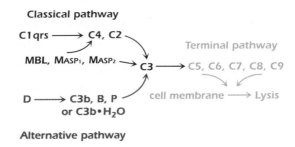

Figure 13.1. Complement activation pathways.

The Classical Pathway

Initiation of the classical pathway occurs when C1 (Clq-r$_2$s$_2$) binds to an activating substance such as an antigen–antibody complex. Clq-r$_2$s$_2$ requires eight Ca^{2+} ions to remain complexed and can be dissociated by ethylenediamine tetraacetic acid (EDTA), ethyleneglycoltetraacetic acid (EGTA), citrate, or other calcium chelators used as anticoagulants. Free Clq can bind to immunoglobulins or other activators, but without the Clr$_2$s$_2$, no activation occurs.

TABLE 13.2. Substances That Activate Human Complement

Substance	C Pathway activated
Antigen–antibody complexes	Classical
β Amyloid (Alzheimer's plaques)	Classical
DNA, polyinosinic acid	Classical
Polyanion–polycation complexes (heparin–protamine)	Classical
C-reactive protein complexes	Classical
Enveloped viruses (some)	Classical
Monosodium urate crystals	Classical
Lipid A of bacterial lipopolysaccharide	Classical
Plicatic acid (from Western red cedar)	Classical
Ant venom polysaccharide	Classical
Mannose-rich bacterial cell walls, etc.	MBL
Inulin	Alternative
Yeast cell walls (zymosan)	Alternative
Sephadex	Alternative
Endotoxin (bacterial lipopolysaccharide)	Alternative
Rabbit erythrocytes	Alternative
Desialylated human erythrocytes	Alternative
Cobra venom factor (CVF)	Alternative
Phosphorothioate backbone oligonucleotides	Alternative
Aggregated immunoglobulins	Classical and alternative
Subcellular membranes (mitochondria)	Classical and alternative
Cell- and plasma-derived enzymes	Classical, alternative, terminal
Plasmin, kallikrein	
Activated Hageman factor (XII)	
Neutrophil elastase, cathepsins	

Binding of C1q to immunoglobulins (Figure 13.2) is through ionic and hydrophobic bonds between the globular head regions of C1q and the Fc region of the immunoglobulin, so the binding is affected by ionic strength: raising the ionic strength above physiologic levels will dissociate the interaction, while decreasing it promotes stronger binding. It requires one IgM molecule bound to antigen, or two closely spaced antigen-bound IgG molecules for the $C1q\text{-}r_2s_2$ to bind in a stable enough configuration to allow C1 activation. Among the human immunoglobulins, the order of ability to bind and activate C1 is IgM > IgG3 > IgG1 $\gg$ IgG2. IgG4, IgA, IgE, and IgD do not bind or activate C1. When two or more C1q globular heads bind to antibodies or other activating substances, the resultant conformational change in $C1q\text{-}r_2s_2$ is reflected in the binding of C1q to $C1r_2s_2$, so that C1r is "released" from constraint and autoactivates to its active enzyme state. It can then cleave C1s to form the enzyme $\overline{C1s}$ (C1-esterase).[2] $\overline{C1s}$ cleaves the N-terminal α-chain of C4 to produce the two fragments C4a and C4b (see Figure 13.3A).

Among serum proteins, only C4, C3, and α_2-macroglobulin possess an internal thiolester bond that allows them to form covalent bonds when activated. The importance of the thiolester will be discussed later. During the activation process, approximately 10% of the C4b binds covalently to the surface of the activating substance and provides a Mg^{2+}-dependent binding site for C2, which can then be cleaved by $\overline{C1s}$ (Figure 13.3B). The C2a fragment formed by this cleavage remains bound to the C4b and contains a protease domain that is expressed in the $\overline{C4b2a}$ complex. This enzyme is the classical pathway **C3 convertase**.

C1 activation is very tightly controlled (Figure 13.4). C1 activity is limited by C1-esterase inhibitor (C1INH or C1-Ina), a member of the serpin (*ser*ine *p*rotease *in*hibitor) superfamily. C1INH forms complexes with $\overline{C1r}$ and $\overline{C1s}$ (Figure 13.5), which are rapidly cleared from the circulation by cells of the reticuloendothelial system. C4a is rapidly inactivated by serum carboxypeptidase N.

$\overline{C4b2a}$ control is effected by C4b-binding protein (C4bp), a member of the **r**egulators of **c**omplement **a**ctivation (RCA) superfamily of proteins. C4bp first binds to $\overline{C4b2a}$, displacing the C2a enzyme moiety, and then acting as a cofactor for factor I-mediated cleavage of the C4b-α' chain as depicted in Figure 13.6. The result of the first cleavage of C4b by factor I is the molecule iC4b, while the second cleavage results in two new fragments: C4c and C4d. Neither iC4b nor the further breakdown products can bind to another C2 molecule and so are hemolytically inactive, but iC4b and C4d are still able to bind to the complement receptors, CR3 (iC3b receptor) and CR2 (C3d,g receptor), respectively. CR1 (C3b -receptor) and membrane cofactor protein (MCP) can serve the same function on cell surfaces as fluid phase C4bp, and decay accelerating factor (DAF) on cells can dissociate $\overline{C4b2a}$, but does not have cofactor activity for factor I. The control of $\overline{C4b2a}$ is complete within 2 to 5 minutes after the initiation of C1 activation in normal serum.

The Lectin Pathway

The lectin pathway is thought to be similar to the classical pathway: MBL binds to carbohydrate residues on the surface of the activating bacteria or other substance and undergoes a conformational change similar to what happens with C1q. MASP1

---

[2]In complement nomenclature, a bar over the symbol for the component indicates the active form of the enzyme: e.g., C1s represents the proenzyme form, and $\overline{C1s}$ represents the active C1-esterase.

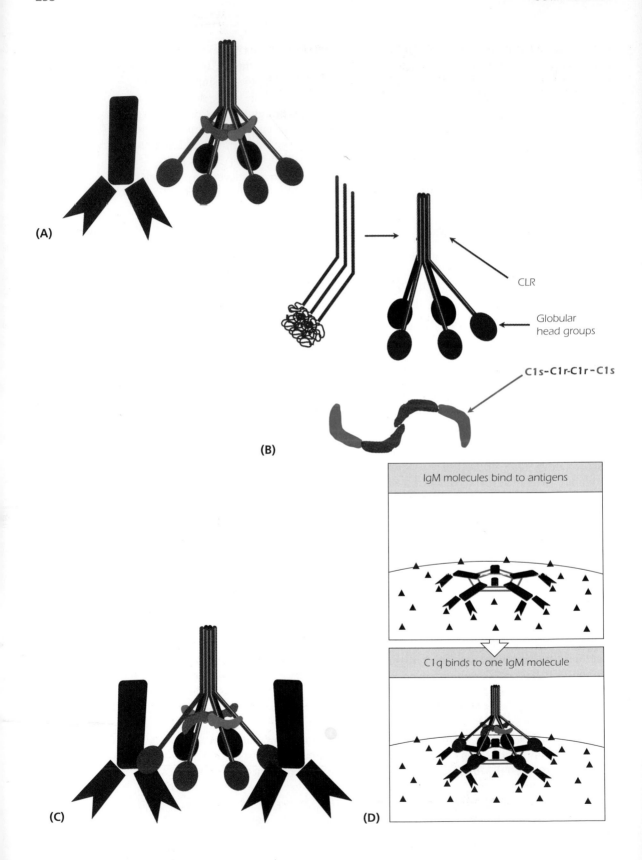

(A)

CLR

Globular
head groups

C1s-C1r-C1r-C1s

(B)

IgM molecules bind to antigens

C1q binds to one IgM molecule

(C)

(D)

becomes active and cleaves C4 and C2 to form $\overline{C4b2a}$, whereas MASP2 appears to be able to cleave C3 directly. More will be learned about this pathway and its control mechanisms during the next few years as experiments are performed using purified components.

The Alternative Pathway

Initiation of alternative pathway activation requires the presence of preformed C3b, or of a form of C3 variably known as "C3b-like C3" or "C3·H₂O," along with factors B and D. Like C4, C3 contains an internal thiolester bond that in the native protein is not exposed to nucleophile attack. There is a slow process called "C3-tickover" in which a few molecules of C3 undergo a spontaneous conformational change that allows water molecules from the external milieu to gain access to the highly reactive thiolester, hydrolyzing the metastable bond (C3*) and forming C3·H₂O. If the C3* is near enough to a suitable acceptor molecule when this conformational change occurs, it can bind to the activator surface instead of water, and form a nucleus for alternative pathway activation.

Figure 13.7 illustrates the molecules and steps required for the alternative pathway. C3·H₂O exhibits the properties of C3b in that it can bind factor B and promote its cleavage by factor D. Preformed C3b, which binds B more efficiently, is created whenever C3 is cleaved by ongoing complement activation or by proteases derived from the coagulation pathways, from inflammatory cells or bacteria. Factor D can cleave B only when the B is bound to $\overline{C3b}$ or $\overline{C3·H_2O}$, and the resulting enzyme, C3bBb (C3·H₂OBb), is the alternative pathway C3 convertase.

The name "C3 convertase" was chosen because, after activation, the electrophoretic mobility of C3 (β-1C) is "converted" to a faster migrating form (β-1A) that we now know as C3c.

Control of the alternative pathway occurs at several levels, as shown in Figure 13.8. The short half-life of C3b* forms a limiting mechanism so that most of the C3 that is cleaved becomes inactive C3bi (i for inactive) in the fluid phase. C3b* has a half-life of about 100 μs. Like C4b, only about 10% of the C3b that is produced becomes bound to the surface of the activator.

←──

Figure 13.2. Interaction of C1 with immunoglobulins. **(A)** The C1 complex is made up of three kinds of subunits: C1q, C1r, and C1s. In each C1qrs complex, there are two molecules each of C1r and C1s, and one of C1q. C1q is produced from six identical subunits, each of which is made of three similar strands. **(B)** Each subunit has a collagen-like tail portion (CLR), and a flexible arm region that ends in a globular head unit. C1r and C1s are single-chain proenzymes that form a tetrameric complex. **(C)** Once the C1q complex has bridged two or more IgG molecules, it undergoes a conformational change that releases C1r and C1s from constraint. **(D)** Unlike IgG, which requires two or more bound antibodies to activate C1, one IgM molecule can bind and activate the C1qrs complex. The C1q binds to the IgM across the joining region of the pentamer, and is thought to be most efficient when the antibody F(ab) regions are bound to the antigen and the Fc-J region is sticking out.

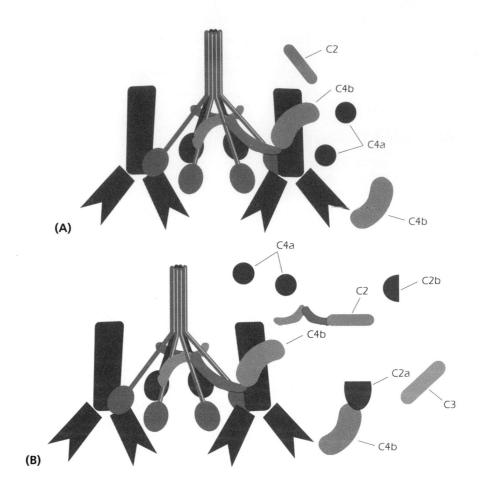

Figure 13.3. Cleavage of C4 and C2 and formation of the classical pathway C3 convertase. **(A)** C4b can form covalent bonds with molecules that are near it when it is formed. This allows it to bind to all kinds of surfaces, including the immune complex or antigen, or another nearby molecule. C4b also participates in the formation of the classical pathway C3 convertase, C4b2a. **(B)** C2b is the smaller fragment of C2, and it may contain the sequence responsible for the C2-kinin activity associated with hereditary angioedema. C2a is the larger fragment, and it contains a serine esterase active site. In order for C2a to act, it must be bound to C4b, and the C4b2a complex is the C3 convertase of the classical pathway.

Two competing mechanisms exist for controlling the activity of $\overline{\text{C3bBb}}$. The first of these (Figure 13.9) is through downregulation in much the same manner as was described for C4b2a: factor H, another member of the RCA family, binds to C3b and displaces Bb. H then serves as a cofactor for cleavage of C3b by factor I, and the resulting fragments, iC3b, C3c, and C3d, are unable to participate in the lytic pathway. As with the inactivation of C4b, the membrane proteins MCP and CR1 can also serve as cofactors for factor I-mediated cleavage of C3b, and DAF can dissociate the $\overline{\text{C3bBb}}$ enzyme complex.

The alternative pathway also has a unique upregulating mechanism that gives it the ability to establish a highly efficient amplification loop (C3-feedback loop

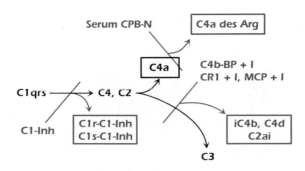

Figure 13.4. Control of the classical pathway.

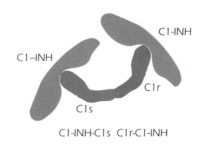

Figure 13.5. Inactivation of C1r and C1s by C1-inhibitor. The active site of C1-INH contains a sequence similar to that recognized by C1r and C1s.

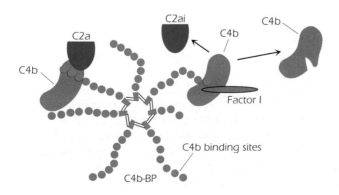

Figure 13.6. Dissociation of C4b2a and inactivation of C4b by C4b-BP and Factor I. C4-binding protein is a spiderlike molecule with 7 arms.

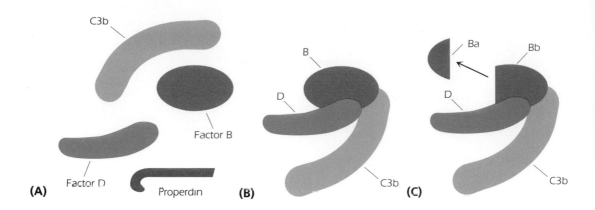

Figure 13.7. Alternative pathway activation. **(A)** The alternative pathway (AP) requires three factors analogous to the classical pathway: Factor D is the equivalent of C1s, factor B is the equivalent of C2, and C3b (C3·H$_2$O, or C3b-like C3) takes the place of C4b. Properdin, unique to the alternative pathway, is required for efficient C3 convertase activity. **(B)** The first step in AP activation occurs when factor B binds to C3b. **(C)** Factor D cleaves the C3b-bound factor B. The Ba fragment is released to the fluid phase, and Bb stays bound to the C3b. C3bBb is the alternative pathway C3 convertase, with the enzymatic activity is in the Bb fragment.

shown in Figure 13.10). Under certain still-undefined conditions related to the surface of the activating substance, properdin can bind to the $\overline{\text{C3bBb}}$ enzyme complex and prevent its dissociation by RCA proteins (Figure 13.11). The $\overline{\text{C3bBbP}}$ complex has a longer half-life than $\overline{\text{C3bBb}}$, and much more C3b is generated in a short time. This provides additional C3b to which factor B can bind, and the activation process continues almost explosively.

Activation of C3 is the central step in all of the complement pathways and the point at which they converge. The structure of C3 is shown by the diagram in Figure 13.12. ***The C3 convertase-mediated cleavage of the C3-α chain creates two fragments: the smaller C3a is a fluid phase anaphylatoxin with proinflammatory properties, while the larger C3b has multiple roles in host defense, inflammation, and immune regulation as well as continuation of the complement-activation cascade.***

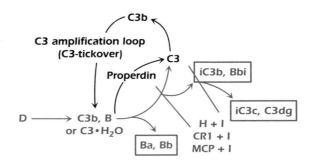

Figure 13.8. Control of the alternative pathway.

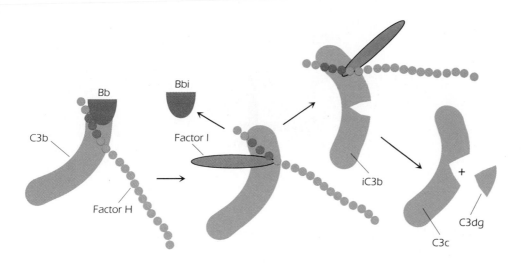

Figure 13.9. Control of the alternative pathway by factors H and I. Factor H binds to C3bBb and displaces the Bb. H acts as a cofactor for I, which cleaves C3b once to produce iC3b, or twice to produce C3c and C3dg. CR1 and MCP can also act as cofactors for I.

The binding of C3b to acceptor carbohydrate or protein molecules was thought for a long time to be random, but recent experiments have shown that there are a limited number of residues to which the thiolester will bind. One result of the short half-life of C3b* is that the C3b deposited on surfaces tends to be located in clusters around the activating enzyme, and some will bind to the C4b or C3b of the enzyme itself. This extra C3b converts the specificity of the C3 convertase to that of C5 convertase by providing a site for C5 to bind to the enzyme: $\overline{C4b2a3b}$, $\overline{C3bBb3b}$ (Figure 13.13).

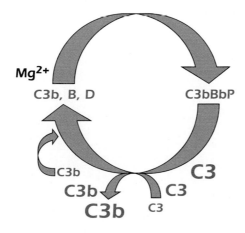

Figure 13.10. The C3 feedback loop.

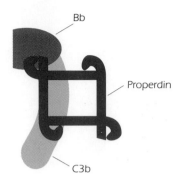

Figure 13.11. Role of properdin. Properdin stabilizes the alternative pathway C3–convertase by binding to C3bBb.

The Terminal Pathway

Cleavage of C5 (Figure 13.14) produces two fragments: C5a has potent anaphyla-toxin properties and is strongly chemotactic for neutrophils and other inflammatory cells, and C5b forms the nucleus for formation of the membrane attack complex (MAC) consisting of complement components C5b-9. MAC can lead to lysis or to formation of the fluid phase terminal complement complex.

The first step in MAC formation occurs when C6 binds to the C5b-α' chain. C7 appears to bind to the C5b-α' chain, as well. C5b67 has affinity for membrane lipid, but the structure at this stage of insertion into the membrane has no lytic capability. The C5b portion is available to aqueous phase probes, while the C6 and C7 appear to be inserted into the outer membrane leaflet. When C8 binds to the C5b67 complex, conformational changes in the C8-α chain allow the complex to penetrate deeper into the lipid bilayer. The C8 can be identified by lipid-soluble labeling methods as the primary membrane-perturbing component.

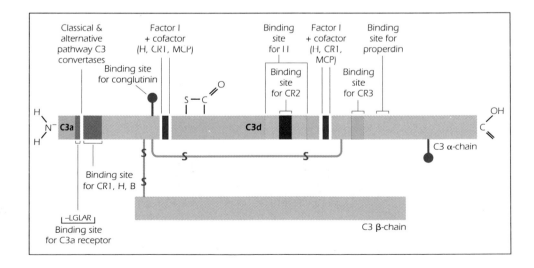

Figure 13.12. Structure and important features of C3.

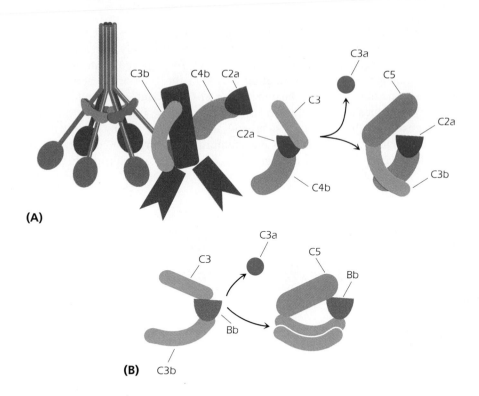

Figure 13.13. Formation of the C5 convertase. **(A)** Cleavage of C3 by either convertase produces newly formed C3b molecules that can bind to the convertase itself, giving the convertase a binding site for C5. The classical pathway C5-convertase is C4b2a3b. **(B)** The alternative pathway C3 convertase is C3bBbC3b.

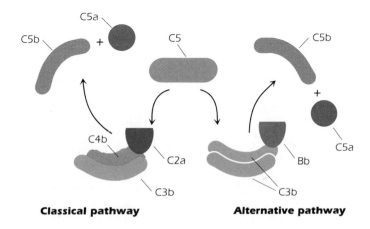

Classical pathway **Alternative pathway**

Figure 13.14. Cleavage of C5 and generation of C5a and C5b.

The C5b-8 complex on a cell membrane serves as a receptor for C9, which binds to the C8-α chain and then unfolds and inserts even more deeply into the membrane. Additional C9 molecules interact with the first to form poly-C9 through C9–C9 interactions. Changes in the conformation of C9 in the membrane attack complex have been demonstrated through the appearance of C9 neoantigenic epitopes, altered susceptibility to proteases, and ultrastructural changes. The lipid bilayer surrounding a MAC is unstable, allowing ions to escape and water to enter the cell that then undergoes osmotic lysis or reacts to the membrane perturbation in various ways, including eliminating the MACs through endo- or ectocytosis. Steps in the formation of the MAC are shown in Figure 13.15.

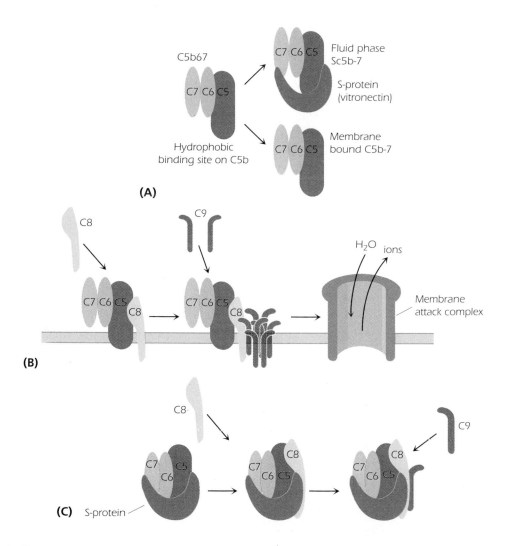

Figure 13.15. The membrane attack complex (MAC) and SC5b-9. (A) C5b, C6, and C7 form a complex that can bind to nearby membranes or to S protein or SP40,40 in the fluid phase. (B) On the cell membrane, the binding of C8 and C9 leads to penetration of the lipid bylayer and destabilization of the membrane integrity. (C) In the fluid phase, S protein or SP40,40 serve as controls for innocent bystander lysis.

The sequential assembly of the MAC provides several steps where regulatory components can interact to prevent damage to "innocent bystander" cells surrounding the area of complement activation. Because the association of C5b with nearby membranes is relatively nonspecific, there are fluid phase and membrane-associated control mechanisms, diagrammed in Figure 13.16, that prevent lysis or damage to cells of self-origin that might otherwise be damaged by "reactive lysis" or "innocent bystander lysis" when complement activation occurs in their vicinity.

One factor that functions to prevent reactive lysis is the surface protein CD59. CD59 is attached to the cell membrane by a glycosylphosphotidylinositol anchor (GPI anchor), and binds to C5b-8 on the cell surface, preventing C9 from polymerizing. A similar widely distributed membrane protein with MAC inhibitory activity called homologous restriction factor (HRF) acts by binding to C8 and C9 and prevents their insertion into the cell membrane.

In the fluid phase, S-protein (vitronectin) or SP-40,40 (clusterin) bind to the hydrophobic regions of C5b6, C5b67, C5b-8, and C5b-9, and prevent interaction with membranes. These soluble forms of C5b complexes can be identified in the circulation after complement activation occurs.

Complement Control Proteins

*The regulators of complement activation (**RCA**) include fluid phase protein factors H and C4bp, along with cell-surface proteins decay accelerating factor (**DAF**), membrane cofactor protein (MCP) and complement receptors 1 and 2 (**CR1, CR2**).* CR1, CR2, DAF, and MCP are RCA membrane proteins found on a wide variety of cells. CR1 (CD35) is the 220-kDa C3b/C4b receptor found on erythrocytes, monocytes, macrophages, eosinophils, neutrophils, B cells, some T cells, follicular dendritic cells, and mast cells. It can also bind to iC3b and C3c, though with lower affinity. CR1 has both decay accelerating and cofactor activities as shown in Figure 13.17. A soluble recombinant form of CR1 (sCR1) has been made by deletion of the transmembrane segment of the protein. This recombinant protein, which has cofactor activity for factor I, is undergoing clinical testing for efficacy as an inhibitor in a variety of inflammatory disorders.

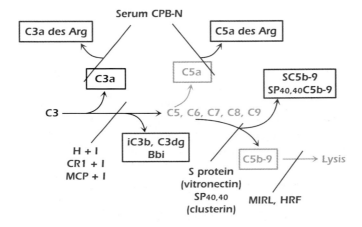

Figure 13.16. Control of the terminal pathway.

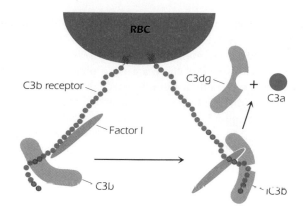

Figure 13.17. Role of the C3b receptor (CR1).

CR2 (CD21) is a 140-kDa membrane glycoprotein expressed on late premature and mature B lymphocytes, some T cells, including thymocytes, and follicular dendritic cells. The CR2 molecule binds C3b, iC3b, and C3d,g fragments of C3. CR2 does not have cofactor activity for factor I.

Other Complement Receptors

CR3 and CR4 are members of the integrin family of leukocyte adhesion molecules. CR3 was the first of these molecules to be described, and has been known by various other names: CD11b/CD18, Mac-1, Mo1, OKM-1, α-M/β-2. Another closely related member of this family, LFA-1 is not a complement receptor. CR3 is expressed on mononuclear phagocytes, natural killer (NK) cells, and granulocytes. It has diverse ligand-binding capability, including coagulation factor X, fibrinogen, lipopolysaccharide, zymosan, ICAM-1, and several bacterial surface molecules as well as iC3b. The number of CR3 molecules per cell is upregulated by inflammatory stimuli, including C3a and C5a, and CR3 facilitates binding of phagocytes to endothelial cells so that extravasation can occur when the cells are responding to a chemotactic signal.

CR4 is expressed on myeloid cells, dendritic cells, activated B cells, NK and some CTLs, and platelets. It has a broad ligand repertoire similar to that of CR3, with iC3b the predominant complement ligand. There is still some question whether this receptor serves primarily as a complement receptor, or if it has an alternative role to play in the inflammatory process.

C1q receptors have been described by several investigators. Of these, the C1qR$_P$ receptor is associated with phagocytosis of C1q- or mannose-binding lectin-coated particles. It is a type I membrane glycoprotein with the capability of transmitting cellular activation signals. The receptors for C3a and C5a have recently been identified as members of the rhodopsin superfamily of receptors, with seven membrane spanning segments coupled to a regulatory G-protein. The C5a receptor (C5aR, CD88) has homology (35%) with the formyl peptide receptor that reacts to N-formyl bacterial chemoattractants. The C3a receptor (C3aR) has a similar structure to the C5aR, with the exception of a large extracellular loop between the first and second transmembrane segments. There has been no receptor identified for C4a at the present time. C3aR and C5aR are widely distributed. C5aR can be found on granulocytes, platelets, mast cells, liver parenchymal cells, lung vascular smooth muscle, endothelium, bronchial and alveolar epithelial cells, and astrocytes and microglial cells in the brain. C3aR are located on platelets, mast cells, macrophages, neutrophils, basophils, eosinophils, monocytes, and endothelial cells. C3aR messenger RNA has also been identified in cells of the thymus, heart, liver, kidneys, colon, small intestine, placenta, testis, ovaries, and several regions of the brain. The widespread distribution of these two receptors suggests that there is a wealth of new information yet to be acquired about the roles of C3a and C5a in a variety of biologic functions.

BIOLOGIC ACTIVITIES OF COMPLEMENT

The complement system has many functions that protect the host. Primary among these is its ability to kill invading microorganisms directly or to enhance ingestion and killing by phagocytic cells. All three pathways are involved in initiating bacterial killing and opsonization, but the alternative pathway is the most efficient at the latter. Individuals that are missing one of the alternative pathway proteins (P, D, B), late components (C3–C9) or one of the control proteins (H or I) tend to get severe infections with pyogenic organisms. They are particularly susceptible to infection by *Neisseria* species, particularly *N. meningitidis*. Deficiencies of the classical pathway components (C1, C4, C2) are also associated with increased risk of infection, though not as strongly as with the alternative pathway or late component deficiencies. Bacteria associated with recurrent infections in these patients include, but are not limited to, *Streptococcus pneumoniae, Haemophilus influenzae*, and *Staphylococcus aureus*. Complement deficiencies are relatively rare (1 in 10,000 people), and are not always associated with disease, since many complement-deficient individuals are diagnosed only after a family member has been identified.

Complement also has the ability to neutralize viruses. C1 can bind directly to and become activated by the surface of several viruses, including the type C retroviruses, lentiviruses, HIV-1, and HTLV-1. MBL also binds and is activated by high mannose residues on the surfaces of HIV-1, HIV-2, and influenza virus. Antibodies against the viruses mediate further binding and activation of the classical pathway on the viral surface. Repeating subunits on the viral capsid or membrane surfaces also activates the alternative pathway. *The binding of complement proteins not only leads to opsonization of the virus and lysis of the virion, but it also interferes with its ability to interact with the membrane of its target cells, and thus blocks its entrance into the cell.*

Complement interaction with viruses has proved to be double-edged sword. While complement clearly plays a role in defense against viral infection, many viruses have evolved to take advantage of complement proteins, both for control of the deposition of complement on their surfaces and for gaining entry to the target cells. Paramyxoviruses (measles virus) use MCP as a receptor for entry into host cells; viruses of the picornavirus family likewise use DAF to infect epithelial cells. The Epstein-Barr virus uses CR2 to gain entry into mononuclear cells, and HIV-1 uses CR1, CR2, and CR3 to infect T cells, B cells, and monocytes. Another sneaky trick of viruses is to capture complement control proteins when the virions bud from host cell membranes. HIV-1, HTLV-1, simian immunodeficiency virus (SIV), and cytomegalovirus (CMV) capture DAF, MCP, and CD59 on their surfaces and are thus protected from complement-mediated lysis in the same way that host cells are protected. As one last ploy, several viruses produce viral proteins that mimic complement inhibitor function. The herpes viruses make several proteins that have DAF- and/or MCP-like activities, or that block C5b-9 formation, and vaccinia virus produces vaccinia control protein (VCP) that contains 4 CCP domains, binds to C3b and C4b and has both decay-accelerating and cofactor activities.

Complement plays a protective role in reproduction. Functional complement is present in the female reproductive tract, and tissues and gametes have abundant regulatory proteins. Spermatozoa are also protected from complement attack by MCP, DAF, and CD59. C3 is secreted by the uterus in response to estrogen, and secretion is blocked by progesterone. MCP, DAF, and CD59 are expressed on trophoblasts early in gestation. MCP and DAF are located variably on fetal tissues, while CD59 is present on all tissues throughout pregnancy. Tissues at the maternal–fetal interface are particularly rich in complement regulatory proteins.

Another very important function of complement is controlling the formation and clearance of immune complexes, as shown in Figure 13.18. When antibodies bind to their appropriate antigens, crosslinking between the molecules and Fc–Fc interactions tend to make the complexes increase in size until they become insoluble. Immunologists have long taken advantage of this property *in vitro* to identify antigens and antibodies by precipitating the immune complexes, either from solution or in agarose gels. *In vivo*, however, it is detrimental to the host for large insoluble complexes to form because they accumulate in tissues such as the skin and kidneys where they cause inflammation and damage to the surrounding cells. Once several antibodies have bound to an antigen and become crosslinked, C1 activation occurs and C4b and C3b are deposited on the molecules of the complex. This has two effects: First, the incorporation of the relatively large complement proteins interferes with further binding of immunoglobulins, and second, the complex can now bind to C3 receptors and be removed from the circulation. If the complex becomes very large in spite of C1 activation, or if the immunoglobulin is of a class that does not bind C1, alternative pathway activation can occur with more C3b deposition. This

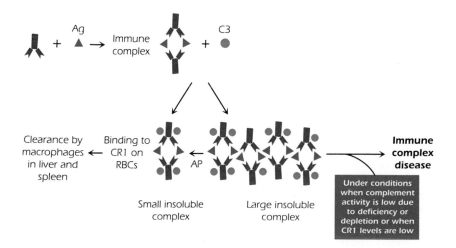

Figure 13.18. Role of complement in clearance of immune complexes.

C3b interferes with the bonding forces that keep the complex together and it starts to break up into smaller pieces that can be cleared by C3 receptors on the cells of the reticuloendothelial system.

One of the most important mechanisms in the clearance of immune complexes is mediated by the CR1 on erythrocytes. Although there are more CR1 molecules per cell on leukocytes, there are far more erythrocytes in the circulation and the majority of available CR1 is on these cells. Small soluble immune complexes with C3b on their surfaces become bound to the CR1 and are carried through the circulation to the liver and spleen. An exchange occurs in which the complex is transferred from the erythrocyte CR1 to macrophage CR3 and Fc receptors, taken into the phagocytes and destroyed. If there is a deficiency in the classical pathway components or CR1, large insoluble immune complexes can form—resulting in disease.

In addition to clearing immune complexes, complement aids the cleanup of debris, dead tissues, and foreign substances. Complement activation at an inflammatory site by membranes altered through oxidation, enzymatic activity, or expression of neoantigens leads to deposition of C4b and C3b that can interact with CR1 and CR3 on phagocytic cells. Subcellular membranes from mitochondria, endoplasmic reticulum, or other organelles directly activate both classical and alternative pathways, making them recognizable by phagocytic cells that have C3 receptors. Unlike cells killed by infection, ischemia, or other means, apoptotic cells do not activate complement.

The anaphylatoxin fragments of C3 and C5, C3a, and C5a, have many physiologic effects at the inflammatory site as shown in Figure 13.19 and 13.20. *C3a and C5a induce contraction in ileal, bronchial, uterine, and vascular smooth muscle in most species studied. Interaction of C3a and C5a with mast cells in the area also leads to the release of additional inflammatory mediators, including histamine.* The induction of vasodilation by these peptides acts to slow local blood flow and increase permeability of vessels. This allows a fresh supply of complement, coagulation, and other proteins from the circulation to permeate the inflamed tissues. Neutrophils and other inflammatory cells that have been attracted by the chemotactic factors and upregulated their surface integrin molecules, have an opportunity to slow down so that they come into better contact with the vessel wall, bind by way of the

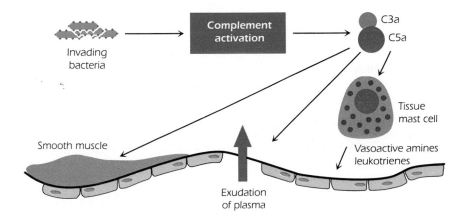

Figure 13.19. Role of complement in inflammation: the anaphylatoxins.

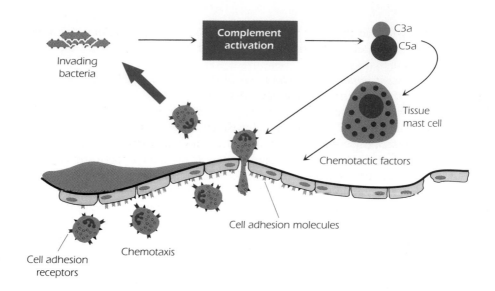

Figure 13.20. Role of complement in inflammation: chemotaxis.

adhesion molecules, and leave the circulation for the site of inflammation. C5a also interacts with monocytes and hepatocytes to cause the release of cytokines and other mediators. IL-6 and C5a induce the acute phase response. Serum carboxypeptidase N (SCP-N, chemotactic factor inactivator, CFI) rapidly cleaves the C-terminal arginine from C3a, C4a, and C5a. The des-Arg forms of the anaphylatoxins are unable to bind productively to their receptors, although $C5a_{des-Arg}$ retains about 2% of its previous chemotactic activity.

C3d,g covalently bound to antigen in immune complexes is taken up by CR2 in cells of the dendritic lineage, providing long-lasting deposits of antigen that stimulate B-cell responses and memory. If a complement-deficient animal is immunized with a T cell-dependent antigen, the immune response made to the antigen is impaired, and the switching of immunoglobulin from IgM to IgG does not occur unless the system is driven by very large amounts of antigen. Studies using strains of mice deficient in C3 or C4 have proved that the enhancing effect of complement on the acquired immune response is dependent on the amount of the components present: an animal that is heterozygous for a complement deficiency will have a response that is intermediate between a normal animal and one that has a complete deficiency.

The complement-dependent enhancement of the immune response is mediated by the binding of CR2 to C3d,g on the antigen, followed by crosslinking of the antigen through surface IgM on the B-cell surface. CR1 is often found with CR2 on the B cell and may bind C3b-bearing immune complexes that can then be processed to C3d,g by the action of factor I, and transferred to the CR2. Human CR2 is also found in a complex with CD19, CD81, and Leu-13 so that transmembrane signals are transmitted via phosphorylation of CD19 when CR2 and mIgM are crosslinked by the C3d,g antigen. Binding of C3d,g to the antigen also appears to alter the enzymatic digestion of the antigen as it is processed by antigen-presenting cells. Antigen-bound C3d appears to have an adjuvant effect, as well.

 ## COMPLEMENT AND DISEASE

There is involvement of complement in the pathogenesis of various disease processes, and complement deficiencies give particular susceptibility to infectious and autoimmune conditions. *Individuals deficient in C1, C4, or C2 have increased risk of developing systemic lupus erythematosus (SLE), although the actual disease presentation may vary somewhat from that of complement normal individuals. This predisposition for SLE appears to be the result of an impaired ability to process and clear immune complexes.* Because large insoluble immune complexes often accumulate along the basement membrane in the kidney, renal involvement is often a result of SLE.

As mentioned above, *patients with complement deficiencies of the alternative pathway and late components are susceptible to recurrent infections with pyogenic organisms. Deficiencies of factors H and I also lead to infections because C3 is depleted when there is uncontrolled activation of the alternative pathway.* There are other acquired conditions where C3 becomes depleted enough to make the patient susceptible to infection. Primary among these is the autoantibody called C3-nephritic factor (C3NeF) found in patients with SLE or partial lipodystrophy. C3NeF binds to the alternative pathway C3 convertase ($\overline{C3bBb}$) in a way that stabilizes it and produces a highly efficient and long-lived fluid phase convertase. If the condition persists, C3 levels can decrease enough to render the patient profoundly C3-deficient.

Deficiencies of the other control proteins also leads to disease. *Hereditary and acquired angioedema (HAE, AAE) result from C1INH deficiency.* Because C1INH is the only control protein for $\overline{C1r}$ and $\overline{C1s}$, uncontrolled cleavage of C2 and C4 results if C1INH levels are inadequate to block $\overline{C1s}$ activity. C1INH also controls the activities of plasmin, kallikrein, and factor XIIa, although it is not the only inhibitor of these enzymes. The actual mediator of edema formation in HAE is not known, but one candidate is a product of secondary C2b cleavage by plasmin, producing the putative C2-kinin. There is also evidence that bradykinin formation is abnormal in HAE patients and may be the cause of the edema formation. AAE results when C1INH levels decrease due to increased utilization. AAE may be a result of abnormal complement activation by lymphoma proteins or cell surface Ig, or by other lymphoproliferative or autoimmune disorders.

Paroxysmal nocturnal hemoglobinuria (PNH) is an uncommon acquired disorder that occurs primarily in young adults. It is characterized by chronic intravascular hemolysis that results in hemolytic anemia and nocturnal hemoglobinuria, venous thrombosis, and inability to produce viable erythrocytes. The condition is due to a somatic mutation in the gene that controls the production of the GPI anchor that attaches type I membrane proteins to the cell surface. This anchor is produced in the endoplasmic reticulum by multiple steps that end with the attachment to the appropriate proteins. The anchored protein is then transported from the Golgi apparatus to the cell surface. In PNH, the anchor is not made properly and the unattached proteins are secreted from the cell into the fluid phase. The defects identified to date are diverse, giving the patients a heterogeneous pattern of expression of cell surface markers. Affected proteins that have been described include DAF, CD59, the Fc-γ

receptor III, urokinase receptor, LFA-3, CAMPATH-1, erythrocyte acetylcholinesterase, and leukocyte alkaline phosphatase. The hemolytic symptoms result from the lysis of unprotected erythrocytes by complement, while the thrombosis may result from abnormal platelet activation by MAC on the platelet surface.

The complement system has been described as an important effector arm of innate and acquired immunity. Activation of complement occurs within a tightly regulated system containing multiple controls for critical steps, but still allows for appropriate amplification leading to the expression of biologic activities that help to protect the host. When the control processes become altered, or genetic deficiencies occur, then activation of the complement system can contribute to the pathogenesis of disease. With the development of modern molecular biologic methods and the increasing availability of transgenic and knockout mice, we will be able to study the impact of the complement proteins on all aspects of immunity. This new understanding of the complement system should also include the development of pharmaceutical agents that can be used to control inappropriate complement activation in human disease.

SUMMARY

1. Complement consists of a group of serum proteins that activate each other in an orderly fashion to generate biologically active molecules, such as enzymes, opsonins, anaphylatoxins, and chemotaxins.

2. Complement can be activated through three pathways: (a) the classical pathway that is initiated by antigen–antibody complexes, (b) the alternative pathway, in which complement components become activated by the cell walls of some bacteria and yeasts, in combination with several serum factors, and (c) the lectin pathway that activates the classical pathway of complement in the absence of C1q.

3. The activation through the classical pathway requires C1q for initiation; the alternative pathway requires C3b, serum factors B and D, and properdin; in the lectin pathway, mannose-binding lectin binds to carbohydrate residues on the surface of the activating bacteria or other substance and undergoes a conformational change similar to what happens with C1q.

4. The level of complement does not increase after immunization.

5. The activity of complement and its components is tightly regulated by various inhibitors including factors H and I.

6. Individuals deficient in C1, C4, or C2 have increased risk of developing systemic lupus erythematosus (SLE). Patients with complement deficiencies of the alternative pathway and late components are susceptible to recurrent infections with pyogenic organisms. Deficiencies of factors H and I also lead to infections because C3 becomes depleted because of uncontrolled activation of the alternative pathway.

REFERENCES

Coca AF (1914): A study of the anticomplementary action of yeast, of certain bacteria and of cobra venom. *Z Immunitaetsforsch* 21:604–622.

Cooper NR, Nemerow GR (1989): Complement and infectious agents: a tale of disguise and deception. *Complement Inflamm* 6:249–258.

Davis AE, III (1988): C1 inhibitor and hereditary angioneuroticedema. *Ann Rev Immunol* 6:595–628.

Fearon DT (1984): Cellular receptors for fragments of the third component of complement. *Immunol Today* 5:105–110.

Flexner S, Noguchi H (1902): Snake venom in relation to haemolysis, bacteriolysis and toxicity. *J Exp Med* 6:277–301.

Gštze O, Mÿller-Eberhard HJ (1971) The C3-activation system: an alternate pathway of complement activation. *J Exp Med* 134:90s–108s.

Hugli TE (1984): Structure and function of the anaphylatoxins. *Springer Semin Immunopathol* 7:193–219.

Ikeda K, Sannoh T, Kawasaki N, Kawasaki T, Yamashima I (1987): Serum lectin with known structure activates complement through the classical pathway. *J Biol Chem* 262:7451–7454.

Law SKA, Reid KBM (1995): Complement: In Rickwood D, Male D (eds): Focus Series, 2nd ed. Oxford, UK: Oxford University Press.

Lepow IH, Pillemer L, Schoenberg MD, Todd EW, Wedgwood RJ (1959): The properdin system and immunity. X. Characterization of partially purified properdin. *J Immunol* 83:428–436.

Marcus RL, Shin HS, Mayer MM (1971): An alternate complement pathway: C3-cleaving activity not due to C4,2a on endotoxic lipopolysaccharide after treatment with guinea pig serum; relation to properdin. *Proc Natl Acad Sci USA* 68:1351–1354.

Matsushita M, Fujita T (1992): Activation of the classical complement pathway by mannose-binding protein in association with a novel C1s-like serine protease. *J Exp Med* 176:1497–1502.

Mayer MM (1961): In Kabat and Mayer's Experimental Immunochemistry, 2nd ed. Springfield, IL: Charles C Thomas, pp133–240.

Mayer MM (1984): Complement: Historical perspectives and some current issues. *Complement* 1:2–26.

Morgan BP (1989): Complement membrane attack on nucleated cells: resistance, recovery and non-lethal effects. *Biochem J* 264:1–14.

Morgan BP (1990): Complement: Clinical Aspects and Relevance to Disease. New York: Academic Press.

Nelson Jr RA (1958): An alternative mechanism for the properdin system. *J Exp Med* 108:515–535.

Nelson Jr RA, Jensen J, Gigli I, Tamura N (1966): Methods for the separation, purification and measurement of nine components of hemolytic complement in guinea pig serum. *Immunochemistry* 3:111–135.

Pangburn MK, Müller-Eberhard HJ (1984): The alternative pathway of complement. *Springer Semin Immunopathol* 7:163–192.

Pillemer L, Blum L, Lepow IH, Ross OA, Todd EW, Wardlaw AC (1954): The properdin system and immunity: I. Demonstration and isolation of a new serum protein, properdin, and its role in immune phenomena. *Science* 120:279–285.

Ross, GD (1986): Immunobiology of the Complement System. New York: Academic Press.

Rother K, Till GO (1988): The Complement System. New York: Springer-Verlag.

Schifferli JA, Paccaud J-P (1989): Complement and its receptor: a physiological transport system for circulating immune complexes. *Contrib Nephrol* 69:1–8.

Schreiber RD (1984): The chemistry and biology of complement receptors. *Springer Semin Immunopathol* 7:221–249.

Volanakis JE, Frank MM (1998): The Human Complement System in Health and Disease. New York: Marcel Dekker.

Whaley K, Loos M, Weiler JM (1993): Complement in health and disease. *Immunol Med Ser* 20:166–194.

REVIEW QUESTIONS

For each question, choose the ONE BEST answer or completion.

1. A patient is admitted with multiple bacterial infections and is found to have a complete absence of C3. Which complement-mediated function would remain intact in such a patient?
   A) lysis of bacteria
   B) opsonization of bacteria
   C) generation of anaphylatoxins
   D) generation of neutrophil chemotactic factors
   E) None of the above.

2. Which of the following screening tests would be most useful for confirming a presumptive diagnosis of a congenital absence of a complement component?
   A) quantitation of serum opsonic activity
   B) quantitation of serum hemolytic activity
   C) quantitation of C3 content of serum
   D) quantitation of C1 content of serum
   E) electrophoretic analysis of patient's serum

3. Complement is required for
   A) lysis of erythrocytes by lecithinase.
   B) NK-mediated lysis of tumor cells.
   C) phagocytosis.
   D) bacteriolysis by specific antibodies.
   E) All of the above.

4. Which of the following is associated with the development of systemic lupus erythematosus (SLE)?
   A) deficiencies in C1, C4, or C2
   B) deficiencies in C5, C6, or C7
   C) deficiencies in the late components of complement
   D) increases in the serum C3 level
   E) increases in the levels of C1, C4, or C2

5. Active fragments of C5 can lead to the following, except
   A) contraction of smooth muscle.
   B) vasodilation.
   C) attraction of leukocytes.

    D) attachment of lymphocytes to macrophages.

    E) All of the above.

6. The alternative pathway of complement activation is characterized by the functions listed below, except

    A) activation of complement components beyond C3 in the cascade.

    B) participation of properdin.

    C) generation of anaphylatoxin.

    D) use of C4.

7. Decay-accelerating factor (DAF) regulates the complement system to prevent complement-mediated lysis of cells. This involves

    A) dissociation of C4b2a or the C3bBb enzyme complex.

    B) blocking the binding of C3 convertase to the surface of bacterial cells.

    C) inhibiting the membrane attack complex from binding to bacterial membranes.

    D) acting as a cofactor for the cleavage of C3b.

    E) causing dissociation of C5 convertase.

8. The following activate(s) the alternative pathway of complement:

    A) lipopolysaccharides

    B) some viruses and virus-infected cells

    C) fungal and yeast cell walls (zymosin)

    D) many strains of gram-positive bacteria

    E) all of the above.

9. Which component(s) of complement could be missing and still leave the remainder of the complement system capable of activation by the alternative pathway?

    A) C1, C2, and C3

    B) C3 only

    C) C2, C3, and C4

    D) C1, C2, and C4

    E) C1, C3, and C4

10. An antigen–antibody immune complex in a C3-deficient individual will still result in

    A) anaphylatoxin production.

    B) depression of factor B.

    C) production of chemotactic factors.

    D) activation of C2.

    E) activation of C5.

Answers to Review Questions

  1. *E* All these functions are mediated by complement components that come after C3 and in its absence cannot be activated.

  2. *B* The hemolytic assay would reveal a defect in any one of the complement components, since all are required to effect hemolysis. The tests for specific components are likely to work only if you happen to pick the right one. They are not useful for screening. Electrophoretic analysis is good for the major serum components (albumin and globulin) but unlikely to give information on many of the complement components.

3. D Complement is required for lysis of bacteria by specific anti-bacteria IgM or IgG. Complement is not required for phagocytosis or lysis of erythrocytes by lecithinase. However, the C3b opsonins, that are generated during complement activation, enhance phagocytosis of the opsonized particle. Although some tumor cells can initiate the alternate pathway of complement activation, complement plays no role in NK-mediated lysis of these cells.

4. A Inherited homozygous deficiency of the early proteins of the classical complement pathway (C1, C4, or C2) are strongly associated with the development of systemic lupus erythematosus (SLE). Such deficiencies probably result in abnormal processing of immune complexes in the absence of a functional classical pathway of complement fixation. Serum levels of C3 or C4 decrease in SLE due to the large number of immune complexes that bind to them. Deficiencies in the late components are associated with recurrent infections with pyogenic organisms.

5. D C5a is an anaphylatoxin, which induces degranulation of mast cells, resulting in the release of histamine, causing vasodilation and contraction of smooth muscles. C5a is also a chemotaxin, attracting leukocytes to the area of its release where the antigen is reacting with antibodies and activates the complement system. It does not promote the attachment of lymphocytes to macrophases.

6. D The alternative pathway of complement activation connects with the classical pathway at the activation of C3. Thus, it does not require C1, C4, or C2. Properdin is essential for the activation through the alternative pathway, since it stabilizes the complex (C3bBb) formed between C3b and activated serum factor B, which acts as a C3 convertase and activates C3. During the activation of the alternative pathway both C3a and C5a are generated; both are anaphylatoxins and cause degranulation of mast cells.

7. A As a cell surface regulator of complement activation, DAF destabilizes both the alternate and classical pathway C3 convertases (C4b2a or C3bBb). Like the other regulators of complement activation (RCA), including CR1, factor H, and C4bBP, these proteins accelerate decay (dissociation) of C3 convertase, releasing the component with enzymatic activity (C2a or Bb) from the component bound to the cell membrane (C4b or C3b).

8. E Each of the pathogens and particles of microbial origin listed can initiate the alternate pathway of complement activation. Parasites (e.g., trypanosomes) and teichoic acid from gram-positive cell walls can also activate complement using this pathway.

9. D C3 is required for the alternative pathway of complement activation, while C1, C2, or C4 are not required.

10. D The immune complex will activate C2 (and C4) but will not activate C3 or any other components. Since the alternative pathway of complement activation also requires C3, this pathway will not be activated. Anaphylatoxins and chemotactic factor generation require C3, while the synthesis of factor B is not related to C3.

14

HYPERSENSITIVITY REACTIONS: ANTIBODY-MEDIATED (TYPE I) REACTIONS

⬤ INTRODUCTION

Under some circumstances, immune responses produce damaging and sometimes fatal results. Such deleterious reactions are known collectively as *hypersensitivity or allergic reactions*; antigens that commonly cause hypersensitivity or allergic reactions are referred to as allergens. It should be remembered that hypersensitivity reactions differ from protective immune reactions only in that they are exaggerated or inappropriate and damaging to the host. The cellular and molecular mechanisms of the two types of reaction are virtually identical.

In the early 1960s, *hypersensitivity reactions were divided into four types*, designated I–IV by Coombs and Gell:

Type I: IgE-mediated reactions are stimulated by the binding of IgE (via its Fc region) to high-affinity IgE-specific Fc receptors (Fc$_\epsilon$RI) expressed on mast cells and basophils. When crosslinked by antigens, the IgE antibodies trigger the mast cells and basophils to release pharmacologically active agents that lead to clinical manifestations, including rhinitis, asthma, and, in severe cases, anaphylaxis. Reactions are rapid, occurring within minutes after challenge, that is, reexposure to antigen. Thus, type I *hypersensitivity is also called immediate hypersensitivity*. In recent years, the term allergy has also become synonymous with type I hypersensitivity

Type II: Cytolytic or cytotoxic reactions occur when IgM or IgG antibodies bind to antigen on the surface of cells and activate the complement cascade, which culminates in destruction of the cells.

Type III: Immune complex reactions occur when complexes of antigen and IgM or IgG antibody accumulate in the circulation or in tissue and activate the complement cascade. Granulocytes are attracted to the site of activation, and damage results from the release of lytic enzymes from their granules. Reactions occur within hours of challenge with antigen.

Type IV: Cell-mediated immunity (CMI) reactions—also called delayed-type hypersensitivity (DTH)—is mediated by T-cell-associated effector mechanisms rather than by antibody. On activation, the T cells release cytokines that cause accumulation and activation of macrophages, which, in turn, cause local damage. This type of reaction has a delayed onset and occurs 1–2 days after challenge with antigen.

This classification system helped to define the initiating mechanisms of allergic reactions and was not meant as an attempt to classify either the pathogenesis of the later stages in the disease process or the actual diseases themselves. As will become apparent in this and the two subsequent chapters on hypersensitivity, certain clinical disorders may represent pure manifestations of individual Coombs and Gell "types" of hypersensitivity, whereas others may be much more complex. Certain clinical conditions that fit the latter, more complex definition, may resist such neat designation within the classical Coombs–Gell scheme.

This chapter deals with type I hypersensitivity. Hypersensitivity types II and III are discussed in Chapter 15; cell-mediated immunity (type IV) is discussed in Chapter 16.

 ## HISTORICAL BACKGROUND

The discovery of the ability of the immune system to cause harm came from studies by Portier and Richet (the latter is a Nobel Prize winner) of the effects of the toxin from a Mediterranean Sea anemone on dogs. Several weeks after an initial administration of the toxin, a second dose was given to determine whether the dogs had developed immunity to it. Some of the dogs, rather than showing increased resistance to the effects of the toxin, experienced excessive salivation, defecation, difficulty in respiration, paralysis of the hind limbs, and death within minutes of receiving the dose. Portier and Richet named this phenomenon anaphylaxis, from the Greek ana, which means "away from," and phylaxis, which means "protection." The term is the antithesis of the phenomenon of prophylaxis ("toward protection"). Subsequent studies revealed that anaphylaxis is the result of hypersensitivity rather than decreased resistance to the toxin.

 ## GENERAL CHARACTERISTICS OF TYPE I HYPERSENSITIVITY

The sequence of events involved in the development of type I hypersensitivity can be divided into several phases: (1) *the sensitization phase*, during which IgE antibody is produced in response to an antigenic stimulus and binds to specific receptors on mast cells and basophils; (2) *the activation phase*, during which reexposure to antigen triggers the mast cells and basophils to respond by release of the contents of their granules; and (3) *the effector phase*, during which a complex response occurs as a result of the effects of the many pharmacologically active agents released by the mast cells and basophils.

SENSITIZATION PHASE

The immunoglobulin responsible for type I hypersensitivity is IgE, formerly called reagin or reaginic antibody. All normal individuals can make IgE antibody specific for a variety of antigens when antigen is introduced parenterally in the appropriate manner. Approximately 50% of the population generates an IgE response to airborne antigens (also referred to as allergens) that are encountered only on mucosal surfaces, such as the lining of the nose and lungs and the conjunctiva of the eyes. However, after repeated exposure to a plethora of these airborne allergens such as plant pollens, mold spores, house dust mites, as well as animal dander, approximately 20% of the general population develops clinical symptoms, resulting in seasonal or perennial allergic rhinitis. An outdated, yet commonly used term used to describe the seasonally airborne allergen-induced clinical symptoms is hay fever.

The term *atopy* (which means "uncommon") is frequently used to refer to IgE-mediated type I hypersensitivity and the term atopic to describe affected patients. Children of atopic individuals often suffer from allergies themselves indicating that familial tendencies are common. Evidence suggests that *IgE responses are genetically controlled by MHC-linked genes* located on chromosome 6 (see Chapter 8). Recently, other IgE regulatory genes have been implicated, including the T_H2 IL-4 gene cluster on chromosome 5 (IL-3, -4, -5, -9, -13) and the high-affinity IgE Fc receptor (FcεRI) gene on chromosome 11.

IgE Antibody Production Is T Cell-Dependent

Several lines of evidence have demonstrated the *T_H2 dependency of IgE responses*. The mechanism by which these cells promote B-cell isotype switching has not been fully elucidated, although it is clear that certain cytokines (IL-4, IL-13) produced by these cells play a pivotal role. *Various studies using experimental animals have demonstrated the importance of IL-4 in IgE responses.* The administration of neutralizing antibodies to IL-4 in mice causes inhibition of inhibits IgE. In addition, IL-4 knockout mice cannot produce IgE following infection with *Nippostrongylus brasiliensis*—a nematode that induces high IgE responses in normal mice. A comparison of IL-4 levels in allergic versus nonallergic people has shown that IL-4 levels are significantly higher in the allergic population. Consistent with this observation is the fact that IgE levels are approximately 10-fold higher in allergic (atopic) individuals as compared with normal subjects. It has been suggested that the low levels of IgE antibody in nonallergic individuals are maintained by suppressor effects mediated by interferon-γ produced by T_H1 cells (see Chapters 10 and 12). *Interferon-γ downregulates IgE production.* Thus, in normal individuals, a balance is maintained between T_H2-derived cytokines, that upregulate IgE responses and T_H1-derived cytokines that downregulate IgE responses. Natural events such as viral infection may disturb this balance and stimulate IgE-producing B cells. Therefore, allergic sensitization may result from failure of a control mechanism leading to overproduction of IL-4 by T_H2 cells and, ultimately, increased IgE production by B cells. Once adequate exposure to the allergen has been achieved by repeated mucosal contact, ingestion, or parenteral injection, and IgE antibody has been produced, an individual is considered to be sensitized. IgE antibody is made in small amounts (its concentration in the blood is the lowest of all immunoglobulins) and very rapidly becomes attached to mast cells and basophils as it circulates past them.

Mast cells, the main effector cells responsible for type I hypersensitivity responses, *are a ubiquitous family of cells generally found around blood vessels in the connective tissue, in the lining of the gut, and in the lungs*. They are large mononuclear cells, heavily granulated and deeply stained by basic dyes (see Figure 14.1). Mast cells are derived from progenitor cells that migrate to the tissue, where they differentiate into mature mast cells. In some species, circulating, polynuclear granulated cells, called *basophils, also take part in type I hypesensitivity responses* and function in much the same way as the tissue-based mast cells. Unlike the mast cells, they mature in the bone marrow and are present in the circulation in their differentiated form. One of *the most important features that mast cells and basophils have in common is that they both have receptors (FcεRI) on their cell membranes that bind with high affinity to the Fc portion of IgE*. Once bound, the IgE molecules persist at the cell surface for weeks, and that cell will remain "sensitized" as long as enough antibody remains attached, and will trigger the activation of the cell when it comes into contact with antigen.

Sensitization may also be achieved passively by transfer of serum that contains IgE antibody to a specific antigen. A procedure of historical interest only, known as

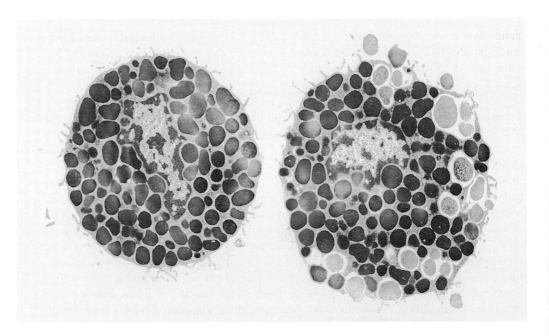

Figure 14.1. Electron micrograph of a normal mast cell illustrating the large monocyte-like nucleus and the electron-dense granules. On the right, a mast cell has been triggered and is beginning to release the contents of its granules, as seen by their decrease in opacity and the formation of vacuoles connecting with the exterior. [Photographs courtesy of Dr. T. Theoharides, Tufts Medical School.]

the **Prausnitz–Küstner (P–K) test**, used to be performed as a test for the antibodies responsible for anaphylactic reactions. In the P–K test serum from an allergic individual was injected into the skin of a normal person. After a lag period of 1–2 days, during which the locally injected antibody diffused toward neighboring mast cells and became bound to them, the site of injection was said to be sensitized, and would respond with an urticarial (hives) reaction when injected with that antigen to which the donor was allergic. Such a reaction in passively sensitized animals is called **passive cutaneous anaphylaxis** (PCA).

 ## ACTIVATION PHASE

IgE-mediated hypersensitivity reactions may be triggered by injection of the specific antigen into the skin of a sensitized individual. This is commonly referred to as the **challenge**. Such challenge, when performed by intradermal injection into the skin, may result in local cutaneous anaphylaxis; when the challenging allergen is distributed throughout the body (such as following intravenous injection), the challenge may trigger systemic anaphylaxis.

The response to intradermal challenge, called **"wheal and flare,"** is characterized by **erythema** (redness due to dilation of blood vessels) and **edema** (swelling produced by release of serum into tissue) (see Figure 16.1A). The reaction is the most rapid of all hypersensitivity reactions and reaches its peak within 10–15 minutes; then it fades without leaving any residual damage.

The size of the local skin reaction observed when an allergic patient is tested or challenged by intradermal injection of a battery of potential antigens (allergens) is roughly indicative of the degree of sensitivity to that particular substance. In addition, if the clinical history of symptoms correlates well with the time of contact with the antigen, then the cutaneous anaphylactic response may be taken as evidence that the symptoms (e.g., sneezing, itchy eyes) are attributable to the allergens of that particular plant pollen or animal dander that engendered the skin response. Other, more quantitative, tests are used as well (see below).

The activation phase of type I hypersensitivity reaction begins with the triggering of the mast cell to release its granules, and their pharmacologically active contents. It requires that at least two of the receptors for the Fc portion of the IgE molecules be bridged together in a stable configuration. In the simplest and immunologically most relevant manner, this linkage is accomplished by a multivalent antigen that can bind a different molecule of IgE to each of several epitopes on its surface, thus cross-linking them and effectively triggering the cell to respond (see Figure 14.2). This linking of receptors may also be accomplished in other experimentally useful ways, such as by addition of an antibody that is specific for IgE molecules (anti-isotype or anti-idiotype antibodies), or for the IgE receptor molecules on the surface of mast cells, exposure to sugar-binding lectins, or even by use of chemical crosslinkers (Figure 14.3). As expected, dimers or aggregates of IgE will also crosslink these Fc receptors and activate mast cells to degranulate. Finally, activation of mast cells can also be achieved using calcium ionophores, which induce a rapid influx of calcium ions into the cell, triggering the signaling cascade leading to degranulation.

It should be pointed out that mast cells may be activated through mechanisms other than IgE Fc receptor crosslinking. The anaphylatoxins C3a and C5a, products

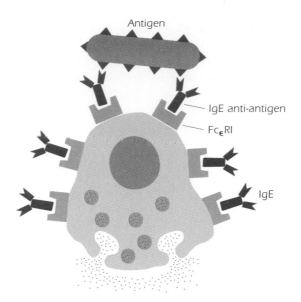

Figure 14.2. Mast cell degranulation mediated by antigen-crosslinking of IgE bound to IgE Fc receptors (FcεRI).

of complement activation (see Chapter 13), as well as various drugs such as codeine, morphine, and iodinated radiocontrast dyes, produce **anaphylactoid reactions**. Physical factors such as heat, cold, or pressure can also activate mast cells, as seen, for example, in cold-induced urticaria (an anaphylactic rash induced in certain individuals by chilling an area of skin). Finally, as noted above, certain lectins (sugar-binding molecules) can also crosslink IgE Fc receptors (see Figure 14.3). High concentrations of lectins are found in certain fruits foods (e.g., strawberries). This might explain the urticaria induced in some individuals after eating these foods.

The triggering of a mast cell by the bridging of its receptors initiates a rapid and complex series of events culminating in the **degranulation of the mast cell and the release of pharmacologically potent molecules**. Because of the ease with which its outcome can be measured, the mast cell has served as a model for the study of activation of cells in general. Among the rapid events known to occur are receptor aggregation, and changes in membrane fluidity, which result from methylation of phospholipids, leading to transient increase in intracellular levels of cyclic adenosine monophosphate (cAMP) followed by an influx of Ca^{2+} ions. The intracellular levels of cAMP and cyclic guanosine monophosphate (cGMP) are known to affect subsequent events and are important in the regulation of those events. In general, a sustained increase in intracellular cAMP at this stage will slow, or even stop, the process of degranulation. Thus, activation of adenylate cyclase, the enzyme that converts adenosine triphosphate (ATP) to cAMP, provides an important mechanism for controlling anaphylactic events.

As noted earlier, type I hypersensitivity reactions are often called immediate hypersensitivity. This term is appropriate in light of the very rapid consequences of IgE FcR crosslinking beginning with movement of mast-cell granules by microfilaments to the cell surface. Once at the cell surface, their membranes fuse with the

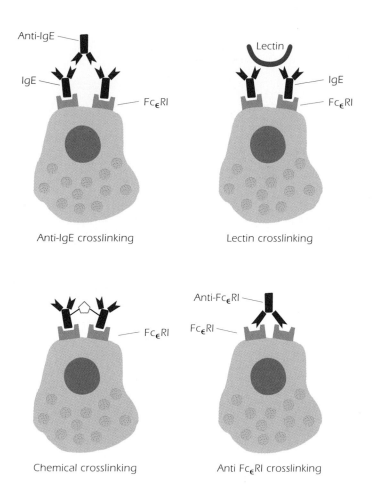

Anti-IgE

IgE

Fc$_\epsilon$RI

Anti-IgE crosslinking

Lectin

IgE

Fc$_\epsilon$RI

Lectin crosslinking

Fc$_\epsilon$RI

Chemical crosslinking

Anti-Fc$_\epsilon$RI

Fc$_\epsilon$RI

Anti Fc$_\epsilon$RI crosslinking

Figure 14.3. Alternate ways in which mast cells can be induced to undergo degranulation.

cell membrane and all the contents are released to the exterior in a process known as *exocytosis* (see Figure 14.1). Depending on the extent of crosslinking on the cell surface, any cell can release some or all of its granules. Furthermore, this explosive release of granules is physiologic and does not imply lysis or death of the cell. In fact, the degranulated cells regenerate and, once the contents of the granules have been synthesized, the cells are ready to resume their function.

EFFECTOR PHASE

The symptoms of IgE-mediated hyperresponsiveness are entirely attributable to the pharmacologically active materials released by the activated mast cells. It is helpful to consider these mediators in two major categories (Figure 14.4). One category consists of basic *preformed mediators*, which are stored in the granules by electrostatic attraction to a matrix protein and are released as a result of the influx of ions, primarily Na$^+$. Cytokines released from mast cells undergoing degranulation includ-

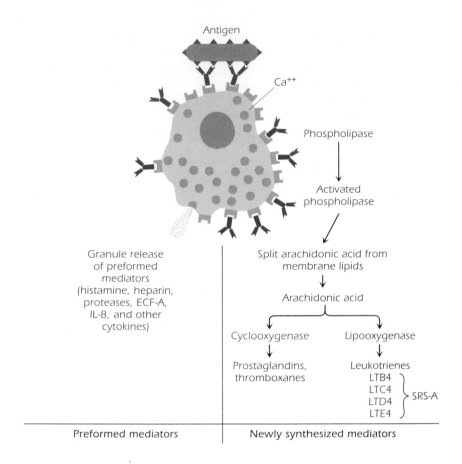

Figure 14.4. Mediators released during activation of mast cells.

ing IL-3, IL-4, IL-5, IL-8, IL-9, TNFα, and GM–CSF, also play a role in attracting and activating inflammatory cells to the site. Inflammatory cells participate in the so-called *late-phase reactions* (described later in this chapter) of type I hypersensitivity in concert with the second category of mast cell mediators—those synthesized de novo. *Newly formed mast cell mediators* consist of substances synthesized, in part, from membrane lipids. Many potent substances are released during degranulation, however, only the most important members of each category are considered here.

Preformed Mediators

Histamine. Histamine is formed in the cell by decarboxylation of the amino acid histidine, and it is stored bound by electrostatic interaction to an acid matrix protein called heparin. When released, *histamine binds rapidly to a variety of cells via two major types of receptor, H1 and H2*, which have different distribution in tissue and that mediate different effects. When histamine binds to H1 receptors on smooth muscles it causes constriction; when it binds to H1 receptors on endothelial cells it causes separation at their junctions, resulting in vascular permeability. H2 receptors are those involved in mucus secretion and increased vascular permeability, as well as in the release of acid from stomach mucosa. All these effects are responsible for some of the major signs in systemic anaphylaxis: difficulty in breathing (asthma) or asphyxiation due to constriction of smooth muscle around the bronchi in the lung, and a drop in blood pressure that results from extravasation of fluid into tissue spaces as the permeability of blood vessels increases. *H1 receptors are blocked by antihistamines*, such as benadryl, by direct competition, and when these drugs are given soon enough, they can counteract the effects of histamine. Blockage of H2 receptors requires other drugs, such as cimetidine. However, some time after the introduction of antihistamines, it was noted that they were ineffective in controlling constriction of smooth muscles that was slower in onset and more persistent than that produced by histamine. This observation led to the discovery of SRS-A, the slow-reacting substance of anaphylaxis (see below), now known to consist of a group of leukotrienes.

Serotonin. Serotonin is present in the mast cells of only certain species, such as rodents. Its effects are similar to those of histamine, in that it causes constriction of smooth muscle and increases vascular permeability.

Chemotactic Factors. A variety of chemotactic factors are released following degranulation of mast cells. These include such cytokines as *GM–CSF, IL-5, and TNFα*. A set of low molecular weight peptides called *eosinophilic chemotactic factors* (ECF) are also released. These produce a chemotactic gradient capable of attracting eosinophils to the site. In addition, the late phase mediators *platelet activating factor* (PAF) and *leukotrienes* (see below) also participate in the chemotaxis of inflammatory cells to the site. Another important inflammatory cell attracted to the site is the neutrophil. Chemotaxis of these polymorphonuclear granulocytes occurs in response to IL-8 (also called neutrophil chemotactic factor) released by activated mast cells. As we shall see later, granulocytes are important in the late phase of IgE-mediated hypersensitivity. Other cells attracted to the site in response to mast cell-derived chemotactic factors include basophils, macrophages, platelets, and lymphocytes.

In type I hypersensitivity reactions, eosinophils appear to serve as a late indicator of the presence of IgE-mediated reactions, especially the late-phase reaction discussed later; they may also release arylsulfatase and histaminase, which destroy several mediators of the hypersensitivity reaction, thus serving as one of the mechanisms to limit the reaction. Eosinophils have an additional function in parasitic worm infections, also discussed later in this chapter.

Heparin. Heparin is an acidic proteoglycan that constitutes the matrix of the granule, and to which basic mediators, such as histamine and serotonin, are bound. Its acidic nature accounts for the metachromatic (high-staining) properties of the mast cell when basic dyes, such as toluidine blue, are applied to it. *Release of heparin causes inhibition of coagulation*, which may be of some use in the subsequent recovery of the mast cell or further introduction of antigen into the reaction area; however, it is not directly involved in the symptoms of anaphylaxis.

Newly Synthesized Mediators

Leukotrienes. When a preparation of smooth muscle, such as a guinea pig uterine horn, is treated with histamine, rapid contraction occurs. The contractions are the basis of a sensitive bioassay for histamine, the **Schultz–Dale reaction**. When the histamine is washed out, rapid relaxation occurs. Addition of an antihistamine to the assay before the addition of histamine inhibits the contraction effect of histamine. If the supernatant solution from a preparation of activated mast cells is also included in the assay, the immediate contraction effect of histamine is blocked by the antihistamine and does not occur; however, a slower prolonged contraction results, and it cannot be easily reversed by washing.

This observation led to the discovery of the **slow-reacting substance of anaphylaxis** (SRS-A), which is so potent and is present in such low concentration that its chemical structure defied analysis for many years. It is now known to consist of **a set of peptides that are coupled to a metabolite of arachidonic acid and are called leukotrienes**. The leukotrienes have been named LTB4, LTC4, LTD4, and LTE4; in minute amounts, they **cause prolonged constriction of smooth muscle**. They are considered to be the cause of much antihistamine-resistant asthma in humans.

Thromboxanes and Prostaglandins. Leukotrienes are only a small part of the complex series of products produced from arachidonic acid released from cell membrane lipids by phospholipases during mast cell triggering. Arachidonic acid is a polyunsaturated, long-chain hydrocarbon that can be oxygenated in two separate pathways (Figure 14.4): by lipoxygenase to give the above-mentioned leukotrienes, and by cyclooxygenase to give prostaglandins and thromboxanes. Many of these latter compounds are vasoactive, causing bronchoconstriction, and are chemotactic for a variety of white cells, such as neutrophils, eosinophils, basophils, and monocytes.

Platelet-Activating Factor. Platelet-activating factor (PAF) induces platelets to aggregate and release their contents of mediators, which include histamine and, in some species, serotonin. Activation of platelets may also induce release of metabolites of arachidonic acid, thus augmenting effects generated by mast cells. PAF itself is one of the most potent causes of bronchoconstriction and vasodilation known, producing shocklike symptoms rapidly in very small doses.

Late-Phase Reaction

As mentioned above, many of the substances released during mast-cell activation and degranulation are responsible for the initiation of a profound **inflammatory response** with infiltration and accumulation of eosinophils, neutrophils, basophils, lymphocytes, and macrophages. Most important, and constituting a large percentage of the cells, are eosinophils and neutrophils that become activated and exacerbate the type I IgE-mediated hypersensitivity. This response often occurs within 4–8 hours and may persist for several days. This is referred to as the late-phase reaction and is shown diagrammatically in Figure 14.5. The mast cell, degranulated by cross-linking of IgE on its surface by antigen, releases eosinophil chemotactic factor (ECF-A) that recruits eosinophils to the reaction area. Their passage, as well as the passage of other leukocytes from the circulation to the tissue, is facilitated by the increased vascular permeability caused by histamine and other mediators. Various cytokines, including GM–CSF, IL-3, -4, -5, and -13 play an important role in eosinophil growth and differentiation, and cell adhesion of certain cell types.

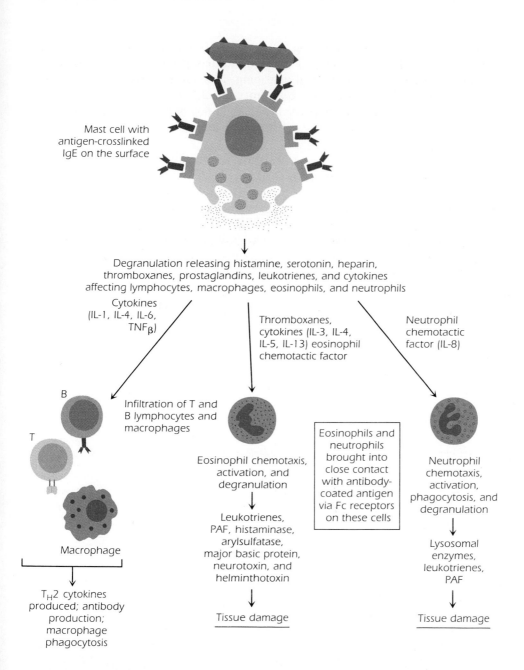

Figure 14.5. A diagrammatic representation of late-phase reaction of type I IgE-mediated hypersensitivity with some of the mediators involved.

Eosinophils can also bind to IgE by virtue of their expression of the low-affinity IgE Fc receptor (FcεRII or CD23). They also express Fc receptors to the Fc portion of IgG. Thus, both IgE- and IgG-bound antigen will bind to their respective Fc receptors on eosinophils, causing these cells to be activated. Like mast cells, once these receptors are triggered they degranulate, releasing leukotrienes that cause muscle contraction. They also release platelet-activating factor (PAF) and major basic protein (MBP). MBP has the ability to destroy various parasites (such as schistosomes) by affecting their mobility and damaging their surface. Also, MBP is toxic to mammalian epithelium of the respiratory tract. Finally, the eosinophilic degranulation releases eosinophilic cationic protein (ECP), a potent neurotoxin and helminthotoxin. All these biologically active substances, while directed toward foreign invaders, cause tissue damage.

Neutrophils recruited to the site in response to chemotactic factors come into close contact with antibody-coated antigen via IgG Fc receptors, which are normally expressed on these cells. Consequently, these cells become activated to phagocitose the antigen−antibody immune complexes. In addition, they release their powerful lysosomal enzymes, which cause great tissue damage. Like degranulation products of eosinophils, degranulation products of neutrophils also include leukotrienes and platelet-activating factor (PAF). Lymphocytes (both T and B) as well as macrophages enter the area, further sensitizing or immunizing the host against the offending antigen or microorganism.

Figure 14.6 illustrates the general mechanism underlying a type I hypersensitivity reaction. This dramatic series of events triggered and mediated by IgE is involved in the elimination of parasites, as described later in this chapter. Unfortunately, the same events take place in certain individuals when the antigen is a harmless

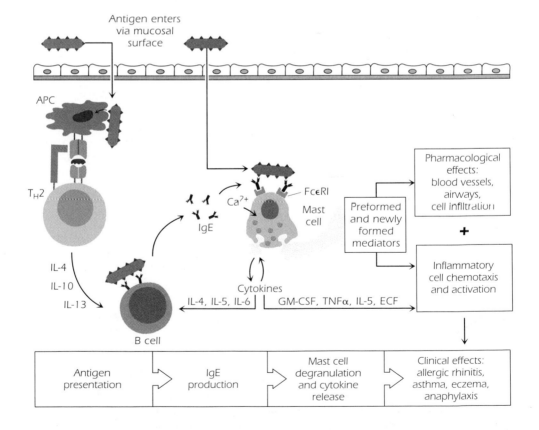

Figure 14.6. Overview of induction and effector mechanisms in type I hypersensitivity.

substance such as pollen, animal dander, or the common dust mite, resulting in tissue damage.

CLINICAL ASPECTS OF TYPE I HYPERSENSITIVITY

The clinical consequences of type I hypersensitivity can range from localized reactions including allergic rhinitis, asthma, atopic dermatitis and food allergies, to severe, life-threatening systemic reactions such as anaphylaxis. It is important to note, however, that, although defined as localized anaphylaxis, asthmatic reactions can also be fatal. Mast cell degranulation is the central mechanism in each of these reactions.

Allergic Rhinitis

Allergic rhinitis (commonly known as hay fever) is the most common atopic disorder worldwide. It is caused by airborne allergens that react with IgE-sensitized mast cells in the nasal passages and conjuctiva. Mediators released from mast cells increase capillary permeability and cause localized vasodilation, leading to the typical symptoms, which include sneezing and coughing.

Food Allergies

Another common atopic disorder (food allergies) is caused by the intake of certain foods (e.g., peanuts, rice, eggs, etc.). When susceptible individuals ingest foods to which they are allergic, this can trigger the crosslinking of allergen-specific IgE on mast cells located in the upper and lower gastrointestinal tract. Mast cell degranulation and mediator release leads to localized smooth muscle contraction and vasodilation often causing vomiting and diarrhea. In some cases, the allergen is absorbed into the bloodstream as a consequence if increased permeability of mucous membranes. Food allergens can then be transported to encounter mast cells present in skin causing wheal and flare reactions (atopic urticaria) commonly known as hives.

Atopic Dermatitis

A form of type I hypersensitivity most frequently seen in young children is ***allergic dermatitis***. This clinical disorder is caused by the development of inflammatory skin lesions induced by mast cell cytokines released following degranulation. These potent inflammatory cytokines released near the site of allergen contact stimulate chemotaxis of large numbers of inflammatory cells—especially eosinophils. The skin eruptions that develop are erythematous and pus (white cell)-filled.

Asthma

Asthma is another common form of localized anaphylaxis. In recent years, the incidence and the severity of asthma have increased dramatically in the United States. Mortality rates have been highest in children living in inner cities. Epidemiologic studies have suggested that the cockroach calyx is a major asthma-inducing allergen in these children. Many other allergens, including airborne pollens, dust, viral antigens, and various chemicals can induce allergic asthma. Alternatively, asthma may be induced by such things as exercise or exposure to cold temperatures independent of allergen exposure, a phenomenon known as intrinsic asthma.

Asthma is a chronic obstructive disease of the lower airways characterized by episodic exacerbations of at least partially reversible airflow limitation. The clinical manifestations of asthma are believed to be the result of three basic pathophysiologic events within the airways: ***(1) reversible obstruction; (2) augmented bronchial responsiveness to a variety of physical and chemical stimuli (airways hyperreactivity); and (3) inflammation.***

Airway inflammation is believed to play a major role in the pathogenesis of this disorder and is therefore a major target for pharmacologic intervention. Cytokine-induced recruitment of large numbers of inflammatory cells, particularly eosinophils, ultimately causes significant tissue injury. Tissue damage is mediated by the many toxic substances released by these inflammatory cells, including oxygen radicals, nitric oxide, and cytokines. These events lead to the development of mucus, buildup of proteins and fluids (edema), and sloughing-off of epithelium, all of which combine to cause occlusion of the bronchial lumen. ***Adhesion molecules*** play a key role in the early events following inflammatory cell recruitment. Various cytokines released by T_H2 cells and by mast cells (e.g., IL-4, IL-13, TNFα) upregulate the expression of leukocyte and endothelial adhesion molecules including intercellular adhesion molecule 1 (ICAM-1), E-selectin, vascular cell adhesion molecule 1, and leukocyte function-associated antigen-1 (LFA-1). Once upregulated, eosinophil–endothelial cell adhesion increases thereby facilitating transendothelial migration and prolonged survival within the lung tissue. Experimental adhesion molecule antagonists (e.g., anti-ICAM-1 monoclonal antibodies) are being investigated as candidate therapies for the treatment of asthma. Promising results using such immuotherapeutic reagents in animal models have stimulated interest in the development of antagonists that can be safely administered to humans.

Detection

In a clinical setting, the degree of sensitivity to a particular allergen is usually determined by the patient's complaints and by the extent of ***skin test reactions***. To avoid serious consequences from intradermal challenge in patients who may be extremely sensitive to certain allergens, a skin-prick test that introduces minute amounts of antigen is given first. Generally the extent of the skin test reaction (*wheal and flare*) observed within 30 minutes of challenge correlates roughly with the degree of sensitivity. We should, however, not forget the possibility of a late-phase reaction, which may occur in some individuals within several hours following the challenge and that sometimes may last 24 hours.

More quantitative assays that correlate, albeit not 100%, with clinical symptoms, are available in the laboratory. One assay, known as the ***radioallergosorbent test*** (RAST), involves covalent coupling of the allergen to an insoluble matrix, such as paper disks or beads. The antigen-coated matrix is then dipped into a sample of the patient's serum and allowed to bind any antibody that is specific for the allergen. After the disk is washed, a radiolabeled antibody specific for IgE is added. The amount of radioactivity bound is a measure of the amount of specific IgE antibody in the serum sample. More commonly, assays to quantitate allergen-specific serum IgE use an approach similar to RAST except that fluorescent or enzyme-linked anti-

IgE is used for the detection of allergen-specific IgE in patient's serum in lieu of radiolabeled antibody.

Intervention

Environmental Intervention. In some cases, the easiest way for individuals to control their allergies is to ***avoid exposure to known allergens***, advice followed infrequently. If some pollens are the cause of the reaction, it may be possible for the patient to go to pollen-free areas during the season when the offending plant is pollinating. Masks and air filters also have a useful role to play, but usually avoidance is difficult for the general atopic population.

Pharmacologic Intervention. Modern pharmaceutical chemistry has provided a host of drugs that are more or less effective at various stages in the evolution of the anaphylactic reaction. In brief, these drugs include

1. ***Cromolyn sodium***, which stabilizes membranes, prevents Ca^{2+} influx, and decreases or prevents mast-cell degranulation when administered before antigen exposure [also, theophylline (and several other substances), which maintains high cAMP levels and inhibits mast-cell degranulation, is given orally or by inhalation to asthmatic patients, it is hoped before exposure to antigen].
2. ***Corticosteroids***, especially when topically applied, which block the metabolic pathways involving arachidonic acid and have general antiinflammatory effects, thus preventing late phase reactions.
3. ***Antihistamines***, which compete with histamine for receptor sites, thereby decreasing or preventing immediate symptoms such as sneezing, itching, and runny nose.
4. ***Sodium cromoglycate***, a drug that is particularly effective in treating allergic asthma, since it prevents both the immediate and late phase responses following bronchial provocation with allergen.
5. ***Epinephrine***, which most effectively treats the life-threatening systemic effects of anaphylaxis. It directly reverses the effects of histamine by relaxing smooth muscle and decreasing vascular permeability.

Immunologic Intervention. For many years, clinical immunologists have practiced a form of ***immunotherapy***, called ***hyposensitization***, whereby patients are injected, over an extended period, with increasing doses of the antigen to which they are sensitive. The improvement in symptoms noted in some patients has been ascribed to several different factors. The most popular rationale is based on the observation that such injections serve to increase the synthesis of IgG antibody specific for the allergen. Such antibody in the circulation presumably binds to and removes the allergen before it has a chance to reach and react with the IgE antibody on the surface of mast cells. Thus, the term ***blocking antibody*** has become associated with this IgG, and there is a rough correlation between titers of this IgG antibody generated and clinical improvement.

Other findings during hyposensitization include an initial increase in levels of IgE antibody, followed by a prolonged decrease on continued therapy. This decrease has been linked to a decrease in intensity of symptoms and is attributed either to induction of tolerance, or to a switch from T_H2 to T_H1 T cells. After repeated sub-clinical doses of the antigen, there is also a progressive decrease in the sensitivity of mast cells and basophils to triggering by antigen. It is likely that the explanation for the apparent benefits of this immunologic therapy encompasses more than one of these demonstrable effects. Whatever the reason, this form of therapy is generally more successful in dealing with allergens that enter the circulation directly, such as bee-sting venom, than for those allergens contacted via mucosal surfaces, such as pollen, where IgG antibody is unlikely to be effective.

Potentially promising experimental immunotherapies for the treatment of IgE-mediated hypersensitivity are being investigated. A promising therapy for the treat-ment of patients with asthma and allergic rhinitis employs the use of anti-IgE hu-manized monoclonal antibody engineered such that it does not cross-link IgE bound to mast cells and basophils. The use of plasmid DNAs encoding a specific antigen (used to induce hyporesponsiveness), as well as cytokines (e.g., IL-12, IL-10), anti-cytokines (e.g., anti-IL-4), or cytokine receptor antagonists (e.g., anti-IL-5 receptor) are also under investigation.

Modified Allergens. Experiments in animals have demonstrated that admin-istration of a chemically altered allergen (e.g., ragweed pollen denatured by urea or coupled to polyethylene glycol) suppresses a primary or established IgE response. The mechanism may involve the induction of suppressor T cells that are both antigen-specific and isotype-specific. The modified allergens do not combine with preexisting IgE antibodies and, therefore, do not trigger anaphylactic responses. Use of such

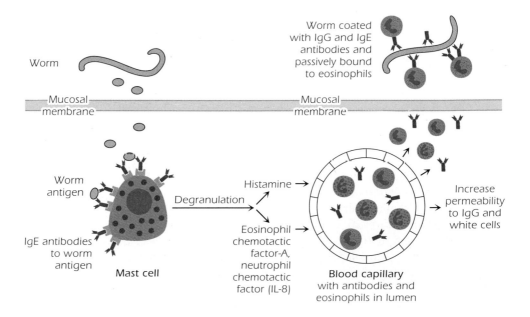

Figure 14.7. A diagrammatic representation of the destruction of a worm by eosino-phils that have migrated to the area and been activated following IgE- and antigen-mediated mast cell degranulation.

modified allergens (allergoids) seems to offer a promising approach to treatment of allergy. Another approach would involve determining the specific epitopes on the allergen to which the helper T cells are directed and to induce tolerance specifically to these epitopes.

THE PROTECTIVE ROLE OF IgE

The *protective effects of type I hypersensitivity* may be seen in situations where the sensitizing antigen is derived from one of many *parasitic worms such as helminths*. The immune response to these worms favors the induction of IgE for reasons that are still not clear. As a consequence of antigens from the worm crosslinking IgE on the surface of mast cells (and eosinophils), histamine, and other mediators associated with the anaphylactic response are released. The effects of increased permeability due to histamine release serve to bring serum components, which include IgG antibody, to the site of worm infestation. The IgG antibody binds to the surface of the worm and attracts the eosinophils, which have migrated to the area as a result of the chemotactic effects of the eosinophilic chemotactic factor (ECF-A). The eosinophils then bind to the IgG-coated worm, by virtue of their membrane receptors for Fc, and release the contents of their granules (Figures 14.7 and 14.8). As noted earlier,

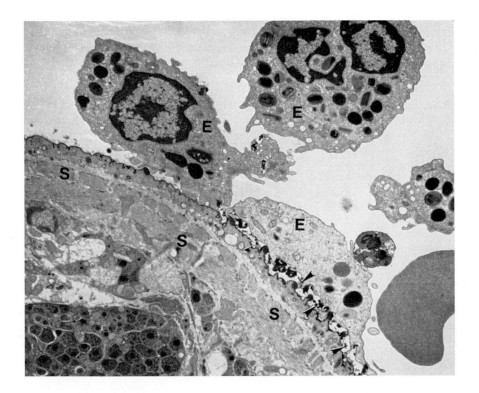

Figure 14.8. Electron micrograph (×6,000) of eosinophils (E) adhering to an antibody-coated schistosomulum (S). The cell on the left has not yet degranulated, but the one on the right has discharged electron-dense material (arrows), which can be seen between the cell and the worm. [Photograph courtesy of Dr. J. Caulfield, Harvard Medical School.]

eosinophils also express the low-affinity Fc receptor for IgE which facilitates the binding of these cells to IgE-coated worms. The major constituent of the contents of the granules released by eosinophils is a major basic protein (MBP), referred to previously, which coats the surface of the worm and leads, in some unknown way, to the death of the worm and its eventual expulsion. Thus, all components of the type I reaction combine to perform this protective function. This beneficial effect of the anaphylactic response in many animals suggests that responses involving *IgE may have evolved to play a role in dealing with worm parasitism*.

SUMMARY

1. Type I hypersensitivity reactions are mediated by IgE antibodies, which bind to specific receptors on the surface of mast cells and basophils. When these receptors are crosslinked by contact with specific antigen, the cell is triggered to respond by releasing its granules and their contents, as well as synthesizing other products from its membrane.

2. IgE responses are T cell-dependent. Allergens stimulate the induction of T_H2 cells, which release cytokines (IL-4, IL-13) that stimulate B-cell class switching to produce IgE.

3. The combined pharmacologic effects of these mediators produce the immediate symptoms typical of this response: increased vascular permeability, constriction of smooth muscles, and influx of eosinophils.

4. A "late-phase" reaction consisting of redness and itching may appear later as a result of the inflammatory response to granule–matrix constituents of the mast cell. Cytokines produced by T_H2 cells also contribute to these inflammatory responses by inducing the recruitment of eosinophils to the site and increasing the expression of various cell adhesion molecules.

5. Clinical manifestations of type I hypersensitivity reactions include localized reactions such as allergic rhinitis, atopic dermatitis, food allergies, and asthma. Systemic reactions can lead to life-threatening anaphylaxis.

6. Despite the dangerous systematic reactions produced by this mode of immune response, its value probably lies in its ability to provide immunity to parasitic infections.

7. Common therapeutic agents used to treat type I hypersensitivity include cromolyn sodium, corticosteroids, antihistamines, sodium cromoglycate, and epinephrine.

REFERENCES

Bevan MA, Metzger H (1993): Signal transduction by Fc receptors: the FcεRI case. *Immunol Today* 14:222.

Coombs RRA, Gell PGH (1963): The classification of allergic reactions underlying disease. In Gell PGH, Coombs RRA (eds): Clinical Aspects of Immunology. Oxford, UK: Blackwell.

Galli SJ, Austin KF (1989): Mast Cell and Basophil Differentiation and Function in Health and Disease. New York: Lippincott-Raven.

Galli SJ, Lantz CS (1998): Allergy. In Paul, WE (ed): Fundamental Immunology, 4th ed. New York: Lippincott-Raven.

Hamawy MM, Mergenhagen SE, Siraganian RS (1994): Adhesion molecules as regulators of mast cell and basophil function. *Immunol Today* 15:62.

Heusser C, Jardieu P (1997): Therapeutic potential of anti-IgE antibodies. *Curr Opinion in Immunology* 9:805.

Ishizaka K (1988): IgE binding factors and regulation of the IgE antibody response. *Annu Rev Immunol* 6:513.

Lichenstein LM (1993): Allergy and the immune system. Sci Am (Sept):126. Marone G (1998): Asthma: recent advances. *Immunol Today* 19:5.

Mygid N (1986): Essential Allergy. Oxford: Blackwell.

Terr AI (1994): Mechanisms of hypersensitivity. In Stites DP, Terr AI, Parslow TG (eds): Basic and Clinical Immunology, 8th ed. E Norwalk, CT: Appleton & Lange.

Terr AI (1994): The atopic diseases. In Stites DP, Terr AI, Parslow TG (eds): Basic and Clinical Immunology, 8th ed. E Norwalk, CT: Appleton & Lange.

Terr AI (1994): Anaphylaxis and urticaria. In Stites DP, Terr AI, Parslow TG (eds): Basic and Clinical Immunology, 8th ed. E Norwalk, CT: Appleton & Lange.

REVIEW QUESTIONS

For each question, choose the ONE BEST answer or completion.

1. The usual sequence of events in an allergic reaction is as follows:
   A) The allergen combines with circulating IgE, and then the IgE:allergen complex binds to mast cells.
   B) The allergen binds to IgE fixed to mast cells.
   C) The allergen is processed by antigen-presenting cells and then binds to histamine receptors.
   D) The allergen is processed by antigen-presenting cells and then binds to mast cells.
   E) The allergen combines with IgG.

2. Epinephrine
   A) causes bronchodilation.
   B) is effective even after anaphylactic symptoms commence.
   C) relaxes smooth muscle.
   D) decreases vascular permeability.
   E) All of the above.

3. A human volunteer agrees to be passively sensitized with IgE specific for a ragweed antigen (allergen). When challenged with the allergen intradermally, he displayed a typical skin reaction due to an immediate hypersensitivity reaction. If the injection with sensitizing IgE was preceded by an injection (at the same site) of Fc fragments of human IgE followed by intradermal injection with allergen, which of the following outcomes would you predict?
   A) No reaction would occur because the Fc fragments would interact with the allergen and prevent it from gaining access to the sensitized mast cells.
   B) No reaction would occur because the Fc fragments would interact with the IgE antibodies making their antigen-binding sites unavailable for binding to antigen.

C) No reaction would occur because the Fc fragments would interact with Fcε receptors on mast cells.

D) The reaction would be exacerbated due to the increased local concentration of IgE Fc fragments.

E) The reaction would be exacerbated due to the activation of complement.

4. The following mechanism(s) may be involved in the clinical efficacy of desensitization therapy to treat patients with allergies to known allergens:

   A) enhanced production of IgG, which binds allergen before it reaches mast cells
   B) skewing of T cell responses from T_H2 to T_H1
   C) decreased sensitivity of mast cells and basophils to degranulation by allergen
   D) decreased production of IgE antibody
   E) All of the above.

5. Immediate hypersensitivity skin reactions

   A) usually occur within 24 hours.
   B) exhibit a raised wheal due to infiltration by mononuclear cells.
   C) exhibit a red flare due to vasodilation.
   D) cannot be elicited by monovalent haptens.
   E) All are correct.

6. Mast cells

   A) are found circulating in the blood.
   B) release their granules following lysis.
   C) are basophilic after complete degranulation.
   D) are very similar to basophils.
   E) All are correct.

7. Antihistamines

   A) bind to receptors for histamine, thereby preventing the histamine from exerting a pharmacologic effect.
   B) are more effective given before, rather than after, the onset of allergic symptoms.
   C) do not influence the activity of leukotrienes.
   D) do not affect binding of IgE to mast cells.
   E) All are correct.

8. In the RAST assay for ragweed pollen

   A) the patient's serum is first mixed with a radiolabeled anti-IgE.
   B) only IgE anti-ragweed antibodies are detected.
   C) the patient's serum competitively inhibits binding of the anti-IgE.
   D) monovalent IgE is used.
   E) complement is utilized.

9. Which of the following statements is *false*?

   A) IL-4 and IL-13 produced by T_H2 cells play a key role in regulating IgE responses.
   B) Interferon-γ produced by T_H1 cells can downregulate IgE responses.
   C) In normal individuals, a balance between T_H1-derived and T_H2-derived cytokines helps to maintain normal levels of IgE.
   D) IL-4 levels are higher in atopic patients.
   E) In IL-4 knockout mice, IgE production is normal following their exposure to parasites due to the regulatory activity of IL-13.

10. Anaphylactic reactions

    A) evolve in minutes and abate within 30 minutes.
    B) may be followed by inflammatory sequelae hours later.

C) are the consequences of released pharmacologic agents.

D) may involve components of mast-cell granule matrix.

E) All of the above.

Case Study

While playing tennis on a warm day, a young man felt a wasp on his arm and brushed it off, but still received a mild sting, which he ignored. Ten minutes later he felt dizzy and began to itch under his arms and on his scalp. When he broke out in hives and felt a tightness in his chest, he headed for the hospital. On the way he felt cold and clammy and collapsed on the seat of the taxi. In the emergency unit his pulse was barely detectable. What happened, and why?

Answers To Review Questions

1. *B* Allergic (also known as atopic) individuals have already made IgE responses to specific allergens. IgE binds passively to cells expressing high-affinity Fc receptors for IgE (e.g., mast cells) and interacts with the allergen when present. This results in crosslinking of the high-affinity FcεR, resulting in mast-cell degranulation. The allergen does not need to be processed by APCs in order to bind to IgE.

2. *E* All are effects of epinephrine and make it useful for treatment of acute anaphylactic symptoms.

3. *C* Since the IgE Fc fragments would bind to the high-affinity FcεR expressed on the surface of mast cells, the allergen-specific IgE would not have access to these receptors and therefore would not bind to these cells. When the allergen is introduced intradermally, while it would bind to the allergen-specific IgE at the site, this would not result in crosslinking of FcεR, which are saturated with soluble IgE Fc fragments. Hence no immediate hypersensitivity reaction would take place.

4. *E* All are considered to be involved to varying degrees in injection therapy.

5. *E* All are correct statements.

6. *D* Mast cells release granules physiologically and not by lysing, they are basophilic before but not after they degranulate, and they are not found circulating freely. Mast cells are similar to circulating basophils.

7. *E* All are correct statements.

8. *B* The RAST assay measures IgE antibody that is allowed to bind to allergen coupled to an insoluble matrix. It detects IgE anti-ragweed antibodies. It does not utilize monovalent IgE, and complement is not utilized in the test.

9. *E* IL-4 knockout mice do not make IgE responses when challenged with parasites, such as *Nippostrongylus brasiliensis*. This finding is consistent with the fact that IL-4 plays a key role in the regulation of IgE responses by B cells.

10. *E* All are true. A and C are true of the classic "wheal and flare" type response, while B and D describe features of the "late-phase" response, which is a complication of some anaphylactic reactions.

Answer to Case Study

This is a classic case of systemic anaphylaxis. In the emergency room epinephrine was promptly administered and the symptoms due to vascular permeability (hives, low blood pressure) and smooth muscle constriction (difficulty in breathing) were reversed. When he revived sufficiently, he revealed that he had been stung by similar-looking insects in the past, the last time 3 months ago, but without any noticeable effects. These stings were apparently the priming injections building up sufficient levels of IgE antibody to sensitize his mast cells. Thus the last sting, despite the fact that little venom was injected, was sufficient to precipitate a systemic reaction. A careful skin test, involving intradermal injection of very dilute wasp venom, should show an immediate "wheal and flare" response, confirming the existence of sensitivity. The young man should be advised to (1) avoid wasps, (2) carry an emergency vial of injectable epinephrine, and (3) undergo desensitization therapy aimed at hyposensitization to the wasp venom antigen.

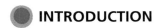

HYPERSENSITIVITY REACTIONS: ANTIBODY-MEDIATED (TYPE II) CYTOTOXIC REACTIONS AND IMMUNE COMPLEX (TYPE III) REACTIONS

INTRODUCTION

Hypersensitivity reactions characterized as type II and type III reactions are mediated by antibodies belonging to the IgG, IgM, and, in some cases, IgA isotypes. It is now clear that these reactions also share certain effector mechanisms. The distinction between these two forms of hypersensitivity lies in the type and location of antigen involved and the way in which antigen is brought together with antibody. Type II hypersensitivity reactions are stimulated by the binding of antibody directly to an antigen on the surface of a cell. Type III reactions are stimulated by antigen–antibody immune complexes. The immune mechanisms that manifest the clinical outcomes of such hypersensitivity reactions are the subject of this chapter.

TYPE II CYTOTOXIC REACTIONS

Introduction

In type II hypersensitivity, *antibodies are formed against target antigens that are either normal or altered cell membrane determinants*. The targeted cell is either damaged or destroyed through a variety of mechanisms. Three different antibody-mediated mechanisms are involved in type II hypersensitivity reactions.

Complement-Mediated Reactions. In complement-mediated type II hypersensitivity reactions, antibodies react with a cell membrane component leading to complement fixation. This activates the complement cascade and leads either to **lysis of the cell** or opsonic effects mediated by receptors for Fc or C3b (Figure 15.1A). **Opsonization** culminates in the phagocytosis and destruction of the cell by macrophages and neutrophils expressing surface receptors for Fc or C3b. Blood cells are most commonly affected by this mechanism. Interestingly, IgG Fc receptor knockout

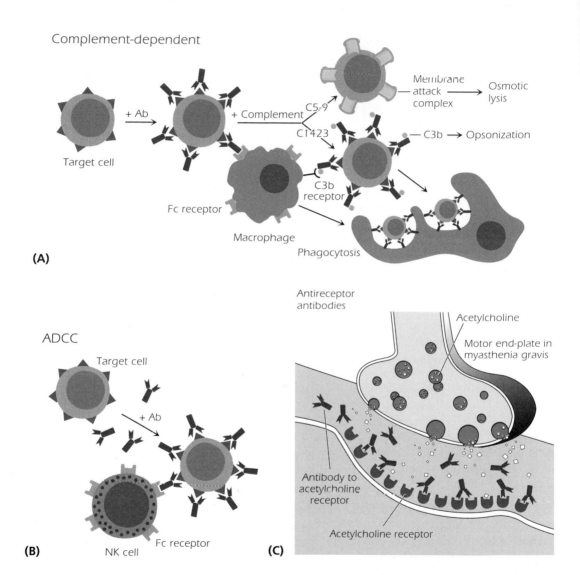

Figure 15.1. Schematic illustration of three different mechanisms of antibody-mediated injury in type II hypersensitivity. **(A)** Complement-dependent reactions that lead to lysis of cells or render them susceptible to phagocytosis. **(B)** Antibody-dependent cell-mediated cytotoxicity (ADCC). IgG-coated target cells are killed by cells that bear Fc receptors for IgG (e.g., NK cells, macrophages). **(C)** Antireceptor antibodies disturb the normal function of receptors. In this example, acetylcholine receptor antibodies impair neuromuscular transmission in myasthenia gravis.

mice fail to mount type II (and type III) hypersensitivity reactions—a finding that underscores the pivotal role played by IgG Fc receptors in initiating these reaction cascades.

Antibody-Dependent Cell-Mediated Cytotoxicity. Antibody-dependent cell-mediated cytotoxicity (ADCC) utilizes IgG Fc receptors expressed on many cell types (e.g., NK cells, macrophages, neutrophils, eosinophils) as a means of bringing these cells into contact with antibody-coated target cells (Figure 15.1B). Lysis of these target cells requires contact but does not involve phagocytosis or complement fixation. In some cases, IgE antibodies are involved in ADCC. In this situation, the low affinity IgE Fc receptor expressed on certain cells (e.g., FcRεII expressed on eosinophils) binds to the Fc portion of IgE antibodies bound to target antigens (e.g., parasites) (see Figure 14.7).

Antibody-Mediated Cellular Dysfunction. Cell surface receptors can also serve as target antigens in type II hypersensitivity reactions. When autoantibodies bind to such receptors they impair or dysregulate function without causing cell injury or inflammation. An example of antibody-mediated cellular dysfunction is seen in ***myasthenia gravis***. Antagonistic autoantibodies reactive with acetylcholine receptors in the motor end plates of skeletal muscles impair neuromuscular transmission causing muscle weakness (Figure 15.1C). Conversely, autoantibodies can serve as agonists in some cases causing stimulation of the target cells. An example of this is seen in ***Graves' disease*** in which antibodies directed against thyroid-stimulating hormone receptor on thyroid epithelial cells stimulates the cells, resulting in hyperthyroidism. These disorders are discussed in more detail in Chapter 17, which deals with the subject of autoimmunity.

Some other examples of clinically important type II hypersensitivity reactions are presented below.

Transfusion Reactions

Transfusion of ABO-incompatible blood results in complement-mediated cytotoxic reactions. As an example, people with type O blood have in their circulation, for reasons that are still not completely clear, IgM anti-A and anti-B antibodies (***isohemagglutinins***), which react with the A and B blood-group substances, respectively. If such a person were to be transfused with type A red blood cells, the immediate consequences could be disastrous. Since there is a considerable amount of IgM anti-A antibody in this person's circulation, all the transfused type A red blood cells will bind some antibody. Because of the efficiency of IgM antibody in activating complement (a single IgM molecule is sufficient to activate many complement molecules; see Chapter 13), and because of the absence of repair mechanisms, red blood cells will be lysed intravascularly by the destructive action of complement on their membranes. Not only does this nullify the desirable effects of the transfusion, but the individual is also faced with the risk of kidney damage from blockage by large quantities of red blood cell membrane, plus the possible toxic effects from the release of the heme complex.

Rh Incompatibility Reaction

A somewhat similar mechanism is exemplified by the *rhesus (Rh) incompatibility reaction* seen in infants born of parents with Rh-incompatible blood groups. Rh antigens are so-named because rabbit antisera raised against rhesus monkey red blood cells (RBC) agglutinate the erythrocytes from approximately 85% of humans tested. RBCs from such individuals are therefore said to be Rh$^+$, whereas cells from the remaining 15% of the population are Rh$^-$. It is now clear that the *D antigen* is by far the strongest immunogen and the most important of all the Rh antigens. Rh$^-$ mothers can become sensitized to Rh antigens during their first pregnancy with a child whose RBCs are Rh$^+$. This occurs as a result of the release of some of the baby's red blood cells into the mother's circulation during birth. If the mother is thereby sufficiently immunized to produce anti-Rh antibody of the IgG isotype, subsequent Rh$^+$ fetuses will be at risk, since, as we saw in Chapter 4, IgG antibody is capable of crossing the placenta. Thus, in second or subsequent pregnancies, when the anti-Rh IgG antibodies have crossed the placenta, they bind to the Rh antigen on the red blood cells of the fetus. Because the density of Rh antigen on the surface of red blood cells is low, these antibodies usually fail to agglutinate or lyse the cells directly. However, the antibody-coated cells are readily destroyed by the opsonic effect of the Fc portions of the IgG, which interact with the receptors for Fc on the phagocytic cells of the reticuloendothelial system. The result is progressive destruction of the fetal or newborn red blood cells, with the pathologic consequences that come from decreased transport of oxygen and result in jaundice from the products of the breakdown of hemoglobin—a condition known as *hemolytic disease of the newborn (erythroblastosis fetalis)*. Prevention of this Rh incompatibility reaction can be achieved with the administration of anti-Rh antibodies to the mother within 72 hours of parturition to effectively block the sensitization phase. This also causes a rapid clearance of Rh$^+$ cells from the mother's circulation. One widely used preparation of anti-Rh antibodies is called *Rhogam* and consists of human IgG against the D antigen.

Autoimmune Reactions

As a consequence of certain infectious diseases, or for other, still unknown, reasons, some people produce an antibody reactive against their own blood cells. When RBCs are the target, binding of anti-RBC autoantibody shortens their life span or destroys them altogether by mechanisms that involve hemolysis or phagocytosis via receptors for Fc and C3b. This may lead to progressive anemia if the production of new red blood cells cannot keep pace with destruction. Occasionally, the antibody only binds effectively at lower temperatures (cold agglutinin), in which case lowering of body temperature, particularly the lower temperature of the arms and legs, leads to effective antibody binding and destruction of the RBCs (see Chapter 17).

Another example of cell destruction by autoantibodies is *idiopathic thrombocytopenia purpura*. In this condition antibodies directed to platelets result in platelet destruction by complement or phagocytic cells with Fc or C3b receptors. Decrease in platelet numbers may lead to bleeding (purpura). Similarly, autoantibodies directed against granulocytes can induce *agranulocytosis* predisposing individuals to various infections. Finally, antibodies may form against other tissue components such as basement membrane collagen, causing ***Goodpasture's syndrome***, and desmosomes, resulting in ***pemphigus vulgaris***.

Drug-Induced Reactions

In some people, certain drugs act as haptens and combine with cells or with other circulating blood constituents and induce antibody formation. When antibody combines with cells coated with the drug, cytotoxic damage results. The type of pathologic injury depends on the type of cell that binds the drug. Thus, for example, Sedormid (a sedative) can bind to platelets causing it to become immunogenic. The resulting antibody response causes lysis of the platelets and resulting thrombocytopenia (low blood platelet count). This disorder, in turn, can give rise to purpura (hemorrage into the skin, mucous membranes, and internal organs), which is the main problem in drug-induced thrombocytopenia purpura. Withdrawal of the offending drug leads to a cessation of symptoms. Other drugs, such as chloramphenicol (an antibiotic), may bind to white blood cells; phenacetin (an analgesic) and chlorpromazine (a tranquilizer) may bind to red blood cells. The consequences of an immune response to these drugs can lead to an agranulocytosis (decrease in granulocytes) in the case of white blood cells and a hemolytic anemia in the case of red blood cells. Damage to the target cell in these examples may be mediated by either of the two mechanisms described above: by cytolysis via the complement pathway or by destruction of cells by phagocytosis mediated by receptors for Fc or C3b.

It should be pointed out that whereas the preceding discussion emphasizes type II reaction induced by drugs, type I, III, and IV reactions may also be induced because of hypersensitivity to drugs. Some reactions are induced by a drug acting as a hapten conjugated to some body components; as discussed in the next chapter, other reactions (type IV) can be induced by the drug acting as a contact sensitizer.

TYPE III IMMUNE COMPLEX REACTIONS

Introduction

In 1903, a French scientist named Arthus immunized rabbits with horse serum by repeated intradermal injection. After several weeks, he noted that each succeeding injection produced an increasingly severe reaction at the site of inoculation. At first a mild erythema (redness) and edema (accumulation of fluid) were noticed within 24 hours of injection. These reactions subsided without consequence by the following day, but subsequent injections produced larger edematous responses, and by the fifth or sixth inoculations the lesions became hemorrhagic with necrosis and were slow to heal. This phenomenon, known as the ***Arthus reaction***, is the prototype of localized type III immune complex reactions or reactions mediated by aggregates of antibody and antigen. It is distinguishable from type III hypersensitivity reactions caused by antigen–antibody immune complexes in the circulation that produce systemic pathogenic effects.

Activation of complement and accumulation of polymorphonuclear leukocytes are important components of immune complex-mediated tissue injury regardless of whether the reaction is a systemic or localized one. The formation of immune complexes can be initiated by exogenous antigens such as bacteria and viruses (or, as in the case of the Arthus reaction described above, by intradermal administration of large amounts of foreign protein). Alternatively, endogenous antigens, such as DNA, can serve as a target for autoantibodies. In the latter case, the clinical outcome is more accurately defined as an autoimmune phenomenon (discussed in more detail in Chapter 17).

Under normal conditions, circulating immune complexes are removed by phagocytic cells of the reticuloendothelial system. In addition, red blood cells that have C3b receptors may bind complexes that have fixed complement and transport them to the liver, where the complexes are removed by Kupffer cells. When large quantities of immune complexes of a certain size are formed in the circulation they can deposit in the tissues and trigger a variety of *systemic pathogenic events*. Alternatively, antigen–antibody complexes can form at extravascular sites as in situ immune complexes resulting in *localized tissue injury*. An example of the latter is seen in a variety of glomerular diseases in which immune complexes are formed in situ on the glomerular basement membrane. The mechanism of injury seen in immune complex-mediated disease is the same regardless of which pattern of immune complex deposition is seen (i.e., systemic versus local). Central to the pathogenesis of tissue injury is the fixation of complement by the immune complexes, activation of the complement cascade, and release of biologically active fragments (e.g., anaphylotoxins C3a and C5a, see Chapter 13). Complement activation results in increased vascular permeability and stimulates the recruitment of polymorphonuclear phagocytes that release lysosomal enzymes (e.g., neutral proteases) that can damage the glomerular basement membrane.

Systemic Immune Complex Disease

The prototype of systemic immune complex disease is *serum sickness*. This term derives from observations made at the turn of the century by von Pirquet and Schick of the consequences of the treatment of certain infectious diseases, such as diphtheria and tetanus, with antisera made in horses. It was well known that the pathologic consequences of infection by both the *Corynebacterium* and the *Clostridium* organisms were due to the secretion of exotoxins that are extremely damaging to host cells. The bacteria themselves are relatively noninvasive and of little consequence. Hence the strategy that evolved to treat these diseases was to neutralize the toxins rapidly, before quantities large enough to kill the host became fixed in tissues. Since active immunization required several weeks before useful levels of antibody were produced, it was necessary to protect the individual through passive immunization by injecting large amounts of a preformed antitoxin antibody as soon as the disease was diagnosed, in order to prevent death by toxin. Horses, which were readily available, easily immunized, and capable of yielding large quantities of useful antisera, were the animals of choice for the production of antitoxin. Today, we know that the administration of large quantities of heterologous serum, from another species, causes the recipient to synthesize antibodies to the foreign Ig, leading to the formation of antigen–antibody complexes that result in the clinical symptoms associated with serum sickness. This form of hypersensitivity is again becoming an important consideration in patients being treated for malignancy, graft rejection, or autoimmune disease with monoclonal antibodies made in mice or rats.

The pathogenesis of systemic immune complex disease can be divided into three phases. In the first phase, antigen–antibody immune complexes form in the circulation. This is followed by deposition of immune complexes in various tissues that initiates the third phase in that inflammatory reactions in various tissues occur (Figure 15.2). Several factors help to determine whether immune complex formation will lead to tissue deposition and disease. The size of the complexes appear to be important. Very large complexes formed under conditions of antibody excess are rapidly removed from the circulation by phagocytic cells and therefore are harmless. Small or intermediate complexes circulate for longer periods of time and bind less avidly to phagocytic cells. Therefore, small to intermediate immune complexes tend to be more pathogenic as compared with large complexes. A second factor that can influence the development of systemic immune complex disease is the integrity of the mononuclear phagocytic system. An intrinsic dysfunction of this system increases the probability of persistence of immune complexes in the circulation. As expected, overloading this phagocytic system with large quantities of immune complexes also compromises its ability to mediate clearance of such complexes from the circulation. For reasons that are not well understood, the favored sites of immune complex deposition are the kidneys, joints, skin, heart, and small vessels. Localization in the kidney can be explained, in part, by the filtration function of the glomeruli.

Localized Immune Complex Disease

Type III hypersensitivity reactions resulting from acute immune complex vasculitis (also known as Arthus reactions) generate localized tissue necrosis. Although it is the prototype for localized type III hypersensitivity reactions, the Arthus reaction is clinically the least commonly seen. It occurs when antigen and antibody meet, at the appropriate concentrations (antibody excess), in or near vessel walls (venules), to form and accumulate as insoluble antigen–antibody complexes much as they would on a gel-diffusion (Ouchterlony) plate (see Chapter 5). Once the complexes are formed, the subsequent events are very similar to those described in the systemic pattern (see Figure 15.2). The end result is rupture of the vessel wall and hemorrhage, accompanied by necrosis of local tissue (see Figure 15.3A,B).

The experimental proof of this course of events involves the demonstration, by the use of fluorescent antibodies, that antigen, antibody, and various complement components can all be detected at the site of damage to the vessel wall. The requirement for complement and granulocytes together was shown in experiments in which animals depleted of complement (by cobra venom factor) or of neutrophils (by specific anti-polymorphonuclear cell serum) formed aggregates of antigen and antibody, but did not produce the characteristic Arthus reactions. More recently, experiments using IgG Fc receptor knockout mice as well as those that have a gene-targeted disruption of the C5a anaphylatoxin receptor (C5aR) demonstrated dominant roles for these receptors in Arthus reactions.

Infection-Associated Immune Complex Disease

In a variety of infections and for as yet unknown reasons, some individuals produce an antibody that cross-reacts with some constituent of normal tissue. Thus, in Goodpasture's syndrome, for example, pulmonary hemorrhage and glomerulonephritis have been shown to be due to an antibody that binds directly to basement membrane in the lung and kidney, activates complement, and causes membrane damage as a

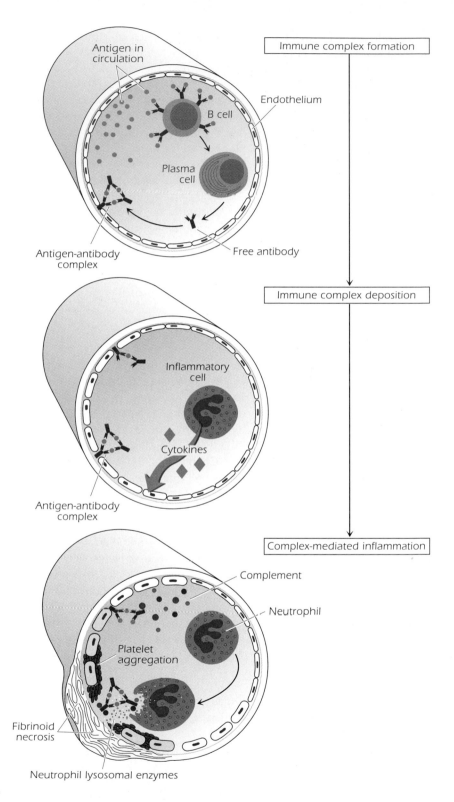

Figure 15.2. Schematic illustration of the three sequential phases in the induction of systemic type III (immune complex) hypersensitivity.

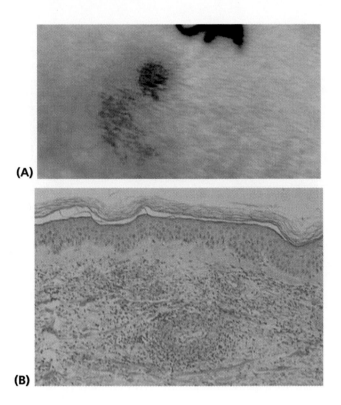

Figure 15.3. Type III hypersensitivity Arthus reaction. **(A)** Gross appearance, showing hemorrhagic appearance (purpura); **(B)** Histologic features of Arthus reaction showing neutrophil infiltrate (courtesy of Dr. M. Stadecker, Tufts University Medical School).

consequence of accumulation of neutrophils and release of degradative enzymes. Goodpasture's syndrome is sometimes considered to be a type II hypersensitivity reaction, since it involves an antibody-mediated cytotoxic effect on normal cells. The distinction between this infection-associated antibody-mediated disease and the immune aggregate disease of serum sickness is that microscopic examination of the lesions reveals a linear, ribbonlike deposit along the basement membrane (see Figure 15.4), as would be expected if an even carpet of antibody were bound to surface antigens. By contrast, in serum sickness the pileup of preformed aggregates on the basement membrane leads to lumpy-bumpy deposits (see Figure 17.2).

Rheumatic fever, a disease that can follow a throat infection with group A streptococci, involves inflammation and damage to heart, joints, and kidneys. A variety of antigens in the cell walls and membranes of streptococci have been shown to be cross-reactive with antigens present in human heart muscle, cartilage, and glomerular basement membrane. It is presumed that antibody to the streptococcal antigens binds to these components of normal tissue and induces inflammatory reactions via a pathway similar to that described above. In rheumatoid arthritis, discussed in Chapter 17, there is evidence for the production of rheumatoid factor, an IgM autoantibody that binds to the Fc portion of normal IgG. These immunoglobulin

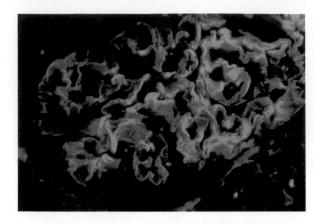

Figure 15.4. Ribbon-like deposit of antibody along the basement membrane revealed by fluorescent antibodies to human Ig. [Courtesy of Dr. A. Ucci, Tufts University Medical School.]

complexes participate in causing inflammation of joints and the damage characteristic of this disease.

In a number of infectious diseases (malaria, some viral infections, leprosy) there may be times during the course of the infection when large amounts of antigen and antibody exist simultaneously and cause the formation of immune aggregates that are deposited in a variety of locations. Thus, the complex of symptoms in any of these diseases may include a component attributable to a type III hypersensitivity reaction.

Occupational Diseases (Hypersensitivity Pneumonitis)

Farmer's lung is an intrapulmonary Arthus-type form of the type III hypersensitivity reactions. It is therefore classified as an occupational disease. In sensitive individuals, exposure to moldy hay leads, within 6–8 hours, to severe respiratory distress or pneumonitis. It has been shown that affected individuals have made large amounts of IgG antibody specific for the spores of thermophilic actinomycetes that grow on spoiled hay. Inhalation of the bacterial spores leads to a reaction in the lungs that resembles the Arthus reaction seen in skin, namely, the formation of antigen-antibody aggregates and consequent inflammation.

There are many similar pulmonary type III reactions that bear names related to the occupation or causative agent, such as pigeon breeder's disease, cheese washer's disease, bagassosis (*bagasse* refers to sugarcane fiber), maple bark stripper's disease, paprika worker's disease, and the increasingly rare thatched roof worker's lung. Dirty work environments, involving massive exposure to potentially antigenic material, obviously lend themselves to the development of this form of occupational disease.

SUMMARY

1. Type II hypersensitivity reactions involve damage to target cells and are mediated by antibody through three major pathways. In the first pathway, antibody (usually IgM, but also IgG) activates the entire complement sequence and causes cell lysis. In the second pathway, antibody (usually IgG) serves to engage receptors for Fc on phagocytic cells, and C3b engages receptors on phagocytic cells with C3b receptors, causing destruction of the antibody and/or C3b-coated target through ADCC. These reactions usually involve circulating blood cells, such as red blood cells, white blood cells, and platelets, and the consequences are those that would be expected from destruction of the particular type of cell. The third pathway leads to dysfunctional cellular consequences caused by the binding of disease-causing antagonistic or agonistic autoantibodies to cell surface receptors (e.g., myasthenia gravis or Graves' disease, respectively).

2. Type III immune complex reactions involve the formation of antigen–antibody complexes that can activate the complement cascade and induce acute inflammatory responses. Release of certain products of complement (C3a and C5a) causes a local increase in vessel permeability and permits the release of serum (edema) and the chemotactic attraction of neutrophils. The neutrophils, in the process of ingesting the immune complexes, release degradative lysosomal enzymes that produce the tissue damage characteristic of these reactions. If the site of reaction is a vessel wall, the outcome is hemorrhage and necrosis; if the site is a glomerular basement membrane, loss of integrity and release of protein and red blood cells into the urine results; and if the site is a joint meniscus, destruction of synovial membranes and cartilage occurs. Multiple forms of this response exist ranging from localized to systemic reactions, depending on the type and location of antigen and the way in which it is brought together with antibody. In all cases, however, the outcome depends on complement and granulocytes as mediators of tissue injury.

REFERENCES

Cotran RS, Kumar V, Robbins SL (1989): The Kidney in Pathologic Basis of Disease. Philadelphia: Saunders.

Dixon FJ, Cochrane CC, Theofilopoulus AN (1988): Immune complex injury. In Samter M, Talmage DW, Frank MM, Austen KF, Claman HN (eds): Immunological Diseases, 4th ed. Boston: Little, Brown.

Fye KH, Sack KE (1994): Rheumatic diseases. In Stites DP, Terr AI, Parslow TG (eds): Basic and Clinical Immunology, 8th ed. E Norwalk, CT: Appleton & Lange.

Hopken UE, Lu B, Gerard NP, Gerard C (1997): Impaired inflammatory responses in the reverse Arthus reaction through genetic deletion of the C5a receptor. *J Exp Med* 29:749

Kumar V, Cotran RS, Robbins SL (1997): Disorders of the immune system. In Basic Pathology, 6th ed. Philadelphia: WB Saunders.

Lawley TJ, Frank MM (1980): Immune complexes and immune complex diseases. In Parker CW (ed): Clinical Immunology, Vol I. Philadelphia: Saunders.

Taki T (1996): Multiple loss of effector cell functions in FcR gamma-deficient mice. *Int Rev Immunol* 13.396.

Terr AI (1994): Immune complex disease. In Stites DP, Terr AI, Parslow TG (eds): Basic and Clinical Immunology, 8th ed. E Norwalk, CT: Appleton & Lange.

Theofilopoulos AN, Dixon FJ (1979): The biology and detection of immune complexes. *Adv Immunol* 28:89.

⬤ REVIEW QUESTIONS

For each question, choose the ONE BEST answer or completion.

1. Which of the following clinical diseases is most likely to involve a reaction to a hapten in its etiology?
   A) Goodpasture's syndrome
   B) hemolytic anemia after treatment with penicillin
   C) rheumatoid arthritis
   D) farmer's lung
   E) Arthus reaction

2. An IgA antibody to a red blood cell antigen is unlikely to cause autoimmune hemolytic anemia because
   A) it would be made only in the gastrointestinal tract.
   B) its Fc region would not bind receptors for Fc on phagocytic cells.
   C) it can fix complement only as far as C1, C4, C2.
   D) it has a too-low affinity.
   E) it requires secretory component to work.

3. The glomerular lesions in immune complex disease can be visualized microscopically with a fluorescent antibody against
   A) IgG heavy chains.
   B) κ light chains.
   C) C1.
   D) C3.
   E) All of the above.

4. The lesions in immune complex-induced glomerulonephritis
   A) are dependent on erythrocytes and complement.
   B) result in increased production of urine.
   C) require both complement and neutrophils.
   D) are dependent on the presence of macrophages.
   E) require all nine components of complement.

5. Serum sickness occurs only
   A) when anti-basement membrane antibodies are present.
   B) in cases of extreme excess of antibody.
   C) when IgE antibody is produced.
   D) when soluble immune complexes are formed.
   E) in the absence of neutrophils.

6. Immune complexes are involved in the pathogenesis of
   A) poststreptococcal glomerulonephritis.
   B) pigeon breeder's disease.

C) serum sickness.

D) an edematous hemorrhagic reaction in the skin of a beekeeper, 2 hours after he was stung for the 20th time.

E) All of the above.

7. The Arthus reaction and farmer's lung differ because

A) only the former is due to antigen–antibody complexes.

B) the mode of contact with the antigen is different.

C) only the former requires complement.

D) only the latter can occur in farmers.

E) the reactions in farmer's lung are much more rapid.

8. The final damage to vessels in immune complex-mediated arthritis is due to

A) cytokines produced by T cells.

B) histamine and SRS-A.

C) the C5, C6, C7, C8, C9 membrane attack complex.

D) lysosomal enzymes of polymorphonuclear leukocytes.

E) cytotoxic T cells.

9. Serum sickness is characterized by

A) deposition of immune complexes in blood vessel walls when there is a moderate excess of antigen.

B) phagocytosis of complexes by granulocytes.

C) consumption of complement.

D) appearance of symptoms before free antibody can be detected in the circulation.

E) All of the above.

10. Type II hypersensitivity

A) is antibody-independent.

B) is complement-independent.

C) is mediated by $CD8^+$ T cells.

D) requires immune complex formation.

E) involves antibody-mediated destruction of cells.

11. A patient is suspected of having farmer's lung. A provocation test involving the inhalation of an extract of moldy hay is performed. A sharp drop in respiratory function is noted within 10 minutes and returns to normal in 2 hours, only to fall again in another 2 hours. The most likely explanation is that

A) the patient has existing T cell-mediated hypersensitivity.

B) this is a normal pattern for farmer's lung.

C) the patient developed a secondary response after the inhalation of antigen.

D) the symptoms of farmer's lung are complicated by an IgE-mediated reactivity to the same antigen.

E) All of the above.

Case Study

A technician in a snake venom-producing farm got careless one day and was bitten by a rare lethal Egyptian cobra. He was rushed to the emergency department, and a call went out immediately for antivenom serum. Fortunately some was located, and within 5 hours he was given 15 ml intravenously. The next day he received another 10 ml, the last available. Within days he was well on the way to recovery and left the hospital a week later. He returned 10 days after leaving the hospital complaining of joint pain, fever, and recurrent itchy hives on his trunk, arms, and legs. What do you suspect is happening, and how would you confirm it?

Answers to Review Questions

1. B Penicillin can function as a hapten, binding to red blood cells and inducing a hemolytic anemia. A, C, and D are examples of immune aggregate (type III) reactions requiring complement and neutrophils for pathologic effects.

2. B Since phagocytic cells have Fc receptors for IgG, bound IgA would not cause engulfment and damage. Thus, A, C, D, and E are false.

3. E The lesions in immune complex disease are dependent on the presence of antigen, antibody, and complement. Hence all can be demonstrated by immunofluorescence at a lesion: A and B, because they are parts of IgG; C and D, because they are the early components of complement activated by the immune aggregated.

4. C Damage by immune complexes requires complement components to attract neutrophils, which are the agents responsible for subsequent tissue damage. Lysis by the final sequence of C6, C7, C8, and C9 is not required.

5. D Anti-basement membrane antibodies may produce damage but can be distinguished from serum sickness lesions by their ribbonlike appearance compared to the lumpy-bumpy appearance of serum sickness lesions. Excess of antibody would clear antigen rapidly with few lesions. IgE antibody is responsible for anaphylactic reactions and neutrophils are required for the lesions typical of serum sickness.

6. E All are examples of type III hypersensitivity reactions: A, by production of antibody, which reacts with normal kidney antigen; B, by inhalation of antigens from pigeon droppings; C, serum sickness is a classical example of an immune complex disease; and D is a description of an Arthus reaction in someone who has been immunized by repeated injection of bee venom.

7. B Both the Arthus reaction and farmer's lung are examples of immune aggregate reactions that require complement and neutrophils. The former involves antigen injected into the skin; the latter involves inhaled antigen.

8. D Neither T cells nor mast cells are responsible for the final tissue damage in immune complex disease. Therefore A, B, and E are eliminated. The final lytic complex of complement is similarly not involved, since complement activation up to C5 is sufficient to bring in the polymorphonuclear leukocytes, whose lysosomal enzymes cause the tissue damage.

9. E All are characteristics of serum sickness.

10. E Type II hypersensitivity reactions occur following development of antibodies against target antigens expressed on normal cells or cells with altered membrane determinants. Antibodies bind to the surface of these cells and mediate damage or destruction by one or more mechanisms, including complement-mediated reactions. CD8$^+$ cytotoxic T cells and immune complexes are not involved in these reactions.

11. D The type III response in farmer's lung and similar occupational diseases has an onset of symptoms usually several hours after exposure. The appearance of breathing difficulties within minutes would create a strong suspicion that a type I anaphylactic response is also present. Presumably the patient made both IgE and IgG antibodies to the actinomycete antigens. A positive wheal and flare reaction on skin testing would provide further confirmation.

Answer to Case Study

Most antivenoms of exotic species such as snake, spider, and scorpion would be made in horses. The horse antiserum neutralized the toxin and saved the patient's life. However, being a foreign protein, it induced an immune response with resultant formation of antigen–antibody complexes and the symptoms of type III hypersensitivity, serum sickness. The localization of these complexes in joints and the activation of complement to give anaphylatoxins were responsible for the joint pain, hives, and itching he experienced. It is possible that he could subsequently develop symptoms of glomerulonephritis as well. Treatment would consist of corticosteroid administration for its general antiinflammatory effects. Confirmatory studies of your diagnosis might include looking for depressed levels of serum C3 and C4 as a result of activation in tissue by the antigen–antibody aggregates. In the convalescent stage one might also find antibody to horse Ig as a final definitive proof of your diagnosis.

16

HYPERSENSITIVITY REACTIONS: T-CELL-MEDIATED, TYPE IV— DELAYED-TYPE HYPERSENSITIVITY

 INTRODUCTION

In contrast to the antibody-mediated hypesensitivity reactions discussed in the previous two chapters, type IV hypersensitivity involves immune responses initiated primarily by antigen-specific T cells. Thus, these responses are an example of ***cell-mediated immunity*** (CMI). When activated by contact with an antigen-presented by antigen-presenting cells, the T cells release cytokines, some of which attract and activate other mononuclear cells that are not antigen-specific such as monocytes and macrophages. This activation is an example of a cascade: the activation of very few, antigen-specific T cells leads to a reaction in which a large majority of recruited, nonantigen-specific mononuclear cells are responsible for the eventual outcome of the reactions. Antigens eliciting this type of response may be foreign tissue (as in allograft reactions), intracellular parasites (e.g., viruses, mycobacteria, or fungi), soluble proteins, or one of many chemicals capable of penetrating skin and coupling to body proteins that serve as carriers.

Unlike antibody-mediated hypersensitivity reactions, which can be transferred from an immunized or sensitized individual to a nonimmune individual via serum, cell-mediated immunity cannot be transferred with serum but can be ***transferred only with T cells***.

The nomenclature for this type of hypersensitivity response has varied over the years, according to historical usage. Originally the response was termed the tuberculin reaction, from the observation by Koch, in 1890, that people infected with *Mycobacterium tuberculosis* gave a positive skin test when injected intradermally with a concentrated lysate of a mycobacterial culture. Subsequently, the delayed nature of the onset of these responses (days, in contrast to minutes or hours for antibody-mediated responses), has led to their collective designation as ***delayed-type hypersensitivity (DTH) reactions***. With the discovery that all these reactions are the consequences of an initial response by T cells, they are now classified as T-cell-mediated or, more simply, cell-mediated immunity (CMI). According to the Gell–Coombs classification of hypersensitivity reactions, DTH or CMI reactions are classified as type IV reactions. This chapter deals with the nature and underlying mechanisms of these reactions.

 ## GENERAL CHARACTERISTICS

Gross Appearance and Histology of the Reaction

A subcutaneous injection of antigen in a sensitized animal or person does not lead to an apparent response until approximately 24–72 hours after challenge. This time course characteristically distinguishes DTH from antibody-mediated reactions, which appear much more quickly (see Chapters 14 and 15). After about 24 hours, evidence of ***erythema*** (redness) and ***induration*** (raised thickening) appear, reaching maximal levels 24–72 hours after the challenge (see Figure 16.1A). The induration can easily be distinguished from edema (fluid) by absence of pitting when pressure is applied. These reactions, even when severe, rarely lead to necrotic damage and resolve slowly.

A biopsy taken early in the reaction reveals primarily mononuclear cells of the monocyte/macrophage series with a few scattered lymphocytes. Characteristically, the mononuclear infiltrates appear as a perivascular cuff before extensively invading the site of deposition of antigen (see Figure 16.1B). Neutrophils are not a prominent feature of the initial reaction. Later biopsies show a more complex pattern, with the arrival of B cells and the formation of granuloma in persistent lesions. The hardness or induration is attributable to the deposition of fibrin in the lesion.

Mechanism of DTH

The mechanisms involved in the sensitization to DTH and the elucidation of the reaction following antigenic challenge are now quite well understood. As in the other types of hypersensitivity reactions, DTH hypersensitivity consists of two main stages, namely, the sensitization stage and the challenge stage, which leads to the reaction. These are shown diagrammatically in Figure 16.2.

In order to mount a DTH reaction, previous ***sensitization*** to the antigen eliciting the response is necessary. This stage lasts 1–2 weeks. Exposure of antigen-specific T cells to peptide–MHC present on antigen-presenting cells results in the activation of the T cell as described in Chapter 10. Once sensitized, the immune system is poised to mount a DTH response following reexposure to the antigen. This ***elicitation phase involves the activation of T_H1 cells***. It should be noted that T cells involved in DTH reactions were formerly referred to as T_{DTH} cells. Only a relatively few antigen-specific T_H1 cells are required to trigger the reaction. These constitute 1–5% of the total cellular, mostly monocytic component of the DTH reaction. Several cytokines are produced by these T_H1 cells, notably chemokines and IFN-γ, which cause chemotaxis and ***activation of macrophages*** (Figure 16.3). It takes approximately 18–24 or even 48 hours from time of antigenic challenge to recruit and

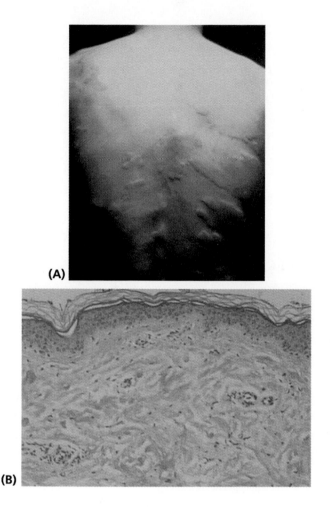

(A)

(B)

Figure 16.1. **(A)** Type IV delayed-type hypersensitivity reaction (tuberculin reaction)—gross appearance showing induration and erythema 48 hours after tuberculin test. [Courtesy of Dr. A. Gottlieb, Tulane University Medical School.] **(B)** Type IV delayed-type hypersensitivity reaction—histologic picture showing dermal mononuclear cell infiltrate and perivascular cuffing. [Courtesy of Dr. M. Stadecker, Tufts University Medical School.]

activate these cells. Cytokines released by all the participating cells are the underlying cause of the DTH reaction. The recruitment and activation of non-antigen-specific cells by antigen specific cells demonstrate the interaction between acquired and innate immunity discussed in Chapter 2. Another cytokine produced by these cells is IL-12. IL-12 suppresses the T_H2 subpopulation and promotes the expansion of the T_H1 subpopulation thereby driving the response to produce more T_H1-synthesized cytokines that activate macrophages. Thus, IL-12 plays an important role in cell-mediated DTH. Table 16.1 summarizes the important cytokines involved in DTH reactions.

DTH reactions can also involve CD8$^+$ T cells, which are first activated and expanded during the induction phase of the response. These cells can damage tissues by cell-mediated cytotoxicity (see Chapter 10). Activation of CD8$^+$ T cells occurs

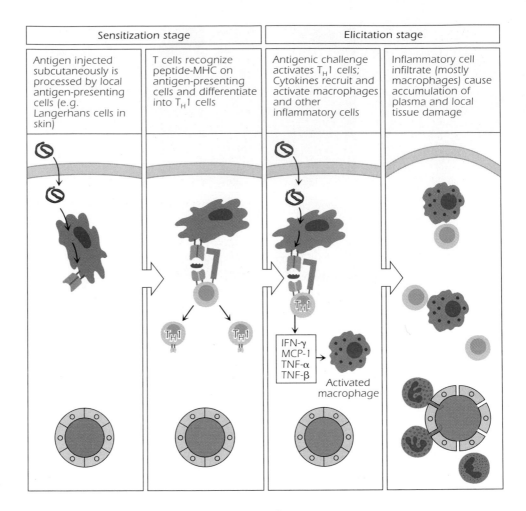

Sensitization stage		Elicitation stage	
Antigen injected subcutaneously is processed by local antigen-presenting cells (e.g. Langerhans cells in skin)	T cells recognize peptide-MHC on antigen-presenting cells and differentiate into T_H1 cells	Antigenic challenge activates T_H1 cells; Cytokines recruit and activate macrophages and other inflammatory cells	Inflammatory cell infiltrate (mostly macrophages) cause accumulation of plasma and local tissue damage

IFN-γ
MCP-1
TNF-α
TNF-β

Activated
macrophage

Figure 16.2. The DTH reaction. Stage of sensitization by antigen involves presentation of antigen to T cells by antigen-presenting cells, leading to the release of cytokines and differentiation of T cells to T_H1 cells. Challenge with antigen involves antigen presentation to T_H1 cells by antigen-presentating cells, leading to T_H1 activation, release of cytokines, and recruitment and activation of macrophages.

as a consequence of the ability of many lipid-soluble chemicals capable of inducing DTH reactions to cross the cell membrane (e.g., pentadecacatechol—the chemical that induces poison ivy). Within the cell, these chemicals react with cytosolic proteins to generate modified peptides that are translocated to the endoplasmic reticulum and then delivered to the cell surface in the context of class I MHC molecules. Cells presenting such modified self-proteins are subsequently damaged or killed by CD8+ T cells.

Consequences of DTH

It should be apparent from the preceding discussion that many of the effector functions in CMI are performed by ***activated macrophages***. In the most favorable cir-

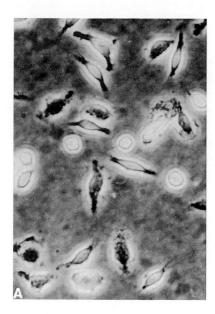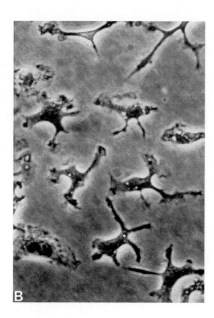

Figure 16.3. The effect of IFN-γ on peritoneal macrophages. **(A)** Normal macrophages in culture as they are just beginning to adhere. **(B)** Macrophages that after activation with IFN-γ have adhered, spread out with development of numerous pseudopodia, and grown larger. More lysosomal granules are also visible. [Courtesy of Dr. M. Stadecker, Tufts University Medical School.]

cumstances, CMI results in destruction of the organism that elicited the response in the first place. This destruction is believed to result predominantly from ***ingestion*** of the organism by macrophages, their activation by IFN-γ, followed by ***degradation*** by ***lysosomal enzymes***, as well as by the by-products of the burst of ***respiratory activity***, such as ***peroxide*** and ***superoxide*** radicals. Foreign tissues, tumor tissue, and soluble or conjugated antigens are dealt with in a similar manner.

In circumstances where the antigen is readily disposed of, the lesion resolves slowly, with little tissue damage. In some circumstances, however, the antigen is

TABLE 16.1. Cytokines Involved in DTH Reactions

Cytokine	Functional effects[1]
IFN-γ	Activates macrophages to release inflammatory mediators
Chemokines	Recruit macrophages and monocytes to the site
MCP-1	
RANTES	
MIP-1α	
MIP-1β	
TNF-α	Causes local tissue damage
TNF-β	Increases expression of adhesion molecules on blood vessels

[1]Additional functional effects are described in Chapter 12.

protected and very persistent; for example, schistosomal eggs and lipid-encapsulated mycobacteria are resistant to enzymatic degradation. In these cases, the response can be prolonged and destructive to the host. Continuous accumulation of macrophages leads to clusters of epithelioid cells, which fuse to form giant cells in **granulomas**. These granulomas, in turn, can be destructive because of their displacement of normal tissue and can result in **caseous (cheesy) necrosis**. The disease process may then be attributable not so much to the effects of the invading organisms as to the persistent attempts of the host to isolate and contain the parasite by the mechanisms of CMI. In diseases such as smallpox, measles, and herpes, the characteristic exanthems (skin rashes) seen are partly attributable to the responses of CMI to the virus, with additional destruction attributable to the attack by cytotoxic T cells on the virally infected epithelial cells.

Variants of DTH

Several known variants of classical DTH or tuberculin reactions have the same basic mechanisms, but have additional features, which are described in the sections that follow.

Contact Sensitivity. *Contact sensitivity* is a form of DTH in which the target organ is the skin, and the inflammatory response is produced as the result of contact with sensitizing substances on the surface of the skin. The prototype for this form of response is **poison ivy dermatitis** (Figure 16.4A,B). The offending substance is **pentadecacatecol**, an oil secreted by the leaves of the poison-ivy vine and other related plants. Pentadecacatecol is a mixture of catechols (dihydroxyphenols) with long hydrocarbon side chains. These features allow it to penetrate the skin by virtue of its lipophilicity (which gives it the ability to dissolve in skin oils) and its ability to couple covalently (by formation of quinones) to some carrier molecules on cell surfaces. Other contact sensitizers are generally also **lipid-soluble haptens**. They have a variety of chemical forms, but all have in common the ability to **penetrate skin** and form **hapten-carrier conjugates**. Experimentally, chemicals such as 2,4-dinitrochlorobenzene (DNCB) are used to induce contact sensitivity. Since virtually every normal individual is capable of developing hypersensitivity to a test dose of this compound, it is frequently used to assess a patients potential for T-cell reactivity. Various metals, such as nickel and chromium, which are present in jewelry and clasps of undergarments, are also capable of inducing contact sensitivity, presumably by way of **chelation** (ionic interaction) by skin proteins.

The induction of contact sensitivity is thought to proceed via presentation of the offending allergen by **Langerhans cells** (antigen-presenting cells in the skin). It is not yet resolved whether the sensitizer couples directly to components on the cell surface of the Langerhans cell or whether it couples first to proteins in serum or tissue that are then taken up by the Langerhans cells. The initial contact results in expansion of the clones of T_H1 cells capable of recognizing the specific contact sensitizer. Subsequent contact with the sensitizer triggers a sequence of events analogous to those described for CMI. In many cases, enough of the sensitizing substance remains at the site of the initial contact so that in approximately one week, when sufficient T-cell expansion takes place, the antigen that persists serves as a challenge and a reaction in this area will flare up without further antigenic challenge. An

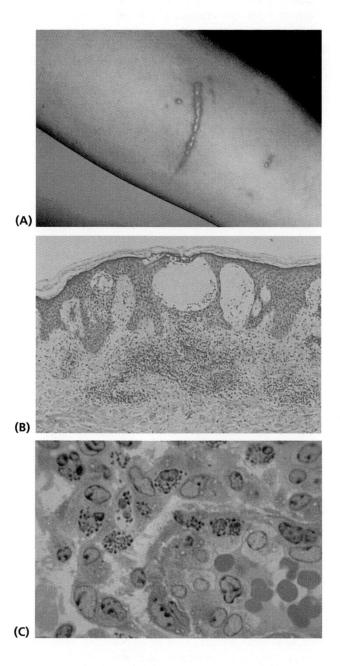

Figure 16.4. **(A)** Type IV contact sensitivity reaction—gross appearance of reaction to poison ivy. [Courtesy of Dr. M. Stadecker, Tufts University Medical School.] **(B)** Type IV contact hypersensitivity reaction—histologic appearance showing intraepithelial blister formation and mononuclear infiltrate in the dermis. [Courtesy of Dr. M. Stadecker, Tufts University Medical School.] **(C)** Cutaneous basophil reaction showing basophils and some mononuclear cells 24 hours after skin test. [Courtesy of Dr. M. Stadecker, Tufts University Medical School.]

additional pathologic component of contact sensitivity reactions in humans is the separation of epidermal cells, *spongiosis*, and *blister* formation (Fig. 16.4B).

The commonly performed procedure for testing for the presence of contact sensitivity is the patch test in which a solution of the suspected antigen is spread on the skin and covered by an occlusive dressing. The appearance, 2–3 days later, of an area of induration and erythema, indicates sensitivity.

Allograft Rejection. As we shall discuss in more detail in Chapter 19, if an individual receives grafts of cells, tissues, or organs taken from an *allogeneic* donor (a genetically different individual of the same species), it will initially be accepted and become vascularized. However, if the genetic difference is at any of the histocompatibility genes, especially genes in the MHC, a rejection process ensues, whose duration and intensity is related to the degree of incompatibility between donor and recipient. The rejection reaction, in general, follows the course described for CMI. After vascularization, there is an initial invasion of the graft by a mixed population of antigen-specific lymphocytes and nonspecific monocytes through the blood vessel walls. This inflammatory reaction soon leads to destruction of the vessels; this deprivation of nutrients is quickly followed by necrosis and breakdown of the grafted tissue.

Cutaneous Basophil Hypersensitivity. An unusual form of delayed reaction has been observed in humans following repeated intradermal injections of antigen. The response is delayed in onset (usually by about 24 hours) but consists entirely of erythema, without the induration typical of classic delayed-hypersensitivity reactions. When this condition was studied experimentally, it was found that the erythema was attended by a cellular infiltrate, but that the predominant cell type was the *basophil* (Fig. 16.4C). Studies in guinea pigs showed that the response was primarily mediated by T cells and was subject to the same MHC restrictions as classic T-cell-mediated responses. When classic delayed hypersensitivity was present, however, infiltrates of basophils were not seen. Thus, cutaneous basophil hypersensitivity (CBH) seemed to be a variant of T-cell-mediated responses, but its exact mechanism was unknown. The picture was complicated still further when it was shown that passive transfer of serum could, under some circumstances, evoke a basophil response.

The function of CBH remained a mystery until it was shown that guinea pigs bitten by certain ticks had severe CBH reactions at the site of attachment of the tick. The infiltration of basophils and, presumably, the release of pharmacologically active materials from their granules resulted in death of the tick and its eventual detachment. Thus, CBH may have an important role in certain forms of immunity to parasites. More recently, basophil infiltrates have also been found in cases of contact dermatitis with allergens such as poison ivy, in cases of rejection of renal grafts, and in some forms of conjunctivitis. These observations indicate that basophils may also play a role in some types of delayed hypersensitivity disease.

TREATMENT OF CELL-MEDIATED IMMUNITY

CMI constitutes a cellular response similar to inflammation (see Chapter 2). It resolves after a period of time (days to weeks) following removal of the antigen.

However, in severe cases or when exposure to antigen persists, corticosteroids, applied either topically or systemically, constitute a very effective treatment.

SUMMARY

1. Delayed-type hypersensitivity (DTH) responses are T-cell-mediated and may be passively transferred with an appropriate quantity of T cells.

2. Unlike type I hypersensitivity, type IV or delayed-type hypersensitivity reactions appear 24–72 hours after antigenic challenge of a sensitized individual.

3. The triggering event for DTH leads to proliferation of T_H1 cells and the release of several cytokines and chemokines, which cause the nonspecific accumulation and activation of monocytes and macrophages. These recruited cells are responsible, in large part, for tissue damage. Cytotoxic $CD8^+$ T cells can also participate in the damage.

4. Macrophages are the major histologic feature of CMI/DTH and account for the protective outcome of CMI such as DTH when pathogens are involved by ingestion and destruction or by released enzymes.

5. CMI is a crucial mode of immunologic reactivity for protection against intracellular parasites, such as viruses, many bacteria, and fungi. However, the nature of the reaction and its mediators also cause delayed-type hypersensitivity reactions.

6. In addition to DTH or tuberculin-type reactions, contact sensitivity and allograft rejection represent variants of the basic mechanism of CMI.

REFERENCES

Adams RM (1989): Occupational Skin Diseases, 2nd ed. Orlando, FL: Grune & Stratton.

Celada A, Nathan C (1994): Macrophage activation revisited. *Immunol Today* 15:100.

Grabbe S, Schwartz T (1998): Immunoregulatory mechanisms involved in elicitation of allergic contact hypesensitivity. *Immunol Today* 19:37.

Kapsenberg ML, Wierenga EA, Bos JD, Jensen HM (1991): Functional subsets of allergen-reactive human $CD4^+$ T cells. *Immunol Today* 12:392.

Mallory SB (1987): Allergic contact dermatitis. *Immunol Allergy Clin N Am* 7:407.

Rosenberg H, Gallin JI (1999): Inflammation. In Paul WE (ed): Fundamental Immunology, 4th ed. New York: Lippincott-Raven.

Sauder DN (1986): Allergic contact dermatitis. In Theiss BD, Dobson AL (eds): Pathogenesis of Skin Disease. New York: Churchill Livingstone. Symposium on Cell-Mediated Immunity in Human Disease (1986): *Hum Pathol* 17:2, 17:3.

Terr AI (1991): Cell-mediated immunity. In Stites DP, Terr AI (eds): Basic and Clinical Immunology, 7th ed. E Norwalk, CT: Appleton & Lange.

Terr AI (1994): Cell-mediated hypersensitivity disease. In Stites DP, Terr AI, Parslow TG (eds): Basic and Clinical Immunology, 8th ed. E Norwalk, CT: Appleton & Lange.

Turk JL (1980): Delayed Hypersensitivity, 3rd ed. Amsterdam: Elsevier.

REVIEW QUESTIONS

For each question, choose the ONE BEST answer or completion.

1. Which of the following does not involve cell-mediated immunity?
   A) contact sensitivity to lipstick
   B) rejection of a liver graft
   C) serum sickness
   D) tuberculin reaction
   E) immunity to chicken pox

2. A positive delayed-type hypersensitivity skin reaction involves the interaction of
   A) antigen, complement, and cytokines.
   B) antigen, antigen-sensitive lymphocytes, and macrophages.
   C) antigen–antibody complexes, complement, and neutrophils.
   D) IgE antibody, antigen, and mast cells.
   E) antigen, macrophages, and complement.

3. Cell-mediated immune responses are
   A) enhanced by depletion of complement.
   B) suppressed by cortisone.
   C) enhanced by depletion of T cells.
   D) suppressed by antihistamine.
   E) enhanced by depletion of macrophages.

4. Delayed skin reactions to an intradermal injection of antigen may be markedly decreased by
   A) exposure to a high dose of X-irradiation.
   B) treatment with antihistamines.
   C) treatment with an antineutrophil serum.
   D) removal of the spleen.
   E) decreasing levels of complement.

5. Patients with DiGeorge syndrome who survive beyond infancy would be capable of
   A) rejecting a bone marrow transplant.
   B) mounting a delayed-type hypersensitivity response to dinitrochlorobenzene.
   C) resisting intracellular parasites.
   D) forming antibody to T-dependent antigens.
   E) All of the above.
   F) None of the above.

6. Which of the following statements is characteristic of contact sensitivity?
   A) The best therapy is oral administration of the antigen.
   B) Patch testing with the allergen is useless for diagnosis.
   C) Sensitization can be passively transferred with serum from an allergic individual.
   D) Some chemicals acting as haptens induce sensitivity by covalently binding to host proteins acting as carriers.
   E) Antihistamines constitute the treatment of choice.

7. Positive skin tests for delayed-type hypersensitivity to intradermally injected antigens indicate that
   A) a humoral immune response has occurred.
   B) a cell-mediated immune response has occurred.

    C) both T cell and B cell systems are functional.

    D) the individual has previously made IgE responses to the antigen.

    E) immune complexes have been formed at the injection site.

8. T cell-mediated immune responses can result in

    A) formation of granulomas.

    B) induration at the reaction site.

    C) rejection of a heart transplant.

    D) eczema of the skin in the area of prolonged contact with a rubberized undergarment.

    E) All of the above.

Case Study

As a member of an anthropologic research team, you have occasion to visit a primitive tribe in the remote reaches of the Amazon jungle. During your visit the natives conduct a ceremony celebrating the rites of passage for young males. This consists, among other things, of covering their bodies with elaborate patterns of stripes and circles using a variety of colors extracted from local plants. On your return 3 weeks later you are asked to look at a young male who has developed alarmingly itchy and weepy red areas of skin that run in sharply demarcated stripes across his back and on one arm. Remembering your introductory course in immunology, you make an educated guess as to the cause. How, under such primitive conditions, could you confirm your diagnosis?

Answers to Review Questions

1. *C* Serum sickness is an example of those reactions mediated by an antibody–antigen complex that involves components of the complement system and neutrophils. All others involve cell-mediated immunity to a significant extent.

2. *B* Cell-mediated reactions result from the triggering of T cells by antigen with recruitment of macrophages. Neither antibody, complement, nor mast cells plays a role in this process, although they do play a role in immediate hypersensitivity responses.

3. *B* Cortisone has a general antiinflammatory effect and is also lytic for some T cells. Complement plays no role, and antihistamines have little effect on this type of response. Depletion of T cells or macrophages would suppress, not enhance, this type of response, since the response is dependent on these cells.

4. *A* High doses of X-irradiation will destroy T cells, which are responsible for initiating the response. Histamine, neutrophils, spleen, and complement do not play a role, and any treatment that affects them would not affect a DTH response.

5. *F* Patients with DiGeorge syndrome have a congenital thymic aplasia and lack all T cell functions. Since A, B, and C are all aspects of a cell-mediated immune response, they would be absent. Additionally, formation of antibody against these antigens is dependent on helper T cells and therefore would not occur in these patients.

6. *D* Patch testing consists of application of the offending allergen under an occlusive dressing, and a positive DTH response after 24–48 hours is considered evidence of sensitivity; thus B is wrong. The allergens involved are those capable of penetrating skin and binding to host carrier proteins; thus D is correct. Oral ingestion of antigen, which, in certain experimental situations, was shown to induce suppression after subsequent induction of contact sensitivity, has not yet been shown to be an effective therapeutic maneuver in humans; thus A is wrong. Corticosteroids, not antihistamines, constitute the treatment of choice for contact sensitivity; thus E is also incorrect.. Passive transfer of cell-mediated immune responses is accomplished with T cells, not with serum, thus C is wrong.

7. *B* A delayed-type hypersensitivity reaction, evidenced by erythema and induration within 24–72 hours of antigen injection, indicates that a cell-mediated reaction has occurred. Such reactions do not involve antibody produced by B cells, thus A, C, D, and E are incorrect.

8. *E* All of these effects are manifestations of cell-mediated immunity. Induration usually takes place at the reaction site. Formation of granulomas is characteristic of a chronic DTH reaction. Rejection of the heart is an example of an allograft response. Some of the chemicals used to cure rubber can induce contact sensitivity after prolonged exposure of the skin to them.

Answer to Case Study

The appearance of the skin lesion and its sharp demarcations and weepy, itchy nature all suggest contact sensitivity. One of the dyes used to paint the body is most likely the sensitizer and, since it persisted on the skin, was also able to provoke a T cell-mediated reaction after the initial expansion of the specific clones. In the absence of sophisticated testing equipment, a simple patch test using samples of the various dyes applied to healthy areas of skin should show a localized contact reaction 24–48 hours later at the site to which the causative dye was applied. (In the laboratory one might also look for an in vitro proliferative response of the patients peripheral blood lymphocytes to added dye. A biopsy of the lesion should reveal an intense infiltrate of mononuclear cells.)

17

AUTOIMMUNITY*

 INTRODUCTION

Tolerance to "self" is an evolutionary device that must remain intact for normal growth, development, and existence. When something occurs to destroy the integrity of self-tolerance (and there are various exogenous as well as endogenous influences that can precipitate such an event), an immune response to self, autoimmunity, may develop.

The consequences of autoimmunity may vary from minimal to catastrophic, depending on the extent to which the integrity of self-tolerance has been affected. Thus, a distinction should be made between autoimmune response and autoimmune disease, in which recognition of self evokes pathologic consequences with the involvement of antibody, complement, immune complexes, and cell-mediated immunity.

In this chapter, some of the more common and better-understood *autoimmune diseases*, together with the mechanisms most probably responsible for them, are discussed in order to present the reader with a framework to view autoimmunity and autoimmune diseases.

 AUTOIMMUNITY AND DISEASE

Several major issues need to be addressed before we discuss specific autoimmune diseases. One concerns the *definition* of autoimmune diseases. A growing number of diseases are suspected of having an autoimmune basis, but the evidence for this may not be straightforward. Criteria used to redefine an idiopathic disease (that is,

---

*This chapter was contributed by Professor Karen M. Yamaga, Department of Tropical Medicine and Medical Microbiology, John A. Burns School of Medicine, University of Hawaii at Manoa.

a disease with unknown origin) to one that has an autoimmune basis will be discussed.

A second issue involves the *etiology* of the disease. Most infectious diseases can be ascribed to a single agent; some genetic diseases are due to a defect in a single gene. By contrast, it is much more difficult to attribute the agent or agents responsible for autoimmune diseases. The most notable quality of autoimmune disease is that the cause is multifactorial, involving both genetic and environmental influences.

A third issue is that some autoimmune phenomena may occur *secondary* to a disease and while significantly contributing to the pathology, the disease should not be considered as a primary autoimmune disease.

CRITERIA FOR AUTOIMMUNE DISEASE

Guidelines have been established for autoimmune disease using three types of evidence.

Direct Proof

Transferring autoantibody or self-reactive lymphocytes to a host and reproducing the disease is the most definitive direct proof. For ethical reasons this criterion has been achieved in only a few circumstances in humans. It can occur when pathogenic antibody is transmitted transplacentally from mother to fetus, in conditions such as neonatal myasthenia gravis, Graves' disease, and polychondritis. T-cell transfer is seldom feasible because MHC molecules of different individuals must be matched. To provide an approach to establishing the pathogenic potential of the T-cell population, severe combined immune-deficient (SCID) mice that lack an immune system can be used as a living "tissue culture flask" for human cells. In fact, peripheral blood lymphocytes from patients with systemic lupus erythematosus (SLE) transferred into these immunologically depleted mice have already been shown to induce immune complex lesions in the kidney of the mice, mimicking human lupus nephritis.

Indirect Evidence

Indirect evidence must be used because of the difficulty in providing direct proof for autoimmune mechanisms. One strategy is to *identify the target antigen in humans, isolate the homologous antigen in an animal model, and reproduce the disease in the experimental animal* by administering the offending antigen. Among the examples in which this approach has succeeded are the induction of thyroiditis with thyroglobulin, myasthenia gravis with acetylcholine receptor, uveitis with uveal S antigen, and orchitis with sperm. Problems arise, however, for those human diseases in which a suitable experimental animal model has not been found, when multifactorial events must occur before the disease arises, when several autoantigens are involved or when the pathogenic antigen is not known.

Another line of indirect evidence that has been used is to *study genetically predisposed animal models*. New Zealand black mice (NZB) spontaneously develop autoimmune hemolytic anemia, while New Zealand white mice (NZW) do not. (NZB × NZW)F_1 animals have been used as a model for human SLE.

The third type of indirect evidence is based on isolating self-reactive antibodies or T cells from the target organs. As examples, antierythrocyte antibodies can be eluted from erythrocytes of autoimmune hemolytic anemia patients, anti-DNA antibodies can be isolated from lupus nephritis patients, and cytotoxic T cells have been found in the thyroid of Graves' disease patients. However, the pathologic significance of these antibodies or T cells has not been easy to establish.

Circumstantial Evidence

Circumstantial evidence is based *on clinical clues that include familial tendency, lymphocyte infiltration, MHC association and, most importantly, clinical improvement with immunosuppressive agents*. For most human diseases, this criterion is used most often to define the disease as autoimmune.

ETIOLOGY OF AUTOIMMUNE DISEASE

As indicated previously, unlike infectious diseases in which the cause can be described to a single organism, autoimmune diseases are multifactorial. A constellation of events must occur before manifestation of the disease becomes apparent. These combinations of events usually encompass both genetic and environmental factors.

Genetic Factors in Autoimmune Disease

The most common evidence for the existence of a *genetic predisposition* to autoimmune disease is in the higher incidence of the disease in monozygotic twins, with a lower but still increased incidence in dizygotic twins and family members when compared with an unrelated population. Although familial tendencies occur, the pattern of inheritance is generally complex and indicates that inheritance is polygenic. This means that no individual gene is sufficient to elicit the disease and many genes may interact with one another. The interaction may result in a synergistic effect, an additive one, or an inhibitory consequence if a gene encodes for a product that cancels out the effect of other genes. Many autoimmune diseases are genetically heterogeneous, that is, the same clinical disease may result from the combined effect of different genes. The fact that predisposing genes are usually common in the general population adds to the difficulty in studying genetic susceptibility. Eliciting the disease may require specific environmental triggers.

One gene family that is associated with autoimmune disease and has been extensively studied is *HLA*, the human MHC. Considering the importance of HLA molecules in shaping the T-cell receptor (TCR) repertoire and their role in recognition by the TCR, this association is not surprising. Specific examples will be discussed later in this chapter in the context of individual autoimmune disease.

In addition, the linkage of non-HLA genes to a number of autoimmune diseases has been found but to date, little is known about their function; the specific genes will be mentioned when individual diseases are discussed below. It will be extremely important to determine the function of these genes in order to understand the complete etiology of the disease.

The mapping of non-MHC genes associated with autoimmune disease has also been described in animal models. For example, as mentioned above, the (NZB ×

NZW)F$_1$ mice develop a disease very similar to human SLE. The NZB mice develop autoimmune hemolytic anemia and glomerulonephritis, while the NZW strain mice have no clinical symptoms. However, when NZB and NZW mice are crossed, the F$_1$ offspring develop a much earlier and more severe form of SLE-like glomerulonephritis than the NZB parent. The NZW mice must therefore contribute some gene(s) that affects the time of onset and severity of the disease. In an SLE-susceptible strain of mice very similar to the NZB × NZW mice, genes on three different chromosomes were found to contribute to lupus glomerulonephritis and anti-double-stranded (ds) DNA antibody formation, traits commonly found in SLE patients.

Environmental Factors

In addition to a genetic predisposition, environmental factors play a role in many autoimmune diseases by triggering the manifestation of the disease. A few autoantigens are protected (*sequestered*) from the immune system (see Chapter 11). Thus, even if some individuals possess autoreactive T and B cells, these cells will not be activated to initiate autoimmunity. The lens and uveal proteins of the eye, the chondrocyte antigens in cartilage, and the antigens of spermatozoa are considered to be examples of sequestered antigens. When they are exposed to the immune system—by some physical accident or due to infection—an autoimmune response may result. Other self-antigens, such as thyroglobulin, IgG, and DNA, which circulate freely, however, also may be involved in autoimmune disease.

In view of all the potentially self-reactive lymphocytes with access to self-antigens, the fact that autoimmune disease is the exception rather than the rule led to the theory that mechanisms exist to hold autoreactive cells in check. Some of these control mechanisms are described in Chapter 11.

The major mechanism that prevents self-reacting T cells from entering into the periphery occurs in the thymus when mature T cells are developing. ***Those T cells that react strongly to self-peptides are deleted.*** This process is an individualized one and some individuals may be more or less efficient in deleting self-reactive T cells. It was recently proposed that an inefficient negative selection process, rather than direct hormonal effects on the immune system (discussed in Chapter 11), may explain the predominance of female sufferers in autoimmune diseases (for example, almost 90% of SLE patients and 95% of Hashimoto's thyroiditis patients are female), but this needs to be demostrated experimentally. Regardless of the reasons why autoreactive immune cells escape to the periphery, control mechanisms must be operating to keep these cells from reacting in normal situations. Some examples of these *peripheral control mechanisms*, and how these control mechanisms are circumvented to lead to autoimmunity, are described below and depicted in Figure 17.1.

Absence of Helper T Cells. Some self-antigens that circulate at low concentrations, such as thyroglobulin, may tolerize self-antigen specific T-helper cells without affecting self-antigen specific B cells (see Chapter 11). Thus, B cells capable of binding thyroglobulin may exist in normal individuals, but they are not triggered to make autoantibody because help by appropriate T cells is not available (see Figure 17.1A).

Several mechanisms have been suggested to explain how the absence or functional inactivation of T helper cells may be overcome to lead to the development of autoimmunity. One suggestion is that autoimmunity develops when an autoreactive

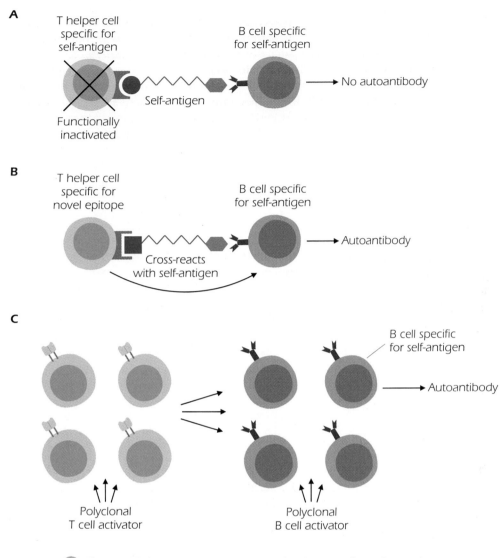

Figure 17.1. Possible mechanisms of induction of autoimmunity.

B cell is activated by T cell help provided by an antigen which contains a **new or altered T cell epitope** (see Fig. 17.1B). This altered epitope activates T cells distinct from those which are tolerant to the self-antigen. Experimentally, such a bypass of tolerance can be achieved by chemical alteration of a self-antigen, or by incorporating it into Freund's complete adjuvant. This may also explain the induction of autoimmune responses following viral infection or after the administration of certain drugs. An autoimmune response can also result following exposure to an antigen cross-reactive with a self-antigen. One example is thyroglobulin derived from a different species, which shares some epitopes with self-thyroglobulin, but also expresses unique epitopes which activate T-helper cells. This results in the activation of self-thyroglobulin specific B cells and the synthesis of autoantibody. In addition, many bacteria, such as streptococci, elicit antibodies that cross-react with normal tissue (heart in the case of streptococcal infection). This *molecular mimicry* can result in autoimmune disease following bacterial infection.

Another possible mechanism involves *polyclonal activators*, which may non-specifically trigger many B-cell clones, including the autoreactive ones, to produce antibody (see Figure 17.1C). Autoantibody synthesis may occur as a consequence of polyclonal T cell activation; for example, by superantigens (discussed in Chapter 10), which activate all T cells expressing a certain $V\beta$, or by grafted, foreign T cells in a graft-versus-host response (see Chapter 19). Alternatively, in the mouse, auto-antibody may be produced as a consequence of stimulation by bacterial lipopoly-saccharide, which directly activates all B cells.

Control by Suppressor T Cells.

Control by Suppressor T Cells. One way by which normal animals may control their immune responses is by induction of cells that function to suppress the immune response, so-called *"suppressor" cells*. Results in some experimental systems have indicated that inhibiting suppressor T cells can result in autoimmunity. This effect may explain why experimentally induced phenomena tend to be acute and self-limiting. Suppressor cells may operate by synthesizing cytokines. As discussed in Chapters 11 and 12, IL-4 inhibits T_H1 activity, whereas IFN-γ inhibits T_H2 activity. Shifting an immune response by preventing IL-4 production may allow the T_H1 activity to remain unchecked resulting in an uncontrolled immunologic response.

In addition to the experimental situations given above, evidence of impaired immunoregulation has been found in several cases of human autoimmune disease, primarily as a deficiency in the functioning of T cells. In some cases, antibodies against suppressor T cells appear, so that the deficiency of these cells may represent a secondary phenomenon.

Absence of MHC Class II Molecules or Secondary Signals on Potential Target Cells.

Absence of MHC Class II Molecules or Secondary Signals on Potential Target Cells. As discussed in Chapters 10 and 11, CD4$^+$ T cells respond to antigen only when presented in association with MHC class II antigens and in the presence of second or costimulatory signals. Thus, certain *APCs that express only MHC class I antigens or lack the costimulatory signal* may not stimulate T cells. It has been shown experimentally that a number of normal cells, such as the endothelial cells in blood vessels and thyroid epithelial cells, may be induced to express MHC class II antigens on their surface by exposure to IFN-γ or other cytokines from activated T cells. These activated cells then become capable, in the absence of specialized APC, of presenting antigens (such as thyroglobulin) to appropriate T cells, thus inducing autoimmune responses. Conceivably, therefore, viral infections of various tissues may lead to induction of MHC class II antigens in relevant cells, triggering a response to some expressed self antigen. Similarly, pancreatic β cells normally do not induce an immune response, but if B7 (CD80/86) antigens are expressed, T cells with the appropriate T cell receptor specificity can become activated by receiving "second signals" through the binding to these molecules via the CD28 interaction.

The study of autoimmune diseases has the potential to be doubly rewarding: in addition to successful treatment of many serious autoimmune diseases, elucidation of the normal control and regulation of the immune response—of which autoimmune disease may represent an aberration—may be better understood.

EXAMPLES OF AUTOIMMUNE DISEASE

The number of autoimmune diseases is growing as circumstantial evidence gives way to more direct proof of the immunologic basis for a number of idiopathic diseases. These autoimmune diseases will be discussed according to their immunopathology and a few examples of diseases that have been reasonably well characterized will be given. A more exhaustive list can be found in references given at the end of this chapter. The diseases are divided into types of effector mechanisms that play a dominant role in the pathogenesis: *antibody, immune complex formation, or effector mechanisms of cell-mediated immunity*. The latter includes effector T cells, (CD4$^+$ T$_H$1 cells, CD8$^+$ T cells, cytotoxic $\gamma\delta$ T cells), and monocyte/macrophage cells. Very little is known about the role of NK cells in these diseases, although NK cells bind antibody through their Fc receptors and may contribute to the pathology by antibody-dependent cell cytotoxicity (ADCC) mechanisms.

Antibody-Mediated Autoimmune Disease

Autoimmune Hemolytic Anemia. Hemolytic anemia is autoimmune *when antibodies react with self-red blood cells*. The cause of a reduction in the number of red blood cells in the circulation is their destruction or removal by antibody directed against an antigen on the surface of the red blood cell. The destruction of the red blood cells can be attributed to two mechanisms. One involves the activation of the complement cascade and eventual *lysis of the red blood cell*. The resultant release of hemoglobin may lead to its appearance in the urine, that is, hemoglobinuria. The second is by the *opsonization* of red blood cells facilitated by antibody and the C3b components of complement. In the latter case, the red blood cells are bound to, and engulfed by, macrophages whose receptors for Fc and C3b attach to the antibody-coated red blood cells.

It is customary to divide the antibodies responsible for autoimmune hemolytic anemia into two groups, on the basis of their physical properties. The first group consists of the *"warm" autoantibodies*, so called because they react optimally with the red blood cells at 37°C. The warm autoantibodies belong primarily to the IgG class, and some react with the Rh antigens on the surface of red blood cells. Because activation of the complement cascade requires the close alignment of at least two molecules of IgG, the relatively sparse distribution of Rh antigens on the surface of the erythrocyte does not favor lysis via the complement pathway. On the other hand, IgG antibodies to these antigens are effective in inducing immune adherence and phagocytosis. Thus, individuals with autoimmune hemolytic anemia can be identified by a Coombs test, which is designed to detect bound IgG on the surface of red blood cells.

A second kind of antibody, *a cold agglutinin*, attaches to red blood cells only when the temperature is below 37°C and dissociates from the cells when the temperature rises above 37°C. Cold agglutinins belong primarily to the IgM class and are specific for I or i antigens present on the surface of red blood cells. Since the cold agglutinins belong to the IgM class, they are highly efficient at activating the complement cascade and causing lysis of the erythrocytes to which they attach. Nevertheless, hemolysis due to cold agglutinins is not severe in patients with autoimmune hemolytic anemia as long as their body temperature is maintained at 37°C. When arms, legs, or skin are exposed to cold and the temperature of the circulating blood is allowed to drop, severe attacks of hemolysis may occur.

Although the cause of autoantibody formation often is not known, some clues are offered by drug-induced anemia. A drug like penicillin, for example, may bind to some protein on the surface of red cells in much the same way as the formation of a hapten-carrier complex and induce formation of antibody. The resulting antibody reacts with the drug (hapten) on the surface of the cell, causing lysis or phagocytosis. In such cases, however, the disease is self-limiting and disappears when drug use is discontinued.

Another example of drug-induced anemia occurs in a small minority of patients using α-methyldopa, an antihypertensive drug. It leads to a disorder that is almost identical to that characterized by warm autoantibodies. Sometimes, cold agglutinins appear after infection by *Mycoplasma pneumoniae* or viruses implicating a role for an infectious disease trigger in genetically susceptible individuals.

Myasthenia Gravis. Myasthenia gravis is another autoimmune disease which involves antibodies to a well-defined target antigen. The target is the *acetylcholine receptor at the neuromuscular junction*. Reaction of the receptor with antibody blocks the reception of a nerve impulse normally carried across the junction by acetylcholine molecules. This blockade results in severe muscle weakness, manifested by difficulty in chewing, swallowing, and breathing, and it eventually leads to death from respiratory failure. It affects individuals of any age, but the peak incidences occur in women in their late twenties and men in their fifties and sixties. The female:male ratio is approximately 3:2.

The disease can be experimentally induced in mammalian animal models by immunization with adjuvant plus acetylcholine receptors purified from torpedo fish or electric eel, which demonstrate significant cross-reactivity with mammalian receptors. The experimental disease, which mimics almost exactly the natural form of the disease, results from the binding of antibodies generated against the foreign receptors to the mammal's acetylcholine receptors. The disease may be passively transferred with antibody. Some babies of myasthenic mothers have transient muscle weakness, presumably because they received sufficient amounts of pathogenic IgG by transplacental passage.

The development of myasthenia gravis may somehow be linked to the thymus, since many patients have concurrent thymoma, or hypertrophy of the thymus, and removal of the thymus sometimes leads to regression of the disease. Molecules cross-reacting with the acetylcholine receptor have been found on various cells in the thymus such as thymocytes and epithelial cells, but whether these molecules are the primary stimulus for the development of the disease is unknown. With regard to genetic predisposition, myasthenia gravis is associated with HLA class II loci.

Graves' Disease. One of the main manifestations of Graves' disease is a hyperactive thyroid gland (hyperthyroidism). This aspect of the disease serves as an example in which *antibodies directed against a hormone receptor may activate the receptor* rather than interfere with its activity, as in myasthenia gravis. For reasons not yet understood, in Graves' disease, patients develop autoantibodies against thyroid cell surface receptors for thyroid-stimulating hormone (TSH). The interaction of these antibodies with the receptor activates the cell in a manner similar to the activation by TSH. The long-lasting stimulation by these antibodies causes hyperthyroidism due to the continuous stimulation of the thyroid gland.

The indirect evidence that Graves' disease is autoimmune includes familial predisposition, genetic association with HLA class II genes, and correlation with antibody titer to TSH receptors and disease severity. However, the best evidence is the transmission of thyroid-stimulating antibodies from a thyrotoxic mother across the placenta, causing transient neonatal hyperthyroidism until the maternal IgG is catabolized. The disease most commonly affects women in their thirties and forties. In nongoitrous areas, the female:male ratio is about 7:1. Genetic factors play a role with a linkage to MHC class II genes, and a familial predisposition. Recently, the International Consortium for the Genetics of Autoimmune Thyroid Disease found a new Graves' disease susceptibility gene on chromosome 20q11.2.

Other Autoantibody-Mediated Diseases. Other examples of autoimmune diseases mediated by autoantibodies are also discussed in Chapter 15. These include ***idiopathic thrombocytopenia purpura*** (antibody specific for a platelet antigen), ***pemphigus vulgaris*** (antibody specific for a skin epidermal antigen), and ***Goodpasture's syndrome*** (antibody specific for basement membrane collagen). In addition, ***rheumatic fever*** occurs as a consequence of antibodies induced in streptrococcal infections cross-reacting with heart muscle. This results in an arthritic condition which damages the joints, and additional problems such as scarring of the heart valves.

Immune Complex-Mediated Autoimmune Disease

Systemic Lupus Erythematosus. SLE presumably gets its name (literally "red wolf") from a reddish rash on the cheeks, which is a frequent early symptom. However, the distribution of the rash resembles the wings of a butterfly rather than the face of a wolf. The designation "wolflike" is thus far-fetched, but the term "systemic" is quite appropriate, since the disease attacks many organs of the body and causes fever, joint pain, and damage to the central nervous system, heart, and kidneys. Kidney lesions, which cause the most mortality from SLE, are the most clearly understood.

Despite the mystery concerning the origin of this disease, details of the immunologic mechanisms responsible for the pathology are partially known. Antibodies to single-stranded and double-stranded DNA are produced in normal individuals, but they are generally low-affinity IgM antibodies. They can, however, undergo isotype switching and somatic mutation resulting in the production of high-affinity IgG antibodies, provided the B cells are given appropriate T-cell help. SLE patients produce ***dangerous levels of anti-DNA antibodies***. Among the possible reasons are: an enhanced activity of $CD4^+$ helper cells, a failure of cells that normally suppress the activation of B cells, or the inability of phagocytic cells to clear immune complexes. Regardless of the reason, patients with SLE produce antibody against several nuclear components of the body (antinuclear antibodies [ANA]), notably against native double-stranded DNA. Occasionally antibodies are also produced against denatured, single-stranded DNA and against nucleohistones, but clinically, the presence of anti-double-stranded DNA correlates best with the pathology of renal involvement in SLE (see below).

These antibodies directed to DNA may form ***circulating soluble complexes*** with DNA derived from the breakdown of normal tissue, such as skin. The abnormal sensitivity of SLE patients to ultraviolet irradiation, which causes prompt exacerbation of symptoms, lends some credence to this idea. As in any immune complex disease (described in Chapter 15), the soluble complexes are filtered out of the blood in the kidneys and get trapped against the basement membranes of the glomeruli, forming characteristic "lumpy-bumpy" deposits. These are shown in Figure 17.2. (Note the difference between the pattern shown in this figure and the "ribbon" pattern depicted in Figure 15.4, which illustrates autoantibody binding to antigen expressed by kidney basement membrane, a characteristic of Goodpasture's syndrome.) Other complexes may be similarly trapped in arteriolar walls and joint synovial spaces. Alternatively, the antigen alone, double-stranded DNA, may become trapped in the glomerular basement membrane through electrostatic interactions with a constituent of the membrane, trapping antibody. These complexes activate the complement cascade and attract granulocytes. In the kidney, the extent of the inflammatory reaction forms the basis of classifying kidney pathology. The resulting damage to the kidneys leads to leakage of protein (proteinuria) and sometimes hemorrhage (hematuria), with symptoms waxing and waning as the rate of formation of immune complexes rises and falls. As the condition becomes chronic, inflammatory $CD4^+$ T_H1 cells enter the site and attract monocytes which further contribute to the pathologic lesions.

Although the antigen that initiates production of these antibodies is unknown, infectious agents have been proposed. SLE may be the result of an immune response made by only a few genetically disposed individuals to some common environmental organism. Other environmental factors include ultraviolet light that exacerbates the disease, the influence of hormones (SLE is 10 times more frequent in women than in men during reproductive years, and exacerbation occurs during pregnancy), and the induction of SLE-like symptoms by drugs, such as penicillamine. Evidence for

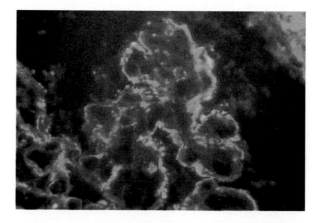

Figure 17.2. "Lumpy-bumpy" staining pattern of fluorescent antibody specific for human Ig: immune aggregate deposits in glomerular basement membrane. [Courtesy of Dr. Angelo Ucci, Tufts University School of Medicine.]

genetic predisposition includes the increased risk of developing SLE among family members, the higher rate of concordance (25%) in monozygotic twins when compared with dizygotic twins (<3%), linkage with HLA class II genes, and the presence of an inherited deficiency of an early complement component in 6% of SLE patients. About 90% of the cases are women of child-bearing age.

T-Cell-Mediated Autoimmune Diseases

Multiple Sclerosis. Multiple sclerosis (MS) *involves demyelinization of central nervous system tissue and leads either to a relapsing–remitting or a chronic progressive paralytic course*. It is considered to be a T-cell-mediated autoimmune disease. The lesions resemble the cellular infiltrates associated with T_H1 cells involved in delayed-type hypersensitivity (see Chapter 16).

It is not clear whether the autoimmune response is due to failure of clonal deletion, from neuroantigen sensitization, or *molecular mimicry to a neuroepitope* following a virus infection. The evidence that MS is an autoimmune disease is indirect and has relied on an experimentally induced model in rodents, namely, experimental allergic encephalomyelitis (EAE). Following immunization of animals with myelin protein in Freund's complete adjuvant, the animals develop many of the characteristics of multiple sclerosis. $CD4^+$ T-cell clones specific for myelin basic protein can transfer the EAE disease. Circumstantial evidence for the autoimmune nature of MS includes the HLA class II association with the disease susceptibility and the finding of a higher T-cell response to myelin components in cerebral spinal fluid of MS patients than in control subjects.

One area of study has established the ability of activated T cells to penetrate the blood-brain barrier that ordinarily prevents cells and macromolecules from entering the central nervous system. Integrins are upregulated in activated T cells, which may allow the T cells to adhere to the vessels near the brain. Activated T cells can also produce metalloproteinases, which disrupt the collagen in the basal lamina allowing T cells to accumulate into the central nervous system. Once there, the T cells must undergo antigenic stimulation (perhaps via microglia) to persist. Chemokines are produced that attract additional inflammatory cells. This results in the accumulation not only of $CD4^+$ T cells, but also macrophages and microglia; all these cells contribute to tissue injury. The inflammatory process induces intense Fas upregulation on oligodendrocytes, making them targets for T cells and microglia expressing FasL and inducing apoptosis.

Familial aggregations occur in MS with a high concordance rate among identical twins (25–30%) as compared with dizygotic twins (2–5%). It is twice as common in females as in males and its peak incidence is at age 35. Recent genetic studies suggest that approximately 12 regions of the human genome may be important for susceptibility to MS. Identifying these genes and determining how they relate to the immune system will aid in understanding the underlying defect and immunopathogenesis of MS.

Type 1 Insulin-Dependent Diabetes Mellitus. Type 1 insulin-dependent diabetes mellitus (IDDM) *involves chronic inflammatory destruction of the insulin-producing β-islet cells of the pancreas*. Genetic factors include several genes in the

HLA class II regions, the insulin gene on chromosome 11 and at least 11 other non-HLA linked diabetes susceptibility genes. Some HLA class II haplotypes are predisposing for the disease and others are protective. For example, approximately 50% of IDDM patients are HLA–DR3/DR4 heterozygotes in contrast to 5% of the normal population. On the other hand, individuals with HLA–DQB1*0602 never develop the disease.

An experimental animal model, the nonobese diabetic (NOD) mouse, shares many key features with the human disease, including the destruction of islet cells by lymphocytes, the association with susceptible MHC genes and transmission by T cells. At least 14 genes contribute to diabetes found in NOD mice. There are, however, notable differences between the human disease and the mouse model. These include the predominance of T cells in NOD mice when compared with IDDM in humans, and a greater bias to incidence of disease in female mice compared to human disease. In IDDM, the major contributors to β cell destruction are cytotoxic T cells, cytokines, and autoantibodies. The pancreatic β cells appear to be particularly susceptible to lysis (as opposed to pancreatic α or δ cells) perhaps because these cells upregulate Fas or costimulatory molecules on their surface during the initial inflammation phase (insulitis). T cells producing FasL can induce apoptosis within the β cells while sparing the other α and δ pancreatic cells lacking Fas.

Hashimoto's Thyroiditis. Hashimoto's thyroiditis is a disease of the thyroid most commonly found in middle-aged women, which **leads to the formation of a goiter or to hypothyroidism and results in the destruction of thyroid function**. There is a greater incidence of other autoimmune diseases in family members of patients with Hashimoto's thyroiditis than in the normal population. The disease is mediated primarily by T cells, but antibodies may contribute to the disease process.

Several target antigens are involved in this disease process, including thyroglobulin, the major hormone produced by the thyroid. Microsomal antigens from thyroid epithelial cells also have been implicated, and antibodies to all these antigens have been found in Hashimoto's disease patients.

The evidence for mediation by T cells is, at best, indirect. The suggestion rests, in part, on the histologic picture that accompanies this disease. There is an infiltration of predominantly mononuclear cells into the thyroid follicles, which is characteristic of other T_H1 reactions. However, the mononuclear infiltrates contain large numbers of B cells in addition to T cells and macrophages, indicating their involvement as well. Progressive destruction of thyroid follicles accompanies the presence of these infiltrates, and the gland attempts to regenerate and becomes enlarged. When destruction of follicles reaches a certain level, the output of thyroid hormone declines and the symptoms of hypothyroidism appear: dry skin, puffy face, brittle hair and nails, and a feeling of being continuously cold.

Further evidence implicating T-cell-mediated responses comes from study of experimental autoimmune thyroiditis, which may be induced in animals either by immunization with thyroglobulin in Freund's complete adjuvant or by passively transferring clones of $CD4^+$ T_H1 cells specific for thyroglobulin. An important distinction between the experimental and the naturally occurring autoimmune disease is that the former is acute and nonrecurring while the latter has a chronic, recurrent course. Thus, the precipitating event in the naturally occurring autoimmune disease is probably some ongoing process, rather than a single immunizing event.

Rheumatoid Arthritis. Rheumatoid arthritis is characterized by *chronically inflamed synovium, densely crowded with lymphocytes, which results in the destruction of cartilage and bone*. The inflamed synovial membrane, usually one cell thick, becomes so cellular that it mimics lymphoid tissue and forms new blood vessels. The synovium is densely packed with dendritic cells, macrophages, T, B, NK cells, and clumps of plasma cells; in some cases the synovium develops secondary follicles. The pathology in its most intense form is probably the consequence of a mixture of immunopathologic mechanisms, specifically, antigen–antibody complexes, complement, polymorphonuclear neutrophils, inflammatory $CD4^+$ T cells, $CD8^+$ cytotoxic T cells, activated macrophages, and NK cells. This "angry mix" releases a variety of cytokines, of which TNF-α and IL-1 are among the earliest, degradative enzymes, and mediators that result in the destruction of the cartilage integrity. Chondrocytes, the cells of the cartilage, become exposed to the immune system and perpetuate the damage by not only serving as potential targets but releasing cytokines and growth factors as well. Synovial fluid often accumulates in the joints of RA patients and contains large numbers of polymorphonuclear neutrophils. After repeated bouts of inflammatory insults, fibrin is deposited, cartilage is replaced by fibrous tissue, and the joint fuses (ankylosis).

It has been suggested that inflammatory processes are initiated by abnormally produced antibody, generally IgM, called rheumatoid factor (RF), which is specific for a determinant on the Fc portion of the patient's own IgG molecules. However, it is unlikely that RF is the common initiator of the disease, since 30% of RA patients do not have detectable levels of RF. The group of patients with RF tends to develop a more aggressive disease. RF serves as a useful marker of disease activity since reduced levels of serum RF are found during remission. The presence of RF contributes to the pathology or RA, but probably does not account for the T-cell response.

The initial insulting trigger may be diverse. A high proportion of RA patients have elevated numbers of B cells infected with Epstein-Barr virus; $\gamma\delta$ T cells from RA patients recognize heat-shock proteins; and bacteria have been associated with RA.

Women are affected three times more often than men and the age of onset is usually during the fourth and fifth decades of life. The association of various genes has been examined in family studies in RA for many different populations. In general, the association of HLA–DR4 alleles and RA has been confirmed in most ethnic groups, although the subtype varies. For example, the HLA–DRB1 association for North American Caucasians is *0401 and *0404, whereas for Israelis, it is *0102 and *0405 and for Yakima Indians, it is *1402. DNA sequencing of these molecules show that they share a segment of the outermost domain of the HLA–DR β chain, called the "shared epitope." Individuals having two different HLA-DRB1 both with shared epitopes had the highest risk for developing RA and expressed the most severe form of the disease. Other genes strongly associated with RA include TNF genes, heat shock protein gene complex, and TCR genes.

Perhaps the most exciting development in rheumatoid arthritis is the clinical use of *TNF-α inhibiting drugs* as a treatment strategy. Two different approaches have been successfully tested: one is a mouse–human *chimeric anti-TNF-α antibody* and the other is a *soluble TNF receptor* genetically linked to the Fc portion of human IgG. Of the cytokine inhibitors tested, these are the first to reach a large-scale market for the treatment of an autoimmune disease. This marks the beginning of a new era in the treatment of rheumatoid arthritis.

Autoimmune Diseases Arising From Deficiency in Components of Complement

Many patients with deficiencies in the early components of complement develop autoimmune diseases such as SLE (see Chapter 13). In addition, specific allotypes of some complement components predispose to the development of autoimmunity.

Both the classical complement pathway and alternative pathway inhibit the formation of large immune complexes. C1, C4, and C2 appear to directly affect the size of immune complexes, whereas C3b plays a key role in both pathways. Incorporation of C3b solubilizes immune complexes. C3b reduces the lattice size of the complex, perhaps by disrupting the capacity of the antibody to bind to the antigens. The addition of C3b to the antigen–antibody complex promotes the binding to C3b receptor on many cell types, including phagocytic cells, and red blood cells. The complexes bound to erythrocytes are rapidly transported to the liver and spleen, and those taken up by phagocytes are degraded.

The inappropriate deposition of immune complexes leading to disease can occur under several different circumstances:

1. Excessive immune complex formation overwhelming the clearance mechanism as in serum sickness (see Chapter 15).
2. Deficient antibody response such that complement is poorly activated.
3. Inherited deficiency of a component of the classical complement pathway. A defect in any one of the C1, C4, or C2 complement components prevents the activation of the classical pathway, and deficiency of C4b and C3b would result in failure to clear immune complexes by macrophages.
4. Abnormalities in complement or Fc receptors on cells also leading to inefficient clearance of immune complexes.

Interestingly, SLE occurs in over 80% of individuals with complete deficiency of C1, C4, or C2. The sera of such patients are markedly deficient in their ability to deposit C3b on immune complexes and "processing" of even normal amounts of these complexes would be altered.

SUMMARY

1. Autoimmunity is a condition in which the body mounts an immune response to one or more of its own constituents.

2. Establishing a disease as autoimmune rests on several types of evidence: (a) direct proof, by transferring autoantibodies or self-reactive lymphocytes into an otherwise healthy individual and reproducing the disease; (b) indirect proof, which requires finding an experimental animal model to mimic the disease; (c) circumstantial evidence based on familial tendency, involvement of immune cells and antibodies, and, most importantly, clinical improvement with immunosuppressive drugs.

3. Initiation of autoimmune diseases usually requires a combination of genetic and environmental events. It is believed that many autoreactive clones of T

and B cells exist normally but are held in check by homeostatic mechanisms. It is the breakdown, by various mechanisms, of these controls that leads to the activation of autoreactive clones and autoimmune disease.

4. A multiplicity of organs and tissues is involved in autoimmune disease, and the type of immune response may involve antibody, complement, T cells, or macrophages.

REFERENCES

De Maria R, Testi R (1998): Fas–FasL interactions: a common pathogenetic mechanism in organ-specific autoimmunity. *Immunol Today* 19:121.

Fauci AS, Braunwald E, Isselbacher KJ, Wilson JD, Martin JB, Kasper DL, Hauser SL, Longo DL (eds) (1998): Harrison's Principles of Internal Medicine, 14th ed. New York: McGraw-Hill.

Feltkamp TEW, Aarden LA, Lucas CJ, Verweig CL, deVries RRP (1999): Genetic risk factors for autoimmune diseases. *Immunol Today* 20:10.

Frank MM, Austen KF, Claman HN, Unanue ER (eds) (1995): Samter's Immunologic Diseases, 5th ed. Boston: Little, Brown.

Hahn BV (1998) Mechanisms of disease: antibodies to DNA. *N Engl J Med* 338:1333.

O'Dell JR (1999): Anticytokine therapy: a new era in the treatment of rheumatoid arthritis? *N Engl J Med* 340:310.

Rose NR (1998): The role of infection in the pathogenesis of autoimmune disease. *Semin Immunol* 10:5.

Rose NR, Bona C (1993): Defining criteria for autoimmune diseases (Witebsky's postulates revisited). *Immunol Today* 14:426.

Sorensen TL, Ransohogg RM (1998): Etiology and pathogenesis of multiple sclerosis. *Semin Neurol* 18:287.

Stewart JJ (1998): The female X-inactivation mosaic in systemic lupus erythematosus. *Immunol Today* 19:352.

 ## REVIEW QUESTIONS

For each question, choose the ONE BEST answer or completion.

1. Most autoimmune diseases are caused by a
- A) single genetic defect.
- B) known infectious organism.
- C) constellation of genetic and environmental events.
- D) hormonal dysregulation.
- E) B-cell defect.

2. Identifying an autoimmune disease in humans is often accomplished by
- A) finding an antibody against self-components.
- B) passively transferring specific T cells from a patient to a healthy individual.
- C) showing that T cells or antibodies are the cause of the tissue damage.

D) circumstantial evidence, such as MHC association and clinical improvement, with immunosuppressive drugs.

E) finding the definitive agent or agents responsible for the disease.

3. The following is/are possible mechanism(s) for the recognition of self-components by the immune system in autoimmune diseases:

A) alteration of a self-antigen so it is recognized as foreign

B) leakage of sequestered self-antigen

C) loss of suppressor cells

D) infection with a microorganism that carries a cross-reactive antigen

E) Any of the above.

4. Rheumatoid factor, found in synovial fluid of patients with rheumatoid arthritis, is most frequently found to be

A) IgM reacting with L chains of IgG.

B) IgM reacting with H-chain determinants of IgG.

C) IgE reacting with bacterial antigens.

D) antibody to collagen.

E) antibody to DNA.

5. The pathology in autoimmune diseases due to antibody may be a result of

A) the formation of antigen–antibody complexes.

B) antibody blocking a cell receptor.

C) antibody-induced phagocytosis.

D) antibody-induced complement mediated lysis.

E) Any of the above.

6. Autoimmune hemolytic anemia:

A) is usually due to warm agglutinins belonging to the IgM class directed against Rh antigens on red blood cells

B) may be due to the production of either cold agglutinins after viral infection or autoantibodies following drug treatment.

C) is the result of cytotoxic T cells lysing red blood cells

D) does not generally involve complement components in red blood cell lysis

E) can be characterized by a negative Coombs test

7. Systemic lupus erythematosus

A) is due to a mutation in double-stranded DNA.

B) is a classic example of a T-cell-mediated autoimmune disease.

C) has multiple symptoms and affects many organs.

D) results from antibodies specific to thyroid.

E) affects only skin epithelial cells.

8. Diseases in which T_H1 cells and cytotoxic $CD8^+$ T cells probably play major roles in their pathology include all of the following *except*

A) myasthenia gravis.

B) Hashimoto's thyroiditis.

C) rheumatoid arthritis.

D) multiple sclerosis.

E) insulin-dependent diabetes mellitus.

9. A patient is found to have a form of diabetes in which his immune system is destroying his pancreatic islet cells. Which is the most likely explanation for this disease state?

A) The patient has an acquired immunodeficiency syndrome.

B) Immune complex formation and complement are the main contributors to insulitis.

C) In the islets of the pancreas, β cells have upregulated MHC class II and Fas molecules, making them susceptible to cell death by immune cells.

D) There is an increase in suppressor cells.

E) CD4^{+} T cells are being destroyed by pancreatic enzymes.

10. Hashimoto's thyroiditis

A) is due primarily to antibodies formed to thyroid-stimulating hormone receptors.

B) mimics an animal model in which the disease is induced by immunization with thyroglobulin.

C) can be transplacentally transmitted causing a neonatal form of the disease.

D) is an autoimmune disease which affects males and females equally.

E) is characterized by immune complex deposition in the thyroid.

Case Study

A 17-year-old boy suffered an injury to his left eye when, during a car crash, a sharp sliver of glass penetrated his eye, damaging his lens and uveal tract. The glass was removed and the injury repaired with complete recovery. However, 3 weeks later he noticed some redness in the left eye and photophobia, followed by pain and severe visual impairment. The left eye was removed, and histologic examination showed an extensively infiltrated uveal tract with abundant lymphocytes and mononuclear cells. Two weeks later the other eye began to show the same symptoms. What is going on, and what could be done?

Answers To Review Questions

1. *C* The etiologies of most autoimmune diseases appear to be multifactorial and require a combination of genetic and environmental events to manifest themselves.

2. *D* For most human autoimmune disease circumstantial evidence is used. Merely finding an antibody to self-components does not imply that there is a disease condition. T cells or antibodies are the cause of tissue damage in many diseases, such as infectious disease, and does not necessarily mean that the disease is an autoimmune one. Passive transfer of T cells is difficult in humans and in most autoimmune diseases, no definitive agent or agents have been identified. The best answer is D.

3. *E* Self-reactive T and B cells may be activated by any of the mechanisms listed.

4. *B* Rheumatoid factor is generally an IgM antibody that reacts with Fc determinants on the H chain.

5. *E* All are possible causes of antibody-induced autoimmune disease.

6. *B* Warm agglutinins belong to the IgG class; cytotoxic T cells are not known to cause autoimmune hemolytic anemia; complement is a frequent participant in lysis or opsonization; the Coombs test is frequently positive for either IgG, IgM or C3 in patients with autoimmune hemolytic anemia.

7. *C* Systemic lupus erythematosus affects skin, kidneys, heart, and joints. Symptoms are due to immune complexes that lodge in those areas and induce damage via activation of complement and infiltration of leukocytes. DNA may be involved as an antigen, but mutation plays no role, and the disease is initiated primarily by antibodies and is not considered a classic T-cell disease.

8. *A* Antibody has been implicated in myasthenia gravis both from experimental animal models and the fact that neonatal form can be transferred through the placenta from mother to baby. The other diseases listed are primarily cell mediated by effector T cells.

9. *C* One of the currently favored mechanisms for type 1 diabetes is an autoimmune response in which CD4$^+$ T$_H$1 cells specific for islet cells which have upregulated the expression of MHC class II molecules become activated and participate in the inflammatory reaction. Cytotoxic T cells and other immune cells cause the death of the β cells leading to insulin-dependent diabetes.

10. *B* Hashimoto's thyroiditis is thought to be a T-cell-mediated disease, some features of which can be found in an experimental model by immunization of animals with thyroglobulin in adjuvant.

Answer to Case Study

The most likely diagnosis is of a rare case of sympathetic ophthalmia, an autoimmune disease in which trauma to uveal, retinal, and lens tissues releases antigens that induce T-cell-mediated responses. Once generated, these T cells attack the damaged eye and induce a granulomatous uveitis. They also have the potential for attacking the healthy eye, producing the same damaging effects. The diagnosis could be confirmed by the appearance of positive delayed-type reactions following skin testing with an extract of bovine uveal tissue, which cross-reacts immunologically with human uveal tissue. A safe procedure would be to look for an in vitro proliferative response of the patient's peripheral blood lymphocytes when exposed to the same antigen.

Immunosuppressive therapy with topical or systemic corticosteroids is useful in mild cases. Removing the damaged eye is the only way to prevent the onset of the autoimmune reaction. In these cases, clinicians must weigh the chances of maintaining useful vision in the injured eye against the risk of an autoimmune reaction with possible loss of both eyes.

18

IMMUNODEFICIENCY AND OTHER
DISORDERS OF THE IMMUNE SYSTEM*

 INTRODUCTION

The immune response is mediated by T cells, B cells (and antibody), phagocytic cells, and complement. As we have seen in previous chapters, interactions among these cells and soluble mediators are tightly controlled. Disorders in the development and differentiation of the cells, synthesis of their products, or interactions between them may lead to immune deficiencies that range in clinical severity from mild to fatal. Although inborn immunodeficiency diseases are rare, it was through astute observations of these "experiments of nature" that the field of cellular immunology emerged. Animal models designed to mimic the different clinical presentations demonstrated the cellular subdivisions of specific immunity into T and B lymphocytes or cell-mediated versus humoral immunity. This approach continues today as these rare syndromes are analyzed on a molecular level to teach us what controls immune cell development, interactions, and intracellular signaling. Noticeably absent from clinical detection are deficiencies where the immune system shows redundancy, such as in the cytokine network. The information gained from studying these diseases is applied, not just to their treatment, but also to treatment of acquired immunodeficiency patients and the development of immunotherapy and chemotherapy for malignancies. Thus, the chapter begins with immune deficiency syndromes, both genetic and acquired, and concludes with a short description of neoplasias of the immune system.

IMMUNE DEFICIENCY SYNDROMES

Immune deficiencies are divided into two major categories: (1) *primary*, which may be hereditary or acquired, in which the deficiency is the cause of disease; and (2) *secondary*, in which the immune deficiency is a result of other disease(s).

*Contributed by Dr. Susan Gottesman, Department of Pathology, SUNY Health Science Center at Brooklyn.

Primary immune deficiencies can be categorized based on clinical presentation, which roughly correspond to the arm of the immune system malfunctioning:

1. **T-cell** or cell-mediated immunity
2. **B-cell** or antibody-mediated immunity
3. both B- and T-cell immunity
4. nonspecific immunity-mediated by **phagocytic cells** and/or **natural killer (NK) cells**
5. **complement** activation

This classification organizes the broad spectrum of immune disorders. Since the expressed immune response is the result of interactions among several cell types, a deficiency of, for example, antibody production and B-cell function, may actually be caused by an underlying problem in T cells or T–B interaction. Nevertheless, classification based on the apparent expressed defect and not necessarily on its underlying cause is a useful framework for diagnosing new patients and comparing with animal models.

Immune deficiency should always be considered in a patient with recurrent infections. The types of infections often facilitate diagnosis. For example, recurrent bacterial otitis media and pneumonia are common in individuals with B-cell (antibody) deficiency; increased susceptibility to fungal, protozoan, and viral infections is seen with T-cell and cell-mediated immune deficiency; systemic infections with bacteria, normally of low virulence, superficial skin infections, or infections with pyogenic (pus-producing) organisms suggest deficiencies in phagocytic cells; and recurrent infections with pyogenic microorganisms are associated with complement deficiencies (Table 18.1). Of particular significance is the occurrence of **opportunistic infections**, diseases caused by microorganisms present in the environment and nonpathogenic in immunocompetent individuals. *Pneumocystis carinii*, cytomegalovirus (CMV), toxoplasmosis, *Mycobacterium avian*, and *Candida* are among the most common organisms involved and are most often associated with deficiencies in cell-mediated immunity.

Primary Immunodeficiency Syndromes

The frequency of primary immune deficiency syndromes is very low, in the order of about 1 in 10,000. Antibody deficiencies constitute approximately 50% of cases; 20% are combined deficiencies in antibody and cell-mediated immunity; 18% are phagocytic disorders; 10% are disorders of cell-mediated immunity alone; and 2% are complement deficiencies.

Severe Combined Immunodeficiency Diseases. Severe combined immunodeficiency diseases (SCID) is a heterogeneous group of diseases in which both cell-mediated immunity and antibody production are defective (Figure 18.1). Originally called Swiss-type agammaglobulinemia, **individuals with SCID are susceptible to virtually any type of microbial infection** (viral, bacterial, fungal, and protozoal), most notably CMV, *Pneumocystis carinii*, and *Candida*. Vaccination with attenuated live virus could prove fatal in these individuals.

TABLE 18.1. The Major Levels of Immune Disorders

Disorder	Associated disease
Deficiency	
B-lymphocyte deficiency — deficiency in antibody-mediated immunity	Recurrent bacterial infections, e.g., otitis media, recurrent pneumonia
T-lymphocyte deficiency — deficiency in cell-mediated immunity	Increased susceptibility to viral, fungal, and protozoal infections.
T- and B-lymphocyte deficiency — combined deficiency of antibody- and cell-mediated immunity	Acute and chronic infections with viral, bacterial, fungal, and protozoal organisms
Phagocytic cell deficiency	Systemic infections with bacteria of usually low virulence; infections with pyogenic bacteria; impaired pus formation and wound healing
NK cell deficiency	Viral infections, associated with several T-cell disorders and X-linked lymphoproliferative symptoms
Complement component deficiency	Bacterial infections; autoimmunity
Unregulated excess	
B lymphocytes	Monoclonal gammopathies; other B-cell malignancies
T lymphocytes	T-cell malignancies
Complement components	Angioneurotic edema due to absence of C1 esterase inhibitor

Patients can be subclassified at initial evaluation according to peripheral lymphocyte subsets. One group has essentially absent T cells and normal or increased numbers of nonfunctioning B cells (T^-B^+). This group may also lack NK cells. A second group has severe lymphopenia due to the absence of both T and B cells (T^-B^-), while a few are T^+B^+. All patients are preferentially treated with T-cell-depleted HLA-matched sibling bone marrow transplantation.

T^-B^+ SUBGROUP

X-Linked SCID. These patients constitute 40–50% of SCID cases and the majority of those showing T^-B^+ lymphopenia. Mutations have been found in the gene encoding the γ chain of the IL-2 receptor, located on the X chromosome. The γ chain is common to the receptors for IL-2, IL-4, IL-7, IL-9, and IL-15 (see Chapter 12 and Figure 18.2A).

In mouse gene knockout models (Chapter 5), IL-2 knockouts show some immune dysfunction, with normal T- and B-cell development and without a scid phenotype. Gamma chain knockouts have defective development of both T and B cell lineages. IL-7 and IL-7R knockouts more closely resemble SCID patients, suggesting that this cytokine is most crucial for T/NK cell development.

Autosomal Recessive SCID. A small subgroup of patients characterized by T^-B^+ lymphopenia show an autosomal recessive (AR) rather than an X-linked pattern of

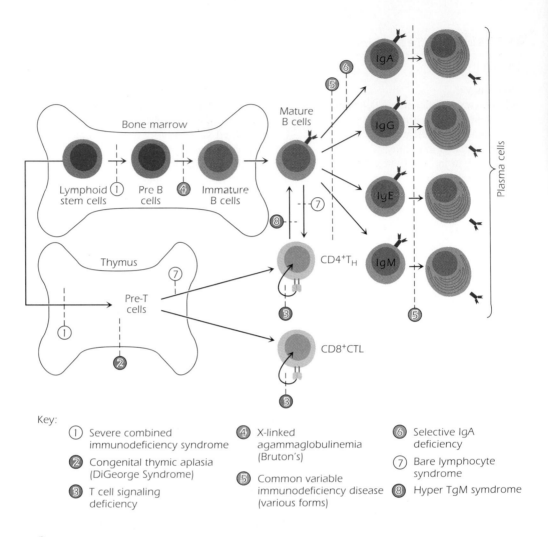

Figure 18.1. Sites of defective lymphopoietic development associated with primary immunodeficiency syndromes.

inheritance. These individuals have an identical phenotype to the X-linked SCID group and cannot be distinguished clinically. Mutations are localized in the gene for **JAK3 tyrosine kinase**, the intracellular molecule responsible for transmitting signals from the γ chain of the receptors (Figure 18.2B). Expression of JAK3 is normally restricted to hematopoietic cells.

T⁻B⁻ SUBGROUP

Adenosine Deaminase Deficiency. Adenosine deaminase (ADA), an enzyme in the purine salvage pathway, is a ubiquitously expressed housekeeping enzyme. ADA deficiency has greatest impact on the immune system, resulting in failure of both T- and B-lymphocyte development. Many patients have an associated characteristic skeletal abnormality. Individuals lacking this enzyme account for approximately 20%

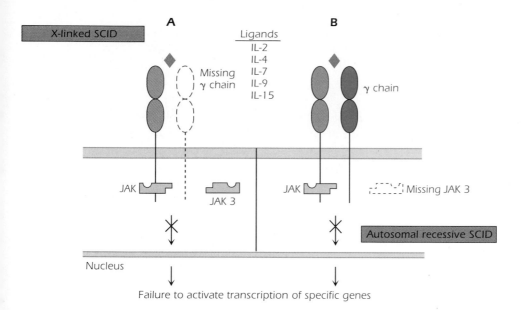

Figure 18.2. **(A)** Cytokine receptors that share the common γ chain fail to generate intracellular signals following ligand binding when this chain is missing. **(B)** Cytokine receptor signaling mediated by the common γ chain is defective when JAK3 tyrosine kinase is missing.

of SCID patients and show an autosomal recessive pattern of inheritance. The deficiency results in buildup of toxic wastes causing symptom progression over time and making early detection and treatment particularly critical in this group. Why these patients do not have more multisystem problems is not completely understood. Investigation of this rare genetic disease has shown the particular importance of the salvage pathway in lymphocyte development and differentiation and led to the development of antileukemic drugs. This is also the first group of patients treated with gene therapy, transfecting a functional gene for ADA in cases lacking a matched sibling marrow donor. Alternative approaches are continuous enzyme supplementation.

Recombinase Deficiencies. Recombination activating genes (*Rag*) 1 and 2 code for enzymes responsible for rearrangement of the immunoglobulin genes in pre-B cells and the T cell receptor genes in pre-T cells (see Chapters 6 and 9). Both appear to be absolutely required for rearrangement, thus mutations in either result in complete absence of T cells, B cells, and immunoglobulin. Maturation stops at the pre-T and pre-B cell stages.

A variant, **Omenn syndrome**, is a "leaky" SCID with reduced but partial *Rag* activity. These patients clinically present similarly to patients with severe graft versus host (GVH) disease (discussed in Chapter 19). Although severely immunodeficient, they are T^+B^-, have massive skin and gastrointestinal infiltration by activated T cells, producing T_H2 type cytokines (see Chapters 10 and 12), and eosinophils. This results in hyper-IgE syndrome and malnutrition due to protein loss. Complete understanding of the clinical picture is still lacking. These patients are difficult to transplant and paradoxically need preparation with immunosuppressive therapy.

T^+B^+ Subgroup

Bare Lymphocyte Syndrome. Although technically comprised of three groups, only those lacking expression of MHC class II molecules, with or without class I expression, consistently show immunodeficiencies. Circulating T and B cell numbers may be normal; however, in the absence of class II molecules, foreign antigen cannot be presented (Figure 18.3). Therefore collaboration does not occur between any of the antigen-presenting cells (B cells, macrophage/monocytes, dendritic cells) and T_H cells. This results in combined immunodeficiency clinically. Most patients have a reversed CD4/CD8 ratio reflecting the requirement for MHC class II expression on thymic epithelial cells for CD4$^+$ T-cell selection (Figure 18.1, defect number 7). The CD4$^+$ T cells present are functional if properly stimulated. Surprisingly, GVH may still occur, thus the requirement for matched bone marrow donors for treatment.

The mutation in this syndrome is not in the MHC class II gene itself, but in the gene encoding an activator required for transcription of class II. One might speculate that a better understanding of this disease could lead to a method for turning off MHC class II expression on transplanted organs thus avoiding rejection.

Few patients deficient in MHC class I expression have been identified and some of these were discovered serendipitously. This is undoubtedly due to the fact that not all individuals show clinically significant immunodeficiency. These patients have a mutation, not in the MHC gene, but in a gene for ***transporter protein (Tap)*** required to place peptide into the MHC class I molecule. (Chapter 8). Occupancy by peptide

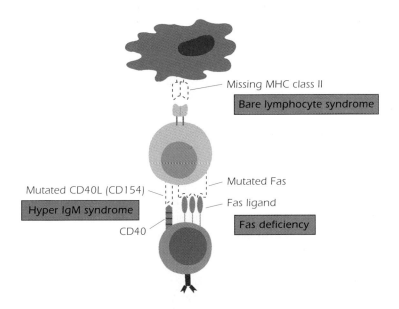

Figure 18.3. Missing cell membrane determinants required for normal T cell–APC interactions result in several primary immunodeficiency syndromes including bare lymphocyte syndrome, hyper IgM syndrome and Fas deficiency.

is required to stabilize and express class I. When symptomatic, these patients have recurrent bacterial pneumonias rather than viral infections as would be expected.

In addition to the combined immunodeficiency diseases already described, there are several which are multisystem inherited disorders.

Wiskott-Aldrich Syndrome. Wiskott-Aldrich syndrome is X-linked and shows a classic triad of bleeding diathesis due to thrombocytopenia (low platelet level in blood), recurrent bacterial infections, and, paradoxically, allergic reactions, eczema, hyper-IgE and food allergies. Longer term patients have increased risk of malignancies, particularly of the lymphoid system. The *WASP* gene on the X chromosome codes for a protein expressed in all hematopoietic stem cells. Current evidence suggests that the protein may normally interact with the cytoskeleton.

The immune defects are variable, but patients characteristically are unable to respond to polysaccharide antigens. Treatment consists of antibiotics and antiviral agents given promptly with each infection. Reconstitution of T and B cells has been reported following bone marrow transplantation. Without treatment, the average lifespan is approximately 3 years. With extension of survival, the incidence of malignancies would be expected to increase.

Ataxia Telangiectasia. Ataxia telangiectasia (AT) is another multisystem genetic disorder in which neurologic symptoms (staggering gait) and abnormal vascular dilation (telangiectasia) accompany lymphopenia, thymic hypoplasia, and depressed levels of IgA, IgE, and sometimes IgG. The immune defect involves both cellular and humoral (T cell-dependent and T cell-independent) immune responses, although T-dependent regions of lymphoid tissues are most severely affected. These children also have greatly increased susceptibility to malignancy, presumably based on a defect in DNA repair or cell cycle arrest following chromosomal damage. AT has been grouped with **Bloom syndrome** and **Faconi's anemia**, both of which similarly show variable immune deficiencies and susceptibility to DNA damage.

Immunodeficiency Disorders Associated With T Cells and Cell-Mediated Immunity. Patients with T-cell-associated deficiency diseases are susceptible to **viral, fungal, and protozoal** infections (Table 18.1). Moreover, because T cells help in the antibody response, these patients also exhibit defects in antibody production. Consequently, T cell-deficient patients may be difficult to distinguish clinically from SCID.

CONGENITAL THYMIC APLASIA (DIGEORGE SYNDROME). DiGeorge syndrome is the most notable T-cell deficiency disease. Defective migration of neural crest cells into the **third and fourth pharyngeal pouches**, which normally takes place during the 12th week of gestation, results in cardiac abnormalities, abnormal facies, and failure of formation of the thymus (**thymic aplasia**) and parathyroids (**hypoparathyroidism**). Newborns therefore present with hypocalcemia (low calcium levels) and congenital cardiac disease. DiGeorge syndrome is not hereditary, occurring sporadically, mostly the result of a deletion in chromosome 22q11. The children suffer from recurrent or chronic infections with viruses, bacteria, fungi, and protozoa. They have either no or very few mature T cells in the periphery (blood, lymph nodes, or spleen) (Figure 18.1, defect number 2).

Although B cells, plasma cells, and serum immunoglobulin levels may be normal, many patients fail to mount an antibody response after immunization. Notably absent is the IgG response, which requires helper T cells. Due to the absence of T cells and abnormal antibody responses, individuals with DiGeorge syndrome should never be immunized with live attenuated viral vaccines!

Formerly, treatment consisted of fetal thymus transplantation, resulting in the appearance of T cells within a week. The fetal thymus used for transplantation needed to be no older than 14 weeks to avoid GVH reactions, which would occur if mature thymocytes were transferred into the immunoincompetent recipient. This donor fetal thymus provided thymic epithelial cells for development of recipient T cells from bone marrow precursors. Although the T cells produced were normal, cell-mediated immunity and help for antibody production were not fully restored. The T cells learned the MHC of the transplanted thymus as "self" and sometimes collaborated poorly with the body's own antigen-presenting cells. Treatment now is mostly in response to symptoms. Some patients have remnants of thymic tissue allowing delayed, though still diminished T-cell maturation. Other disorders associated with the syndrome (such as congenital heart disease) add to the overall poor prognosis.

T-Cell Deficiencies With Normal Peripheral T-Cell Numbers. A number of patients have been identified with functional, rather than numerical, defects in their T cells. Clinically they present with opportunistic infections and a strikingly high incidence of autoimmune disease. Family studies show autosomal recessive pattern of inheritance. Molecular analysis demonstrates that the underlying cause is heterogenous, with deficient expression of CD3ε, CD3γ, or ZAP 70 tyrosine kinase. ZAP 70 is required for intracellular transduction of signal after T cell receptor binding (see Chapter 10). This latter group lacks CD8$^+$ T cells, suggesting that the ZAP 70 molecule is also required for CD8$^+$ T-cell differentiation in the thymus (Figure 18.1, defect number 3).

Chronic Mucocutaneous Candidiasis. Chronic mucocutaneous candidiasis, an infection of skin and mucous membranes by the *fungus Candida albicans*, which is normally present but nonpathogenic, is a poorly defined collection of syndromes associated with a *selective defect in the functioning of T cells*.

Patients usually have normal T cell-mediated immunity to microorganisms other than *Candida* and normal B cell-mediated immunity (antibody production) to all microorganisms including *Candida*. This disorder affects both males and females, particularly children, and there is some evidence that it may be inherited.

B-Cell or Immunoglobulin-Associated Immunodeficiency Disorders.
B-cell or immunoglobulin-associated immune diseases range from those having defective B-cell development with complete absence of all immunoglobulin classes to those associated with deficiencies in a single class or subclass of immunoglobulin. Patients suffer from recurrent or chronic infections beginning in infancy (Bruton's agammaglobulinemia) to young adulthood. Evaluation includes analysis of B cell number and function and immunoelectrophoretic and quantitative determinations of immunoglobulin class and subclass.

X-Linked Infantile Agammaglobulinemia. First described in 1952 by Bruton, X-linked infantile agammaglobulinemia (XLA) is also called *Bruton's agam-*

maglobulinemia. The disorder is relatively rare (1/100,000). It is first noticed at approximately 5–6 months, when the infant has lost the maternally derived IgG that had passed through the placenta. At that age, the infant presents with serious and repeated bacterial infections due to a severe depression or virtual *absence of all Ig classes*.

The major defect is the inability of pre-B cells, present at normal levels, to develop into mature B cells. The *BTK gene*, which is mutated in XLA, normally codes for a tyrosine kinase enzyme residing in the cytosol. BTK seems to be essential for signal transduction from the pre-B cell receptor on developing B cells. Without this signal, the cell develops no further (Figure 18.1, defect number 4). All mature B cells from female carriers of the mutant gene have only the nonmutated X chromosome active. XLA is therefore one of several inherited immunodeficiency diseases described in which a mutation in a cytoplasmic tyrosine kinase is responsible. The JAK3 form of SCID and ZAP 70 form of T-cell deficiency were described above.

Analysis of the blood, bone marrow, spleen, and lymph nodes of XLA patients reveals near *absence of mature B cells and plasma cells*, explaining the depressed Ig levels. The limited number of B cells generated appear normal in their ability to become plasma cells. Infants with X-linked agammaglobulinemia have recurrent bacterial otitis media, bronchitis, septicemia, pneumonia, arthritis, meningitis, and dermatitis. The most common etiologic agents are *Hemophilus influenzae* and *Streptococcus pneumoniae*. Frequently, patients also suffer from malabsorption due to infestation of the gastrointestinal tract with *Giardia lamblia*. The infections do not respond well to antibiotics alone. Treatment therefore consists of periodic injections of *intravenous gamma globulin* (IVGG) containing large amounts of IgG (discussed further in Chapter 21). Although this passive immunization has maintained some patients for 20–30 years, the prognosis is guarded, as chronic lung disease due to repeated infections often supervenes.

TRANSIENT HYPOGAMMAGLOBULINEMIA. At approximately 5–6 months of age, passively transferred maternal IgG disappears and synthesis by the infant begins to rise. Premature infants may have transient IgG deficiency if they are not yet able to synthesize immunoglobulins. Occasionally, a full-term infant may also fail to produce appropriate amounts of IgG, even when levels of IgM or IgA are normal. This appears to be due to a deficiency in number and function of T helper cells. Transient hypogammaglobulinemia may persist for a few months to as long as 2 years. It is not sex-linked and can be distinguished from the X-linked disease by normal numbers of B cells in the blood. Although treatment is usually not necessary, infants need to be identified since immunizations should not be given during this period.

COMMON VARIABLE IMMUNODEFICIENCY DISEASE. Patients with common variable immunodeficiency disease (CVID) have markedly decreased serum IgG and IgA levels, with normal or low IgM and normal or low peripheral B-cell numbers. The cause of the disease, which affects both males and females, is not entirely clear and is probably not uniform. Onset may occur at any age, with two peaks between 1 to 5 years and 15 to 20 years. Affected individuals suffer from recurrent respiratory and gastrointestinal infections with *pyogenic bacteria* and, paradoxically, *autoimmune diseases* such as hemolytic anemia, thrombocytopenia, and systemic lupus erythematosus, which are associated with autoantibodies. Many also have disorders of cell-mediated immunity. Long-term, these patients have a high incidence of **cancer**, particularly lymphomas and gastric cancer.

CVID is characterized by a failure of maturation of **B cells into antibody secreting cells** (Figure 18.1, defect number 5). This defect may be due to an inability of the B cells to proliferate in response to antigen; normal proliferation of B cells without secretion of IgM; secretion of IgM without class switching to IgG or IgA (due to intrinsic B-cell or T-cell abnormality); or failure of glycosylation of heavy chains of IgG. In most cases, the disorder appears to be the result of diminished synthesis and secretion of immunoglobulins. The disease is familial or sporadic with unknown environmental influences triggering onset.

Treatment depends on severity. For severe disease, with many recurrent or chronic infections, IVGG therapy is indicated. Treated patients can have a normal life span. The women have normal pregnancies, although, of course, no maternal IgG is transferred to the fetus.

Selective Immunoglobulin Deficiencies. Several syndromes are associated with selective deficiency of a single class or subclass of immunoglobulins. Some are accompanied by compensatory elevated levels of other isotypes, as exemplified by increased IgM levels in cases of IgG or IgA deficiency.

IgA DEFICIENCY. **IgA deficiency** is the most common immunodeficiency disorder in the Western world, with an incidence of approximately 1 in 800 (Figure 18.1, defect number 6). The cause is unknown, but appears to be associated with decreased release of IgA by B lymphocytes. IgA deficiency may also occur transiently as an adverse reaction to drugs. Patients may suffer from recurrent sinopulmonary viral or bacterial infections, celiac disease (defective absorption in the bowel), or may be entirely asymptomatic.

Treatment of symptomatic patients consists of wide-spectrum antibiotics. Therapy with immune serum globulin is not useful because commercial preparations contain only low levels of IgA, and because injected IgA does not get to the local secretory areas where IgA is normally the protective antibody. Furthermore, the patients may mount their own IgG or IgE response to IgA in the transferred immune serum, causing hypersensitivity reactions. In general, however, the prognosis is good, with many patients surviving normally.

IgM DEFICIENCY. There are selective deficiencies in other immunoglobulin isotypes. An example is **IgM deficiency**, a rare disorder, in which patients suffer from recurrent and severe infections with polysaccharide-encapsulated organisms, such as pneumococci and *Haemophilus influenzae*. Selective deficiencies in subclasses of IgG have been described but are very rare.

Disorders of T–B Interactions. There are at least two diseases in which the T and B lineages appear to mature normally but interactions between them are abnormal. Although both are due to underlying T-cell abnormalities, the predominating clinical symptoms are in the B-cell or humoral immune response. These diseases are hyper IgM syndrome and X linked lymphoproliferative disease.

HYPER-IgM SYNDROME. Patients with X-linked hyper-IgM syndrome (XHIM) present with recurrent respiratory infections at 1–2 years of age. These boys have very low serum IgG, IgA and IgE with normal to elevated IgM (Figure 18.1, defect number 7). Their B cells, which are normal in number, function in culture and will isotype switch when stimulated. The T cells are also normal in number, subset distribution and proliferative response to mitogen. A mutation in the **CD40L gene** on the X chromosome results in absence of CD40 ligand (CD154) on T_H cells (Figure 18.3). CD40L costimulates the B cell through its CD40 molecule (see Chapter 10). This signaling rescues the B cell from apoptosis and appears important, if not necessary, for isotype switching. Recruitment of B cells into follicles does not occur, resulting in lack of germinal center formation. The children also have a partial block in neutrophil differentiation and subtle changes in T-cell function. This may explain their propensity for opportunistic infections, particularly *Pneumocystis carinii* pneumonia (PCP) and poorer prognosis than XLA. Those patients with similar presentations to XHIM but with an autosomal recessive pattern of inheritance may have a B-cell defect, possibly in CD40.

Interestingly, a mutation in a structurally related molecule, Fas, which is required for apoptosis (discussed in Chapter 11), causes massive lymphoid hyperplasia, abnormal T cells and autoimmune disease but no increased susceptibility to infection (Figure 18.3).

X-LINKED LYMPHOPROLIFERATIVE DISEASE OR DUNCAN'S SYNDROME. X linked lymphoproliferative disease (XLP) is rare. Patients are clinically healthy with normal T- and B-cell numbers prior to exposure to **Epstein-Barr virus** (EBV), which results in a severe or fatal course of infectious mononucleosis (caused by EBV). Survival of infection is frequently followed by malignant lymphoma or dysgammaglobulinemia. The latter two may also occur without prior EBV. The lymphomas are predominantly aggressive B-cell lymphomas at extranodal sites, particularly the gastrointestinal tract. Burkitt's lymphoma, the most frequent type, is associated with EBV in endemic areas (see below). Although the pattern of lymphomas is similar to those in AIDS patients, the incidence is much greater in individuals with XLP. An inability of T cells to regulate B-cell growth is considered to be a major part of the underlying defect. Prognosis is extremely poor. This syndrome was observed in six maternally related males of the Duncan family, thus its name.

Phagocytic Dysfunctions. Polymorphonuclear leukocytes and macrophages/monocytes play an important role in both innate and acquired immunity, acting either alone or in concert with lymphocytes. Phagocytic dysfunction may be secondary, caused by **extrinsic factors**, such as drugs, systemic diseases like diabetes, or caused by defects in other arms of the immune system. Inherited deficiencies have helped identify the molecules required for each step of phagocytic cell action leading up to elimination of the pathogen: migration and adhesion (LAD), phagocytosis and lysosomal fusion (CHS), and respiratory burst for killing (CGD) (Figure 18.4).

LEUKOCYTE ADHESION DEFICIENCY. Leukocyte adhesion deficiency (LAD) is a group of disorders in which leukocyte interaction with vascular endothelium is disrupted. In order for leukocytes to arrive at sites of infection they must first leave the bloodstream. This is accomplished initially by slow rolling of the cell along the endothelium through the interaction of selectins on endothelium and **selectin ligands** on leukocytes (see Figure 12.2). Chemoattractants then cause the cell to stop rolling. They adhere more firmly, followed by transendothelial migration. These latter steps

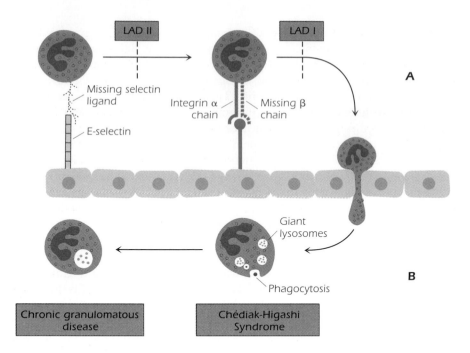

Figure 18.4. **(A)** Defects in cell adhesion disrupts the ability of leukocytes to interact with vascular endothelium causing impairment of migration of these cells from the blood to sites of infection. **(B)** Impairments in mechanisms required for phagocytosis results in defective intracellular killing of microorganisms.

involve the interaction of ***integrins*** on leukocytes and their ligands on endothelial cells.

LAD I. ***LAD I*** is an autosomal recessive disease mapping to chromosome 21. Patients have a defect in the β subunit of integrin molecules, preventing their expression. The β subunit is common to three integrins: LFA-1(CD11a/CD18), Mac-1 (CD11b/CD18) and p150,95 (CD11c/CD18) found on granulocytes, monocytes, and lymphocytes. Therefore adhesion and migration of all white blood cells are impaired (Figure 18.4). LAD I individuals suffer from recurrent soft tissue bacterial infections, with increased white blood cells, but without pus formation, and impaired wound healing. Newborns have delayed separation of umbilical cord. As expected, lymphocyte function is also affected due to the lack of LFA-1 expression.

LAD II. Individuals with ***LAD II*** have a defect in selectin ligands, thus cells from these patients cannot roll along the endothelial surface, the first step for migration. Although the immunodeficiency symptoms are milder, the underlying defect in fucose metabolism results in other developmental abnormalities. In both LAD forms, because there is no or little pus formation the children do not show classical clinical signs of severe infection (Figure 18.4).

CHÉDIAK-HIGASHI SYNDROME. Chédiak-Higashi Syndrome (CHS) is an autosomal recessive disease characterized by abnormal giant granules and organelles in the cells (Figure 18.4). Particularly affected are the lysosomes and melanosomes, resulting in defects in pigmentation, neutrophil and NK cell function, platelet function, and neurologic abnormalities. There is defective degranulation and fusion of lysosomes with phagosomes resulting in diminished intracellular killing of organisms. With time, patients develop massive lymphohistiocytic infiltrates in the liver, spleen, and lymph nodes. Pyogenic organisms such as streptococcus and staphylococcus cause recurrent, sometimes fatal infection. Prognosis is poor.

CHRONIC GRANULOMATOUS DISEASE. In chronic granulomatous disease (CGD), the final step in killing of ingested organisms is defective (Figure 18.4). Their intracellular survival results in granuloma formation. Normally, activated neutrophils and mononuclear phagocytes have a respiratory burst, consuming oxygen and generating hydrogen peroxide and superoxide radicals used for killing organisms. Mutations in any of the subunits of NADPH oxidase can result in CGD. The most common form is due to a mutation in the *CYBB* gene located on the X chromosome and coding for *cytochrome b*$_{245}$. The other subunits are coded for by autosomal genes.

Symptoms appear during the first two years of life. Patients have enhanced susceptibility to infection with organisms that are normally of low virulence, such as *Staphylococcus aureus, Serratia marcescens*, and *Aspergillus*. Associated abnormalities include lymphadenopathy (increase in lymph node size) and hepatosplenomegaly due to the chronic and acute infections. Treatment consists of aggressive immunization and therapy with wide-spectrum antibiotics, antifungal agents, and interferon-γ.

In addition to CGD, disorders with reduced or absent levels of **glucose-6 phosphate dehydrogenase, myeloperoxidase**, and **alkaline phosphatase** result in decreased intracellular killing of organisms.

INTERFERON-γ RECEPTOR DEFICIENCY. A mutation in *IFNγR1* gene results in an inability of the monocytes to respond to IFN-γ with secretion of TNF-α. The patients are selectively susceptible to weakly pathogenic mycobacterium, suggesting that the other effects of IFN-γ are compensated for. These individuals serve to demonstrate the importance of IFN-γ in controlling mycobacterial infections. Immunization with live bacillus Calmette-Guérin (BCG), common in some parts of the world, is dangerous in these patients with this defect.

Natural Killer Cell Deficiency. Very little is known about natural killer (NK) cell deficiency in humans, and only a few such cases have been reported. Animal studies suggest that NK cell deficiency impairs allograft rejection and is linked to higher susceptibility to viral diseases and increased metastatic tumors. NK cell defects are seen in severe combined immunodeficiency disorders, in some T and phagocytic cell disorders, and in X-linked lymphoproliferative syndrome.

Diseases Due to Abnormalities in the Complement System. Complement is important in the killing of bacteria, **opsonization**, chemotaxis, and B-cell activation (see Chapter 13). They also participate in the elimination of antigen−antibody complexes, preventing **immune complex** deposition and subsequent disease. Deficiencies in complement are inherited as autosomal traits, with heterozygous individuals having half the normal level of a given component. For most components this is sufficient to prevent clinical disease. The half-life of activated complement components is also normally carefully controlled by inhibitors which break down the products or dissociate the complexes.

DEFICIENCIES OF EARLY COMPLEMENT COMPONENTS. The early components are most important in opsonization with C3 being the pivotal molecule. Thus patients with *deficiencies of C1, C4, C2*, and particularly *C3* have increased infections with encapsulated organisms (*S. pneumonia, S. pyogenes, H. influenza*) and rheumatic diseases due to improper clearance of immune complexes (Figure 18.5). In fact, systemic lupus erythromatosus (SLE) is the most common presenting symptom of some complement deficiencies. SLE in these individuals is of earlier onset and more

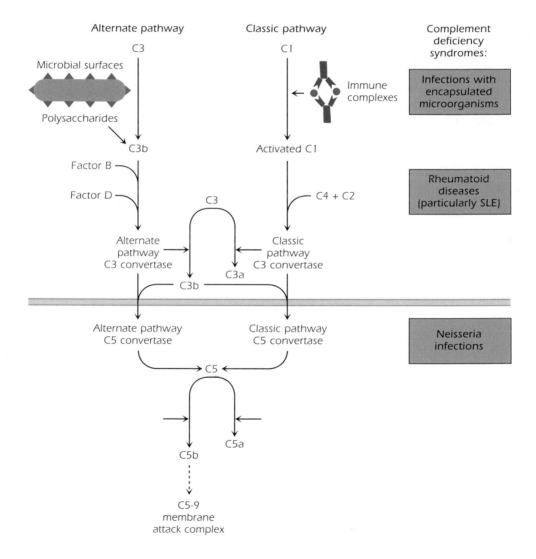

Figure 18.5. Complement cascade showing that deficiencies in early phase complement components predispose individuals to infections caused by encapsulated microorganisms and rheumatoid syndromes. Late phase complement deficiencies are associated with *Neisseria* infections.

severe than without this association and frequently occurs without anti-DNA antibodies.

Since the alternative pathway can also activate C3, bypassing the need for C1,4, and 2, deficiencies of C3 itself are associated with the most severe symptoms, particularly infectious complications.

DEFICIENCIES OF LATE COMPLEMENT COMPONENTS. Deficiencies of the later complement components, C5–C9 interfere with the generation of the membrane attack complex (MAC). MAC is directly lytic and the primary defense against gram-negative bacteria, particularly *Neisseria meningitidis* (Figure 18.5).

DEFECTIVE CONTROL OF COMPLEMENT COMPONENTS

Hereditary Angioedema. In hereditary angioedema, patients lack a functional ***C1 esterase inhibitor***. Without this inhibitor, the action of C1 on C4, C2 and the kallikrein system is uncontrolled, generating large amounts of vasoactive peptides. These peptides cause increased blood vessel permeability. Patients suffer from localized edema, which becomes life-threatening when it occurs in the larynx, obstructing the airway passage. Treatment includes avoidance of precipitating factors, usually trauma, and infusion of C1 esterase inhibitor.

Paroxysmal Nocturnal Hemoglobulinuria. In paroxysmal nocturnal hemoglobulinuria (PNH), patients have a defect in the glycosyl phosphatidyl inositol anchor of a family of proteins which attach to the cell membrane. These proteins include those that normally inactivate complement. ***Decay accelerating factor*** (DAF or CD55) and CD59 dissociate bound C3 convertase thus preventing lysis. Without these surface molecules, granulocytes, platelets, and particularly red blood cells, are susceptible to spontaneous lysis. Intravascular hemolysis occurs, more prominently in the kidney at night where the acidic environment activates the alternative pathway.

PNH may be an acquired somatic mutation in a pleuripotential hematopoietic stem cell and may evolve into acute leukemia. During its chronic course, patients show symptoms of severe anemia, thrombotic events, and chronic infections.

Secondary Immunodeficiency Syndromes

Secondary immune deficiency diseases are the consequence of other diseases. By far the most common cause of immunodeficiency disorders worldwide is malnutrition. In developed countries it is more often iatrogenic, caused by the use of ***chemotherapeutic agents*** in cancer therapy or deliberate ***immunosuppression*** for organ transplantation as well as for autoimmune disease. Secondary immunodeficiencies are also seen in untreated autoimmunity and with overwhelming infections by bacteria.

 ## ACQUIRED IMMUNODEFICIENCY SYNDROME (AIDS)

Initial Description and Epidemiology

In 1981 several cases of an unusual *Pneumocystis carinii* pneumonia (PCP) were reported in homosexual males in the San Francisco area. This was followed by the recognition of an aggressive form of Kaposi's sarcoma in a similar population in New York City. Since those first recognized cases of AIDS until today over 12 million people have died worldwide and over 30 million are currently infected.

Infection with human immunodeficiency virus (HIV) is the cause of AIDS. The virus is transferred through blood and body fluids. Blood, semen, vaginal secretions, breast milk, and, to a small extent, saliva of an infected individual contain free virus or cells containing virus. Thus HIV can be transmitted through sexual contact, sharing of needles, transfusion of blood or blood products, placental transfer, passage through birth canal, and breast feeding.

Although first recognized in sexually active homosexual males in large U.S. cities, the infection and the disease have no sexual preference. Worldwide, heterosexual transmission is most common. In the United States, although homosexual males and intravenous drug abusers still constitute the major infected groups, the largest increase in rate of AIDS incidence is in heterosexual women and minorities, African-Americans and Hispanics. Transmission of the virus through transfusion of blood and blood products has been virtually eliminated in this country through screening of donors, testing of units, and heat inactivation of clotting factor concentrates. A dangerous "window period" still exists; the reasons will become clear later. Efficiency of transmission from mother to infant, which accounts for over 80% of the pediatric cases, can be greatly diminished by antiviral therapy of the mother and avoidance of vaginal childbirth and breast feeding. In spite of these positive statements they exist as almost a footnote to an epidemic that continues to spread worldwide without signs of abating, particularly in Africa and Southeast Asia.

Human Immunodeficiency Virus

Human immunodeficiency virus (HIV) is an enveloped human retrovirus of the lentivirus family. Two strains of HIV have been described, HIV-1 and HIV-2, the latter found mostly in Western Africa. HIV-1 is the more virulent strain.

The viral core contains two identical single strands of genomic RNA and three enzymes; integrase, protease, and reverse transcriptase (Figure 18.6). The envelope, which is derived from the host cell membrane displays viral glycoproteins, including gp120 and gp41, which are critical for infection.

Gp120 has high affinity for CD4, therefore cells expressing CD4, such as CD4$^+$ T cells, and macrophages/monocytes and dendritic cells which also express low levels of surface CD4, are potential targets for the virus. After binding to the CD4, gp120 must also bind a coreceptor. Two *chemokine receptors* (see Chapter 12) can fulfill this role depending on the tropism of the HIV. This tropism is determined by the variant of the gp120 molecule. *Macrophage tropic HIV* uses CCR5 and requires only a low level of CD4 on the host cell. CCR5 is expressed by macrophage, dendritic cells and CD4$^+$ T cells. *Lymphotropic HIV* uses CXCR4 found on T cells and requires a high density of CD4 on the cell surface. Both coreceptors are G-coupled proteins with seven transmembrane spanning domains. CCR5 normally binds RANTES, MIP-1α and MIP-1β. CXCR4 binds stromal derived factor-1.

CCR5 seems to be the major coreceptor for establishing primary infection since individuals with mutations in CCR5 appear to be at least partially protected. Development of drugs directed at chemokine receptors is thus an active area of research. It is suggested that if an individual is first infected by sexual contact with a macrophage tropic variant, the virus will be established in the mucosal associated lym-

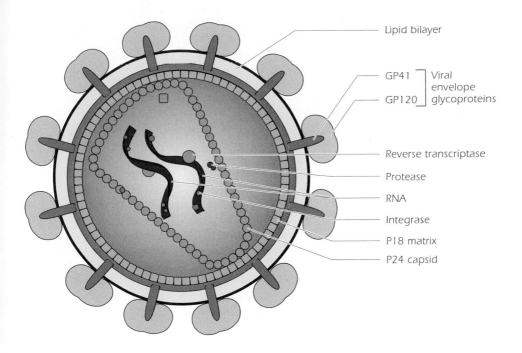

Figure 18.6. Structure of human immunodeficiency virus-1 (HIV-1) showing two identical RNA strands (the viral genome) and associated enzymes including reverse transcriptase, integrase, and protease packaged in a cone-shaped core composed of p24 capsid protein with surrounding p18 protein matrix, all surrounded by a phospholipid membrane envelope derived from the host cell. Virally encoded membrane proteins (gp41 and gp120) are bound to the envelope

phoid tissue where macrophage and dendritic cells in particular will then provide a reservoir. Exposure to antigen promotes viral replication, a switch to the lymphotropic form and further rapid dissemination in the body. The tropism of the virus changes within the infected individual.

Following binding of gp120 to CD4 and its coreceptor, gp41 allows fusion of the viral envelope and cell membrane with viral entry. In the host cell, viral RNA is replicated to a cDNA copy by its enzyme, reverse transcriptase. cDNA then enters the nucleus where it is integrated into the host genome as a provirus with the help of the viral enzyme, integrase. The virus may remain in this relatively latent form for years.

The HIV genome has a long terminal repeat region (LTR) at each end (Figure 18.7). The LTR is required for viral integration and has binding sites for regulatory proteins. When the T cell is activated by antigen, a cascade of reactions results in an increase in NF-κB transcription factor. NF-κB binds to a promoter region in LTR activating transcription of the provirus by host RNA polymerase.

The long mRNA transcript is spliced at alternative sites for protein synthesis. The first two proteins made are Tat and Rev. Tat returns to the nucleus, acting as a transcription factor itself, binding to LTR and increasing the rate of viral transcription. Rev also acts in the nucleus, binding to the Rev responsive element in the viral mRNA transcript and increasing RNA transport rate to the cytoplasm. When the

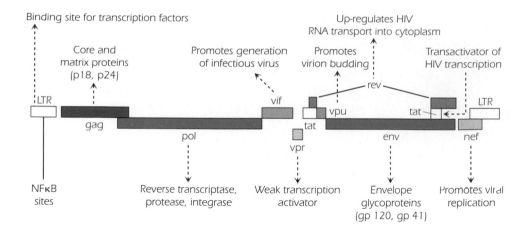

Figure 18.7. The genes and proteins of HIV-1. The HIV-1 RNA genome is flanked by long terminal repeats (LTR) required for viral integration and regulation of the viral genome. Several viral genes overlap resulting in different reading frames thus allowing the virus to encode many proteins in a small genome. The known functions of the gene products shown are listed.

mRNA is transported more rapidly, less splicing occurs in the nucleus. Thus the second wave of proteins made are structural components of the viral core and envelope. In the third wave, unspliced RNA serves as the RNA for the new viral particles and for the translation of gag and pol. Pol codes for the viral protease, which cleaves the product of env to produce gp120 and gp41, reverse transcriptase, and integrase.

Release of virus from CD4$^+$ T cells frequently results in lysis of the cell, whereas the macrophage serves as a reservoir, transporting virus to other parts of the body (lymphoid tissue and central nervous system) and producing a small number of particles without cytopathic consequences.

Azidothymidine (AZT), also called Zidovudin, is an inhibitor of reverse transcriptase and was the first promising drug used in HIV infection. Protease inhibitors form a second class of agents in use. HIV is capable of an amazing rate of spontaneous mutation during the course of an infection in a single individual. This is as a result of lack of fidelity of the reverse transcriptase and RNA polymerase. In consequence, drug resistance develops rapidly.

Clinical Course

Acute Infection. The clinical course can be divided into three phases. Upon initial infection with HIV, many patients are asymptomatic. Others show a flulike illness, characterized by fever, sore throat, and general malaise starting 2 to 4 weeks after infection and lasting 1 to 2 weeks. During this time there is a viremia (virus in peripheral blood) and a precipitous drop in the circulating CD4$^+$ T cells. The immune system responds by generating cytotoxic T cells and antibodies specific for the virus. The CTL are partially responsible for the drop in CD4$^+$ T cells, killing virally infected cells. At this point the patient has seroconverted, expressing detectable antibody to HIV proteins. The number of CD4$^+$ T cells in the peripheral blood then recovers.

Chronic Latent Phase. Although the immune response seems standard for a viral infection, it merely contains rather than eradicates the virus. The extremely high rate of mutations may explain the ineffectiveness of the immune response. A latent phase is established which may last as long as 15 years.

During this relatively asymptomatic period, a low level of viral replication continues, associated with a gradual decline in CD4$^+$ T-cell number. HIV, therefore, never has a truly latent phase. The number of virally infected T cells in the peripheral blood is extremely low during this phase. The lymph nodes are the predominant location of infected cells. Macrophages act as a reservoir. Follicular dendritic cells function not only as a reservoir but also to present virus captured on their surface. This allows continuous presentation of virus to T and B cells, resulting in the intense follicular (germinal center) hyperplasia and lymphadenopathy typical of this phase.

The T cells are undergoing a slow rate of lysis, which eventually results in involution of the lymph node. This T-cell death seems to be the result of a combination of factors. First, production of virus in the cells themselves causes lysis. Second, the infected cell seems to be more susceptible to apoptosis. Third, CTLs kill some of the infected cells. Finally, uninfected T cells may be killed in an ADCC like mechanism due to binding of soluble gp120 and anti-gp120 antibody to CD4 molecules expressed on their surface.

Patients have traditionally been followed during this phase by their peripheral CD4$^+$ T-cell counts and CD4/CD8 cell ratio. The ratio, which is normally approximately 2, is reversed with CD8 cells outnumbering CD4 cells. This can be seen in other viral infections; however, in those cases the reversal is often due to an increase in CD8$^+$ cells. In HIV, CD4$^+$ T cells are diminished. As these cells reach progressively lower values, the patient becomes symptomatic, entering the final phase, AIDS.

Crisis Phase. AIDS was originally recognized by the clinical appearance of unusual infections and malignancies that continue to be the hallmarks of full-blown AIDS. The Centers for Disease Control (CDC) have listed those illnesses that are considered AIDS-associated (Table 18.2). They fall into three categories: opportunistic infections, unusual malignancies, and neurologic syndromes, reflecting the primary effects of HIV on the immune system and CNS.

What initiates this symptomatic or crisis phase appears to be several factors acting concurrently. The gradual drop in CD4$^+$ T cells eventually results in an immunodeficient state, leaving the individual susceptible to opportunistic infections, as is seen in patients with primary immunodeficiency and in immunosuppressed transplant patients. Activation of virally infected T cells by antigen results in stimulation of viral transcription and progeny formation. This leads to accelerated T-cell death, exacerbating the immunodeficient state. Rapid viral replication also increases the mutation rate, allowing escape from any immune controls that might remain.

The patterns of infections and *malignancies* may partially reflect the risk factors for a particular patient. This is suggested by differences seen between AIDS patients and other immunosuppressed individuals and among AIDS patients with different modes of exposures. Thus some individuals have not only been infected with HIV but also with other sexually transmitted diseases. *Human papillomavirus* (HPV) is associated with the development of cervical cancer in women. Exposure to HPV,

● **TABLE** 18.2. AIDS-Associated Diseases Defined by CDC

Infections — frequently disseminated
    Fungal
        Pneumocystis
        Candidiasis
        Cryptococcosis
        Histoplasmosis
        Coccidioidomycosis
    Parasitic
        Toxoplasmosis
        Cryptosporidiosis
        Microsporidiosis
        Leishmaniasis
    Bacterial
        Mycobacteriosis, including "atypical" Salmonella
    Viral
        Cytomegalovirus
        Herpes simplex virus
        Varicella zoster virus
Neoplasms
    Sarcoma
        Kaposi's sarcoma
    Lymphoma
        Burkitt's lymphoma
        Diffuse large B-cell lymphoma
        Effusion based lymphoma
        Primary CNS lymphoma
    Cancer
        Invasive cancer of the uterine cervix

combined with the individual's immunodeficient state, may be responsible for a markedly increased incidence of ***invasive cervical cancer*** in HIV$^+$ women. The CDC has now included invasive cervical cancer in the AIDS-associated malignancies.

The aggressive form of ***Kaposi's sarcoma*** (KS) is virtually unique to AIDS patients, particularly male homosexuals, in whom it may occur early in the course of the disease. This abnormal proliferation of small blood vessels normally presents as a slow-growing tumor on the lower extremity skin of elderly men. ***Human herpes virus 8*** (HHV-8) has been identified in KS from AIDS patients. Whether these vessels grow in response to the virus or the virus is directly oncogenic is unknown. This virus is also associated with an unusual form of aggressive lymphoma seen in AIDS patients, primary effusion lymphoma. Again this malignancy is more common in male homosexual AIDS patients and some have both the lymphoma and KS concurrently.

Aggressive ***B-cell lymphomas***, mostly ***EBV-associated***, are seen at an incidence similar to that seen in immunosuppressed transplant patients. These lymphomas are usually ***Burkitt's lymphoma*** (see below) or diffuse large B cell and are often found outside the lymph nodes (extranodal). In AIDS, the CNS is a frequent site of primary lymphoma.

The *infectious diseases* in AIDS reflect the patient's markedly depressed cell-mediated immune system. As in any T cell-immunodeficient patient, *Pneumocystis carinii* pneumonia (PCP) is a major infectious complication. *Candidiasis* is seen relatively early in AIDS. In addition, the B cells are chronically stimulated, resulting in polyclonal hypergammaglobulinemia (elevated serum immunoglobulins), circulating immune complexes, and markedly increased plasma cell production. In spite of this apparent B-cell activity, patients are unable to mount an effective antibody response to new antigens, perhaps due to the T-cell defect, however they also have particular difficulty with encapsulated organisms. Normally not a human pathogen, *Mycobacterium avian* can cause overwhelming infection.

The CNS is infected with HIV presumably via transport by macrophage. The virus infects microglia cells, which are of the macrophage lineage, oligodendrocytes and astrocytes. The CNS is susceptible to infection by *cryptococcus, toxoplasmosis*, and *CMV*. In addition, AIDS-related dementia and progressive encephalopathy has been frequently documented. In total, up to 50% of AIDS patients show CNS symptoms and over 70% have CNS changes at autopsy.

Severe diarrhea may be caused by any one of a number of organisms infecting the gastrointestinal tract. *Cryptosporidia*, mycobacterium avian, and CMV are among the most common. Although these patients have reason enough for weight loss and fatigue, it appears that cachetic or wasting symptoms are out of proportion with known associated conditions. It is suggested that the virus alters the cytokine profile from the macrophage.

Prevention, Control, and Therapy of HIV Infection

Prevention and control of HIV is best accomplished by avoiding unprotected contact with blood and body fluids from infected individuals. Education and public awareness of both what to avoid and what is safe (casual contact) is required to control the disease and contain possible panic.

Starting in 1985, all blood donations in the United States were tested for antibodies to HIV. This still leaves a window period of several weeks following recent exposure and infection and preceding the appearance of an antibody response. Blood donors are therefore screened by an interview process and asked direct questions orally and in writing about high-risk behavior. Testing for viral RNA is proposed for the near future. The viremia following infection precedes the immune response. Detection of RNA, which includes a polymerase chain reaction (PCR) amplification step, is very sensitive and will decrease the window period but not entirely eliminate it.

HIV$^+$ pregnant women are placed on AZT to decrease viral load and thereby diminish risk of transplacental virus transfer. Caesarean section is performed to eliminate infection during passage through the birth canal. Finally, exposure through breast milk is avoided.

Immediately following accidental exposure to infected products, AZT is administered to prevent establishment of infection.

Diagnosis of HIV infection is generally by detection of antibodies by ELISA and confirmed by Western blot analysis. Patients have been monitored by following their absolute CD4$^+$ T-cell count in the peripheral blood. Correlations have shown that opportunistic infections generally are not seen with CD4 counts above 500/μl.

The CDC has designated CD4 counts below $200/\mu l$ as an indicator of full-blown AIDS.

Therapy with AZT had been used for individuals whose CD4 counts were decreasing below the 500 mark. Currently, individuals who are HIV-positive, but asymptomatic, are placed on triple-agent antiviral therapy with inhibitors directed against reverse transcriptase, protease, and nucleoside. This therapy prevents infection of new cells; however, infected cells remain until lysed. Patients are now monitored for viral load by quantitative analysis of viral RNA following PCR. The fall in viral titers is rapid and dramatic, but a small baseline titer almost always remains. Discontinuation of the drugs results in a resurgence of virus as one would expect. Unfortunately, mutations allow escape from control by these agents, thus the push to develop an extensive armory of drugs. The therapy is not without side effects, particularly suppression of hematopoietic cells. Additional time is needed to see how successful this approach will be.

Extension of life span and improvement in quality of life was first made by aggressive, even prophylactic treatment of infections, particularly PCP. Infection still remains the major immediate cause of death in AIDS patients.

Although infectious diseases have traditionally been controlled by vaccine, HIV presents a serious challenge to vaccine development. Witness the ability of the virus to escape eradication in spite of both an antibody and cytotoxic T-cell response in recently infected individuals. Both the virus' ability to hide out and its high mutation rate need to be overcome. The question of which arm of the immune system (cell-mediated immunity or antibody production) is desirable has not even been answered.

The greatest hope would be to have the immune response ready before exposure, as is done in most other vaccines. However, animal models are limited, the best being the simian monkey, which develops a similar disease after infection with simian immunodeficiency virus (SIV). Human testing is fraught with many ethical difficulties. Understanding the molecular biology and structure of all viral components will be essential for development of a safe vaccine.

NEOPLASMS OF THE IMMUNE SYSTEM

Throughout this chapter a common theme has been that dysregulation of the immune system can result in the emergence of neoplasms. This is seen in patients with primary immunodeficiency diseases, AIDS, and immunosuppressed transplant patients. In these circumstances the malignancies are most often aggressive B-cell lymphomas, frequently associated with EBV infection. Although malignant transformation of any element of the immune system can occur without clinical immunodeficiency, as these tumors are analyzed at the molecular level, dysregulation in the malignant clone or surrounding cells becomes obvious.

Lymphoid leukemias and lymphomas were originally categorized by cell morphology and clinical outcome. A *leukemia* designation implies the malignant cells are predominantly in the circulation and/or bone marrow. A *lymphoma* presents as solid masses either in the lymph nodes, spleen, thymus or extranodal organs. Sometimes the same malignant cell type can show either presentation.

In 1996 WHO recommended a classification system based on cell of origin (B vs T) and stage of differentiation (immature or precursor vs mature or peripheral) (Table 18.3). These tumors are outgrowths of a transformed lymphoid cell which

⬤ T A B L E 18.3. World Health Organization Classification for Lymphoid Neoplasms

B-cell neoplasms
  Precursor B-cell lymphoblastic leukemia/lymphoma
  Mature B-cell neoplasms
    Chronic lymphocytic leukemia/small lymphocytic lymphoma/prolymphocytic leukemia
    Follicular lymphoma
    Mantle cell lymphoma
    Marginal zone lymphoma of mucosa-associated lymphoid tissue (MALT) type
    Nodal marginal zone lymphoma
    Splenic marginal zone lymphoma
    Hairy cell leukemia
    Diffuse large B-cell lymphoma (including subtypes: mediastinal, primary effusion, intravascular)
    Burkitt's lymphoma
    Plasmacytoma
    Plasma cell myeloma
    Lymphoplasmacytic lymphoma
T-cell neoplasms
  Precursor T-cell lymphoblastic leukemia/lymphoma
  Mature T/NK cell neoplasms (selected)
    T-cell large granular lymphocytic leukemia
    NK cell leukemia
    Peripheral T-cell lymphoma (unspecified)
    Mycosis fungoides
    Sézary syndrome
    Primary cutaneous anaplastic large cell lymphoma
    Systemic anaplastic large cell lymphoma
    Extranodal NK/T-cell lymphoma, nasal type
    Intestinal T-cell lymphoma
    Hepatosplenic $\gamma\delta$ T-cell lymphoma
    Adult T-cell leukemia/lymphoma
Hodgkin's lymphoma
  Nodular lymphocyte predominant Hodgkin's lymphoma
  Classical Hodgkin's lymphoma
    Nodular sclerosis
    Mixed cellularity
    Classical, lymphocyte-rich
    Lymphocyte-depleted

appears frozen in development. They have the same surface markers and many of the same properties as the corresponding normal cells at that stage. The malignant cells, however, do not continue to mature, accumulate in large numbers, and all originate from a single clone (monoclonal).

Southern blot analysis of DNA extracted from a B- or T-cell neoplasm will show a single band for the immunoglobulin gene or T-cell receptor gene, respectively. This demonstrates that all the tumor cells have the same rearrangement for these genes and defines the lymphoid growth as monoclonal. PCR may be used before the Southern blot to detect a small population of monoclonal cells. For some lymphoid neoplasms, a unique molecular abnormality, which at least contributes to the transformation of that cell, has been identified. Those will be highlighted here.

B-Cell Neoplasms

Precursor B-Cell Lymphoblastic Leukemia/Lymphomas. B acute lymphoblastic leukemia (B-ALL) corresponds to the pro-B, pre-B, or immature B-cell stages of development as demonstrated by surface CD markers and extent of immunoglobulin gene rearrangement in the individual patient's leukemia. Similar to the normal pro-B and pre-B cell, corresponding ALLs (L1 and L2) express terminal deoxynucleotidyl transferase (TdT) in their nucleus. Chemotherapy has been successful in treating children with these leukemias. ALL L3 is the leukemic counterpart of Burkitt's lymphoma (see below) and corresponds to a mature B cell that is just entering the periphery. Many have the translocation described.

Burkitt's Lymphoma. Burkitt's lymphoma is characterized by a translocation that places the *c-myc oncogene* next to the immunoglobulin heavy chain gene or one of the two light chain genes [t(8;14), t(8;22), or t(2,8)] (Figure 18.8). The myc protein is normally involved in activating genes for cell proliferation when a resting cell receives a signal to divide. Translocation to the immunoglobulin genes leads to increased expression of c-myc and increased cell proliferation. Possibly antigenic stimulation of the B cell initiates the overexpression of c-myc, now under the control of the immunoglobulin gene.

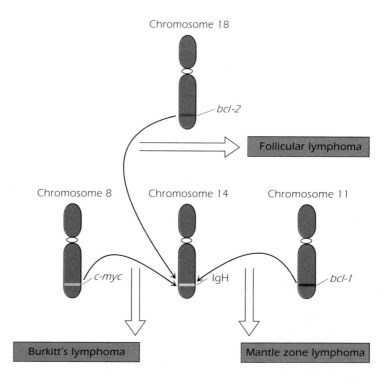

Figure 18.8. Several B-cell neoplasms are associated with translocations of genes to the chromosomal locus encoding the immunoglobulin heavy chain gene on chromosome 14.

In equatorial Africa, this lymphoma is endemic and is associated with EBV infection of the cells. Burkitt's lymphoma is one of the malignancies seen in immunosuppressed patients in whom EBV is also found.

Follicular Lymphoma. These lymphomas represent transformation of the B cells normally found in lymph node follicles (Figure 18.9). In a normal germinal center, B cells are stimulated by antigen. They can respond by proliferating and undergoing affinity maturation, isotype switching, and changing into memory or plasma cells. If their antibody is a poor match for that antigen or of low affinity, the cell undergoes apoptosis or cell death. In follicular center lymphomas, the ***bcl-2*** gene, which produces a protein that interferes with apoptosis is translocated to the immunoglobulin heavy chain gene [t(14;18)] (Figure 18.8). This results in continuous expression of bcl-2 protein, preventing death of the cells. In fact, these B-cell neoplasms have only a low rate of proliferation and a long chronic clinical course.

Mantle Cell Lymphoma. The normal germinal center is surrounded by a collar of small quiescent B cells which have not yet seen antigen (Figure 18.9). A neoplasm of these mantle zone cells has the same B-cell phenotype as their normal counterpart. Many have a translocation of the ***bcl-1*** gene to the immunoglobulin heavy-chain gene [t(11;14)], resulting in overexpression of cyclin D1 (Figure 18.8). Cyclin D1 protein is normally responsible for promoting cell cycle progression from G1 to S phase leading to cell division. This lymphoma has a more aggressive course than the follicular center lymphomas.

MALToma or Marginal Zone Lymphoma. MALToma or marginal zone lymphomas arise in the mucosal-associated lymphoid tissue (MALT) and, interestingly, may be associated with chronic antigenic stimulation or autoimmune disease of that organ. For example, chronic *Helicobacter pylori* infection of the stomach may lead to the development of gastric lymphoma, presumably preventable by antibiotic treatment for the organism. Autoimmune thyroiditis or ***Hashimoto's disease*** and autoimmune disease of the salivary glands or ***Sjörgen's syndrome*** have a high incidence of this B-cell lymphoma in the corresponding organ.

These associations suggest two interesting, not mutually exclusive, hypotheses. First, that chronic antigenic stimulation, particularly of a limited number of specificities, provides fertile ground for the development of a B-cell lymphoma. B cells, which continue to undergo somatic mutation of their immunoglobulin genes, may accumulate transforming mutations with continuous stimulation. The second hypothesis is that a defect in the regulation of the B cells, whether intrinsic or due to lack of T-cell downregulation, lead to both autoimmune disease and eventually lymphoma.

Chronic Lymphocytic Leukemia/Small Lymphocytic Lymphoma. Chronic lymphocytic leukemia (CLL) (or small lymphocytic lymphoma [SLL]) is a malignant transformation of $CD5^+$ B cells. B-CLL is the most common leukemia in North America and Western Europe, seen mostly in older individuals. These patients are extremely susceptible to infection, suggesting that their nonmalignant cells are not functioning properly. Autoimmune antibodies are common, particularly against red blood cells, resulting in autoimmune hemolytic anemia. This leukemia/lymphoma again suggests a neoplasm arising in the setting of or causing an immune dysregulation. CLL has a long clinical course but eventually there is massive involvement of every organ, peripheral blood and bone marrow by leukemic cells.

Plasma Cell Neoplasms. Neoplastic growths of plasma cells may be solitary resulting in a ***plasmacytoma*** or may be at multiple sites, predominantly throughout the bone and called ***multiple myeloma*** or ***plasma cell myeloma***. They may be a mixture of cells appearing as lymphocytes, plasma cells, or something in between, lymphoplasmacytoid cells (***lymphoplasmacytic lymphoma*** or ***Waldenström's macroglobulinemia***). These are still the product of a single clone. The cells may produce and secrete their immunoglobulin product and this monoclonal protein can cause more difficulties for the patient than the cells themselves. Free light chain deposits called ***amyloid*** can result in organ failure, especially in the kidneys. Excreted in the urine, these free light chains called ***Bence-Jones proteins*** provided a means to study light chain structure. In Waldenström's macroglobulinemia, overproduction of IgM may be so great as to slow blood flow and clog vessels (hyperviscosity syndrome).

The monoclonal protein is detected in the serum and sometimes in the urine as an M spike (seen in the M region) in electrophoretic evaluation. All other normal immunoglobulins are severely decreased and the patients are therefore immunosuppressed with respect to antibody production. Before the appearance of full-blown myeloma, patients may have a small amount of monoclonal immunoglobulin for many years. Many individuals remain at this stage, never progressing to disease.

As for normal plasma cells, IL-6 functions as an autocrine growth factor for myeloma cells. IL-6 is also overproduced by the stromal bone marrow cells in these patients.

T-Cell Neoplasms

Precursor T-cell Acute Lymphoblastic Leukemia/Lymphoma. This neoplasm of immature T cells has characteristics identical to those of thymocytes frozen in their immature state. They are frequently double positive for CD4 and CD8 and

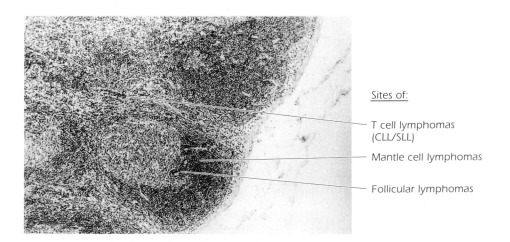

Sites of:

T cell lymphomas (CLL/SLL)

Mantle cell lymphomas

Follicular lymphomas

Figure 18.9. A section through a normal lymph node showing sites where T- and B-cell lymphomas may arise.

have little or no CD3 on their surface. They have not yet completed rearrangement of their T cell receptor genes and still express TdT. T-ALL presents as a leukemia or as a thymic mass. Treatment has not been as successful as for B-ALL.

Peripheral T-Cell Neoplasms. Peripheral T-cell lymphomas have a varied presentation. They go wherever T cells are normally found; skin, lung, vessel wall, gastrointestinal tract, lymph nodes. They seem to have a more aggressive course than B-cell lymphomas. A particular T-cell neoplasm of the skin, ***mycosis fungoides*** may also have a leukemic phase (***Sézary syndrome***).

Adult T-Cell Leukemia/Lymphoma. Adult T-cell leukemia/lymphoma (ATLL) is an aggressive T-cell leukemia that was described in 1970 in a region of Japan where it is endemic. It is also found in the Caribbean and a small region of the United States. ATLL is a neoplasm of mature $CD4^+$ T cells. In early attempts at treatment, the neoplasm was found to respond temporarily (few months) to administration of anti-Tac antibody. Tac was later found to be the α chain of the IL-2 receptor, and IL-2 is an autocrine growth factor for these cells.

ATLL is caused by the retrovirus human T-cell lymphotropic virus 1 (HTLV-1), which was described and isolated before recognition of AIDS and HIV. The proviral genomic structure is similar in HTLV-1, containing a LTR region and encoding for structural and regulatory proteins as well as viral enzymes, reverse transcriptase, integrase, and protease. Tax, its protein that transactivates HTLV-1 transcription by binding to LTR, also activates host genes, including those coding for IL-2, IL-2R α chain, and a parathyroidlike hormone. Therefore activation of proviral transcription is associated with activation and proliferation of the host cell. Patients with ATLL frequently have extreme elevations in serum calcium levels due to the PTH-like hormone.

Transmission of the virus is similar to HIV, associated with blood and body fluids, with greater transfer in breast milk. Thus many are infected during infancy. The incubation period of this virus is long, typically 20 to 40 years. The virus also infects $CD4^+$ T cells and the nervous system, and patients may present with neurologic disease.

Fortunately, only approximately 1% of infected patients develop ATLL. What initiates its development after so many years is unknown. The $CD4^+$ T cells harbor the virus in a quiescent state. Unlike HIV, the virus is not cytolytic for these cells once activated, to the contrary HTLV-1 leads to transformation of the T cells. Once diagnosed with ATLL, survival is generally 6 months to 1 year. The blood supply of the United States and Great Britain is screened for HTLV-1 infection.

Hodgkin's Disease

Hodgkin's disease is a lymphoma characterized by the presence of relatively small numbers of large binucleate malignant cells named Reed-Sternberg cells in a reactive background of small T cells, eosinophils, plasma cells, and fibrosis. This reactive milieu is the result of abundant cytokine production, particularly IL-5, by either the tumor cells, background cells, or both. The patients show clinical signs of increased cytokine production with fevers, night sweats, and weight loss.

The lineage origin of the Reed-Sternberg cell, which expresses only CD15 and CD30, has been the subject of much debate. Currently evidence showing rearrangements found in the immunoglobulin genes using molecular techniques on single cells suggest that the Reed-Sternberg cell may derive from a postgerminal center B cell.

SUMMARY

1. Immune deficiency disorders are called *primary* when the deficiency is the cause of disease and *secondary* when the deficiency is a result of other diseases or the effects of treatment regimens.

2. Immune deficiency diseases may be due to disorders in the development or function of B cells, T cells, phagocytic cells, or components of complement.

3. Immune deficiency disorders predispose patients to recurrent infections. The infection type is sometimes characteristic of the underlying deficiency.

4. Immune deficiencies constitute one type of defect or disorder of the immune system. Another aspect of such disorders is the unregulated proliferation of B lymphocytes, T lymphocytes, phagocytes, and their products, or the unregulated activation of components of the complement system. This may account for the association of immune deficiencies with autoimmune disease and malignancies.

5. HIV, by infecting and killing $CD4^+$ lymphocytes, causes a massive immunosuppressive illness known as the acquired immune deficiency syndrome (AIDS).

6. Neoplasms of the immune system are uncontrolled monoclonal proliferations that can be related to their normal cell counterparts and stage of differentiation. Many have specific chromosomal translocations causing dysregulation of cell proliferation and death. Some are associated with viral infections such as EBV and HTLV-1.

REFERENCES

Ammann AJ (1994): Mechanisms of immunodeficiency. In Stites DP, Terr Al, Parslow TG (eds): Basic and Clinical Immunology, 8th ed. E Norwalk, CT: Appleton & Lange.

Anderson DC, Springer TA (1987): Leukocyte adhesion deficiency: an inherited defect in Mac-1, LFA-1, and p150, 95 glycoproteins. *Annu Rev Med* 38:175.

Baltimore D, Feinberg MB (1989): HIV revealed: towards a natural history of the infection. *N Engl J Med* 132:1673.

Clerici M, Shearer GM (1994): The T_H1-T_H2 hypothesis of HIV infection: new insights. *Immunol Today* 14:107.

Fahey JL (1993): Update on AIDS. *Immunologist* 1:131.

Fauci AS (1993): Multifactorial nature of human immunodeficiency virus disease: implications for therapy. *Science* 262:1011.

Green WC (1993): AIDS and the immune system. *Sci Am* (Sept): 99.

Helbert MR, L'Age-Stehr J, Mitchison NA (1993): Antigen presentation, loss of immunologic memory and AIDS. *Immunol Today* 14:340.

Kohler H, Muller S, Nara P (1994): Deceptive imprinting in the immune response against HIV-1. *Immunol Today* 15:475.

Lusso P, Gallo RC (1995): Human herpes virus 6 in AIDS. *Immunol Today* 16:67.

Ochs HD, Smith CIE, Puck JM (1999) Primary Immunodeficiency Diseases. New York: Oxford University Press. Orkin SH (1989): Molecular genetics of chronic granulomatous disease. *Annu Rev Immunol* 7:277.

Rosenberg ZF, Fauci AS (1990): Immunopathogenic mechanisms of HIV infection: Cytokine induction of HIV expression. *Immunol Today* 11:176.

 REVIEW QUESTIONS

For each question, choose the ONE BEST answer or completion.

1. An 8-month-old baby has a history of repeated gram-positive bacterial infections. The most probable cause for this condition is that
   A) the mother did not confer sufficient immunity on the baby in utero.
   B) the baby suffers from erythroblastosis fetalis (hemolytic disease of the newborn).
   C) the baby has a defect in the alternative complement pathway.
   D) the baby is allergic to the mother's milk.
   E) None of the above.

2. A 50-year-old worker at an atomic plant who previously had a sample of his own bone marrow cryopreserved was accidentally exposed to a minimal lethal dose of radiation. He was subsequently transplanted with his own bone marrow. This individual can expect
   A) to have recurrent bacterial infections.
   B) to have serious fungal infections due to deficiency in cell-mediated immunity.
   C) to make antibody responses to thymus-independent antigens only.
   D) All of the above.
   E) None of the above.

3. Which of the following immune deficiency disorders is associated exclusively with an abnormality of the humoral immune response?
   A) X-linked agammaglobulinemia (Bruton's agammaglobulinemia)
   B) DiGeorge syndrome
   C) Wiskott-Aldrich syndrome
   D) chronic mucocutaneous candidiasis
   E) ataxia telangiectasia

4. A sharp increase in levels of IgG, with a spike in the IgG region seen in the electrophoretic pattern of serum proteins is an indication of
   A) IgA or IgM deficiency.
   B) multiple myeloma.
   C) macroglobulinemia.
   D) hypogammaglobulinemia.
   E) severe fungal infections.

5. Patients with DiGeorge syndrome may fail to produce IgG in response to immunization with T-dependent antigens because
   A) they have a decreased number of B cells that produce IgG.
   B) they have increased numbers of suppressor T cells.

    C) they have a decreased number of helper T cells.

    D) they have abnormal antigen-presenting cells.

    E) they cannot produce IgM during primary responses.

6. A 2-year-old child has had three episodes of pneumonia and two episodes of otitis media. All the infections were demonstrated to be pneumococcal. Which of the following disorders is most likely to be the cause?

    A) an isolated transient T-cell deficiency

    B) a combined T- and B-cell deficiency

    C) a B-cell deficiency

    D) transient anemia

    E) The child has AIDS.

7. A healthy woman gave birth to a baby. The newborn infant was found to be HIV-seropositive. This finding is most likely the result of

    A) the virus being transferred across the placenta to the baby.

    B) the baby is making anti-HIV antibodies.

    C) the baby's erythrocyte antigens cross-reacting with the virus.

    D) the mother's erythrocyte antigens cross-reacting with the virus.

    E) maternal HIV-specific IgG being transferred across the placenta to the baby.

8. Immunodeficiency disease can result from

    A) a developmental defect of T lymphocytes.

    B) a developmental defect of bone marrow stem cells.

    C) a defect in phagocyte function.

    D) a defect in complement function.

    E) All of the above.

9. A 9-month-old baby was vaccinated against smallpox with attenuated smallpox virus. He developed a progressive necrotic lesion of the skin, muscles, and subcutaneous tissue at the site of inoculation. The vaccination reaction probably resulted from

    A) B-lymphocyte deficiency.

    B) reaction to the adjuvant.

    C) complement deficiency.

    D) T-cell deficiency.

    E) B- and T-lymphocyte deficiency.

10. The most common clinical consequence(s) of C3 deficiency is (are)

    A) increased incidence of tumors.

    B) increased susceptibility to viral infections.

    C) increased susceptibility to fungal infections.

    D) increased susceptibility to bacterial infections.

    E) All of the above.

Case Study

A 4-year-old child who just moved to a new town with his mother is brought to a pediatrician's office with a complaint of the child's failure to thrive, including loss of appetite, weight loss, and persistent cough. On physical examination the child appears pale and sickly, has a low-grade fever, but no other physical signs. His past history is unremarkable except for a fractured leg at 1 year of age that required a blood transfusion during surgery, but it healed without complication. A battery of tests are performed to arrive at a diagnosis. X-ray examination showed some bilateral pulmonary infiltrates. Blood count is normal, with slightly reduced white cell numbers. An ELISA to detect serum immunoglobulins showed elevated IgG, IgM, and IgA. Skin tests performed with mumps, tetanus, and candida antigens were negative. Antibiotic therapy was started, but on the next visit the child was sicker and now had enlarged lymph nodes, spleen, and liver. What diagnosis should the physician be thinking of at this point and how could it be confirmed?

Answers to Review Questions

1. E None of the above is likely to be the underlying cause for the history. The baby is probably hypogammaglobulinemic. Hypogammaglobulinemia leads to recurrent bacterial infections. Viral and fungal infections are controlled by cell-mediated immunity, which is normal in hypogammaglobulinemic individuals. Answer A is incorrect because the mother's IgG, which passed through the placenta, would have a half-life of 23 days, and would therefore not be expected to remain in the baby's circulation for 8 months. At this age any Ig present in the baby's circulation is synthesized by the baby. Answer B is irrelevant, since erythroblastosis fetalis is caused by the destruction of the newborn's Rh$^+$ erythrocytes by the Rh$^-$ mother's antibodies to Rh antigen. Answer C is unlikely since the classical complement pathway would still be protective; moreover, a defect in the alternative pathway would not result in the selective inability to protect from only gram-positive bacterial infections. Answer D is incorrect since, even if allergic to the mother's milk, the baby should not suffer from increased frequency of bacterial infections.

2. E The autologous bone marrow cells, which contain stem cells, will replicate, differentiate, and repopulate the hematopoietic-reticuloendothelial system, rendering the individual immunologically normal. As such, the individual is not expected to have bacterial, viral, or fungal infections or to respond to antigens differently from a normal individual.

3. A The only immune deficiency disorder that is associated with an abnormality exclusively of the humoral response is Bruton's agammaglobulinemia or X-linked agammaglobulinemia. DiGeorge syndrome results from thymic aplasia, where there is a deficiency in T cells that may influence the IgG responses, which require helper T cells. Wiskott–Aldrich syndrome is associated with several abnormalities. Ataxia telangiectasia is a disease with defects in both cellular and humoral immune responses although T-cell-dependent areas of lymphoid tissues are most severely affected. Chronic mucocutaneous candidiasis is a poorly defined collection of syndromes associated with a selective defect in the functioning of T cells.

4. B This pattern is characteristic of multiple myeloma (IgG myeloma). Multiple myeloma may be recognized by the synthesis of large amounts of homogeneous antibody of any one isotype. Although patients with multiple myeloma may suffer from a decreased synthesis of other Ig isotypes, the electrophoretic pattern is not necessarily an indication of IgA or IgM deficiency.

5. C Patients with DiGeorge syndrome have a decreased number of T cells—in particular, helper T cells, which are essential for the IgG response to T-dependent antigens. These patients have normally functioning B cells and are capable of responding to T-independent antigens, or with only IgM responses (primary responses) to T-dependent antigens.

6. C The cause for the described case history is very likely due to B-cell deficiency, which is characterized by recurrent bacterial infections leading to otitis media and pneumonia. T-cell deficiency would usually result in viral, fungal, and protozoal infections. The same is true for combined T- and B-cell deficiency. Answer D (transient anemia) is irrelevant in this case—anemia is not generally associated with increased infections. It is unlikely that with a history of only pneumococcal infections the child would have AIDS. The latter syndrome is associated more with characteristic infections such as with *Pneumocystis carinii* and various viral infections.

7. *E* The most likely explanation is that the "healthy" mother has been infected with HIV-1 and is making anti-HIV IgG, which is transferred to the fetus and newborn transplacentally. While it is possible that the HIV was transferred to the infant across the placenta, this would not cause the newborn to make antibodies to the virus at this young age—thus answers A and B are incorrect. Answers C and D are false because this unlikely situation would result in the recognition of the viral antigen as "self" and the individual would not make anti-self antibodies.

8. *E* All are correct. Immunodeficiency disorders may result from defects in the development of bone marrow stem cells into lymphocytes and other cells that participate in the immune response. They can also result from defects in phagocyte functions, which are important in phagocytosis and presentation of antigen. Immunodeficiency disorders may also result from defects in complement function—an absence or malfunction of one or more of the complement components, their activators, or regulators.

9. *D* T-cell deficiency would result in the absence of the crucial immunologic defenses against viral infection, that is, cell-mediated immunity. Cell-mediated immunity plays the major role in immunity to viral infections, much greater than the roles of antibody or complement. In fact, individuals with impaired T-cell-mediated immunity should not be vaccinated with live virus, which, even if attenuated, may cause a serious infection.

10. *D* Deficiency in C3 is associated with increased susceptibility to bacterial infections, since C3 plays an important role in the destruction of bacteria and their increased opsonization, by participating in the classical and the alternative pathways of complement activation. Cell-mediated immunity (CMI) is generally more important in the resistance of the host to viral and fungal infections. Also, in general, CMI is considered to be more important than complement in the resistance of the host to tumors.

Answer to Case Study

This is a possible case of childhood AIDS, presumably attributable to the earlier transfusion with blood obtained from a blood bank. Although present-day tests to screen blood from donors are highly reliable, there are still isolated cases of HIV transmission by blood transfusion. Following a long incubation period the child presented with a slightly lowered white cell count, somewhat elevated immunoglobulin levels, but a seriously compromised T-cell function. The latter was determined by the absence of skin reactions to mumps, tetanus toxoid, and candida antigens, all of which elicit T-cell-mediated delayed-type hypersensitivity reactions in normal individuals. A follow-up test of the levels of circulating $CD4^+$ and $CD8^+$ cells revealed a ratio of 0.4, indicating that helper $CD4^+$ cells, the target of the HIV virus, have declined markedly. Further study of the lung infiltrate, which failed to respond to antibiotic therapy, would be done by bronchoscopy and lavage. Microscopic examination of the washings would probably show an opportunistic organism such as *Pneumocystis carinii*, a common cause of death in patients with AIDS. Final confirmatory evidence would come from an examination of the child's serum for the presence of antibody to HIV antigens, a clear indication of an infection with HIV, and from the use of an HIV-specific PCR to ascertain the presence the viral genes.

19

TRANSPLANTATION IMMUNOLOGY

INTRODUCTION

The immune response has evolved as a way of discriminating between *"self"* and *"nonself."* Once "foreignness" has been established, the immune response proceeds toward its ultimate goal of destroying the foreign material, be it a microorganism or its product, a substance present in the environment, or a tumor cell. The triggering of the immune system in response to such foreign substances is, of course, of great survival value.

The same discriminating power of the immune response between "self" and "nonself" is undesirable in instances that are highly artificial, such as the transplantation of cells or organs from one individual to another for therapeutic purposes. Indeed, results of such transplantations were formerly disastrous, culminating in the rejection of the transplanted tissue.

With the current understanding of the mechanisms involved in transplant rejection and the advent of effective immunosuppressive therapies, transplantation of various organs and tissues for therapeutic purposes has become commonplace (Table 19.1). For example, over 10,000 kidneys are transplanted annually worldwide with a high degree of success. Transplantations of heart, lungs, cornea, liver, and bone marrow that were considered spectacular and were widely publicized as recently as 25 years ago, have now become commonplace. Although rejection episodes have been significantly reduced due to the use of immunosuppressive therapies, they have not been eliminated. Thus, transplantation immunology continues to be a major area of research. Later in this chapter, we will briefly describe the experience of one of us (E.B.) who has undergone a heart transplantation.

RELATIONSHIP BETWEEN DONOR AND RECIPIENT

Various gradations in relationships of transplantation from donor to recipient are shown in Figure 19.1 and are described below.

⬤ T A B L E 19.1. Transplantation of Specific Organs and Tissues

Organ/Tissue	Clinical uses	Comments
Skin	Burns, chronic wounds, diabetic ulcers, venous ulcers	Commonly autologous grafts; increasing use of artificial skin consisting of stromal elements and cultured cells of allogeneic or xenogeneic origin
Kidney	End-stage renal failure	Graft survival now exceeds 85% at one year even with organs from unrelated donors.
Liver	Hepatoma and biliary atresia	Successful in about two-thirds of recipients at 1 year.
Heart	Cardiac failure	Survival rates in excess of 80% at 1 year.
Lung	Advanced pulmonary or cardiopulmonary diseases	Sometimes performed together with heart transplantation
Bone marrow	Incurable leukemias and lymphomas, congenital immunodeficiency diseases	Risk of GVHD a unique feature of bone marrow transplantation; increasingly, transplantation of hematopoietic stem cells being used.
Cornea	Blindness	HLA matching not advantageous since this is a "privileged" site that normally lacks lymphatic drainage.
Pancreas	Diabetes mellitus	Pancreas and kidney transplantation sometimes performed together. Success rates approaching that seen with kidney transplants.

1. An *autograft* is a graft or transplant from one area to another on the same individual such as would occur in the transplantation of normal skin from one area of an individual to a burned area of the same individual. The graft is recognized as *autochthonous* or *autologous* ("self"), and no immune response is induced against it. Barring technical difficulties in the transplantation process, the graft will survive or "take" in its new location.

2. An *isograft* or *syngraft* is a graft or transplantation of cells, tissue, or organ from one individual to another individual who is *syngeneic* (genetically identical) to the donor. An example of an isograft is the transplantation of a kidney from one identical (homozygotic) twin to the other. As in the case of an autograft, the recipient who is genetically identical to the donor recognizes the donor's tissue as "self" and does not mount an immune response against it. The two individuals (i.e., donor and recipient), are described as *histocompatible*.

3. An *allograft* is a graft, or transplant, from one individual to a genetically dissimilar individual of the same species. Since all individuals of a given outbred species, except monozygotic twins, are *allogeneic* (genetically dissimilar), regardless of how closely they may be related, the graft is recognized by the recipient as foreign and is immunologically rejected. The donor and recipient, in this case, are *nonhistocompatible* or *histoincompatible*.

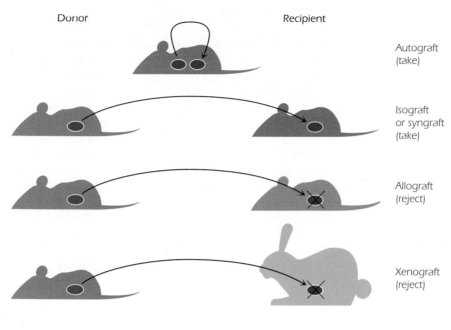

Donor   Recipient

Autograft
(take)

Isograft
or syngraft
(take)

Allograft
(reject)

Xenograft
(reject)

Figure 19.1. Situations of tissue transplantation.

4. A *xenograft* is a graft between a donor and a recipient from different species. The transplant is recognized as foreign, and the immune response mounted against it will destroy or reject the graft. Donor and recipient are again *histoincompatible*.

THE ROLE OF THE IMMUNE RESPONSE IN ALLOGRAFT REJECTION

The most direct evidence that the immune response is involved in graft rejection is provided by experiments in which skin is transplanted from one individual to a genetically different individual of the same species, namely, between allogeneic donor and recipient. Mouse skin with black hair transplanted onto the back of a white-haired mouse appears normal for 1 or 2 weeks. However, after approximately 2 weeks, the transplant begins to be rejected, and is completely sloughed off within a few days. This process is called *first-set rejection*. If, after this rejection, the recipient is transplanted with another piece of skin from the same initial donor, the process of *rejection is accelerated*, and the graft is sloughed quicker, within about a week of the second transplant. This accelerated rejection is termed a *second-set rejection*. By contrast, a piece of skin from a genetically different strain grafted onto this same mouse is rejected with first-set kinetics. Thus, second-set rejection is an expression of specific *immunologic memory* for antigens expressed by the graft. The participation of T cells in the rejection response can be shown by transferring T cells from an individual sensitized to an allograft into a normal syngeneic recipient. If the second recipient is transplanted with the same allograft that was used on the original

T-cell donor, a second-set rejection ensues. This establishes that T cells primed in the initial grafting mediate the accelerated rejection in the second host.

Many other lines of evidence establish the immunologic nature of graft rejection. For example, (1) histologic examination of the site of the rejection reveals *lymphocytic and monocytic cellular infiltration* reminiscent of the delayed-type hypersensitivity reaction (see Chapter 16); both CD4$^+$ and CD8$^+$ cells are present at the site (and, as we shall see later, both play a crucial role in graft rejection); (2) individuals that lack T lymphocytes (such as athymic, or "nude," mice or humans with DiGeorge syndrome; see Chapter 18) do not reject allografts or xenografts; and (3) the process of rejection slows down considerably or does not occur at all in immunosuppressed individuals. It has also been demonstrated that in a normal individual, *T cells* and *circulating antibodies* are induced to the antigens expressed by an allograft or a xenograft.

CLINICAL CHARACTERISTICS OF ALLOGRAFT REJECTION

Clinically, allograft rejections fall into three major categories: (1) *hyperacute rejection*, (2) *acute rejection*, and (3) *chronic rejection*. The following are descriptions of the rejection reactions as might be observed, for example, after transplantation of a kidney; they also apply for rejection of other tissues.

Hyperacute Rejection

Hyperacute rejection occurs within a few minutes to a few hours of transplantation. It is a result of destruction of the transplant by *preformed antibodies* to incompatible MHC antigens and, in some cases, to carbohydrates expressed on transplanted tissues (e.g. on endothelial cells). In some cases, these preformed antibodies are generated as a result of previous transplantations, blood transfusions, or pregnancies. These cytotoxic antibodies activate the *complement* system, followed by platelet activation and deposition causing *swelling* and *interstitial hemorrhage* in the transplanted tissue, which decrease the flow of blood through the tissue. *Thrombosis* with *endothelial injury* and *fibrinoid necrosis* are often seen in cases of hyperacute rejection. The recipient may have *fever, leukocytosis*, and produce *little or no urine*. The urine may contain various cellular elements, such as erythrocytes. Cell-mediated immunity is not involved at all in hyperacute rejection.

At present there is no therapy for successful prevention or termination of hyperacute rejection.

Acute Rejection

Acute rejection is seen in a recipient who has not previously been sensitized to the transplant. Cell-mediated immunity mediated by T cells is the primary cause of acute rejection. It is the common type of rejection experienced by individuals for whom the transplanted tissue is a mismatch, or who receive an allograft and insufficient immunosuppressive treatment to prevent rejection. For example, an acute rejection reaction may begin a few days after transplantation of a kidney, with a complete loss of kidney function within 10–14 days. Acute rejection of a kidney is accompanied by a rapid *decrease in renal function. Enlargement and tenderness* of the grafted kidney, a *rise in serum creatinine level, a fall in urine output, decreased renal blood flow*, and presence of **blood cells** and **proteins in the urine** are characteristic. Histologically, cell-mediated immunity, manifested by intense infiltration of lymphocytes and macrophages, is taking place at the rejection site. The acute rejection reaction may be reduced by immunosuppressive therapy, for example, with corticosteroids, cyclosporine, and other drugs, as we shall see later in this chapter.

Chronic Rejection

Chronic rejection caused by both antibody and cell-mediated immunity occurs in allograft transplantation months or years after the transplanted tissue has assumed its normal function. In cases of kidney transplantation, chronic rejection is characterized by **slow, progressive renal failure**. Histologically, the chronic reaction is accompanied by **proliferative inflammatory lesions** of the small arteries, **thickening of the glomerular basement membrane**, and **interstitial fibrosis**. Because the damage caused by immune injury has already taken place, immunosuppressive therapy at this point is useless, and little can be done to save the graft.

While the preceding example is for kidney transplantation, it is important to point out that the rate, extent, and underlying mechanisms of rejection may vary, depending on the transplanted tissue and site of the transplanted graft. The recipients circulation, lymphatic drainage, expression of strong antigens on the graft, and several other factors determine the rejection rate. For example, bone marrow and skin grafts are very sensitive to rejection compared to heart, kidney, and liver grafts.

 HISTOCOMPATIBILITY ANTIGENS

Antigens that evoke an immune response associated with graft rejection are referred to as **transplantation antigens**, or **histocompatibility antigens**. These antigens are cell-surface molecules encoded by histocompatibility genes (H genes) situated at a histocompatibility locus (H locus). Since different alleles encoding allelic forms of the histocompatibility antigens exist at each H locus in different individuals, the antigens are also referred to as alloantigens.

If there were only one H locus with two alleles, for example, A and B, the possible genotypes and phenotypes of the alloantigens would be

Genotype	Phenotype
AA	A
AB	AB
BB	B

Transplantation between individuals with the above genotypes are accepted or rejected as follows:

Donor	Recipient	Accept/Reject Reason
1) AA → AA	Accept	A recognized as self
2) BB → AA	Reject	B recognized as foreign
3) AB → AA	Reject	B recognized as foreign
4) AA → BB	Reject	A recognized as foreign
5) BB → BB	Accept	B recognized as self

Donor	Recipient	Accept/Reject Reason
6) AB → BB	Reject	A recognized as foreign
7) AA → AB	Accept	A recognized as self
8) BB → AB	Accept	B recognized as self
9) AB → AB	Accept	A or B recognized as self

In reality, there are many H loci containing many alleles. For example, in mice there are about 40 H loci. However, while transplantation antigens may be encoded by various loci, each species contains one major region that is of prime immunologic importance for that species. This region is the ***major histocompatibility complex (MHC)***. It codes for major transplantation antigens; minor transplantation antigens are encoded by other loci. As described in Chapter 8, in the mouse, this region is called H-2. It consists of a segment of chromosome 17, and contains the genes encoding for class I molecules encoded by K, D, and L genes and class II molecules encoded by I region genes. In humans, the MHC that is located on chromosome 6 is known as ***HLA*** (for human leukocyte antigen), since it contains genes encoding these antigens.

As we have already seen in Chapter 8, the human HLA gene complex consists of several closely linked genes (loci), known as A, B, C (MHC class I), and DP, DQ, and DR (MHC class II). Each locus has many different alleles. The particular combination of alleles at closely linked loci on the same chromosome is termed the ***haplotype***: two haplotypes, one from each parent, constitute the genotype of the individual. In a sense, the haplotype is the genotype of linked loci on each of the parental chromosomes.

Recalling the structure and genetics of MHC class I and class II molecules (Chapter 8), class I molecules consist of an α chain encoded by the MHC and $\beta2$ microglobulin, encoded on chromosome 15. The A, B, and C loci in humans (K, D, and L loci in mice) code for the α chain (heavy chain) of MHC class I molecules, which contain a variable region. This accounts for the polymorphism exhibited by MHC class I molecules.

The DP, DQ, and DR genes of the D region in humans (the I region in mice) code for class II molecules that may be expressed on the surface of such cells as ***B lymphocytes, monocytes, Langerhans cells*** of the skin, and certain ***endothelial*** cells. Again, as described in Chapter 8, each class II molecule consists of an α chain and a β chain. Both chains exhibit extensive allelic variability, although the β chain has more extensive variability than the α chain.

The structure and major function of class I and class II molecules in the presentation of antigen to T cells have been discussed in Chapters 8 and 10. In the present chapter, we shall discuss their role in inducing transplantation reactions.

MHC Class I and Class II Molecules as Targets in Allograft Rejection

As we have seen, graft rejection is the consequence of a T-cell-dependent immune responses and, in many cases, cytotoxic antibodies play a role too: the recipient's T cells are activated by antigen, in particular by the nonself (foreign) MHC molecules expressed on the graft. The key initiating event in graft rejection is the direct activation of the recipients CD4$^+$ T cells by nonself MHC class II molecules expressed on specialized cells of the graft. (These nonself MHC molecules may have peptides derived from either the graft or the recipients proteins bound in their peptide-binding groove.) The recipient's CD8$^+$ T cells may also be directly activated by nonself MHC class I molecules expressed on many cells in the graft.

Nonself MHC molecules are highly potent transplantation antigens, activating an enormous number of T-cell clones in the recipient. It is estimated that up to 5% of all clones in the body may respond to a nonself MHC molecule, orders of magnitude higher than the response to a conventional protein antigen. Presumably, the combination of nonself MHC molecule plus bound peptides cross-reacts with T cell receptors on many different T cells. As we described in Chapters 9 and 10, the "everyday" specificity of the T cell within an individual is restricted by self-MHC, the allelic specificity seen in the thymus during T-cell differentiation. Thus, the exposure of an individual to nonself MHC molecules expressed on the graft represents an artificial but clinically relevant situation. Another mechanism that contributes to host T-cell activation is that the antigen-presenting cells of the recipient that encounter the graft take up the alloantigens (major and minor), process the molecules, present the resulting peptides on self (recipient) MHC molecules to T cells, and activate them.

Sensitization of the recipient by donor-cell antigens activates the immune response by triggering both CD4$^+$ and CD8$^+$ cells. As a result, cytokines are synthesized and T cells cytotoxic for the graft are activated. The most important cytokines generated are IL-2, IFN-γ, and TNF-β as happens in delayed-type hypersensitivity (see Chapter 16). IL-2 is important for T-cell proliferation and differentiation into cytotoxic T lymphocytes (CTL) and T cells participating in DTH (T$_H$1), IFN-γ is important for the accumulation and activation of macrophages in the graft area, and TNF-β is cytotoxic to the graft. Moreover, IFN-α, -β, and -γ as well as TNF-β and TNF-α increase the expression of class I molecules, while IFN-γ increases the expression of class II molecules on allograft cells, thus amplifying the reaction and enhancing graft rejection.

The MHC class II molecules or antigens coded by the DR locus play the most important role in tissue rejection, so much so that there is a good agreement among transplant immunologists that the better the match (parity) in HLA-DR antigens between donor and recipient, the higher the probability of graft survival. In general, the graft does not survive if the donor and recipient do not share any HLA-DR haplotype.

It should be pointed out that although molecules coded for by the MHC are mainly responsible for graft rejection, weak antiallograft reactions may be generated by minor transplantation antigens, and the combined response to several minor antigens may result in eventual graft rejection. In fact, as we will discuss later in this chapter, minor transplantation antigens appear to be important in bone marrow transplantation and have been implicated in graft-versus-host (GVH) disease (discussed later in this chapter) in cases of HLA-matched bone marrow transplantations.

Xenogeneic Transplantation

It is estimated that more than 50,000 people who need organ transplants die each year while waiting for a compatible donor. To address the critical shortage of donated human organs for transplantation, studies are under way in the use of nonhuman organs. For ethical and practical reasons, species closely related to the human, such as the chimpanzee, have not been widely used. Attention has focused on the pig, some of whose organs are anatomically similar to the human. Interestingly, the human T-cell response to xenogenic MHC antigens is not as strong as to allogeneic MHC molecules.

The major problem with using pig organs, and organs from other species, in human recipients, however, is the existence of natural or preformed antibodies to carbohydrate moieties expressed on the graft's endothelial cells. As a consequence, the activation of the complement cascade occurs rapidly and hyperacute rejection ensues. Finally, another concern that has stimulated debate about the safe use of xenografts concerns the possibility that animal organs and tissues may harbor viruses that might infect humans. This fear is underscored by the possibility that the HIV pandemic may have been caused by the transmission of a virus from monkeys to humans. In the United States, the Centers for Disease Control and Prevention and other public health agencies have drafted guidelines to monitor patients who receive xenografts using sensitive assays to detect viruses that may be present.

TESTS FOR HISTOCOMPATIBILITY ANTIGENS

Tissue typing consists of the analysis of histocompatibility antigens of donor and recipient and allows a determination of the degree of foreignness between the two individuals, thus serving to predict the outcome of a transplant procedure. With the advent of new and better immunosuppressive drugs and modalities, analysis of histocompatibility antigens and attempts to match donor and recipient by the similarity of their HLA antigens is becoming less and less essential. Nevertheless in many instances, such as bone marrow transplantation, HLA analyses are being performed and are therefore discussed below.

There are several ways to determine the degree of parity or disparity between transplantation antigens. One way is the serologic detection of cell-surface antigens; the other way is by measuring the reaction between leukocytes from the donor and recipient [primarily detecting differences (or showing parity) of class II antigens].

Serologic Detection of Transplantation Antigens

A panel of antisera that react differently with different histocompatibility antigens is used to define transplantation antigens. The antisera are obtained from people who have had multiple transplantations or transfusions and from multiparous (multiple birth) women. Monoclonal antibodies are also used for defining HLA antigens. These antisera and monoclonal antibodies are used in a *lymphocytotoxicity test* in which the sera, in the presence of complement, are monitored for ability to damage the target cells, which are lymphocytes. Thus, lymphocytes of the donor and recipient, which carry MHC class I and class II antigens, are reacted with a panel of antibodies. The reaction with the various antibodies establishes the *serologic type* of each transplantation antigen on the cells. Similarity of donor and recipient transplantation antigens is indicated by similarity in the specific antisera with which the two sets of cells react (or do not react).

Serologic *tissue typing* provides a fairly reliable measure of parity (or disparity) between transplantation antigens of the donor and the recipient. However, because the number of antisera available for such a test is finite, there is always the possibility that, although the panel of sera shows a "match" (i.e., the identity of antigens on the donors and recipients leukocytes) differences would be found if the panel of antisera were enlarged.

Genotyping of Transplantation Epitopes

A relatively new approach to tissue typing is to type epitopes on HLA molecules rather than the entire molecule. Such comparison may be performed serologically, or better yet, on the genomic level. Thus, DNA segments are amplified by the polymerase chain reaction (PCR) to obtain DNA quantities that afford sequencing oligonucleotides and sequence comparison. This highly sensitive, rapid, and accurate method is far more accurate than serologic typing because it can detect differences on the level of a single amino acid. Indeed, typing on the genomic level has shown differences in instances where complete "match" has been shown by serologic means.

Detection of Transplantation Antigens by Mixed Leukocyte Reaction

In the *mixed leukocyte reaction* (MLR), leukocytes from donor and recipient are cultured together for several days. The donor leukocytes contain T cells with specificity directed against the alloantigens on the recipient cells, and those *T cells* will therefore be triggered to *proliferate* in the presence of these antigens (see Table

T A B L E 19.2. Cases of Mixed Lymphocyte Reaction Associated With Different Transplantation Situations

Transplantation situation	HLA relationship	Treatment of reacting leukocytes	MLR
Tissue between identical twins	HLA identical (syngeneic)	No treatment	(−) No reaction
Tissue between nonrelated donor and recipient	HLA different (allogeneic)	No treatment	(+) Reaction intensity depends on the degree of HLA difference between donor and recipient
Tissue between nonrelated donor and recipient	HLA different (allogeneic)	Donor's cells are treated with a mitotic inhibitor, thus testing reactivity of only recipient cells (performed to test for donor–recipient match)	(+) This is a one-way MLR; reaction intensity depends on the degree of HLA difference between donor and recipient
Bone marrow transplantation, or tissue grafting to an immunoincompetent recipient	HLA different (allogeneic)	Recipient's cells are treated with a mitotic inhibitor, thus testing reactivity of only donor's cells (performed to avoid graft-versus-host reaction)	(+) This is a one-way MLR; reaction intensity depends on the degree of HLA difference between donor and recipient

19.2). The same is true for recipient leukocytes, which will proliferate in the presence of alloantigens on the donor cells. The proliferation is usually measured by introducing a radioactively labeled precursor to DNA, such as *³H-thymidine*, into the culture. The greater the extent of proliferation, the more DNA is synthesized by the proliferating cells, and the more radioactivity is incorporated into the cells' DNA. The radioactivity incorporated in DNA is then calculated to provide a measure of the proliferative response.

In most cases, it is essential to ascertain whether the recipient lymphocytes will react against the donor histocompatibility antigen (rather than whether the donor lymphocytes will react against the recipient alloantigens). For this purpose, an MLR is set up in which the donor cells have been treated with mitomycin C or X-irradiation to prevent their proliferation. In this way, the only cells with the ability to proliferate are the recipient leukocytes. Such a reaction is called a ***one-way mixed leukocyte reaction***. In this one way MLR CD4$^+$ cells proliferate to foreign MHC class II molecules and CD8$^+$ cells develop into T cytotoxic cells specific for the foreign class I molecules.

In comparison to the serologic test, which defines the specific antigens of the MHC of the donor and recipient, the MLR measures the total parity (or disparity) between donor and recipient cells, a parameter that is important for transplantation: the stronger the MLR (the greater the extent of proliferation), the higher the disparity between donor and recipient. Conversely, an MLR in which cellular proliferation is not induced, indicates complete parity or histocompatibility between donor and recipient, as when it is performed on cells from identical twins (see Table 19.2). It is important to emphasize that disparity in MHC class II antigens is the most important factor in transplant rejection.

The MLR is also performed when transplants are to be made into an immunosuppressed individual. It is essential that such transplantation be performed between well-matched individuals in order to avoid a reaction by any inadvertently transplanted immunocompetent cells directed against the recipients tissue, a few of which can produce an intense graft-versus-host (GVH) reaction, which we will discuss later. As we shall see toward the end of this chapter, when bone marrow, which may contain immunocompetent T cells, is transplanted into an immunologically incompetent host, it is essential to remove all competent mature T cells before transplantation to avoid this reaction.

Although MLR testing for histocompatibility is a highly effective indicator of the degree of parity between donor and recipient, it is a lengthy procedure and requires several days, whereas the serologic test takes only a few hours. Thus, the use of MLR and/or serologic testing is dictated by the speed with which an organ must be transplanted after its removal from the donor. While transplantation of organs from a living donor can await the results of the MLR test, sufficient time for this test may not be available in cases of organs obtained from recent cadavers. This is one reason why organ banks are set up to select the best-matched recipient when an organ becomes available.

As has been pointed out earlier, tissue or organ transplantation is relying more and more on immunosuppressive agents to prolong graft survival and less and less on tissue typing. In fact, recent results comparing graft survival with immunosuppressive agents show that, depending on the transplanted tissue, there is little difference in graft survival regardless of whether tissue typing or cross matching indicated a "match" between donor and recipient, as long as an effective immunosuppressive regimen was used.

PROLONGATION OF ALLOGRAFT SURVIVAL

A major clinical issue in transplantation immunology is to determine how the components and regulatory interactions involved in graft rejection might be manipulated to allow allograft (or xenograft) acceptance. Nonspecific approaches using immunosuppressive drugs that reduce the overall immunocompence of the recipient to all foreign antigens have been used with success to achieve this goal. However, given the need to treat patients chronically with these drugs to maintain the immunosuppressed state, such individuals are predisposed to opportunistic infections as well as malignancies. Accordingly, chemoprophylaxis is given to patients undergoing nonspecific, generalized immune suppression to help reduce the incidence of infections. The potential malignancy problem is one that cannot be addressed prophylactically.

More recently, experimental strategies that seek to prevent responses only to the antigens of a particular donor have been investigated. The ultimate goal of this approach is to achieve tolerance, which is lasting and ensures donor-specific nonresponsiveness. As discussed in Chapter 11, there are several mechanisms by which T-cell and B-cell tolerance to self-antigens is achieved. These include clonal deletion, anergy, and suppression. Although clinical trials have begun in which tolerance-inducing strategies are combined with conventional immunosuppressive therapies (discussed below), none of these strategies have been used to replace such chronic therapy in clinical transplantation.

Several of the standard and experimental immunosuppressive agents used in transplantation cases are discussed below. Commonly they are used in various combinations with each other to prevent graft rejection in transplantation of heart, kidney, lungs, liver, and other organs and tissues.

Antiinflammatory Agents

Corticosteroids, such as prednisone, prednisolone, and methylprednisolone, are powerful antiinflammatory agents. As pharmacologic derivatives of the glucocorticoid

TABLE 19.3. Standard and Experimental* Immunosuppressive Drugs Used in Transplantation

Inhibitors of lymphocyte gene expression	Corticosteroids
	Cyclosporine (Neoral)
	FK-506
Inhibitors of cytokine signal transduction	Anti-CD25*
	Rapamycin*
	Leflunomide*
Inhibitors of nucleotide synthesis	Azathioprine (Imuran)
	Mercaptopurine
	Chlorambucil
	Cyclophosphamide

family of steroid hormones, their physiologic effects result from their binding to intracellular steroid receptors that are expressed on almost every cell of the body. The immunosuppressive action of corticosteroids is due to several effects, most of which are a consequence of corticosteroid-induced regulation of gene transcription. Corticosteroids downregulate the expression of several genes that code for inflammatory cytokines. These include IL-1, IL-2, IL-3, IL-4, IL-5, IL-8, TNF-α, and GM-CSF. Cortocosteroids also inhibit expression of adhesion molecules causing inhibition of leukocyte migration to sites of inflammation. They therefore inhibit the activity of inflammatory cells. In addition, they promote the release of cellular endonucleases leading to the induction of apoptosis in lymphocytes and eosinophils. Moreover, they reduce phagocytosis and killing by neutrophils and macrophages and reduce expression of MHC class II molecules. In this way, cortocosteroids inhibit T-cell activation and T-cell function.

It is important to acknowledge that despite these beneficial antiinflammatory effects, corticosteroids also have potent toxic effects including fluid retention, weight gain, diabetes, thinning of the skin, and bone loss. Therefore, the efficacy of corticosteroids in the control of disease involves the judicious use of these agents to strike a careful balance between their beneficial and toxic effects. As will be discussed below, given the growing arsenal of immunosuppressive therapies, corticosteroids are often used in combination with other panimmunosuppressive agents in an effort to keep the dose and toxic side effects to a minimum.

Cytotoxic Drugs

Antimetabolites that suppress the immune response include the purine antagonists *azathioprine* and *mercaptopurine*, which interfere with the synthesis of RNA and DNA by inhibiting inosinic acid, the precursor for the purines adenylic and guandylic acids. *Chlorambucil* and *cyclophosphamide*, compounds that alkylate DNA, also have antimetabolic activity and interfere with the metabolism of DNA. These agents were originally developed to treat cancer. The observation that they are also cytotoxic to lymphocytes led to their use as immunosuppressive therapeutic agents. As expected, however, they have a range of toxic effects since they interfere with DNA synthesis in many tissues in the body. Consequently, in addition to their immunosuppressive activity, they can also cause anemia, leukopenia, thrombocytopenia, intestinal damage, and hair loss. Indeed, fatal reactions to these cytotoxic drugs have also been reported. As noted above, the availability of other immunosuppressive agents, allows them to be used in combination therapies at lower, less toxic doses.

Cyclosporine, FK-506 (Tacrolimus), and Rapamycin (Sirolimus)

Several relatively new supplements to immunosuppressive antimetabolite and cytotoxic drugs are now available. The three described here (cyclosporin A, FK-506, and rapamycin) exert their pharmacologic effects by binding to immunophilins B, a family of intracellular proteins involved with lymphocyte signaling pathways. Upon binding to immunophilins, these agents interfere with signal transduction pathways needed for clonal expansion of lymphocytes.

Cyclosporine is a compound that has become important and widely used for immunosuppression during allotransplantation. In many instances, enhancement in survival of an allograft between "unmatched" donor and recipient cyclosporine was almost as effective as when transplantation was performed between "matched" individuals. Cyclosporine is a cyclic peptide derived from a soil fungus (*Tolypocladium inflatum*). It greatly enhances graft survival by interfering with cytokine gene transcription in T cells. The complex of cyclosporine and its cytoplasmic receptor cyclophilin binds to and blocks the phosphatase activity of calcineurin, which is an intracellular signaling protein that is essential for transcriptional activation of the IL-2 gene. It also suppresses production IL-4, and IFN-γ as well as the synthesis of IL-2 receptors (CD25). In addition, it is known to induce the synthesis of TGF-β a cytokine that has immunosuppressive activity. Cyclosporine is effective when administered before transplantation but is ineffective in suppressing ongoing rejection. Recent evidence indicates cyclosporine is nephrotoxic and is also associated with an increased risk of cancer in patients who take this drug long-term. It has been suggested that these and other side effects are largely due to the TGF-β-inducing property of cyclosporine.

FK-506 or *tacrolimus* is also used widely to treat transplant patients. It is a macrolide compound obtained from the filamentous bacterium *Streptomyces tsukabaenis*. Macrolides are compounds that have a multimembered lactone ring to which is attached one or more deoxy sugars. Although its structure is considerably different from that of cyclosporine, its biologic and immunosuppressive activities are similar. Like cyclosporine its affect is on T-cell activation by blocking calcineurin activity and the accompanying cytokine production.

Rapamycin or *sirolimus* is an experimental macrolide antibiotic with immunosuppressive activity. It is derived from the bacterium *Streptomyces hygroscopicus* and, like cyclosporin A and FK-506, it inhibits T-cell activation. However, it does this using a different pharmacologic mechanism. Thus while cyclosporin A and FK-506 block calcineurin activity, rapamycin inhibits T-cell activation by blocking signal transduction mediated by IL-2 and other cytokines not by inhibiting IL-2 production.

Leflunomide, another experimental drug, also targets the signal transduction machinery of T cells by blocking the activity of tyrosine kinases associated with cytokine receptors. It also prevents T-cell proliferation by inhibiting de novo pyrimidine synthesis.

Antibody Therapy and Blocking of Costimulatory Molecules

For many years, *antilymphocyte globulin (ALG)* prepared in horses immunized with human lymphocytes has been used to treat acute graft rejection. While this therapeutic approach can effectively remove unwanted lymphocytes, treatment of humans with large amounts of foreign horse protein has the disadvantage of inducing a serum sickness caused by the formation of immune complexes (see Chapter 15). Nevertheless, ALG is still used today to treat acute graft rejection. Clearly, the challenge for those attempting to develop new antibody-based therapies for transplant patients is to develop less immunogenic antibodies with more specifically targeted effects. To this end, monoclonal antibodies are gaining use as somewhat more target-specific (not transplantation-antigen-specific) than the immunosuppressants. The advent of chimeric mouse–human and other engineered antibodies (e.g., "humanized" mouse monoclonal antibodies) has helped to reduce the limitations of alloantibody therapy by minimizing the antigenicity of these proteins (see Chapter 5). Since the effector cells responsible for allograft rejection are T cells, all of which express CD3 as part of the TCR, this cell membrane determinant has been used with success as a target in antibody-mediated immunosuppressive therapy. OKT3, a mouse monoclonal antibody directed against the CD3 antigen of humans, has been used in clinical transplantation.

Antibodies to the IL-2 receptor (CD25) expressed on activated T cells and antibodies to CD4 are also being used to prevent graft rejection. In addition, the use of antibodies to several other molecules important for T-cell adhesion (e.g., anti-ICAM-1) and T-cell activation are currently under investigation. Among the latter category of T-cell determinants, a humanized mouse antibody against human CD154 (also known as CD40 ligand) has recently been shown to prevent acute renal allograft rejection in nonhuman primates. Other target antigens include the costimulatory molecules B7.1 (CD80) and B7.2 (CD86). As discussed in Chapter 10, binding of B7.1 or B7.1 to CD28 initiates a cascade of T-cell activation events. Just how these costimulatory antigen–antibody duos sidetrack the immune system from attacking mismatched donor organs remains unknown. Conversely, binding of CTLA-4, an alternate ligand for these costimulatory molecules, delivers inhibitory signals to the responding T cells. In light of the importance of these costimulatory molecules in regulating the functional activities of T cells, experiments were performed to assess the effects of antibodies that block their ability to bind to their natural ligands. As predicted, blocking CD28 ligation interferes with the transmission of signals needed for gene expression and T-cell activation. Thus, antibodies that interfere with costimulatory molecule-mediated T-cell activation may have efficacy in transplant patients. It should be noted that a related experimental approach uses the inhibitory ligand, CTLA-4, to suppress the function of these costimulatory molecules. In animal studies, injection of soluble CTLA-4 has been found to allow the long-term survival of certain grafted tissues. Evidence suggests that the mechanism responsible for the beneficial effect of CTLA-4 involves the blocking of costimulation of the T cells that recognize donor antigens thus inducing a state of unresponsiveness (anergy).

It should be clear from the above that several experimental approaches are being taken with the hope of finding immunosuppressive agents that will be less toxic and will not leave the recipient helpless to opportunistic infections in the absence of a fully competent immune response. However, it should be stated that with all the experimental approaches mentioned above the main agents that are most commonly used for clinical immunosuppression are corticosteroids (e.g., prednisone), cyclosporin A (Neoral), FK506, and azathioprine.

BONE MARROW TRANSPLANTATION

Transplantation of bone marrow constitutes a special transplantation situation because it is performed mostly between an immunocompetent donor and an immunoincompetent recipient. Usually these immunoincompetent patients have severe combined immunodeficiency (SCID), Wiskott-Aldrich syndrome (see Chapter 18), or advanced leukemia, and they receive bone marrow from identical siblings. Today such transplantations are performed with a fair degree of success. In the past few years, transplantation of bone marrow from donors who are nonidentical but who are HLA-matched or partially matched is gaining success and acceptance. Specifically, haploidentical bone marrow (parental bone marrow that is only half MHC-identical) has been successfully used. Indeed, such bone marrow transplantation is the treatment of choice for children with SCID.

Although bone marrow transplantation between identical twins can be performed with relatively low immunologic risk, transplantation of bone marrow from an immunocompetent donor to an HLA-nonmatched or partially matched recipient is highly risky due to the presence of competent T cells in the donor's marrow, which may result in a graft-versus-host reaction (see below). To reduce this risk, it is imperative to remove the T cells from the transferred bone marrow. This removal, which can be achieved by a number of methods (e.g., treatment with monoclonal anti-T-cell antibodies and complement), widens the choice of bone marrow donors.

 GRAFT-VERSUS-HOST REACTIONS

Transplantation of immunocompetent lymphocytes from a donor to a genetically different recipient can result in a reaction mounted by the grafted lymphocytes against the recipient's tissue. This *graft-versus-host (GVH)* reaction is particularly important in cases where immunocompetent lymphoid cells are transplanted into individuals who are *immunologically incompetent* and therefore cannot reject the transplanted cells. This situation is best exemplified in cases where immunocompetent cells are transferred into individuals with various immunodeficiency disorders or in cases of bone marrow transplantation into an immunosuppressed recipient. It is interesting that GVH disease may occur in bone marrow transplant recipients even if the donor and recipient are perfectly HLA-matched. This is probably due to minor, non-HLA-coded, transplantation antigens recognized by donor T cells.

In experimental animals, a *GVH reaction may lead to a wasting syndrome* in the recipient; in humans, GVH reactions may produce *splenomegaly* (enlarged spleen), *enlarged liver and lymph nodes, diarrhea, anemia, weight loss,* and other disorders in which the underlying causes are inflammation and destruction of tissue. The GVH reaction is initiated by the transferred T lymphocytes from the donor, which recognize the recipient's transplantation antigens as foreign. Donor T cells thus become activated as in an allograft response. In GVH disease, however, most of the inflammatory cells that participate in the reaction, and that are mainly responsible for destruction of tissue, are host cells recruited to the site of the reaction by cytokines released by the donor's lymphocytes.

 FETAL–MATERNAL RELATIONSHIP

A puzzling phenomenon associated with allograft rejection is why the fetus, which expresses maternal and paternal histocompatibility antigens, is not rejected by the mother as an allograft. It is clear that the mother can mount an antibody response against fetal antigen, as exemplified by anti-Rh antibodies produced by Rh⁻ mothers. More importantly, women who experienced multiple births have antibodies to the father's MHC. It appears, however, that in most cases the antibodies are harmless to the fetus, and what is important is the mother's ability—or, rather, inability—to respond with the production of cytotoxic T cells against the fetus. There is evidence that fetal trophoblast cells that constitute the outer layer of the placenta that come in contact with maternal tissue do not express polymorphic MHC class I or class II molecules but express only the nonpolymorphic class Ib MHC molecule, HLA-G. Thus, the fetal trophoblast does not prime for a cellular immune response associated with allograft rejection.

It has been suggested that the major function of HLA-G is to provide a ligand for the killer cell inhibitory receptors (KIR) on maternal NK cells, thus preventing them from killing the fetal cells (see Chapter 2). HLA-G is also expressed in thymic medullary epithelium, where it might ensure T-cell tolerance to this molecule. Finally, no cells expressing large amounts of MHC class II molecules (e.g., dendritic cells) have been found in the placenta.

Other factors that affect the immune response and may be involved in the fetal-maternal relationship include cytokines, complement inhibitory proteins, and other as yet unknown factors. Another factor that appears to operate in the survival of the fetus—the "allograft"—is ***α-fetoprotein***, a protein synthesized in the yolk sac and fetal liver. α-Fetoprotein has been demonstrated to have immunosuppressive properties. All in all, the fetus and several other tissues in the body that do not initiate an immune response or are not affected by immune components are termed ***immunologically privileged*** sites. Overall, it appears that multiple factors are responsible for one of the most spectacular immunologically privileged sites: the fetus.

HEART TRANSPLANTATION: A PERSONAL STORY

It is strictly coincidental and not associated with any deliberate pedagogic exercise that one of us (E.B.) has recently undergone a heart transplant, which is briefly described here.

The realization that one requires a heart transplant as a last resort comes as a shock in spite of years of cardiomyopathy. Before being accepted into the transplant program at the University of California San Diego Medical Center, dozens of tests, some of which are uncomfortable and painful, had to be performed to ensure that a healthy heart would not be transplanted into a "sick" body or a body that may develop malignancies as a result of immunosuppression (e.g., intestinal polyps, which may become malignant).

Having undergone all the necessary tests and having been accepted into the program, the long wait for a suitable heart began. I was kept in the cardiac intensive care unit waiting for a blood group- and Rh-matched donor heart for 2 months. My awareness of time became blurred, and I nearly forgot why I was there and what I was waiting for. While some patients less moribund may wait at home until a suitable heart becomes available, the wait may range from a few days or weeks to many months. Not all patients survive the wait.

Finally, and rather unexpectedly, the transplant coordinator brought the "good news": a suitable heart was available. This was one of the most emotional moments of the transplantation process. Despite all the rationalization that the donor did not die for my sake, the realization that the precious gift of the heart of someone who died tragically in a car accident would be transplanted into me was a very emotional experience.

In the hands of a very competent heart transplant surgeon, the surgical procedure is almost routine. Immediately before surgery, I was given a cocktail of immunosuppressive agents (cyclosporin [Neoral] or FK506, prednisone, and azathioprine) along with a host of antibiotics, antiviral and antifungal agents, and other medications to help prevent infections due to nonspecific immunosuppression that I, like all other organ allograft recipients, will continue to take for the rest of my life. The immunosuppressive agents have severe side effects. The blood level of cyclosporine is routinely monitored and the side effects of other medications are evaluated periodically. The fact that I am capable of writing and retelling my story testifies to their effectiveness.

It is hoped that in the future less "brutal" nonspecific or, better yet, specific immunosuppressive agents will become available to make allotransplantation, or even xenotransplantation, less dangerous. We remain confident that with continued research in this arena, the hope for an even higher quality of life for patients following transplantation will become a reality.

SUMMARY

1. Transplantation rejection is immunologically mediated.

2. Both T cells and circulating antibodies are induced against allografts and xenografts. While antibodies are responsible for hyperacute rejection, T cells are mainly responsible for the rejection of most other tissue.

3. The most important transplantation antigens, which cause rapid rejection of the allograft, are found on cell membranes and are encoded by genes in the major histocompatibility complex (MHC), which is called HLA in humans and H-2 in mice. The structures encoded by these genes, MHC class I and class II molecules, are involved in discriminating between "self" and "nonself" and in cellular interactions.

4. The degree of histocompatibility between donor and recipient can be determined serologically, by recombinant DNA technology, or by the mixed leukocyte response (MLR).

5. Survival of nonmatched allografts is prolonged by antiinflammatory agents, cytotoxic agents, antimetabolites, and other modalities aimed at immunosuppressing the recipient. These approaches to enhance graft survival are gaining acceptance and wide use in human tissue and organ transplantation.

REFERENCES

Armitage JO (1994): Bone marrow transplantation. *N Engl J Med* 330:827.

Auchincloss H Jr, Sachs D (1998): Xenogeneic transplantation. *Annu Rev Immunol* 16:433.

Auchincloss H Jr, Sykes M, Sachs D (1998): Transplantation immunology. In Paul WE (ed): Fundamental Immunology, 4th ed. New York: Lippincott-Raven.

Charenoud L (1998) Tolerogenic antibodies and fusion proteins to prevent graft rejection and treat autoimmunity. *Mol. Med. Today* 4:25.

Charlton B, Auchincloss H Jr, Fathman CG (1994): Mechanisms of transplantation tolerance. *Annu Rev Immunol* 12:707.

Ferrara JLM, Deeq HJ (1991): Graft versus host disease. *N Engl J Med* 324:667.

Garovoy MR, Stock P, Baumgardner G, Keith F. Linker C (1994): Transplantation. In Stites DP, Terr AI, Parslow TG (eds): Basic and Clinical Immunology, 8th ed. E Norwalk, CT: Appleton & Lange.

Hunt JS (1992): Immunobiology of pregnancy. *Curr Opin Immunol* 4:591.

Kirk, AD (1999): Treatment with humanized monoclonal antibody against CD154 prevents acute renal allograft rejection in nonhuman primates. *Nat Med* 5:686.

Lechler RI, Lombardi G, Batchelor JR, Reinsmoen N, Bach FH (1990): The molecular basis for alloreactivity. *Immunol Today* 11:83.

Roopenian DC (1992): What are the minor histocompatibility loci? A new look at an old question. *Immunol Today* 13:7.

Schreiber SL, Crabtree GR (1992): The mechanism of action of cyclosporin A and FK-506. *Immunol Today* 13:136.

Sherman LA, Chattopadhyay S (1994): The molecular basis of allorecognition. *Annu Rev Immunol* 11:385.

Suthanthiran M, Strom TB (1994): Renal transplantation. *N Engl J Med* 331:365.

Winkelstein A (1994): Immunosuppressive therapy. In Stites DP, Terr AI, Parslow TG (eds): Basic and Clinical Immunology 8th ed. E Norwalk, CT: Appleton & Lange.

● REVIEW QUESTIONS

For each question, choose the ONE BEST answer or completion.

1. Kidney transplantation was performed using a kidney from a donor who was matched to the recipient by serologic tissue typing. However, within a few months the kidney was rejected. Assuming no technical problems with the surgical procedure, one reason for the rejection may be that
   A) there was insufficient blood supply to the graft.
   B) there could have been a mismatch, which would have been detected by a mixed lymphocyte reaction.
   C) the recipient developed blocking antibodies.
   D) the recipient also suffered from Wiskott–Aldrich syndrome.
   E) the donor was agammaglobulinemic.

2. Currently, the best indicator for predicting compatibility for transplantation of tissue from donor A to recipient B is obtained by
   A) one-way mixed leukocyte reaction between B cells and mitomycin C-treated A cells.
   B) one-way mixed leukocyte reaction between A cells and mitomycin C-treated B cells.
   C) serologic typing and cross-matching of A and B cells.
   D) two-way mixed leukocyte reaction between A and B cells.
   E) matching for blood group antigens.

3. The MHC contains all of the following except
   A) genes that encode transplantation antigens.
   B) genes that encode immunoglobulins.
   C) genes that regulate immune responsiveness.
   D) genes that encode some components of complement.
   E) genes that encode class I and class II antigens.

4. The most common serologic test used for the detection of HLA antigens on lymphocytes is

A) the complement fixation test.
B) double gel diffusion.
C) complement-dependent cytotoxicity test.
D) mixed lymphocyte reaction.
E) radioimmunoassay.

5. Which of the following statements regarding GVH disease is *incorrect*?

A) GVH can result from MHC differences between donor and recipient.
B) GVH requires immunocompetent donor cells.
C) GVH may result from infusion of blood products that contain viable lymphocytes into an immunologically incompetent recipient.
D) GVH requires natural killer cells.
E) GVH may occur in an immunosuppressed individual.

6. Transplant rejection may involve

A) cell-mediated immunity.
B) type III (immune complex) hypersensitivity.
C) complement-dependent cytotoxicity.
D) the release of IFN-γ.
E) All of the statements are correct.

7. Which of the following statements concerning the mixed leukocyte reaction (MLR) is correct?

A) Specific responding cells are B lymphocytes.
B) MLR results in clonal expansion of specific, alloantigen-reactive cells.
C) MLR between unrelated individuals who differ according to HLA serology is usually negative.
D) Stimulation of proliferation is controlled primarily by the HLA-A region alleles.
E) All of the statements are correct.

8. In clinical transplantation, cytotoxic antibodies reactive against antigens expressed on the grafted tissue

A) cause delayed rejection of the transplant.
B) are responsible for hyperacute rejection.
C) cause rejection when present in the donor.
D) are not usually directed against HLA antigens.
E) activate cytotoxic T cells, which then cause hyperacute rejection.

9. Serologic testing before kidney transplantation reveals that the leukocytes of a prospective recipient are killed by the following anti-HLA antibodies in the presence of complement: anti-B27, anti-A1, and anti-A3. You can conclude that

A) the prospective recipient expresses the B27, A1, and A3 HLA specificities.
B) the prospective recipient does not express the B27, A1, and A3 HLA specificities.
C) the potential donor and the prospective recipient are not siblings.
D) the potential donor and the prospective recipient are not identical twins.
E) the prospective recipient should not receive a kidney graft that expresses these HLA specificities.

10. A clinical trial investigating the efficacy of a humanized anti-CD28 monoclonal antibody in prolonging kidney allograft survival shows that patients treated with this biologic reagent have significantly fewer episodes of chronic rejection. The probable mechanism responsible for this effect is best explained by

A) the binding of anti-CD28 to B cells, which blocks their interaction with B7.1 and B7.2 expressed on T cells.

B) the formation of circulating CD28-anti-CD28 immune complexes.

C) the binding of anti-CD28 to T cells, which interferes with signal transduction needed for T-cell activation.

D) the binding of anti-CD28 to suppressor T cells, which then become activated.

E) the binding of anti-CD28 to B and T cells which interferes with signal transduction and activation of both populations.

Case Study

A child is brought to the hospital suffering from an aplastic bone marrow after ingestion of benzene. All blood elements are at low levels and death is imminent. The child and a sibling were rapidly typed as both being A^+ Rh^+, HLA-A3,7: B4,8, and bone marrow was transfused. Within a few days the RBC count rose, indicating a successful take. However, 3 weeks later the child began to experience diarrhea and a skin rash on the palms and soles of the feet, spreading to the trunk. This was followed by jaundice and enlarged liver and spleen. Administration of an anti-CD3 monoclonal antibody plus cyclosporine produced some improvement. What went wrong, and why?

Answers To Review Questions

1. B The most probable reason for the rejection is that, although serologically the donor and recipient were matched, this was an incomplete measure. The accuracy of serologic matching is predicated on the number of sera used in the test. There is always the possibility that a mismatch would have been detected if additional sera were used. In genotyping by PCR, the transplantation epitope is highly sensitive and accurate. Even the mixed leukocyte reaction is more reliable, since it can detect mismatches that may not be detected serologically. Answer A is not correct, since it is stated that there were no problems due to the surgical procedure. Answer C is incorrect since blocking antibodies, if indeed developed by the recipient, would be expected to enhance the survival of the transplant. Answer E is incorrect because the immune status of the kidney donor is, in this case, irrelevant to the outcome of the transplantation.

2. A Compatibility can be reliably predicted by the one-way mixed leukocyte reaction between the recipient's B cells and mitomycin C-treated cells from the donor. In this test, only the reactivity of the recipient cells against the donor antigens is measured. The reverse—that is, reaction between A cells and mitomycin C-treated recipient B cells—is of no practical importance, because A is not the recipient. Serologic typing and cross-matching of A and B are of value, since those tests are more rapid than the MLR. However, there is always the possibility that the panel of antisera used is not complete and that if more antisera were used a mismatch would be found. The two-way MLR is important in assessing the total degree of parity (or disparity) in transplantation antigens, but it does not determine if the reaction is that of the donor to the recipient cells, or of the recipient to donor cells, or both. Matching for blood group antigens is imperative but not sufficient. Nevertheless, if you answered D, it is also acceptable.

3. B The MHC complex contains all genes mentioned except genes that encode immunoglobulins. They are on different chromosomes.

4. *C* The most common serologic test used for detection of HLA antigens on lymphocytes is the complement-dependent cytotoxicity test. The mixed leukocyte reaction, especially the one-way MLR, is an excellent test for HLA-D antigens, but it is a test based on cellular reactions and not on the reaction of serum antibodies.

5. *D* The GVH disease is caused by the destruction of cells or tissue of an immunoincompetent recipient by immunocompetent lymphoid cells transferred from a histoincompatible donor. The GVH reaction does not require natural killer cells.

6. *E* All are correct. The important process in the rejection of an allotransplant is cell-mediated immunity. Here, T cells, which recognize the alloantigens, become activated; the T cells release cytokines, one of which is IFN-γ, which recruits and activates phagocytic cells that, together with cytotoxic T cells, destroy the graft. However, the reaction to the allotransplant may also involve antibodies (IgM and IgG), which can cause damage to tissue via activation of complement and the recruitment of polymorphonuclear cells to the site of the reaction. The polymorphonuclear cells would damage the graft by the release of their lysosomal enzymes.

7. *B* The MLR results in the clonal expansion of specific T cells, which recognize the alloantigens in the D region of the HLA. Although clones of B cells may also expand, the major cellular expansion is that of the T cells. The MLR between unrelated individuals who differ according to HLA serology is usually positive (rather than negative). Thus only choice B is correct.

8. *B* Cytotoxic antibodies, such as IgM and IgG, cause hyperacute rejection by complement-mediated cell lysis or by opsonization and subsequent destruction of the transplant by phagocytic cells. The cytotoxic antibodies may be directed against blood group antigens or to HLA antigens on transferred cells (e.g., leukocytes); thus answer D is incorrect. The presence of cytotoxic antibodies in the donor is usually of no clinical importance since, even if they are transferred to the recipient with the donor's blood, they become highly diluted in the recipient. Choice E is incorrect because cytotoxic antibodies play no role in activation of cytotoxic T cells. Thus, choice B is correct.

9. *A* The demonstration that leukocytes are killed in the presence of complement when exposed to antibodies specific for the HLA specificities listed indicates that the cells express these determinants. Killing is due to complement-mediated cytotoxicity. Since no information regarding the HLA phenotype of any siblings is given, choices C and D are incorrect. Choice E is also incorrect, since it would be desirable to graft the prospective recipient with a kidney graft that expresses these determinants. Thus, choice A is correct.

10. *C* Experimental models have demonstrated that injection of allografted mice with anti-CD28 monoclonal antibody does, indeed, prolong survival of the allograft. Blocking CD28 ligation interferes with the transmission of signals needed for gene expression (e.g., IL-2 synthesis) and T-cell activation. B7.1 and B7.2 are costimulatory molecules that ligate CD28 expressed on antigen-presenting cells leading to T-cell activation.

Answer to Case Study

The symptoms are typical of GVH disease. The hasty matching presumably involved serologic typing only and matching for MHC class II molecules by PCR genotyping, or by MLR, was not done. In addition, care was not taken to deplete the donor bone marrow of mature T cells. Presumably, histoincompatibility between the donor and recipient triggered the donor's T cells to attack the recipient's cells, resulting in the symptom complex seen. Therapy aimed at destroying or inhibiting activated donor T cells is not as effective as eliminating them in the first place.

20

TUMOR IMMUNOLOGY

 INTRODUCTION

The existence of an immune response against a tumor is based on changes in the surface components of the malignant cell that do not occur in its normal counter part that give rise to structures that are antigenic. In 1943 Gross observed that when tumor cells were transplanted into the skin of syngeneic (genetically identical), histocompatible mice, the cells formed nodules that grew for a few days and then regressed. When identical tumor cells were reinjected into the mice, they did not produce nodules or grow. These findings were interpreted to mean that the mice that rejected the tumor did so because they had become immunologically resistant—or immune—to the tumor. Subsequently, *tumor-specific transplantation antigens* (TSTAs), or *tumor rejection antigens* (TRAs), which have the ability to induce antitumor immune responses, have been demonstrated for many tumors in a variety of animal species, including humans.

The goals of tumor immunology are (1) to elucidate the immunologic relationship between the host and the tumor and (2) to utilize the immune response to tumors for the purpose of *diagnosis, prophylaxis*, and *therapy*. In the present chapter we discuss various approaches to meeting these goals.

TUMOR ANTIGENS

Advances in immunologic and molecular biologic methodology have greatly facilitated the identification of tumor antigens capable of eliciting immune reactions. The majority of human tumor antigens now known have been identified by the transfection of genomic DNA or cDNA libraries into cells expressing the appropriate MHC molecule, followed by the identification of transfectants using assays that measure

T cell antitumor reactivity. More recently, a technique that is not dependent on the prior availability of antitumor T cells has been described. This approach, called serologic analysis of recombinant cDNA expression libraries (SEREX), uses diluted serum from cancer patients to detect the presence of antibodies to a range of novel antigens from tumor-derived cDNA libraries. Using this approach, at least one tumor antigen (NY-ESO-1) has been identified and shown to be reactive with $CD8^+$ cytotoxic T cells and other candidate antigens are being studied.

In principle, there are three possible mechanisms that may lead to the appearance of unique tumor antigens: mutation, gene activation, and clonal amplification. Some of these antigens may consist of structures that are unique to the cancerous cells and are not present on their normal counterparts. Other tumor antigens may represent structures that are common to both malignant and normal cells but are "masked" on the normal cells and become "unmasked" on malignant cells. Still other antigens on tumor cells represent structures that are qualitatively not different from those found on normal cells but that are "overexpressed"—present at significantly increased numbers on the cancer cell as products of cellular oncogenes. An example is the high levels of human epidermal growth factor receptor (HER) due to increased expression of the ***HER-2/neu-1*** oncogene (e.g., in certain breast and ovarian cancers), and the elevated ***RAS*** oncogene products present on some human prostate cancer cells. Still other antigens on malignant cells represent structures that are present on fetal or embryonic cells, but disappear from normal adult cells. These latter antigens are referred to as ***oncofetal antigens***. Normal genes that were previously silent may also be activated by carcinogens. It is generally assumed that unique tumor antigens on tumors induced by carcinogens are products of mutated genes with "hot spots" for mutations.

There is little or no cross-reactivity between carcinogen-induced tumors. This absence of cross-reactivity is probably due to the ***random mutations*** induced by the chemical or physical carcinogens, leading to a large array of different antigens. For example, if the chemical carcinogen methylcholanthrene is applied in an identical manner to the skin of two genetically identical animals, or on two similar sites on the same individual, the cells of the developing tumors (sarcomas) will exhibit antigens unique to each tumor, with no immunologic cross-reactivity between the tumors. As with chemically induced tumors, there is little or no cross-reactivity between physically induced tumors, such as those induced by ultraviolet light or by X-irradiation.

Carcinogens can also cause ***clonal amplification*** of single cells expressing a particular normal antigen and convert an otherwise nonimmunogenic molecule to an immunogenic antigen. The carcinogen-induced transformation event(s) that cause the emergence of such expanded clones most likely affects the genes that possess mutation-sensitive hot spots while sparing the genes responsible for other normal proteins. When these normal proteins are clonotypic (i.e., only expressed by single clones of cells), their expression is dramatically amplified therefore making them targets for immune responses, assuming tolerance can be broken. As an example, the idiotypes of antigen-specific receptors expressed by B or T cells may not be sufficient to elicit a response in the normal host, but may serve as target antigens for tumor cells bearing the same idiotype.

In summary, chemical or physical carcinogens often induce tumors that express antigens that exhibit a ***unique antigenic specificity*** either as a consequence of gene mutations or clonal amplification. Cells of a given tumor, arising from a single transformed cell, all share common antigens, but different tumors, even if induced by the same carcinogen, are antigenically distinct from one another.

CATEGORIES OF TUMOR ANTIGENS

Tumor antigens may be classified into several major categories (Table 20.1). The categories differ in both the factors that induce the malignancy and the immuno-chemical properties of the tumor antigens.

Normal Cellular Gene Products

Some tumor antigens are derived from normal genes that, under normal circum-stances, are programmed to be expressed only during embryogenesis. Examples of these *oncodevelopmental tumor antigens* include the melanoma-associated antigen (MAGE) family of proteins that are not expressed in any normal adult tissues except for the testes (an immunologically privileged site). MAGE antigens are candidate tumor vaccine antigens because their expression is shared by many melanomas. An-other example of tumor antigens in this category are those expressed as a conse-quence of phenotypic changes associated with cellular differentiation.

Another example of an oncofetal antigen is the *carcinoembryonic antigen* (CEA), found primarily in serum of patients with *cancers of the gastrointestinal*

 T A B L E 20.1. Categories of Tumor Antigens

Category		Type of antigen	Name of antigen	Types of cancer
Normal cellular gene products	Embryonic	Oncofetal antigens	MAGE-1	Several
			MAGE-2	Several
			CEA	Lung
				Pancreas
				Breast
				Colon
				Stomach
			AFP	Liver
				Testis
	Differentiation	Normal intracellular enzymes	PSA	Prostate
			Tyrosinase	Melanoma
		Oncoprotein	HER-2/neu	Breast
				Ovary
		Carbohydrate	Lewis	Lymphoma
	Clonal amplification	Immunoglobulin idiotype	Specific antibody of B cell clone	Lymphoma
Mutant cellular gene products	Point mutations	Oncogene product	Mutant RAS proteins	Several
		Suppressor gene product	Mutant p53	Several
		Cycline-dependent kinase (CDK)	Mutant CDK-4	Melanoma
Viral gene products	Transforming viral gene	Nuclear proteins	E6 and E7 proteins of HPV	Cervical

tract, especially cancer of the colon. Elevated levels of CEA have also been detected in the circulation of patients with some types of **lung cancer, pancreatic cancer**, and some types of **breast and stomach cancer**. However, it should be noted that elevated levels of CEA have also been detected in the circulation of patients with nonneoplastic diseases, such as emphysema, ulcerative colitis, and pancreatitis, as well as in the sera of alcoholics and heavy smokers.

Another oncodevelopmental antigen is **α-fetoprotein** (AFP), which is normally present at high concentrations in fetal and maternal serum but absent from serum of normal individuals. AFP is rapidly secreted by cells of a variety of cancers and is found particularly in patients with **hepatomas** and **testicular teratocarcinomas**.

Finally, amplified clones of malignant B or T cells that express antigen-specific receptors represent yet another example of how normal cellular gene products can be characterized as tumor antigens. The idiotype of the particular immunoglobulin or TCR expressed by the transformed B or T cell, respectively, effectively identifies that clone as a unique population of malignant cells.

Mutant Cellular Gene Products

The genetic origins of several unique tumor antigens that are products of mutated genes have been identified. In every case, the antigen was caused by a somatic mutation (i.e., by a genetic change absent from autologous normal DNA). Often, these mutations occur in genes that code for functionally important parts of the expressed protein. For example, the mutation in the cycline-dependent kinase-4 (CDK-4) reduces the binding to its inhibitor (p16INK-4), which happens to be a tumor-suppressor protein. This mutation is found in many cases of familial melanoma. Another example of a tumor antigen that is generated as a result of a mutant cellular gene is the mutant p53 protein. The p53 mutation generates common conformational changes in p53—a protein that normally acts as a suppressor of cellular growth. Mutations in p53 are among the most common seen in tumors of human and experimental animals. They typically occur in evolutionarily conserved regions of the p53 gene and result in overproduction of the protein, which then serves as an antigen for B and T cells. Antibody and T-cell responses are also seen when mutations occur in RAS oncogene-encoded proteins. Mutant RAS proteins, resulting from a glycine substitution at position 12 of RAS, represent one of the most common mutations in human cancers.

The potential use of mutated proteins as immunologic targets for therapy is best illustrated by experimental evidence showing that tumor immunity in vivo can be induced by vaccination against mutant p53 peptides if given with interleukin-12. Because p53 is commonly expressed in cancer cells, T cells directed against normal p53 might preferentially destroy tumor cells. Furthermore, p53 knockout mice can be induced to generate cytotoxic T cells specific for normal p53 that, on adoptive transfer into p53 wild-type mice, can eradicate p53-overexpressing tumors without signs of autoimmunity to the host.

Tumor Antigens Encoded by Viral Genes

Animal studies have shown that tumors induced by DNA or RNA oncogenic virus exhibit **extensive immunologic cross-reactivity**. This is because any particular oncogenic virus induces the expression of the same antigens in a tumor, regardless of the tissue of origin or the animal species. For example, in animals, DNA viruses such as polyoma, SV40, and Shope papilloma virus induce tumors that exhibit extensive cross-reactivity within each virus group. Many leukemogenic viruses, such as Rauscher leukemia virus, induce the formation of tumors that exhibit cross-reactivity not only within each virus group but also between some groups. In this connection, there is considerable evidence to suggest that several human cancers, such as ***Burkitt's lymphoma, nasopharyngeal carcinoma, T-cell leukemia***, and ***hepatocellular carcinoma*** are caused by viruses.

As might be expected, the viral proteins, which ultimately serve as unique tumor antigens, are expressed intracellularly as predominantly nuclear proteins. In order for cytotoxic T lymphocytes (CTL) to recognize these antigens, they must be processed and presented as MHC-associated peptides. Studies using SV40-specific CTL have confirmed that these cells can recognize processed fragments of proteins that are primarily located intracellularly. The unique tumor antigens of cells transformed by SV40 and several other viruses, including polyoma virus, adenovirus, and human papilloma virus (HPV) have been studied extensively and, in many cases, shown to be clearly related to the transformed phenotype and the establishment of malignancy. Such viruses have so-called early region genes designated E1A/E1B and E6/E7, that are transcribed during early stages of viral replication and in transformed cells. Like other categories of tumor antigens, these proteins are candidate targets for therapy.

Immunologic Factors Influencing the Incidence of Cancer

In the late 1950s, a hypothesis emerged to help explain the primary reason for development of T-cell-mediated immunity during the evolution of vertebrates. It was proposed that the main function of the T-cell-mediated arm of the immune system was to provide specific defense against altered self or neoplastic cells. The term ***immunosurveillance*** was coined to describe the concept of immunologic resistance against the development of cancer. We now know that T-cell immunity is necessary for resistance to a variety of infections, most notably, viral infections. Animal studies as well as epidemiologic and immunologic studies of patients with various immunodeficiencies (primary, secondary, or acquired) have now provided evidence to support this hypothesis but only with regard to cancers associated with viruses or, in some cases, UV exposure. By contrast, most common forms of cancer are not increased in immunoincompetent individuals. However, patients with immunodeficiency are usually susceptible to viral infections and certain malignant neoplasms (Table 20.2). The absence of immunosurveillance of spontaneous cancers or those induced by carcinogens does not imply that such tumors are not antigenic. Indeed, there is sufficient evidence to support the conclusion that these tumor cells, like those induced by viruses, are sensitive to immunologic destruction. Nevertheless, the natural development of immunologic responses usually fails to prevent cancer from developing. It is hoped that the successful manipulation of such responses (e.g., vaccination with unique tumor antigens) will serve as a viable option for the prevention or treatment of cancer in the future.

Effector Mechanisms in Tumor Immunity

Until recently most of the information concerning antitumor immune effector mechanisms and their capacity to destroy tumor cells has been derived from experiments

TABLE 20.2. Malignant Neoplasms With an Increased Incidence in Immunodeficiency Patients

Type of immunodeficiency	Cancer	Associated virus
Primary (congenital)	Hepatocellular carcinoma	HBV
	B-cell lymphoma	EBV
Secondary drug-induced	B-cell lymphoma	ERV
	Squamous cell carcinoma (skin)	HPV
	Hepatocellular carcinoma	HBV
	Cervical carcinoma	HPV
AIDS	Cellular carcinoma	HBV
	Cloagenic or oral carcinoma	HPV
	B-cell lymphoma	EBV

EBV, Epstein-Barr virus; HBV, hepatitis B virus; HPV, human papilloma virus; UV, ultraviolet light.

with transplantable tumors in animals or from in vitro experiments. There is now ample evidence to suggest that adaptive and innate immune response play important roles in the relationship between the host and the tumor in humans as well.

Immune effector mechanisms that are potentially capable of destroying tumors in vitro are summarized in Table 20.3. In general, destruction of tumor cells by these mechanisms is more efficient in the case of **dispersed tumors** (i.e., when the target tumor cells are in single-cell suspension) than in the case of solid tumors, probably because dispersed cells are more accessible to immune action.

B-Cell Responses

Lysis of Tumor Cells Mediated by Antibody and Complement. Both **IgM** and **IgG** antibodies have been shown to destroy tumor cells in vitro in the

TABLE 20.3. Effector Mechanisms in Cancer Immunity

Effector mechanism	Comments
Antibodies and B cells (complement-mediated lysis, opsonization)	Role in tumor immunity poorly understood
T cells (cytolysis, apoptosis)	Critical for rejection of virally and chemically-induced tumors
NK cells (cytolysis, ADCC, apoptosis)	Tumor cells not expressing one of the MHC class I alleles are effectively rejected by NK cells
Lymphokine-activated killer (LAK) cells (cytolysis, apoptosis)	Antitumor responses seen in certain human cancers following adoptive transfer of LAK cells
Macrophages and neutrophils (cytostasis, cytolysis, phagocytosis)	Can be activated by bacterial products to destroy or inhibit tumor cell growth
Cytokines (apoptosis, recruitment of inflammatory cells)	Growth inhibition can occur using adoptively transferred tumor cells transfected with certain cytokines (e.g., G-CSF)

presence of complement. Several studies conducted with mice indicate that, in the presence of complement, antitumor antibodies are effective in vivo in destroying some leukemia and lymphoma cells and in reducing metastases in several other tumor systems. Other studies in vivo and in vitro, however, show that the same antibodies, in the presence of complement, are ineffective in destroying the cells of the same tumor in a solid form.

Destruction of Tumor Cells by Opsonization and Phagocytosis. Destruction of tumor cells by phagocytic cells has been demonstrated in vitro, but only in the presence of antitumor immune serum and complement. The relevance of this finding in vivo is unknown.

Antibody-Mediated Loss of Adhesive Properties of Tumor Cells. It appears that metastatic activity of certain kinds of tumors requires the adhesion of the tumor cells to each other and to the surrounding tissue. Antibodies directed against tumor cell surfaces may interfere with the adhesive properties of the tumor cells. The relevance of this mechanism in vivo is also unknown.

Cell-Mediated Responses

Direct Destruction of Tumor Cells by Cytotoxic T Lymphocytes. Destruction of tumor cells in vitro by specific immune T lymphocytes has been demonstrated numerous times for a variety of tumors, both dispersed and solid. Moreover, from many studies with experimental animals (primarily but not exclusively mice), there is good evidence that tumor-specific, cytotoxic T cells are responsible for destruction of virally-induced tumors in vivo. Although helper T cells participate in the induction and regulation of cytotoxic T cells, the destruction of the tumor cell is achieved by the $CD8^+$ *CTL* with specificity for the antigens on the surface of the tumor cell.

Antibody-Dependent, Cell-Mediated Cytotoxicity. Antibody-dependent, cell-mediated cytotoxicity (***ADCC***) involves (1) the binding of tumor-specific antibodies to the surface of the tumor cells; (2) the interaction of various cells, such as granulocytes and macrophages, which possess surface receptors for the Fe portion of the antibody attached to the tumor cell; and (3) the destruction of the tumor cells by substances that are released from these cells that carry receptors for the Fe portion of the antibody. The importance of this mechanism in the destruction of tumor cells in vivo is still not clear.

Destruction of Tumor by Natural Killer Cells and Lymphokine-Activated Killer Cells. *Natural killer (NK) cells* are a distinct subpopulation of lymphocytes that, without prior sensitization and without MHC restriction, can kill certain tumor cells. Tumor cells that fail to express at least one of the MHC class I molecules are targets for NK cells (see Chapter 2, Figure 2.5). These cells can lyse a variety of target cells, such as virally infected cells, antibody-coated cells, undifferentiated cells, and cells from a number of different tumors. NK cells have receptors for the Fc region of IgG (CD16) and, as we have seen in Chapter 4, can participate in ADCC. Like activated macrophages, NK cells secrete TNF-α that induces hemorrhage and tumor necrosis; however, the exact mechanism by which NK cells recognize and kill the tumor cells is still not clear.

Lymphokine-activated killer (LAK) cells are tumor-specific killer cells obtained from the patient. The cells are grown in vitro in the presence of IL-2 and then adoptively transferred back to the same patient. LAK cells constitute a heterogeneous population of lymphocytes that include NK cells. However, their activity cannot be attributed solely to NK cells since they can kill, in vitro, tumor cells that are not killed by NK cells. Although the natural biologic function of LAK cells is still obscure, they are now being tested for efficacy in tumor immunotherapy in humans (a topic discussed later in this chapter). A more recent innovation is the use of T cells isolated from the tumor and expanded and activated with IL-2. These *tumor-infiltrating lymphocytes* (TIL) show promise of greater specificity.

Destruction of Tumor Cells by Activated Macrophages and Neutrophils. Macrophages and neutrophils are generally not cytotoxic to tumor cells in vitro. They can be activated by bacterial products in vitro to cause selective cytostasis or cytolysis of malignant cells. Macrophages may also become highly cytotoxic (Figs. 20.1 and 20.2) when they are activated by cytokines, most notably IFN-γ produced by an activated population of T lymphocytes, which, by themselves, are not cytotoxic. These T lymphocytes (CD4$^+$) are tumor-specific: they release IFN-γ

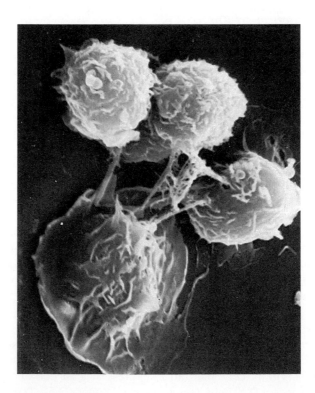

Figure 20.1. A scanning electron micrograph showing an activated macrophage with filopodia extending to the surface of three melanoma cells. ×4,500. [Photograph courtesy of Dr. K.L. Erickson, School of Medicine, University of California, Davis; reproduced with permission of Lippincott/Harper and Row.]

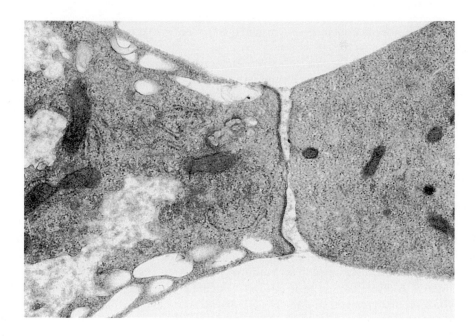

Figure 20.2. "The kiss of death." An electron micrograph showing a contact point between an activated macrophage (left) and a melanoma cell after 18 hours of coculture leading to cytolysis of the melanoma target cell. Flocculent material is found between the cells; a dense plate is associated with the cell membranes of the macrophage process; microtubules also appear in these projections. ×26,000. [Photograph courtesy of Dr. K.L. Erickson, School of Medicine, University of California, Davis; reproduced with permission of Lippincott/Harper and Row.]

after activation by tumor antigen. Other cytokines released by these antigen-activated T lymphocytes attract macrophages to the area of the antigen. IFN-γ also prevents migration of macrophages away from the antigen. The mechanism of activation of macrophages by T cells specific for tumor antigen, leading to destruction of tumor cells, is similar to mechanisms involved in delayed-type hypersensitivity reactions in allograft rejection or in the killing of microorganisms: antigen-specific T cells become activated by antigen, and they release cytokines, which attract and activate macrophages. These activated macrophages are cytotoxic to the microorganism, to tumor cells, and even to "self" cells in the vicinity of the activated macrophages. The damaging and killing activity of activated macrophages is due to several products that they release, notably *lysosomal enzymes* and *tumor necrosis factor alpha* (TNF-α) . Mounting evidence to indicate that destruction of tumor cells by activated macrophages occurs in vivo includes the following observations:

1. Resistance to a tumor can be abolished by specific depletion of macrophages.
2. Increased resistance to tumor accompanies an increase in the number of activated macrophages.
3. Administration of TNF-α into tumor-bearing animals causes hemorrhage and tumor necrosis.

4. Activated macrophages are frequently found at the site of regression of a tumor.

However, the relationship between the tumor and the tumor-associated macrophages is quite complex. On one hand, macrophages can and, indeed, do kill tumor cells. In addition, macrophages and tumor cells have been shown to produce reciprocal growth factors, leading to an almost symbiotic relationship. Thus, changes in the delicate balance between macrophages and tumor cells may drastically affect the fate of the tumor.

 ## CYTOKINES

As discussed above, cytokines can have a variety of ancillary functions that facilitate immune effector mechanisms in cancer immunity. It is important to note that, depending on the cytokines produced, immune effector mechanisms may be stimulated or inhibited. Consequently, the result may either be stimulation or inhibition of the growth of premalignant or malignant cells by acquired and/or innate immunity. The growth-promoting effects of cytokines is seen in the case of certain tumor cells that produce and respond to cytokines in an autocrine fashion. Similarly, production of TGF-β by some tumor cells promotes tumor growth due to the angiogenic properties of this cytokine.

Cytokines such as TNF and IFN-γ have antitumor effects because, among other functions, they upregulate MHC class I and class II antigens on some tumor cells. Decreased expression of these antigens allows tumor cells to evade the actions of cytotoxic T cells and NK cells. Cytokine upregulation of MHC antigens thereby facilitates important cell-mediated effector mechanisms. The effects of sustained high levels of certain cytokines have been studied using tumor cells transfected with cytokine genes. Transfection with genes coding for cytokines IL-1, IL-7, and IFN-γ followed by adoptive transfer of such cells into tumor-bearing mice has been shown to significantly inhibit the growth of tumors.

 ## LIMITATIONS OF THE EFFECTIVENESS OF THE IMMUNE RESPONSE AGAINST TUMORS

There is no question that an immune response can be induced against tumors. Why, then, in spite of the immune response, does the tumor continue to grow in the host? Several possible mechanisms may be operational either alone or in combination with each other. As shown in Table 20.4, *tumor-related and host-related factors may influence the escape of tumor cells from destruction by the immune system*. Tumor-related factors include those that relate to defective immunosensitivity and range from the lack of an antigenic epitope to resistance of tumor cells to tumoricidal effector pathways. Defective immunogenicity of the tumor may also account for a tumor's escape from immunologic destruction. Here, again, the lack of an antigenic epitope heads the list of possible mechanisms. Several other mechanisms, including lack of expression of costimulatory molecules by tumor cells and shedding of tumor antigens, and subsequent tolerance induction may also contribute to the failure of such cells to induce immune responses. Finally, the stromal environment is critical

TABLE 20.4. Mechanisms of Tumor Escape from Immunologic Destruction

Tumor-related	*Failure of the tumor to provide a suitable target*
	(a) Lack of antigenic epitope
	(b) Lack of MHC class I molecule
	(c) Deficient antigen processing by tumor cell
	(d) Antigenic modulation
	(e) Antigenic masking of the tumor
	(f) Resistance of tumor cell to tumoricidal effector pathway
	Failure of the tumor to induce an effective immune response
	(a) Lack of antigenic epitope
	(b) Decreased MHC or antigen expression by the tumor
	(c) Lack of costimulatory signal
	(d) Production of inhibitory substances (e.g., cytokines) by the tumor
	(e) Shedding of antigen and tolerance induction
	(f) Induction of T-cell signaling defects by tumor burden
Host-related	*Failure of the host to respond to an antigenic tumor*
	(a) Immune suppression or deficiency of host including apoptosis and signaling defects of T cells due to carcinogen (physical, chemical), infections, or age.
	(b) Deficient presentation of tumor antigens by host antigen-presenting cells
	(c) Failure of host effectors to reach the tumor (e.g., stromal barrier)
	(d) Failure of host to kill variant tumor cells because of immunodominant antigens on parental tumor cells

for preventing or permitting the immunologic destruction of tumor cells. Under certain circumstances, the stroma is the site for paracrine stimulatory loops that cause rapid malignant growth and thereby impede immunologic destruction.

Host-related mechanisms that promote the evasion of tumors from immunologic destruction are also summarized in Table 20.4. Immune suppression, deficient presentation of tumor antigens by APCs, and failure of host effectors to reach the tumor due to stromal barriers or the possible privileged-site setting of the tumor may facilitate immune evasion. Finally, studies have shown that expression of an immunodominant tumor antigen tends prevent sensitization to other tumor antigens, thus preventing immune attack on variants.

Nonspecific suppression mediated by tumor cells can also allow tumors to escape from immunologic destruction. Certain types of tumors synthesize various compounds, such as **prostaglandins**, which reduce many aspects of immune responsiveness. However, the role of this mechanism in the escape of tumors from destruction by the immune response is still unclear.

Finally, the immune response and its various components have a finite capacity for the effective destruction of tumors (or, for that matter, of invading microorganisms). Thus, while immunization may result in effective protection against an otherwise lethal dose of tumor cells, it is ineffective if the dose of tumor cells is sufficiently large. The progression of the growth of a tumor in an immunocompetent host, in the face of an immune response, may be due to a rapid increase in the mass of the tumor, which outstrips the increase in immune responsiveness, until the large mass of the tumor overwhelms any effects of the immune response.

● IMMUNODIAGNOSIS

Immunodiagnosis of tumors may be performed to achieve two separate goals: (1) the immunologic detection of **antigens** specific to tumor cells, and (2) the assessment of the host's **immune response** to the tumor. Immunodiagnosis is predicated on immunologic cross-reactivity, and immunologic methods may be used to detect tumor antigens and other "markers" in cases where tumor antigens exhibit similarities from individual to individual. In the presence of such immunologic cross-reactivity, antibody or lymphocytes from individuals with the same type of tumor would be expected to react with the cross-reactive tumor antigens, regardless of the individual from which they have been derived.

Tumor cells may express cytoplasmic, cell-surface, or secreted products that are different in nature and/or quantity from those produced by their normal counterparts. Because of the generally weak antigenicity of the tumor-specific markers, such differences, either qualitative or quantitative, have generally been demonstrated by the use of antibodies produced in xenogeneic animals. In the past few years, the use of **monoclonal antibodies** has greatly enhanced the specificity of immunodiagnosis of tumor cells and their products. Monoclonal antibodies are currently gaining use not only in the detection of antigens and products associated with the presence of tumor cells but also for their efficacy in the localization and **imaging** of tumors. Injection of **radiolabeled** tumor-specific antibodies (radioimmunoconjugates) into the tumor-bearing individual permits **visualization** by computer-assisted tomography (CAT) of the radiolabeled antibodies attached to the tumor. This method allows the detection of small metastases as well as the primary tumor mass. Some of the most widely used and reliable immunodiagnostic procedures for the detection of malignancies are described below.

Detection Of Myeloma Proteins Produced By Plasma Cell Tumors

Abnormally high concentration in serum of monoclonal immunoglobulins of a certain isotype, or the presence of light chains of these immunoglobulins (**Bence-Jones proteins**) in the urine, is indicative of **plasma cell tumors**. The concentration of these **myeloma proteins** in the blood or urine is a reflection of the mass of the tumor. Consequently, the effectiveness and duration of therapy for this tumor may be monitored by measurement of the concentration of myeloma proteins in the serum and urine.

Detection of α-Fetoprotein

α-Fetoprotein (AFP) is a major protein in fetal serum. After birth, the level of AFP falls to approximately 20 ng/ml. Levels of AFP are elevated in patients with **liver cancer**, but they are also elevated in noncancerous hepatic disorders such as cirrhosis and hepatitis. Nevertheless, concentrations of AFP of 500–1000 ng/ml are generally indicative of the presence of a tumor that is producing AFP, and monitoring AFP levels is indicative of regression or progression of the tumor.

Carcinoembryonic Antigen

Carcinoembryonic antigen (CEA) is a term applied to a glycoprotein produced normally by cells that line the gastrointestinal tract, in particular the colon. If the cells become malignant, their polarity may change, so that CEA is released into the blood instead of the colon. Concentrations in the blood of CEA exceeding 2.5 ng/ml are generally indicative of malignancy, and monitoring CEA levels is helpful in monitoring tumor growth or regression. Here again, however, higher than normal levels of CEA in blood may be due to noncancerous diseases, such as cirrhosis of the liver or inflammatory diseases of the intestinal tract and lung.

Detection of Prostate-Specific Antigen

Prostate-specific antigen (PSA) is currently widely used for screening and early detection of prostate cancer. Levels above 8–10 ng/ml blood are suggestive of prostate cancer. Confirmatory tests are required since prostatitis and benign prostate hypertrophy also may result in the release into the bloodstream of the prostate-specific antigen derived from glandular prostate epithelium. The test is especially useful for monitoring significant increases or decrease of blood levels of PSA that correlate with increase or decrease of tumor size.

There are other ''markers'' associated with malignancies, such as enzymes and hormones, that can be detected by immunologic methods. Qualitative as well as quantitative determinations of all tumor markers are useful in monitoring the extent of malignancy and the effect of therapy on it.

 ## TUMOR IMMUNOPROPHYLAXIS

Immunization against an oncogenic virus would be expected to provide prophylaxis against the virus and, hence, against the subsequent induction of tumor by the virus. Indeed, this approach has been successful in the protection of chickens against *Marek's disease*, and a significant degree of protection against *feline leukemia* and *feline sarcoma* has been achieved by immunizing cats with the respective oncogenic viruses. Immunization against the tumor itself requires that the tumor possess specific antigens and that these antigens cross-react immunologically with any prepared vaccine. There are literally thousands of reports of effective immunization against transplantable animal tumors, using as immunogens (1) sublethal doses of live tumor cells, (2) tumor cells in which replication has been blocked, (3) tumor cells with enzymatically or chemically modified surface membranes, and (4) extracts of antigens from the surface of tumor cells, either unmodified or chemically modified. Despite these reported successes in the protection of experimental animals against transplantable tumors, the efficacy of immunoprophylaxis for protection of humans and animals against spontaneous tumors has not been sufficiently evaluated. This lack of complete study relates to the need for appropriate immunogens and the danger of inducing the production of immunologic elements that may, in fact, enhance metastasis, and thus be detrimental to the host.

 ## IMMUNOTHERAPY

Leonardo da Vinci (1452–1519) wrote that "the supreme misfortune is when theory outstrips performance." Unfortunately, this is a fairly accurate characterization of the current state of cancer immunotherapy. Numerous attempts have been made to treat cancers in animals and humans by immunologic means. Although reports of successful immunotherapy in human cancers are increasing in the literature, to date, immunotherapy has not been proved to be an effective treatment of cancer, either when used as the sole treatment or as an adjunct to other forms of therapy such as chemotherapy, radiotherapy, or surgery.

Currently, a wide range of strategies in experimental immunotherapy of tumors are in use (Figure 20.3). Tumor-specific monoclonal antibodies (e.g., anti-CD20 for the treatment of certain lymphomas; anti-Her2/neu-1 for the treatment of certain patients with breast and ovarian cancers) can mediate cytolysis either by engaging NK cells via Fc receptors (ADCC), or by complement activation. Trials of cancer immunotherapy are underway in which toxins, such as ricin, or radioactive isotopes attached to tumor-specific antibodies are delivered specifically to the tumor cells for direct killing. The extent to which these "immunotoxins" will prove effective in the treatment of cancer remains to be established. Xenogeneic antibodies (e.g., mouse anti-human monoclonal antibodies) that have been molecularly engineered using recombinant DNA technology to "humanize" their constant regions (see Chapter 5) are also being tested as candidates for immunotherapy. Bispecific antibody constructs designed to bring immune effector cells into contact with tumor cells and to simultaneously stimulate the cytotoxic activity of effector cells are also under investigation. Examples include antibodies that recognize unique tumor antigens and IgG Fc receptors (CD16) to activate NK cells. Similarly, bispecific antibodies constructs containing Fabs specific for tumor antigens and CD3 have also been studied. A relatively new approach involves the creation of recombinant fusion proteins con-

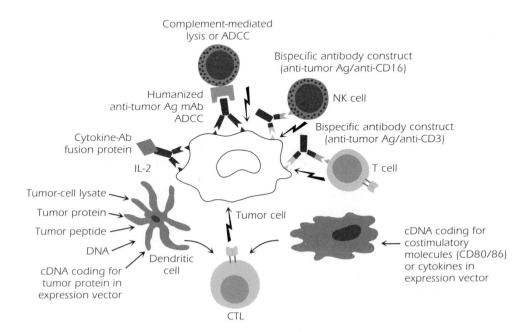

Figure 20.3. Current strategies in experimental immunotherapy.

sisting of antitumor antibodies and cytokines (immunocytokines). Such fusion proteins are designed to concentrate cytokine-mediated immune effector functions at the tumor site. Several approaches are designed to stimulate or bolster the function of tumor-specific CTLs. CTLs can be activated against tumor antigens by tumor cells rendered immunologic by expression of either costimulatory molecules such as CD80/CD86 or cytokines. A highly effective method for stimulating tumor-specific CTLs involves the presentation of MHC class I tumor antigen peptides by dendritic cells. Dendritic cells are either directly loaded with peptides or exposed to tumor cell lysates, tumor proteins, or transfection of tumor-derived cDNA in an expression vector.

For tumor antigens that have been molecularly characterized, active vaccination using recombinant vaccines have been developed using vaccinia, *Listeria*, or virus-like particles. Active immunization has also been studied by injection of naked DNA plasmid constructs (DNA vaccines) with the goal of having the unique tumor antigen encoded and expressed by muscle cells. In some studies, the genes encoding cytokines (e.g., GM-CSF) are or immune-enhancing cytokines such as IL-2 and IL-12 also introduced to improve the presentation of the tumor antigen by dendritic cells at the site of injection.

Attempts at immunotherapy of animal and human malignancies have also been aimed at the augmentation of specific anticancer immunity, utilizing nonspecific enhancement of the immune response. In particular, stimulation of macrophages, using BCG (bacille Calmette-Guerin) or *Corynebacterium parvum* has been successfully used in some cases. One example is the use of BCG for treating patients with residual superficial urinary bladder cancer. Repeated instillation of live mycobacteria into the bladder by way of catheter after surgery has become the treatment of choice for superficial bladder cancer.

Trials are also in progress on the effects of various cytokines, such as ***interferon-α, β, and γ, IL-1, IL-2, IL-4, IL-5, IL-12, tumor necrosis factor***, and others either singly or in combination on tumor regression. To date, these trials are mostly inconclusive. The clinical use of ***lymphokine-activated killer (LAK) cells*** and ***tumor-infiltrating lymphocytes*** (TIL) have also been applied to the treatment of cancer with variable results. LAK cells are produced in vitro by cultivation of the patient's own peripheral lymphocytes with IL-2. Upon reinfusion into the patient, dramatic improvement has been recorded in a number of cases. In the latter case, a documented success has been reported using TIL adoptively transferred to patients with melanoma. These lymphocytes, removed from a tumor biopsy, expanded in vitro with IL-2 and given back to the tumor-bearing individual, have an antitumor activity many times higher than LAK cells, thus less is needed for therapy.

Our growing understanding of cancer and of the immune system continues to fuel the development of new immunotherapeutic strategies. In all cases, such strategies must be evaluated in preclinical models for their potential usefulness. The great promise that the immune system can be exploited for the treatment and prevention of cancer must be tempered by the few examples of documented efficacy that have emerged. Nevertheless, given the rapid advances in biotechnology and the molecular identification of human tumor antigens, we are entering a new era of cancer immunotherapy. At the present time, we can say with certainty that tumor immunology has clearly yielded significant improvements in the diagnosis of cancer and it is likely that immune-based diagnostic methods will continue to offer useful new ways to detect tumor cells and monitor their growth.

SUMMARY

1. Tumor immunology deals with (a) the immunologic aspects of the host—tumor relationship and (b) the utilization of the immune response for diagnosis, prophylaxis, and treatment of cancer.

2. Tumor antigens induced by carcinogens do not cross-react immunologically. On the other hand, extensive cross-reactivity is exhibited with virally-induced tumor antigens. Several types of tumors produce oncofetal substances, which are normally present during embryonic development.

3. The immune response to tumors involves both humoral and cellular immune responses. Destruction of tumor cells may be achieved by: (a) antibodies and complement; (b) phagocytes; (c) loss of the adhesive properties of tumor cells caused by antibodies; (d) cytotoxic T lymphocytes; (e) Antibody-dependent, cell-mediated cytotoxicity (ADCC); and (f) activated macrophages, neutrophils, NK cells, and LAK cells.

4. The role of the immune response to tumors appears to be important in the host—tumor relationship, as indicated by increased incidence of tumors in immunosuppressed hosts and by the presence of immune components at sites of tumor regression. However, the immune response to a tumor may not be effective in eliminating the tumor because of a variety of tumor- and host-related mechanisms.

5. Immunodiagnosis may be directed toward the detection of tumor antigens or the host's immune response to the tumor.

6. Immunoprophylaxis may be directed against oncogenic viruses or against the tumor itself.

7. Immunotherapy of malignancy employs various preparations for the augmentation of tumor-specific as well as nonspecific immune responses. Approaches include: (a) active immunization; (b) passive therapy with antibodies; (c) local application of live bacterial vaccines (BCG); (d) use of cytokines; and, (e) adoptive transfer of effector cells.

REFERENCES

Alexandroff AB, Robins RA, Murray A, James K (1999): Tumour immunology: false hopes —new horizons? *Immunol Today* 19:247.

Epenetos AA, Spooner RA, George AJT (1994): Application of monoclonal antibodies in clinical oncology. *Immunol Today* 15:559.

Jager E, Chen YT, Drifhout JW (1998): Simultaneous humoral and cellular immune response against cancer-testis antigen NY-ESO-1: definition of human histocompatibility leukocyte antigen (HLA)-A2-binding peptide epitopes. *J Exp Med* 187:265.

Mantovani A, Bottazzi B, Colatta F, Sozzani S, Ruco L (1992): The origin and function of tumor associated macrophages. *Immunol Today* 13:265.

Marshall JL, Hawkins MJ, Tsang KY, Richmond E, Pedicano JE, Zhu MZ, Schlom J (1999): Phase I study in cancer patients of a replication-defective avipox recombinant vaccine that expresses human carcinoembryonic antigen. *J Clin Oncol* 17:332.

Melief CJ, Offringa R, Toes RE, Kast WM (1996): Peptide-based cancer vaccines. *Curr Opin Immunol* 8:651.

Noguchi Y, Richards EC, Chen YT, Old LJ. (1995): Influence of interleukin-12 on p53 peptide vaccination against established Meth A sarcoma. *Proc Natl Acad Sci USA* 92:2219.

Ockert D, Schmitz M, Hampl M, Rieber EP (1999) Advances in cancer immunotherapy. *Immunol Today* 20:63.

Rosenberg, SA (1997): Cancer vaccines based on the identification of genes encoding cancer regression antigens. *Immunol Today* 18:175.

Rosenberg SA (1999) A new era for cancer immunotherapy based on the genes that encode cancer antigens. *Immunity* 10:281.

Rosenberg, SA, Yang, JC, White, DE, Steinberg, SM (1998): Durability of complete responses in patients with metastatic cancer treated with high-dose interleukin-2: identification of the antigens mediating response. *Ann Surg* 228:307.

Schreiber H (1999): Tumor immunology. In Paul WE (ed): Fundamental Immunology, 4th ed. New York: Lippincott-Raven.

Stockert E, Jager E, Chen YT (1998): A survey of the humoral immune response of cancer patients to a panel of human tumor antigens. *J Exp Med* 187:1349.

Vitteta ES, Thorpe PE, Uhr JW (1993): Immunotoxins: magic bullets or misguided missiles? *Immunol Today* 14:252.

● REVIEW QUESTIONS

For each question, choose the ONE BEST answer or completion.

1. The appearance of many primary lymphoreticular tumors in humans has been correlated with

   A) hypergammaglobulinemia.
   B) acquired hemolytic anemia.
   C) BCG treatment.
   D) resistance to antibiotics.
   E) impairment of cell-mediated immunity.

2. Tumor antigens have been shown to cross-react immunologically in cases of

   A) tumors induced by chemical carcinogens.
   B) tumors induced by RNA viruses.
   C) all tumors.
   D) tumors induced by irradiation with ultraviolet light.
   E) tumors induced by the same chemical carcinogen on two separate sites on the same individual.

3. Which of the following is *not* considered a mechanism by which cytokines mediate antitumor effects?

   A) They enhance the expression of MHC class I molecules.
   B) They activate LAK and TIL cells.
   C) They have direct antitumor activity.
   D) They induce complement-mediated cytolysis.
   E) They increase activity of cytotoxic T cells, macrophages, and NK cells.

4. Rejection of a tumor may involve which of the following?

    A) T-cell-mediated cytotoxicity
    B) ADCC
    C) complement-dependent cytotoxicity
    D) destruction of tumor cells by phagocytic cells
    E) All are correct.

5. Immunotoxins are

    A) toxic substances released by macrophages.
    B) cytokines.
    C) toxins completed with the corresponding antitoxins.
    D) toxins coupled to antigen-specific immunoglobulins.
    E) toxins released by cytotoxic T cells.

6. It has been shown that a B-cell lymphoma could be eliminated with anti-idiotypic serum. The use of this approach to treat a plasma cell tumor would not be warranted because

    A) plasma cell tumors have no tumor-specific antigens.
    B) plasma cell tumors are not expected to be susceptible to ADCC.
    C) plasma cell tumors can be killed in vivo only by cytotoxic T lymphocytes that bear the same A, B, and C transplantation antigens.
    D) the plasma cells do not have surface Ig.
    E) the idiotype on the plasma-cell surface is different from that on the B-cell surface.

Case Study

A patient suffering from a rare cancer is treated with a cocktail of cytokines, which includes IL-2 and IL-12 and shows improvement as measured by a reduced tumor burden, despite various side effects of the therapy. Various functional parameters of the patient's peripheral blood cells were tested before, during, and after therapy. An assay designed to measure macrophage phagocytic activity indicates a significant increase in phagocytosis of antibody-opsonized bacteria one day following injection of the cocktail. Explain what might account for this observed effect. How could you confirm your hypothesis? Discuss how this increased phagocytic activity could be responsible for the patient's improvement.

Answers To Review Questions

1. *E* There is a nearly 100-fold increase in the incidence of lymphoproliferative tumors in individuals with impaired immunity, in particular with impaired cell-mediated immunity. Hypergammaglobulinemia, acquired hemolytic anemia, or resistance to antibiotics are not correlated with increases in lymphoproliferative tumors; neither is BCG treatment, which in some instances has even been shown to influence favorably the course of some leukemias.

2. *B* Immunologic cross-reactivity has been demonstrated only in cases of virally induced tumors (caused by either RNA or DNA viruses). Tumors induced by chemical or physical carcinogens do not exhibit cross-reactivity, even if induced by the same carcinogen on separate sites on the same individual.

3. *D* Interferon-α, β, and γ enhance the expression of class I MHC molecules on tumor cells that makes them more vulnerable to killing by CTLs. IL-2 activates LAK and TIL cells. TNF-α and β both have direct antitumor activity. IFN-γ increases the activity of CTLs, macrophages, and NK cells, each of which plays an important role in tumor cell destruction. Cytokines play no role in the activation of complement, therefore D is incorrect.

4. *E* All are correct. Destruction of tumor cells may be mediated by T-cell-mediated cytotoxicity, by antibody-dependent cell-mediated cytotoxicity (ADCC), by complement-mediated cytotoxicity, and by phagocytic cells, which are attracted to the tumor by T-cell lymphokines and/or complement components, and become activated by the lymphokines or perform enhanced phagocytosis as a result of the present of opsonins on the target cells.

5. *D* Immunotoxins consist of toxic substances (or radioactive atoms) conjugated to immunoglobulin molecules specific for tumor cells or other target cells.

6. *D* The only relevant statement is that plasma cells do not have surface immunoglobulins and would therefore not be susceptible to treatment with antiidiotypic antibodies. Plasma cell tumors do have tumor-specific antigens and would be susceptible to ADCC with antibodies to these antigens. Statement C is not correct.

Answer to Case Study

Therapeutic infusion of cytokine cocktails can cause a variety of immunomodulatory effects. IL-12 is known to induce increased IFN-γ production by T cells, which, in turn, increases the activity of cytotoxic T lymphocytes, macrophages, and NK cells. Each of these cell populations plays a role in the immune response to tumors. The probable reason why the patient's macrophages showed increased phagocytic activity when exposed to antibody-opsonized bacteria is that IFN-γ also increases macrophage Fc receptor expression. Their ability to bind to antibody-coated bacteria would therefore be greatly facilitated—thus, phagocytosis would be enhanced. One way to confirm this hypothesis would be to measure IFN-γ levels in the patient's peripheral blood following cytokine cocktail infusions. Assuming this mechanism were confirmed, it would help to explain the patient's improvement, since increased Fc receptor expression would also be expected to increase ADCC activity directed against tumor antigens. Thus, if the patient had serum antibody specific for tumor antigens, this antitumor mechanism probably functioned in concert with the cytokine-enhanced tumoricidal activities of macrophages and NK to reduce the tumor burden.

21

RESISTANCE AND IMMUNIZATION TO INFECTIOUS DISEASES*

 INTRODUCTION

The primary function of the immune system is to defend the body against invasions by microorganisms. Historically, infectious diseases have been the leading cause of death for human populations and most deaths from infection occurred in infancy and childhood. There have been many catastrophic epidemics in history. For example, the bubonic plague caused by the bacterium *Yersinia pestis* killed one quarter of the European population in the mid-1300s. Hence infectious diseases have provided tremendous selective pressures for the evolution of the immune system. Host defenses are characterized by a considerable amount of layering and redundancy. Layering refers to defense in depth and includes physical barriers such as the skin and mucosal membranes and innate and adaptive immune mechanisms. Redundancy is exemplified by the fact that there are several types of phagocytic cells, antigen-presenting cells, cytokine-producing cells, opsonins, and so on, such that for many immune functions, multiple mechanisms are in place to achieve the desired end. The redundancy of the immune system allows some hosts to survive for prolonged times despite severe immune impairment. For example, some individuals with advanced HIV infection have significant infection-free intervals despite profound CD4$^+$ T-cell deficiencies.

Microbes differ in their pathogenicity and virulence. Only a small minority of all microorganisms are pathogens. In general, most pathogens have special characteristics that distinguish them from nonpathogenic microbes and allow them to overcome host defenses and cause disease. Pathogenicity refers to the ability of a microbe

*Contributed by Dr. Arturo Casadevall, Department of Microbiology and Immunology, Albert Einstein College of Medicine.

to cause disease and virulence is the degree of pathogenicity. Pathogenicity depends on microbial characteristics and the immune status of the host. In patients with intact immune systems, microbes must be sufficiently virulent to establish themselves and cause infection. However, in patients with weakened immune systems, low virulence microbes can cause serious infections. Those microbes that are pathogenic in individuals with weakened immune systems are often referred to as "opportunistic" pathogens. Hence the microbial properties of pathogenicity and virulence are associated with, and partially dependent on, the immune status of the host.

Human hosts are colonized with many species of microbes. These microbes are known as commensals. In circumstances of normal immune function commensal microorganisms are not harmful and can serve an important role for the host by such as the manufacture of vitamin K by gut bacteria. However, commensals can become pathogens in circumstances where the normal host defenses are breached. For example, both *Staphylococcus epidermitis* and *Candida albicans* are part of the normal skin flora but can cause life-threatening infections in patients with intravenous catheters that provide a break in the skin. Some therapies for cancer produce immune suppression, which leaves patients at risk for serious infections with low-virulence microbes, such as commensals.

In this chapter we will discuss how mammalian hosts protect themselves against various types of pathogens and discuss how the immune system can be primed for antimicrobial defense through active and passive immunization.

INNATE AND ADAPTIVE IMMUNE DEFENSES

A microbial infection is an attempt by the microbe to establish itself in the environmental niche defined by the host that results in damage to the host. For an infection to be successful, the microbe must breach barriers and overcome mechanical and chemical mechanisms that interfere with entry and attachment. Mechanical defenses include epithelial surfaces, mucous secretions, and cilia, which move microbes and prevent their attachment. The secretions found in mucosal surfaces, such as saliva, tears, and mucus, contain enzymes, iron-binding proteins, and antibodies that are antimicrobial. The overwhelming majority of microbes that come into contact with the host are contained by innate immune mechanisms that include complement, neutrophils, and macrophages (see Chapter 2). The fact that most individuals suffer only a few significant infections in their lifetime is testament to the enormous efficacy of innate defense mechanisms in preventing microbes from establishing themselves in the host. When pathogenic microbes establish themselves in the host humoral and cellular mechanisms are required for containment and eradication of infection (Chapters 1 and 2). Although practically all microbial pathogens elicit both humoral and cellular immune responses, the relative efficacy of these host defense mechanisms varies depending on the type of pathogen and the mechanism of pathogenesis. The initial interaction of the microbe with immune cells produces cytokines that promote the differentiation of $CD4^+$ T cells into either the T_H1 or T_H2 subsets, which differ depending on the cytokines that they produce. As discussed in Chapter 12, T_H1-associated cytokines promote inflammation whereas T_H2-associated cytokines promote B-cell proliferation and the development of strong antibody responses. The polarization of the $CD4^+$ T cells into T_H1 or T_H2 subsets can have profound consequences for the type of response made and for its efficacy against individual pathogens. For example, T_H1 responses are thought to be critical for the containment and clearance of mycobacteria and fungal pathogens by activating macrophages. On the other hand, certain parasites require the production of IgE for eradication, which implies the importance of T_H2 responses in those infections. T_H2 cells promote iso-type immunoglobulin switching and may be involved in somatic hypermutation. However, this view of immunity (T_H1-T_H2 paradigm) is probably a simplification of a very complex process, which has nevertheless provided a useful working model for dissecting the types of immune responses in infection. For most pathogens it is likely that close collaboration between humoral and cellular immune responses is essential for effective defense against most pathogens. However, for some pathogens one arm of the adaptive immune response may be more important in host defense than the other.

 ## HOST DEFENSE AGAINST THE VARIOUS CLASSES OF MICROBIAL PATHOGENS

The effective immune response to a particular microbe varies with the type of path-ogen and the microbial strategy for pathogenesis. Viruses, bacteria, parasites, and fungi each use different strategies to establish themselves in the host, and, conse-quently, the effective immune response for each of these classes of microbial path-ogens is different. Although each pathogen is different, certain themes emerge when one considers immune responses to the various classes of pathogens.

Immunity to Viruses

All viruses are obligate intracellular pathogens and many have evolved to have highly sophisticated mechanisms for cellular invasion, replication, and evasion of the im-mune system. Host defenses against viral infections aim to first slow viral replication and then to eradicate infection. The antiviral response can be complex, with several factors affecting the outcome of the host–pathogen interaction, such as the route of entry, site of attachment, aspects of pathogenesis by the infecting virus; induction of interferon; antibody response; and cell-mediated immunity. An important early de-fense mechanism consists of the production of various types of interferons (IFN), including IFN-α by leucocytes, IFN-β by fibroblasts, and INF-γ by T and NK cells. Interferons are antiviral proteins or glycoproteins produced by several different types of cell in the mammalian host in response to viral infection (or other inducers such as double-stranded RNA). Interferons serve as an early protective mechanism. IFN-α and IFN-β produced by virally infected cells diffuse to adjoining cells and activate genes that interfere with viral replication. These interferons also stimulate production of MHC class I molecules and proteasome proteins that enhance the ability of virally infected cells to present viral peptides to T cells. Furthermore, IFN-α and IFN-β activate NK cells that recognize and kill host cells infected with viruses thus limiting viral production. NK cells are characterized by their ability to kill certain tumor cells in vitro without prior sensitization and constitute an early cellular defense against viruses. Later in the course of infection, when antibodies to viral antigens are available, NK cells can eliminate host cells infected with virus through antibody-dependent cell-mediated cytotoxicity (ADCC). NK cells also produce INF-γ, a potent activator of macrophage function that helps to prime the immune system for producing an adaptive immune response. Complement system proteins damage the envelope of some viruses that may provide some measure of protection against certain viral infections.

While IFNs, NK cells, and possibly complement function to slow and partially contain many viral infections, the infection may progress and trigger an immune response. The humoral response results in the production of antibodies to viral proteins. Some antibodies can prevent viruses from invading other cells and these are called *neutralizing* antibodies. IgG appears to be the most active isotype against viruses. Opsonization represents a convergence of humoral and cellular immune mechanisms. IgG, which has combined, through its Fab portion, with viral antigens on the surface of infected host cells, links also to Fc receptors on several cell populations including NK cells, macrophages, and polymorphonuclear cells (PMNs). These cells then can phagocytose and/or damage the virus-infected cell—a phenomenon termed antibody-dependent cell-mediated cytotoxicity (ADCC) (see Chapter 5). Antibodies to viral proteins can prevent infection by interfering with the binding of virus to host cells. The production of secretory IgA can protect the host by preventing infection of epithelial cells in mucosal surfaces. Antibodies can also interfere with the progression of viral infection by agglutinating viral particles, activating complement on viral surfaces, and promoting phagocytosis of viral particles by macrophages. The production of an antibody response serves to limit viral spread and facilitates the destruction of infected host cells by ADCC. Hence the effective antibody response to viruses include the production of antibodies that

1. neutralize (or impede) the infectivity of viruses for susceptible host cells.
2. fix complement and promote complement damage to virions.
3. inhibit viral enzymes.
4. promote opsonization of viral particles.
5. promote ADCC of virus-infected cells.

Different types of antibodies may be necessary for the control of specific types of viral infections. Consider the case of influenza and measles virus infections. Infection of the epithelium of the respiratory tract by influenza virus leads to production of virus in epithelial cells and spread of the virus to adjacent epithelial cells. An appropriate and sufficient immune response would involve the action of antibody at the epithelial surface. This action might be effected through locally secreted IgA, or local extravasation of IgG or IgM. On the other hand, some viral diseases, such as measles or poliomyelitis, begin by infection at a mucosal epithelium (respiratory or intestinal, respectively) but exhibit their major pathogenic effects after being spread hematogenously to other target tissues. Antibody at the epithelial surface could protect against the virus, but circulating antibody could do likewise.

However, once a virus has attached to a host cell, it is usually not displaced by antibody. Hence an effective antibody response is usually not sufficient to eliminate a viral infection, particularly when the virus has established itself in host cells. The eradication of a viral infection usually requires an effective cell-mediated response. The cellular adaptive response results in the production of specific CD4$^+$ and CD8$^+$ T cells that are essential for clearance of viral infections. CD4$^+$ T cells are believed to be intimately involved in the generation of effective antibody responses by facilitating isotype class switching and affinity maturation. CD4$^+$ T cells also produce important cytokines to stimulate inflammatory responses at sites of viral infection and activate macrophage function. Cytotoxic $CD8^+$ T cells (CTLs) are the principal effector T cells against viruses. They are generated early in viral infection and they usually appear before neutralizing antibody. $CD8^+$ T cells can recognize viral antigens in the context of MHC class I molecules and can kill host cells harboring viruses. Since MHC class I molecules are expressed by most cell types in the host, $CD8^+$ T cells can recognize many types of infected cells and thus represent a critically important component of the host adaptive response against viral infections.

In summary, innate immune mechanisms initially interfere with viral infection through the production of IFNs and the killing of infected cells by NK cells. These early defenses buy time until powerful adaptive immune responses are generated. The adaptive immune responses produce neutralizing antibodies that reduce the number of viral particles and cytotoxic T cells that kill infected cells.

Immunity to Bacteria

Host protection against bacterial pathogens is achieved through a variety of mechanisms that include both humoral and cellular immunity. Antibacterial defenses include bacterial lysis, via antibody and complement, opsonization, and phagocytosis, with elimination of phagocytosed bacteria by the liver, spleen, and other components of the reticuloendothelial system. The relative efficacy of the various immune mechanisms depends on the type of bacteria and the cell surface of the bacteria. Bacterial pathogens can be roughly divided into four classes: gram-positive, gram-negative, mycobacteria, and spirochetes, depending on their cell wall and membrane composition. Some gram-positive and gram-negative bacteria have polysaccharide capsules. Another crucial distinction between bacterial pathogens is whether they are intracellular or extracellular pathogens. Intracellular bacterial pathogens reside in cells and are partially shielded from the full array of host immune defenses. In general, humoral immunity is very important for protection against extracellular bacteria, whereas cellular immunity tends to be the primary immune mechanism for the control and eradication of intracellular bacteria.

Gram-Positive Bacteria. *Gram-positive bacteria* have thick electron-dense cell walls composed of complex crosslinked peptidoglycan that allow them to retain the stain crystal violet (hence gram-positive). In addition to a thick layer of peptidoglycan, the cell wall of gram-positive bacteria contains teichoic acids, carbohydrates, and proteins. Teichoid acids are immunogenic and constitute major antigenic determinants of gram-positive bacteria. This type of cell wall provides the gram-positive bacteria with a thick layer of protection that makes them resistant to lysis by the complement system. Defenses against gram-positive bacteria include specific antibody responses to provide opsonins and phagocytic cells, such as neutrophils and macrophages, to ingest and kill them. Opsonization and phagocytosis involve the action of IgG and IgM alone or in concert with C3b. The alternative complement pathway may be triggered directly by the gram-positive bacterial cell wall, resulting in the deposition of complement opsonins in the cell surface and the production of mediators of the inflammatory response. Although the complement system does not lyse gram-positive bacteria directly, it provides opsonins and mediators of inflamation that are critical for host defense.

Gram-Negative Bacteria. *Gram-negative bacteria* do not retain crystal violet stain and have a layered cell wall structure composed of outer and inner membranes separated by a thin layer of peptidoglycan in the periplasmic space. Hence gram-positive and negative bacteria have major differences in their cell wall structure. The outer membrane of gram-negative bacteria contains lipopolysaccharide (LPS), which is also known as *endotoxin*. The polysaccharide portion of LPS has antigenic determinants that confer antigenic specificity. Many gram-negative bacterial species include variants with different LPS structure that can be identified serologically as serotypes. LPS is highly toxic to humans and can produce cardiovascular collapse, hypotension, and shock, during infection with gram-negative bacteria. The alternative complement pathway may be activated directly by the LPS found in the walls of gram-negative bacteria or by the polysaccharide capsule of gram-negative bacteria acting on C3. Activation of the alternative pathway leads to the generation of the chemotactic molecules C3a and C5a, the opsonin C3b, and can result in bacteriolytic action by the C5–C9 membrane attack complex (see Chapter 13). The ability of the complement system to lyse some gram-negative bacteria directly is an important distinction from gram-positive bacteria that are impervious to complement mediated lysis because of the thick peptidoglycan layer. Defenses against gram-negative bacteria include the complement system, specific antibody and phagocytic cells.

Mycobacteria. *Mycobacteria* have cell walls distinct from gram-positive and gram-negative bacteria. Mycobacterial cell walls are characterized by a high lipid content, which makes the bacteria difficult to stain. Another property of the mycobacterial cell wall is *acid fastness*, which allows them to retain certain dyes after being treated with acid. Mycobacteria grow slowly and have hydrophobic surfaces that make them clump. Mycobacterial cell wall components elicit strong immune responses during infection, including delayed hypersensitivity reactions that form the basis for the tuberculin test. Hypersensitivity reactions to mycobacterial proteins may be involved in the pathogenesis of mycobacterial infections. Mycobacteria elicit strong antibody responses but the role of humoral immunity is uncertain. The primary defense mechanisms against mycobacteria are macrophages and cell-mediated immunity.

Spirochetes. *Spirochetes* are thin helical microorganisms and include the etiologic agents of syphilis (*Treponema pallidum*) and Lyme disease (*Borrelia burgdorferi*). Spirochetes lack cell walls such as those found in gram-positive, gram-negative, and mycobacteria. Instead they have a thin outer membrane that contains few proteins. Spirochetes are thin, fragile, and require special techniques for visualization in the microscope such as dark-field microscopy or immunofluorescence. Important host defenses against spirochetes include complement, specific antibody, and cell-mediated immunity.

Immunity to Parasites

The parasites are a diverse group of complex pathogens that include the protozoa and helminths. Many parasites have different tissue stages that may differ in cellular location and antigenic composition thus providing a difficult problem for the immune system. Some parasites are *protozoa*, single-celled eukaryote organisms that may exist in either a metabolically active form called a trophozoite or a dormant tissue form known as a cyst. The protozoal diseases include amebiasis, malaria, leishmaniasis, trypanosomiasis, and toxoplasmosis. Host defenses against protozoa include both humoral and cellular mechanisms, but their relative importance may vary with the individual pathogen. For some protozoal infections, such as amebiasis, malaria, and trypanosomiasis, humoral immunity in the form of antibody has been shown to mediate protection against infection. However, for other protozoal infections such as leishmaniasis and toxoplasmosis, cellular immunity is more important. Other parasites are multicellular worms called **helminths**. Unlike other pathogenic microorganisms the helminths are large pathogens that can range from 1 cm to 10 m. Large size poses particular problems for host defenses and the control of helminth infections require a complex interplay between tissue and immune responses. The helminths are notorious for causing chronic infections that can elicit intense immune responses to worm antigens. There is general agreement that eosinophils are important effector cells against helminths but many aspects of the host response to worms remain obscure. Specific IgE to helminth antigens is believed to be important for host defense by priming eosinophils for ADCC. Worm infections are often accompanied by an increase in blood eosinophils and serum IgE levels.

Immunity to Fungi

Fungal pathogens are eukaryotes that tend to cause serious infections primarily in individuals with impaired immunity. Fungi cause tissue damage by the elaboration of proteolytic enzymes and inducing inflammatory responses. Some fungi like *Histoplasma capsulatum* survive inside macrophages and are intracellular pathogens. One fungal pathogen, *Cryptococcus neoformans* has a polysaccharide capsule, which is required for virulence. Fungi differ from bacteria in having a different type of cell wall composed of crosslinked polysaccharides. Fungal cells are generally impervious to lysis by the complement system. The host response to fungal infections include both humoral and cellular responses. The primary form of host defense against fungal pathogens is widely acknowledged to be cell-mediated immunity. The need for intact T-cell function in resistance to fungi is particularly evident in the predisposition of patients with AIDS to life-threatening infections with such fungi as *Histoplasma capsulatum* and *Cryptococcus neoformans*. Historically, antibody-mediated immunity was not thought to be very important against fungi, but several protective monoclonal antibodies have been described in recent years against *C. albicans* and *C. neoformans*. Hence it is likely that both cellular and humoral immune mechanisms contribute to protection against fungi.

 ## MECHANISMS BY WHICH PATHOGENS EVADE THE IMMUNE RESPONSE

Despite the formidable defenses of the immune system some microorganisms manage to establish themselves in the host and cause life-threatening infections. Many pathogenic microbes have special adaptations that allow them to evade the immune system. Learning about the mechanisms by which microbial pathogens evade the host immune response is important because it can teach us about the efficacy and limitations of host defense mechanisms. Furthermore, a better understanding of the strategies used by microbes to survive immune attack can be used to design new therapies and vaccines to fight infection.

Encapsulated Bacteria

Polysaccharide capsules are important virulence determinants of several human pathogens, including *Streptococcus pneumoniae* (pneumococcus), *Haemophilus influenzae*, *Neisseria meningitidis* (meningococcus), and *Cryptococcus neoformans*. These capsules are antiphagocytic and thus protect the pathogen from ingestion and killing by host phagocytic cells. Some capsules also interfere with the action of the complement system. Polysaccharide molecules are often weakly immunogenic and infection by encapsulated pathogens may not necessarily elicit high titer antibody responses. Infants and young children are particularly vulnerable to life-threatening infections with encapsulated bacteria because their immature immune systems do not mount adequate antibody responses. Other individuals at high risk are those with inherited or acquired deficiencies in antibody production and those that lack normal spleen function. Because the opsonized and phagocytosed bacteria are cleared by the spleen, anatomically or functionally asplenic patients are particularly vulnerable to encapsulated bacteria. The mechanism of antibody action against encapsulated pathogens involves providing opsonins for phagocytosis and killing by neutrophils and macrophages. Antibodies to capsular polysaccharide function by promoting phagocytosis directly through Fc receptors or, indirectly, by activation of the classical complement pathway.

Toxins

For some bacterial infections the manifestations of disease are caused by toxins. Bacterial toxins are proteins that produce their physiologic effects at minute concentrations. Examples include *Corynebacterium dipththeriae* and *Clostridium tetani*, the causes of diphtheria and tetanus, respectively. The relationship of the toxin function to bacterial invasion and evasion of the immune response is variable and may differ for each pathogen. Some toxins such as tetanus and botulinum toxin do not appear to injure the immune response directly. Other toxins such as the streptolysins produced by streptococci are toxic to neutrophils. Diphtheria toxin may promote bacterial infection by damaging the mucosa. The interaction of certain toxins with the immune system can have major immunologic consequences when they are able to bind the T cell receptor of large numbers of T cells. These toxins are known as superantigens and include the staphylococcal toxic shock syndrome toxin (see Chapter 10). Superantigens stimulate large numbers of T cells to proliferate, synthesize cytokines and then die by apoptosis resulting in the loss of important immune cells.

Most toxins are highly immunogenic and elicit strong humoral and cellular immune responses. Specific antibodies can bind to and neutralize bacterial toxins. Protection against toxins is predominantly associated with IgG, although IgA may also be important in neutralization of certain exotoxins such as cholera enterotoxin. Because the exotoxins bind firmly to their target tissue, they generally cannot be displaced by subsequent administration of antitoxin. Hence in toxin-mediated diseases (e.g., diphtheria) prompt administration of antitoxin is necessary to prevent attachment of (additional) exotoxin and the damage caused by the exotoxin. This can be illustrated by the effectiveness of antitoxin given at varying times as protection against the lethal effects of diphtheria toxin in humans (Table 21.1). As the infection progresses the effectiveness of administration of diphtheria antitoxin is significantly reduced. Some bacterial toxins are enzymes, such as the lecithinase of the bacterium

TABLE 21.1. Protection of Humans by Diphtheria
Antitoxin Given on Indicated Day of Disease

Day	Number of cases	Fatality rate
1	225	9
2	1,445	4.2
3	1,600	11.1
4	1,276	17.3
5 (or later)	1,645	18.7

From Pappenheimer AM Jr (1965): The diphtheria bacilli and the
dipththeroid. In Dubos RJ, Hirsch JG (eds): Bacterial and Mycotic
Infections of Man, 4th ed. Philadelphia: Lippincott, with permission.

Clostridium perfringens or snake venom. However, antibodies that bind the toxin
may not necessarily inhibit the enzymatically active sites of toxin.

Antigenic Variation

Pathogens can escape the immune system by generating variants with different antigenic composition. This mechanism for evasion of host defenses is known as ***antigenic variation***. Classical examples of pathogens that evade the host response by
antigenic variation are influenza virus, HIV, *Streptococcus pneumonia*, trypanosomes,
and Group A streptococcus. Influenza virus generates antigenic variation because it
has a segmented RNA genome that can be resorted to yield virions expressing new
combinations of the two main surface antigens: the hemagglutinin and neuraminidase
surface proteins. Antigenic variation for influenza virus occurs through both antigenic
drift and antigenic shift. ***Antigenic drift*** is the result of point mutations in the influenza virus genome, which produce antigenic changes in the hemagglutinin and neuraminidase. ***Antigenic shift*** occurs when influenza virus expresses a new allele of
hemagglutin or neuraminidase protein that results in a major antigenic change and
results in the emergence of a new viral strain. The result of antigenic drift and
antigenic shift for influenza virus is that the virus changes rapidly such that one
influenza infection does not confer protection against subsequent infection. HIV undergoes rapid antigenic variation in vivo because it has an error prone reverse transcriptase that produces mutations that translates into antigenic changes in surface
proteins. Other pathogens such as *Streptococcus pneumoniae* (pneumococcus) present the host with antigenic variation as a result of existing in multiple serotypes,
each of which has a different antigenic composition. There are over 80 pneumococcal
serotypes and infection with one serotype does not confer protection against infection
with subsequent infection with a different serotype. Hence the host must deal with
infection by each pneumococcal serotype as if it was an infection by a different
microbe. Pathogens may also encode for antigenic variation in their genomes. Trypanosomes cause chronic infections by the emergence of new antigenic types during
infection that express different variant surface glycoproteins (VSG). In a trypano-
some infection the host mounts an antibody response to the VSG being expressed
by the majority of parasites and this clears most parasites. However, in every typanosome infection there are small numbers of organisms that express a different VSG

antigen that is not recognized by the antibody response. As the antibody response helps to clear the original typanosome population, the remaining organisms expressing a different VSG then proliferate while at the same time generating a new subpopulation of antigenic variants that can survive the new antibody response. The cycle then repeats itself. Since there are many VSG genes, trypanosomes are able to cause persistent infections by producing escape variants that differ in antigenic composition in every generation. The M protein of Group A streptococcus provides another example of antigenic variation. The M protein is required for virulence and functions by preventing phagocytosis through a mechanism that involves deposition of fibrinogen on the bacterial surface. M proteins elicit protective antibody but are antigenically variable such that streptococcal infection with one strain does not elicit resistance to other strains.

Intracellular Survival

Some microorganisms are taken up by phagocytic cells but manage to survive in the intracellular environment. These pathogens include the bacteria *Mycobacterium tuberculosis* and *Listeria monocytogenes*, the fungus *Histoplasma capsulatum*, and the protozoa *Toxoplasma gondii*. In general, protection against intracellular microorganisms is the domain of cell mediated immunity although for several pathogens antibody responses also contribute to host defense. Granulomatous inflammation is a tissue manifestation of cell-mediated immunity associated with containment of several intracellular pathogens.

Although phagocytic cells are generally efficient antimicrobial cells, microbes capable of intracellular survival use any of several strategies to avoid being killed after phagocytosis. *M. tuberculosis* and *Chlamydia* block the fusion of lysosomes with the phagocytic vacuole. *H. capsulatum* interferes with acidification of the phagolysosomal vacuole. *Listeria monocytogenes* produces bacterial products that allow it to escape from the phagolysosomal vacuole to the cell cytoplasm, which presumably provides a more nutritionally favorable niche. Other bacteria like *Shigella flexneri* may promote their survival inside phagocytic cells by triggering apoptosis and death of the phagocytic cell. *Toxoplasma gondii* generates its own vacuole where its remains insulated from host lysosomes and this avoids triggering recognition of infected cells by the immune system.

Suppression of the Immune System

Some pathogens insure their survival in a mammalian host by actively suppressing the immune response. Many viruses include genes capable of modulating the immune response. For example, Epstein-Barr virus encodes a gene which produces a protein that is a homolog of IL-10 that downregulates the immune response. Other viruses like herpes simplex have virally encoded Fc and complement receptors that interfere with the function of antibody and complement. Herpes simplex virus can also interfere with recognition of infected cells by the immune system through a mechanism that inhibits MHC class 1 molecule presentation on the infected cell and blocks its interaction with virally derived peptides. The fungus *Cryptococcus neoformans* sheds large amounts of capsular polysaccharide that interfere with the formation of inflammatory responses in tissue. HIV infects a variety of cells, including CD4 T cells and hence is able to directly interfere with the cells necessary for an effective immune response. HIV-induced CD4 T-cell depletion produces a spiraling deterioration of immune function that culminates in AIDS and leaves the patient vulnerable to many opportunistic infections.

Extracellular Enzymes

Some bacteria produce enzymes that degrade immune molecules. For example, *Neisseria meningitidis* and *Neisseria gonorrhoeae* produce IgA proteases that destroy IgA in mucosal surfaces. Streptococci produce hemolysins, which are believed to aid the organism in dissemination and some elaborate a peptidase that cleaves the C5a complement protein.

Expression of Antibody Binding Proteins

Some bacteria such as streptococci express cell surface proteins that can bind immunoglobulins through their Fc region. Examples of these proteins are protein A and protein G. The ability of these proteins to bind immunoglobulin molecules is exploited in immunologic research by using them in affinity chromatography to purify IgG.

 ## PRINCIPLES OF IMMUNIZATION

Protection against infectious diseases by the use of vaccines represents an immense, if not the greatest, accomplishment of biomedical science. One disease, smallpox, has been totally eliminated by the use of immunization, and the incidence of other diseases has been significantly reduced, at least in areas of the world where immunization can be practiced correctly.

If a large enough number of individuals can be immunized, "herd immunity" is achieved, and the transmission of communicable diseases between persons is interrupted. Although deliberate immunization alone can sometimes reduce the incidence of a disease to a very low level, successful immunization programs require the intelligent practice of other measures, both hygienic and sanitary, which contribute to general improvements in public health.

Immunization can be either *active* or *passive*. *Active immunization* generally refers to the administration of a vaccine that can elicit a protective immune response. *Passive immunization* refers to the administration of antibodies or lymphocytes, which then provide protection in the recipient host. Active and passive immunizations are exemplified in Table 21.2.

 ## OBJECTIVES OF IMMUNIZATION

The objective of active immunization is to provide the individual with long lasting immunologic protection against exposure to infectious agents. Many vaccines are given in childhood to protect against infections that are usually acquired early in life. The objective of passive immunization is provide transient protection against a particular infection. For example, an individual bitten by a rabid animal may be given an injection of immune globulin to rabies virus to protect against infection

● TABLE 21.2. Examples of Active and Passive Immunization

Type of immunity	How acquired
Active	
Natural (unintended)	Infection
Artificial (deliberate)	Vaccination
Passive	
Natural	Transfer of antibody from mother to infant in placental circulation or colostrum
Artificial	Passive antibody therapy (serum therapy, administration of immune human globulin)

with this virus. Protection against the development of disease can also be conferred by postexposure immunization. For example, an individual exposed to the rabies virus can be protected against this lethal infection by administration of both rabies vaccine and immune globulin against rabies virus. Other examples of postexposure immunization include the use of toxoid and antitoxin against diphtheria, vaccination with tetanus toxoid after trauma, and administration of immune serum globulins against HAV and hepatitis B virus (HBV) after exposure. Great effort is currently aimed at the development of therapeutic vaccines that will forestall the relentless progression of AIDS in HIV-infected individuals.

The potential for use of vaccines to prevent certain cancers in humans is discussed in Chapter 20. Nevertheless, some cancers may be prevented by vaccines that prevent infections associated with the subsequent development of carcinoma. For example, there is a strong association between primary carcinoma of the liver and infection by hepatitis B virus (HBV). Hence the use of the recombinant HBV vaccine in high-risk groups may provide protection against both hepatitis and the subsequent development of hepatoma.

● HISTORICAL ASPECTS OF IMMUNIZATION

Protective active immunity (immunoprophylaxis) may result from either natural, unintended, or deliberate exposure to infectious agents or their components. This was evident to the ancient inhabitants of Asia, who intentionally exposed people to the scabs and fluid from the lesions of smallpox, a disease known in the Western world as "variola major." The practice, termed variolation, was introduced into England and its American colonies in 1721. Protection against smallpox was dependent on the presence of viral antigens in the lesions. The crudeness of the preparation assured the presence not only of inactive virus, but also of active (and virulent) virus in sufficient concentration to produce smallpox, so that some unfortunate individuals died of the disease. As a result, the practice was soon discontinued in the West.

Later in the eighteenth century it was noted that milkmaids who were exposed to cowpox (vaccinia), a disease of cattle, appeared to escape infection with smallpox. Jenner, an English physician, showed that deliberate administration of lymph from a cow with cowpox to humans led to protection against smallpox. It is evident from this cross-protection by vaccinia that the viruses of smallpox and cowpox share an antigen(s) that can induce a protective immune response. (The vaccinia virus used in modern times is known to differ genetically from the cowpox virus.)

Approximately a century later (1879) Roux, working in Pasteur's laboratory, demonstrated that bacteria that caused chicken cholera or anthrax could be weakened (*attenuated*) by certain cultivation practices in the laboratory, so that they could no longer cause disease but still retained enough antigenicity to induce immunity. Pasteur and his collaborators also showed that storage in the laboratory of tissue infected with rabies virus yielded an agent that was markedly less virulent than the parent rabies virus, but still antigenic. Pasteur called these protective antigens "vaccines" in commemoration of Jenner's work on the use of vaccinia to protect against smallpox.

Toward the end of the nineteenth century, it was discovered that certain bacteria caused disease (diphtheria, tetanus) by the release of potent exotoxins. Fortuitously, it was demonstrated that treatment of these (protein) exotoxins with formaldehyde and other chemicals eliminated their toxicity but left their antigenic properties unaffected. Formaldehyde appears to effect this change by providing methylol derivatives at the amino groups. These modified toxins, or "toxoids," have been the mainstays of immunization for many decades.

Successful cultivation of viruses in the laboratory, in in vitro conditions, was not achieved until the 1930s, when tissue-culture techniques permitted replication and attenuation of the yellow fever virus so that it could be used for a vaccine. The most significant advance, however, followed the discovery, in 1949 by Enders, Weller, and Robbins (all Nobel laureates), that poliomyelitis virus could be grown in vitro in human embryonic cells or monkey kidney cells. Recovery of sufficient quantities of virions permitted preparation of inactivated (noninfective) polio vaccine and, later, modified, attenuated viral vaccines. "Subunit" vaccines, which contain particular fractions of viruses (or bacteria), have been introduced more recently. Moreover, recent advances in vaccine technology discussed later in this chapter will, undoubtedly, result in additional effective vaccines against many infectious diseases afflicting humans and domestic animals.

 ## ACTIVE IMMUNIZATIONS

Recommended Immunizations

The usual recommended schedule in the United States for active immunization at various ages is shown in Table 21.3. In recent years a *H. influenzae* type b polysaccharide–diphtheria toxoid conjugate was added to the vaccination schedule of young children (first dose at 2 months of age). The use of this vaccine has resulted in a dramatically reduction in *H. influenzae* type b infections in vaccinated children. The vaccination schedule in the United Kingdom is similar for children, except that the age at which vaccines are administered may be slightly different, and BCG (bacille Calmette-Guérin, attenuated *Mycobacterium bovis*) vaccine is recommended for the 10 to 14-year-old age group.

In other parts of the world, the immunization schedule may be different. The World Health Organization, for example, recommends administration of BCG and oral polio vaccines at the time of birth, and measles vaccine as soon as possible after the ninth month of age (see the section Age and Timing of Immunizations below).

● TABLE 21.3. Schedule for Active Immunization of Children and Adults

Age	Vaccine
Birth	Hepatitis B (Hep B)
1–2 months	Hep B
2 months	Diphtheria and tetanus toxoids and acellular pertussis (DTP), *Haemophilus influenzae* type b (Hib), inactivated polio (IPV)
4 months	DTP, Hib, IPV, rotavirus (Rv)
6 months	Hep B, DTP, Hib, IPV, Rv
12–15 months	Oral poliovirus vaccine (OPV), measles, mumps, rubella (MMR), varicella vaccine for susceptible children
4–6 years	DTP, OPV, MMR
11–12 years	Hep B, MMR, varicella
25–64 years	Measles, rubella
>65 years	Influenza, pneumococcal disease

Adapted from JAMA, Vol 281:601–603, with permission.

Use of Vaccines in Selected Populations

In addition to the usual schedule of immunizations shown in Table 21.3, some individuals receive additional vaccinations as shown in Table 21.4. Influenza virus (inactivated) is given to persons over 60 years of age and to those with cardiorespiratory ailments. Hepatitis B vaccine (viral protein produced by recombinant DNA technology) is given to health care and emergency workers who are exposed to human blood. Hepatitis A (inactivated virus) has been approved for use in children and adults. Varicella (attenuated) is given to patients with acute lymphocytic leukemia and has recently been approved for broader use in healthy individuals. Adenovirus vaccines are used to prevent outbreaks of respiratory infections in military recruits. Vaccination against smallpox is no longer recommended for civilians but is still given to selected military personnel.

Several vaccines against bacterial infections are also used in specific populations. A polyvalent vaccine consisting of several antigenic types of capsular polysaccharides from *Streptococcus pneumoniae* is given to individuals with cardiorespiratory ailments, to anatomically or functionally asplenic individuals, and to patients with sickle-cell anemia, renal failure, alcoholic cirrhosis, or diabetes mellitus. These individuals have limited capability to mount the antibody/complement/phagocytic activity required against the encapsulated bacteria such as *S. pneumoniae*. Unfortunately, this vaccine may not be as effective in persons at high risk for pneumococcal pneumonia as in normal individuals because the immune defects preclude the generation of strong antibody responses. *S. pneumoniae* polysaccharide–protein conjugate vaccines has proven effective in preliminary clinical studies and may be available soon for protection of pneumococcal infection. *Neisseria meningitidis* vaccine (several serogroups of capsular polysaccharide) is given to military recruits and to children in high-risk regions. Both live attenuated and a polysaccharide vaccines are available for protection against *Salmonella typhi*, the cause of typhoid fever. Because of some unique needs or limited efficacy, some vaccines are recommended only under limited circumstances. A vaccine against Lyme disease has recently been li-

T A B L E 21.4. Selective Use of Vaccines Under Limited Circumstances

Occupational or other exposure	Vaccine
Susceptible health-care personnel, homosexual males, intravenous drug users	Hepatitis B
Susceptible health-care personnel	Measles, mumps, influenza, varicella, rubella
Health-care personnel in close contact with tuberculosis patients	BCG
Veterinarians, animal handlers, and animal bite victims	Rabies
Handlers of imported animal hides, furs, bonemeal, wool, and animal bristles	Anthrax
Military personnel	Meningococcus, yellow fever, anthrax
Includes individuals who live and work in grassy and wooded regions containing ticks infected with *Borrelia burgdorferi*	Lyme
Travelers to certain areas	Meningococcus, yellow fever, cholera, typhoid fever, plague, Japanese B encephalitis, polio

censed for use in persons at high risk for infection. Concern about the potential use of anthrax spores in biologic warfare has led the United States military to require vaccination of all personnel. These vaccines and appropriate circumstances are described in Table 21.4.

BASIC MECHANISMS OF PROTECTION

Anatomic Location of Host Immune Response

There are differences in the intravascular–extravascular distribution of immunoglobulins (see Table 4.1). For example, local synthesis of secretory IgA in the lamina propria, beneath a mucous membrane, yields antibody at the epithelial surface (respiratory or intestinal), an area through which certain pathogens or their toxins may enter. IgA is the predominant Ig in secretions of the nasal, bronchial, intestinal, and genitourinary tracts, and in saliva, colostrum, and bile. Oral administration of attenuated polio virus (**Sabin vaccine**) leads to demonstrable IgA to polio in nasal and duodenal secretions, whereas parenteral injection of inactivated polio virus (**Salk vaccine**) does not. The local antibodies generated by the Sabin vaccine provide the advantage of intercepting of the polio virus at the portal of entry. However, some IgG and IgM may be found in local secretions, so that serum Ig may also play a role at an epithelial surface (while IgM appears to have restricted access to extravascular areas, both IgG and IgM can be found in inflammatory exudates). In addition, the hematogenous (viremic or bacteremic) stage of several infections that are acquired through a mucous membrane can lead to an encounter between infectious agent and antibody in the circulation as well as the extravascular fluid. Thus, the Salk vaccine given parenterally induces immunity to polio virus during its viremic stage.

There are some unique, but still poorly understood, differences in the partitioning of immunoglobulins in serum and secretions. For example, while IgG_4 represents only 3.5% of the plasma IgG, it constitutes 15% of IgG in colostrum. In the cerebrospinal fluid, IgG and IgM may be found as a result of local production in the central nervous system due to the stimulus by infectious agents.

Significance of the Primary and Secondary Responses

The rapidity of the anamnestic response to a reencounter with antigen provides the host with potential protection upon repeated exposures to an infectious agent. This anamnestic response is relevant in at least two significant ways in the application of immunoprophylaxis. First, it may be of particular importance in those infections with a relatively long incubation period (>7 days), as is illustrated in Figure 21.1. Thus, an individual infected by agent A, which causes disease after a 3-day incubation period, would produce a primary immune response some time (e.g., 7–14 days) after onset of the infection. On a second encounter with agent A, the individual may again develop disease, because an anamnestic response may not be sufficiently rapid to

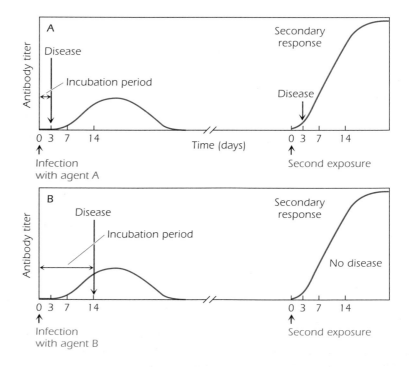

Figure 21.1. The relationship between the primary and secondary immune responses and disease produced by infection with agent A or B. Infection caused by agent A has shorter incubation period than infection caused by agent B.

inhibit agent A (Figure 21.1A). The individual infected with agent B, which causes disease after a 14-day incubation period, would produce a primary response (e.g., some 7–14 days after infection). On a second encounter with agent A, the anamnestic response occurring within 7 days would be sufficient to reduce the severity or prevent the disease with the 14-day incubation period (Figure 21.1B).

The second influence of the anamnestic response concerns the level to which the immune response has been raised. In the example cited above, agent B, which causes disease in 3 days, may be prevented from causing disease after a reexposure if there is a persisting high enough level of antibody. Such a level can be achieved deliberately by a series of immunizations (especially applicable with nonviable antigens). Thus, it is customary to give several injections of tetanus toxoid (as DTP) over a period of 6 months in childhood immunizations. Such a "primary series" of injections generates anamnestic secondary responses that successively raise the concentration of antitoxin to protective levels, which are sustained in the serum for 10–20 years.

Protective Effect of the Immune Response

Acquired immune responses may exert their effects essentially independently of certain innate defense mechanisms (for example, neutralization of bacterial exotoxin by antitoxic antibody). Alternatively, these acquired responses may function in concert with other components of the host defense apparatus, (for example, when antibody functions to opsonize infectious particles, or when antibody interacts with complement and an infectious agent leading to lysis of the agent).

Age and Timing of Immunizations

The various mechanisms involved in protection, described in the preceding section, can be affected by several factors, including nutritional status, presence of underlying disease (which affects levels of globulin or cell-mediated immunity), and age. The timing of childhood immunization is driven largely by the fact that the efficacy of certain vaccines is variable depending on the age of the child.

In utero, the human fetus normally appears well insulated from antigens and most infectious agents, although certain pathogens (e.g., rubella virus) can infect the mother and seriously injure the fetus. The immunity of the mother protects the fetus by permitting interception and removal of infectious agents before they can enter the uterus, or it protects the newborn by virtue of transplacental or mammary gland antibody.

The fetus and neonate have poorly developed lymphoid organs, with the exception of the thymus, which at the time of birth is largest in size relative to the body size at any age. The fetus appears capable of synthesizing mainly IgM, which becomes apparent after 6 months of gestation. Levels of IgM gradually increase to about 10% of the adult level at the time of birth.

IgG becomes detectable in the fetus at about the second month of gestation, but it is IgG of maternal origin. The level of IgG increases significantly at about 4 months of gestation and markedly in the last trimester. At the time of birth the concentration of IgG slightly exceeds the maternal concentration of IgG. Thus, the fetus is provided with maternally synthesized IgG antibodies, which can provide antitoxic, antiviral, and some kinds of antibacterial protection. The levels of these maternal antibodies gradually decline as the infant begins to synthesize its own antibodies, so that total IgG at 2–3 months of age is less than 50% of the level at birth. The serum concentrations of immunoglobulins during human development are shown in Figure 21.2.

Some aspects of the immune response of the newborn, for example, against some infectious agents (*Toxoplasma*, *Listeria*, herpes simplex virus) in which cell-mediated immunity is critical, are not well developed. But the newborn can produce antibody to various antigens, such as parenterally administered toxoid, inactivated poliomyelitis virus, orally administered attenuated poliomyelitis virus, and others. However, administration of pertussis vaccine very soon after birth not only fails to induce a protective response but also creates an impaired response (tolerance?) to the vaccine when it is given again later in infancy. Therefore, in most industrialized countries the initial administration of vaccines is deferred until the child is 2 months old. However, the WHO recommends earlier commencement of immunization (at 6 weeks) in developing countries.

Maternal antibody, while capable of providing protection to the neonate against a variety of infectious agents or their toxins, may also reduce the response to antigen. For example, a sufficient quantity of maternal measles antibody persists in the 1-year-old infant to interfere with the active response of the infant to the vaccine, so that vaccination is usually delayed until the child is at least 1 year of age.

Children less than 2 years of age have a general inability to produce adequate levels of antibody in response to injection of bacterial capsular polysaccharides, such as those of *Haemophilus influenzae* type b, various serogroups of *Neisseria meningitidis*, and *Streptococcus pneumoniae* serotypes. It has been suggested that this inability arises because infants do not respond to T-independent antigens, despite their early (in utero) capacity to generate IgM. Chemical linkage of polysaccharide to T-dependent antigens, such as diphtheria toxoid, or to *N. meningitidis* outer membrane protein, has improved the immunogenicity such that children under 2 years of age respond to polysaccharides. An effective conjugate vaccine is already available against *H. influenzae*, which has virtually eliminated this infection in vaccinated

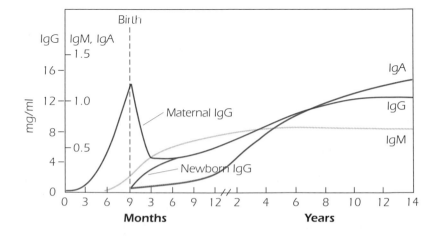

Figure 21.2. Concentration of immunoglobulin in the serum during human development. [After Benich H. Johanssen SGO (1971): *Adv Immunol* 13:1, with permission.]

children. Conjugate vaccines against *S. pneumoniae* are in advanced clinical development, which will, it is hoped, provide protection against this important bacterial pathogen.

At the other end of the age spectrum—in people older than 60 years of age—there also appears to be a reduced capability to mount a primary response to some antigens, such as influenza virus vaccine, but the elderly retain the ability to mount a secondary response to antigens to which they have been previously exposed. The healthy elderly also respond well to bacterial polysaccharides, so that administration of pneumococcal polysaccharide vaccine can usually induce protective levels of antibody. Other groups, besides the elderly, who are especially susceptible to pneumococcal pneumonia (see the section Active Immunization in this chapter) should also be immunized. The same groups as those who have enhanced susceptibility to the encapsulated respiratory pathogen *Streptococcus pneumoniae* and to persons at high risk of exposure (e.g., residents of nursing homes and medical personnel) should also receive influenza vaccines.

Use of Mixed, Multiple Antigens

Routine immunization against some infectious agents is simplified by their having a single antigenic type (e.g., the toxins of diphtheria and tetanus, polysaccharide of *Haemophilus influenzae* type b, and various viruses such as measles, mumps, and rubella). However, immunization against other agents (e.g., poliovirus and pneumococci) must provide protection against several antigenic types. The host can be vaccinated simultaneously with several antigens and still generate adequate responses, although in some instances the generation of sufficient immunity requires repeated (booster) administration of antigen(s). The usual, initial immunizations of children entails the injection of hepatitis B, diphtheria and tetanus toxoids, acellular *Bordetella pertussis*, *Haemophilus influenzae* type b conjugate vaccine, inactivated polio virus, and rotavirus vaccines. The estimated 10^{12} lymphoid cells in the human body are capable of responding to a huge array of antigens without significant competition. Although there is a possibility that a live viral vaccine may inhibit the immune response to a second live viral vaccine given a few days later, this interference does not appear to be of practical importance. Thus, it has been ascertained that simultaneous injection of measles, mumps, and rubella vaccines provides a protective response to all three of these viruses.

 PRECAUTIONS

Site of Administration of Antigen

The usual site of parenteral (intradermal, subcutaneous, intramuscular) administration of vaccines is the arm, in particular the deltoid muscle. Studies have shown a suboptimal response to hepatitis B vaccine when given by intragluteal injection, as compared with injection in the arm. The parenteral administration of inactivated polio vaccine may induce a higher antibody response in the serum than the attenuated oral polio vaccine, but the response to the latter, which includes secretory IgA, affords adequate protection.

Some vaccines may provide a greater antibody response when given by the respiratory route than when given by injection (e.g., attenuated measles vaccine), but administration via the respiratory route remains an investigational method.

Hazards

There are potential hazards associated with the use of some vaccines. Vaccines made from attenuated agents (e.g., measles, mumps, rubella, oral polio, bacille Calmette-Guérin) have the potential for causing progressive disease in the immunocompromised patient or in the patient on immunosuppressive therapy. In rare cases, reversion of attenuated poliovirus type III to virulence in the intestine of the vaccinated individual has caused paralytic polio; for this reason, some investigators favor the use of inactivated polio vaccine, which is used exclusively in some countries. Concern about vaccine-associated paralytic polio has resulted in a change in recommendations for vaccination against polio virus such that the inactivated poliovirus vaccine is now given first followed by the live attenuated vaccine.

Live attenuated organisms should ordinarily not be given to pregnant women because of potential damage to the fetus. (The virions in rubella vaccine have been transmitted to the fetus, although without any recognized injurious effect.) Live attenuated vaccines are generally contraindicated for patients with severe immune disorders that may not be able to control the weakened pathogen in the vaccine preparation. Vaccination against smallpox is no longer carried out (except in some military personnel) since the disease has been eradicated; however, if vaccinia should be utilized in the future as a carrier for other antigens (discussed in a subsequent section), care must be taken because this virus can cause serious problems, not only in immunocompromised individuals but also in individuals with certain cutaneous lesions. Contact between vaccinated and vulnerable individuals must be avoided until the vaccinia lesions have healed.

Arthritis and arthralgia are common but transient complications following vaccination with attenuated rubella virus, particularly in adult women. Of the inactivated vaccines, the killed *Bordetella pertussis* bacterial vaccine in DTP was associated with some serious side effects, including encephalopathy in the infant. Although serious side effects were relatively rare and the benefits of the pertussis vaccine outweighed any of alleged risks of immunization, the killed bacteria vaccine was replaced by an acellular vaccine containing inactivated pertussis toxin and one or more antigenic components (e.g., filamentous hemagglutinin and fimbriae). The acellular pertussis vaccine has significant fewer side effects than the earlier vaccine while retaining efficacy.

Tetanus and diphtheria toxoids may provoke local hypersensitivity reactions. Because an adequate initial series of immunizations in childhood appears to give immunity that lasts some 10 years, the use of "booster" injections of tetanus toxoid should be guided by the nature of an injury and the history of immunization. The increased hypersensitivity to diphtheria toxoid of adolescents and adults necessitates use of a smaller dose of diphtheria toxoid than is used for children. Because influenza virus is cultivated in chick embryos, allergy to egg protein is a contraindication to vaccination against this virus. Whole influenza virus vaccine is used in adults but gives side effects in children, so a split-virus component vaccine is recommended for persons under 13 years of age. Some vaccines contain preservatives, such as the organomercurial compound thimerosal (Merthiolate), or antibiotics, such as neomycin or streptomycin, to which the vaccinated individual may be allergic.

RECENT APPROACHES TO PRODUCTION OF VACCINES

Advances in recombinant DNA technology and in the technology of rapid, automated synthesis of peptides and other areas of bioengineering (e.g., monoclonal antibodies) hold promise for improvements in available vaccines and new approaches to the production of vaccines.

Vaccines Produced by Recombinant DNA

Recombinant DNA technology provides the means for expressing protein antigens in large amounts for vaccine use. An example of the successful application of recombinant DNA technology to vaccine production is provided by the experience with the hepatitis B vaccine. Hepatitis B is a major cause of liver infection and is associated with a long term risk of hepatocellular carcinoma. An effective vaccine against hepatitis B was developed in the 1970s by purifying viral antigen from the blood of chronically infected donors. In the 1980s, the HIV epidemic heightened awareness about transmission of blood borne pathogens and there were concerns that this vaccine could transmit disease. Although several studies showed the plasma-derived vaccine was safe, an alternative was developed by expressing the hepatitis B antigen in yeast using recombinant DNA technology. This recombinant vaccine simplified the production of antigen by avoiding reliance on human blood plasma and eliminated any potential hazard arising from inadvertent contamination of vaccine antigen with bloodborne pathogens. Recombinant DNA technology has also been used to generate the first effective vaccine against Lyme disease. Other vaccines produced by recombinant DNA technology are in various stages of clinical testing. Some of these molecular approaches may provide practical, safer and more effective means of immunization than are currently available.

Conjugated Polysaccharides

Conjugated polysaccharide vaccines have revolutionized the approach to vaccination against encapsulated bacterial pathogens. Humoral immunity is critical for protection against encapsulated pathogens but most microbial polysaccharides are T-independent antigens, which are usually poorly immunogenic. Another problem with polysaccharide vaccines is that young children tend not to mount antibody responses to polysaccharide antigens. Children are at high risk for infection with encapsulated bacteria such as *Streptococcus pneumoniae* and *Haemophilus influenzae*. Conjugation of polysaccharide to a protein (e.g., tetanus or diphtheria toxoid) results in a molecule that behaves as a T-dependent antigen and elicits strong antibody responses to the polysaccharide moiety. Conjugation of such (bacterial) polysaccharides or oligosaccharides (e.g., of *Haemophilus influenzae*), to proteins such as diphtheria toxoid has provided vaccines that are effective in this age group. In fact, use of *Haemophilus influenzae* type b conjugate vaccine has led to a virtual elimination of this infection in vaccinated children. A conjugated polysaccharide vaccine against certain serotypes of *Streptococcus pneumoniae* may be available soon. Conjugated polysaccharide vaccines are under development for other pathogens including meningococci, group B streptococci, *Salmonella typhi* and *Shigella* species. Conjugated polysaccharide vaccines are protective by eliciting strong antibody responses to the polysaccharide portion of the conjugate.

Synthetic Peptide Vaccines

The premise underlying synthetic peptide vaccine development is to use immunogenic peptides to elicit a protective immune response. Synthetic peptide vaccines are designed using the knowledge of the amino acid sequence of the protein antigen that elicits a protective immune response. In theory, synthetic peptide vaccines have the advantage that highly purified peptides may be made in large quantities and their simpler antigenic composition may afford protection with fewer side effects. The general approach is to identify potential epitopes in a protective protein antigen using various algorithms, synthesize a series of peptides corresponding to the amino acid sequence, and test these for immunologic activity. One problem with peptide vaccines is that peptides are poorly immunogenic due to their small size and require conjugation to carrier proteins. Several synthetic peptide vaccines are currently in clinical testing. A word of caution: if the vaccine consists of a peptide comprising an epitope recognized by B cells and a carrier recognized by T cells, no anamnestic (memory) response should be expected when the immunized individual encounters the B-cell epitope on a different carrier such as, for example, on the natural antigen from which the B-cell epitope has been taken (the carrier effect, described in Chapter 10).

Blocking of Specific Receptors

Since many pathogens must attach to specific host receptors to cause infection, immune responses that block the ligand–receptor interaction may be protective. Several vaccines that can block access to the receptors, such as by molecular mimicry of the ligand on the pathogen, are currently in development.

Anti-Idiotype Vaccines

An antibody (idiotype) induced to a specific epitope of an antigen has a combining site that structurally fits the epitope. If that antibody, in turn, is used as an immunogen to induce an antibody (an anti-idiotype) that reacts with the antigen-combining site of the idiotype, the anti-idiotype may structurally mimic the epitope. This structural mimicry is referred to as an "*internal image*." Because of the resemblance of the anti-idiotype and the original antigen epitope, its internal image (anti-idiotypic antibody) can be used as an immunogen to induce antibodies against the original epitope (Figure 21.3).

An example is an immunogen consisting of antibodies made in mice against a monoclonal mouse antibody to hepatitis B surface antigen. Immunization with these anti-idiotypic antibodies that contain the "internal image" of an epitope on the hepatitis B surface antigen induces antibodies to that epitope. When the toxic effects of certain biologic toxins preclude their use as antigens, anti-idiotypic antibodies can be used to elicit an antitoxic response.

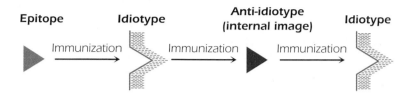

Figure 21.3. A representation of an anti-idiotype (internal image) immunogen.

Virus-Carrier Vaccine

It is possible to introduce into a live virus, such as vaccinia, adenovirus, or poliovirus by means of a vector, a gene from another organism that codes for a desired antigen. The vaccinia virus construct replicates in the host, expresses the foreign gene and then serves as a vaccine to that particular antigen. This approach is useful provided that the vaccinia virus is not hazardous to the host (as it may be to an immunocompromised individual). This virus-carrier vaccine has the additional advantage in that it can potentially induce both cell-mediated and antibody-mediated immunity to the incorporated antigen.

Bacterium-Carrier Vaccine

Attenuated bacteria such as strains of *Salmonella typhimurium*, *Escherichia coli*, and BCG can also serve as carriers for pathogen genes in an effort to elicit pathogen specific responses. These bacteria are altered by recombinant techniques, which introduce a foreign gene that can express the antigens of pathogenic microbes and induce immune responses. *S. typhimurium*, an intestinal pathogen, could be used to induce mucosal immunity to the foreign antigens.

DNA Vaccines

Recently it was discovered that vaccination with a plasmid encoding the DNA sequence for a protective antigen linked to a strong mammalian promoter could elicit an immune response to the protein. DNA vaccines are thought to work by allowing the expression of the microbial antigen inside host cells that take up the plasmid. DNA vaccines function by generating of the desired antigen inside cells and this has the advantage that it may facilitate MHC presentation. Other advantages of DNA vaccines are the absence of infection risk, greater stability relative to protein vaccines, and the possibility of delivering the antigen to cells that are not usually infected by the pathogen for better modulation of the immune response. DNA vaccines could be useful for immunizing young children who still have maternal antibody. The feasibility of DNA immunization has now been demonstrated against several viral, bacterial, and protozoal infections in laboratory animals. One concern with DNA vaccines is the possibility that they could be mutagenic by integrating in host DNA. At this time DNA vaccines are the subject of intense experimental study.

Toxoids

Toxins can be inactivated to produce toxoids for vaccination. Toxoids are among the earliest and most successful vaccines. Administration of toxoids prepared from inactivated tetanus, botulism or diphtheria toxin elicit antibody responses that prevent disease. Toxoids are effective despite the fact that natural infection does not always confer long-lasting immunity, presumably because the amount of toxin produced in infection may not be sufficient to elicit a strong immune response. Hence a bout of tetanus or diphtheria does not confer immunity to recurrent infection but vaccination with a toxoid provides full protection.

 PASSIVE IMMUNIZATION

Passive immunization results from the transfer of antibody or immune cells to one individual from another individual who has already responded to direct stimulation by antigen. Passive immunization differs from active immunization in that it does not rely on the ability of the host's immune system to make the appropriate response. Hence passive immunization with antibodies results in the immediate availability of antibodies that can mediate protection against pathogens. Passive immunization can occur naturally as is the case during transfer of antibodies through the placenta or colostrum or therapeutically when preformed antibody is administered for the prophylaxis or therapy of infectious diseases.

Passive Immunization Through Placental Antibody Transfer

The developing fetus is passively immunized with maternal IgG as a result of placental transfer of antibody. Such antibodies are present at birth and protect the infant against those infections for which IgG is sufficient and for which the mother had immunity. For example, transfer of antibody to toxins (tetanus, diphtheria), viruses (measles, poliovirus, mumps, etc.) and certain bacteria (*Haemophilus influenzae* or *Streptococcus agalactiae* group B) can provide protection to the child in the first months of life. Hence adequate active immunization of the mother is a simple and effective means of providing passive protection to the fetus and infant. (However, some premature infants may not acquire the maternal antibodies to the extent that full-term infants do.) Toxoid vaccination can elicit IgG responses that cross the placenta to provide protection to the fetus and newborn. This protection is extremely important in areas of the world where an unclean obstetric environment can lead to tetanus neonatorum (of the newborn).

Passive Immunization via Colostrum

Human milk contains a variety of factors that may influence the response of the nursing infant to infectious agents. Some of these factors are natural selective factors that can affect the intestinal microflora, namely, by enhancement of growth of desirable bacteria and by nonspecific inhibitors of some microbes, by the action of lysozyme, lactoferrin, interferon, and leukocytes (macrophages, T cells, B cells, and granulocytes). Antibodies (IgA) are found in breast milk, the concentration being higher in the colostrum (first milk) immediately postpartum (Table 21.5). The pro-

● T A B L E 21.5. Levels of Immunoglobulin in Colostrum[a]

Class	Day postpartum				Approximate normal adult
	1	2	3	4	
IgA[b]	600	260	200	80	200
IgG[c]	80	45	30	16	1,000
IgM	125	65	58	30	120

[a]After Michael JR, Ringenback R, Hottenstein S. (1971): *J Infect Dis* 124:445.
[b]80% of this is secretory IgA.
[c]IgG$_4$ represents 15% of colostral IgG and 3.5% of serum IgG.

duction of antibody is the result of B cells that are stimulated by intestinal antigens and migrate to the breast where they produce immunoglobulin (the "enteromammary system"). Thus, organisms colonizing or infecting the alimentary tract of the mother may lead to production of colostral antibody, which affords mucosal protection to the nursing infant against pathogens that enter via the intestinal tract. Antibody to the enteropathogens *Escherichia coli*, *Salmonella typhi*, *Shigella* species, poliomyelitis virus, and coxsackievirus and echovirus have been demonstrated. Feeding a mixture of IgA (73%) and IgG (26%) derived from human serum to low-birth-weight infants who could not have access to mothers' breast milk protected them against necrotizing enterocolitis. (Antibodies to nonalimentary pathogens have also been demonstrated in colostrum—e.g., tetanus and diphtheria antitoxins, and antistreptococcal hemolysin.)

Tuberculin-sensitive T lymphocytes are also transmitted to the infant through the colostrum, but the role of such cells in passive transfer of cell-mediated immunity is uncertain.

Passive Antibody Therapy and Serum Therapy

The administration of specific antibody preparations was one of the first effective antimicrobial therapies. Antibody against particular pathogens could be raised in animals such as horses and rabbits (heterologous antibody) and administered to humans for treatment of various infections as *serum therapy*. Serum from individuals recovering from infection is rich in antibodies and can also be used for passive antibody therapy (homologous antibody). In recent years, some monoclonal antibodies made in the laboratory have been used for passive antibody therapy of infectious diseases. This is an area of great research activity and it is likely that more antimicrobial therapies based on antibody administration will be developed in the future.

The active agent in serum therapy is specific antibody. In the preantibiotic era (before 1935) serum therapy was often the only therapy available for the treatment of infection. Serum therapy was used for the treatment of diphtheria, tetanus, pneumococcal pneumonia, meningococcal meningitis, scarlet fever, and other serious infections. For example, in World War I tetanus antitoxin produced in horses injected with tetanus toxoid was used to treat the wounded British troops and resulted in prompt reduction in cases of tetanus. This experience allowed the determination of the minimum concentration of antitoxin needed to provide protection and also showed that the period of protection in the human was brief. The basis for the latter

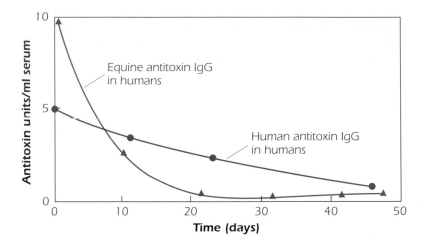

Figure 21.4. Serum concentration of human and equine IgG antitoxin following administration into humans.

is shown schematically in Figures 21.4 and 21.5. The heterologous equine antibody in the human undergoes dilution, catabolism, immune complex formation, and immune elimination. By contrast, the homologous human antibody, which reaches a peak level in the serum about 2 days after subcutaneous injection, undergoes dilution and catabolism with a reduction to half the maximal concentration in about 23 days (the half-life of human IgG_1, IgG_2, and IgG_4 is 23 days; that of IgG_3 is 7 days). The protective level of the human antibody is thus sustained considerably longer than that of the equine antibody. Heterologous antibody, such as that from the horse, can cause at least two kinds of hypersensitivity reaction: type I (immediate, anaphylaxis) or type III (serum sickness from immune complexes). If no other treatment is avail-

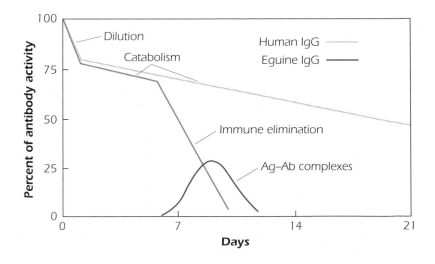

Figure 21.5. The fate of human and equine IgG following administration into humans.

able, it is possible to use the heterologous antiserum in an individual with type I sensitivity by administration of gradually increasing but minute amounts of the foreign serum, given repeatedly over several hours. Some preparations of heterologous antibody [e.g., equine diphtheria antitoxin and antilymphocyte serum (ALS)] are still used in humans. In recent years advances in hybridoma and recombinant DNA technology provide the means to synthesize human immunoglobulins for therapy and we are no longer dependent on animal sources for therapeutic antibodies. Human antibodies have significantly longer half life and reduced toxicity in humans.

Monoclonal and Polyclonal Preparations

Hybridoma technology that allows the production of monoclonal antibodies was discovered in 1975 (see Chapter 5). Polyclonal preparations result from the antibody response to immunization or recovery from infection in a host. In general, antibody to a specific agent is only a small fraction of the total antibody in a polyclonal preparation. Furthermore, polyclonal preparations usually contain antibodies to multiple antigens and include antibodies of various isotypes. Monoclonal antibody (mAb) preparations differ from polyclonal antibody preparations in that a mAb has one specificity and one isotype. As a result the activity of mAb preparations is considerably greater for the amount of protein present than polyclonal preparations. Another advantage of monoclonal preparations is that they are invariant and do not have the lot-to-lot variability associated with polyclonal preparations that are dependent on quantitative and qualitative aspects of the immune response for their potency. However, polyclonal preparations have the advantage that, by including antibodies with multiple specificities and isotypes, they encompass a higher biologic diversity. Several mAb and polyclonal antibody preparations are currently used for human therapy.

Preparation and Properties of Human Immune Serum Globulin

The use of immune globulin from human serum began in the early 1900s, when serum of patients convalescing from measles was given to children who had been exposed to measles but had not yet developed symptoms. Additional attempts in 1916, and later, showed that early administration of serum obtained from individuals who had recovered from infection with measles virus, could protect against the emergence of clinically apparent measles. In 1933 human placentae were also recognized as a source of measles antibody. A problem with using serum for passive therapy is that it contains relatively little antibody in a large volume. In the early 1940s Cohn and colleagues devised a method for the separation of the "gammaglobulin" (γ-globulin) fraction from human serum by precipitation with cold ethanol. This "Cohn fractionation" represented a practical and safe method for production of homologous human antibody for clinical use. Plasma is collected from healthy donors or placentae. The plasma or serum from several donors is pooled and the preparation is termed immune serum globulin (ISG) or human normal immunoglobulin (HNI). If the plasma or serum is from donors who are specially selected after an immunizing or booster dose of antigen, or after convalescence from a specific infection, the specific immune globulin preparation is designated accordingly [e.g., tetanus immune globulin (TIG), hepatitis B (HBIG), varicella-zoster (VZIG), or rabies (RIG)]. Large quantities can be obtained by plasmapheresis—removal of the plasma while returning the blood cells to the donor. The fraction containing antibody globulin(s) is precipitated by cold ethanol. The resultant preparation (1) is theoretically free of hepatitis virus and HIV, (2) concentrates many of the IgG antibodies about 25-fold, (3) is stable for years, and (4) can provide peak levels in blood approximately 2 days after intramuscular injection. Preparations that are safe when administered intravenously (called IVIG or IVGG) involve cold alcohol precipitation followed by various other treatments, including fractionation using polyethylene glycol or ion exchangers; acidification to pH 4–4.5; exposure to pepsin or trypsin; and stabilization with maltose, sucrose, glucose, or glycine. Such stabilization reduces aggregation of the globulins that can trigger anaphylactoid reactions (see the section Precautions). In these newer intravenous preparations, IgG is present in about one-third to one-fourth its concentration in the intramuscular immune globulin preparations and there is only a "trace" of IgA and IgM (see Table 21.6).

Indications for the Use of Immune Globulin

Antibody to RhD antigen (Rhogam) is given to Rh$^-$ mothers within a 72-hour perinatal period to prevent their immunization by fetal Rh$^+$ erythrocytes that could affect future pregnancies. As discussed in Chapter 15, Rhogam administration protects by promoting the removal of Rh$^+$ fetal cells to which the mother is exposed during parturition, and thus avoids the sensitizing of the Rh$^-$ mother by Rh$^+$ antigens. Tetanus immune globulin (TIG) (antitoxin) is used to provide passive protection after certain wounds and in the absence of adequate active immunization with tetanus toxoid. Varicella-zoster immune globulin (VZIG) is given to leukemics who are highly vulnerable to the varicella-zoster (chickenpox) virus and to pregnant women and their infants exposed to or infected with varicella virus. Cytomegalovirus human immune globulin (CMV-IGIV) is used prophylactically for recipients of bone marrow or renal transplants. Rabies immune globulin (RIG) is given together with active immunization with human diploid cell rabies vaccine to individuals bitten by potentially rabid animals (human RIG is not universally available so equine antibody may be necessary in some areas). Hepatitis B immune globulin (HBIG) may be given to a newborn child of a mother with evidence of hepatitis B infection, to medical personnel after an accidental stick with a hypodermic needle, or after sexual contact with an individual with hepatitis B. (ISG may also be used against hepatitis B; see below.) Vaccinia immune globulin is given to eczematous or immunocompromised individuals with intimate exposure to others who have been vaccinated against small-

⬤ T A B L E 21.6. Comparison of Human Immune Serum Globulin

Source	Immunoglobulin (mg/100 ml)		
	IgG	IgA	IgM
Whole serum	1,200	180	200
Immune serum globulin	16,500	100–500	25–200
Intravenous immunoglobulin	3000–5,000	trace	trace
Placental immune serum globulin	16,500	200–700	150–400

pox by live attenuated vaccinia vaccine. Such compromised individuals can develop destructive progressive disease from the attenuated vaccine.

IVIG has been used in certain circumstances for its antimicrobial properties. IVIG has had significant success against group B streptococcal infections in premature neonates, echovirus induced chronic meningoencephalitis, and against Kawasaki's disease, a condition of unknown etiology. IVIG administration can reduce bacterial infections in patients with hematopoietic malignancies, such as chronic B-cell lymphocytic leukemia or multiple myeloma. Chronic IVIG administration has been useful in children with immunosuppressive conditions and in premature infants; in hypogammaglobulinemia and primary immune deficiency disease repeated injections of ISG are required. IVIG also has therapeutic value in a variety of autoimmune conditions. For example, in immune idiopathic thrombocytopenic purpura (ITP), IVIG presumably blocks the Fc receptors on phagocytic cells and prevents them from phagocytosing and destroying platelets coated with autoantibodies. IVIG has also been used with varying success in other immune cytopenias.

Precautions on the Use of Immune Therapy

The preparations of globulin other than IVIG have to be given by the intramuscular route, since intravenous administration is contraindicated because of possible anaphylactoid reactions. These are probably due to aggregates of Ig formed during the fractionation by ethanol precipitation. These aggregates activate complement to yield anaphylatoxins (IgG$_1$, IgG$_2$, IgG$_3$, and IgM by the classical pathway; IgG$_4$ and IgA, by the alternative pathway) or crosslink Fc receptors directly leading to the release of inflammatory mediators. The IVIG safe for intravenous administration has been increasingly used, particularly when repeated administration is required as in agammaglobulinemia.

One unique contraindication to the use of the usual immune globulin preparations is in cases of congenital deficiency of IgA. Since these patients lack IgA, they recognize it as a foreign protein and respond by making antibodies against it, including IgE antibodies that can lead to a subsequent anaphylactic reaction. The IVIG preparations with only a trace of IgA may pose less of a problem.

 IMMUNOTHERAPY

Historically, the major form of immunotherapy (treating an existing disease) used for the treatment of infectious diseases was serum therapy, which was largely abandoned in the early 1940s because of the toxicity of heterologous sera and the introduction of antimicrobial chemotherapy. For many years, postexposure passive immunization described above, was the major application of immunotherapy to the treatment of infectious diseases. In recent years there has been renewed interest in the potential of immunotherapy because of several developments including a marked increase in the prevalence of drug-resistant microbes, increasing numbers of individuals with chronic immune suppression as a consequence of the HIV epidemic and medical advances, and the emergence of new infectious agents for which there is no effective therapy.

Antibody Therapies

The use of immunoglobulin preparations for postexposure prophylaxis has already been mentioned. In general, antibody administration is more effective if given before infection than after the onset of clinical symptoms. Nevertheless, there is a large body of evidence that, in some circumstances, antibody can be given to treat established infection. In this regard, serum therapy for pneumococcal and meningococcal infections was highly effective in reducing mortality in the pre-antibiotic era. Recently, antibody therapy has been shown to be effective against human respiratory syncytial virus and cryptosporidium infections. Antibody preparations are now available for therapy of RSV infections in children. Antibody therapies have the advantage that they provide the host with a natural product that can enhance immune function. However, antibody preparations are usually very expensive and require intravenous administration for the treatment of systemic infections. Many antibody preparations against infectious agents are currently under development and one can anticipate that more will be available in the future.

Antibody directed against cytokines that produce undesirable effects in certain clinical situations may provide a useful immunotherapeutic modality. For example, septic shock is a physiologic response of the host to microbial products. This response leads to the release of cytokines, arachidonic acid derivatives, kinins, and other substances that can affect endothelial, myocardial, and other cells, with resultant organ dysfunction, such as oliguria (scanty urination), hypotension, and altered mental status. Administration of antibodies that neutralize microbial products or host-produced cytokines may interrupt the sequence of events leading to septic shock and thus provide a useful adjunctive therapy in the management of certain infections.

Colony Stimulating Factors

Colony stimulating factors (CSFs), as discussed in Chapter 12, are host proteins that stimulate the development and maturation of white blood cells. Granulocyte-colony-stimulating factor (G-CSF), granulocyte-macrophage colony stimulating factor (GM-CSF) and macrophage-colony stimulating factor (M-CSF) have been cloned by recombinant DNA technology and are now available for clinical use. CSFs have proven to be useful in accelerating the recovery of bone marrow cells in patients who have undergone myelosuppressive therapy for cancer or organ transplantation. In these patients neutrophil depletion (neutropenia) is a major predisposing factor for severe infection. By shortening the period of neutropenia CSFs can reduce the incidence of serious infections in patients receiving myelosuppressive therapy. CSFs also enhance leukocyte function and there is encouraging preliminary information suggesting that these proteins may be useful as immunotherapy for enhancing host defenses against various pathogens.

Several other cytokines are powerful activators of the immune system and there is great interest in learning how to use them as adjunctive therapy against infectious diseases. IFN-γ is a powerful activator of macrophage function, which has been shown to reduce the incidence of severe infections in patients with chronic granulomatous disease. IFN-γ has shown encouraging results as adjunctive therapy for some infections, including drug-resistant *Mycobacterium tuberculosis* infection and several unusual fungal infections.

SUMMARY

1. To cause disease microbes must gain entry and survive in the host and cause damage.

2. The effective host defenses against individual pathogens depend on the type of pathogen.

3. Pathogens use a variety of strategies to escape host defenses including: polysaccharide capsules, antigenic variation, intracellular survival, proteolytic enzymes, and active suppression of the immune response.

4. In general, an effective host response to a pathogen utilizes components of both humoral and cellular immunity. However, for some pathogens, one arm of the immune system may provide the primary protection.

5. Protection against diseases may be achieved by active as well as passive immunization.

6. Active immunization may result from previous infection or from vaccination, while passive immunization may occur by natural means, such as the transfer of antibodies from mother to fetus via the placenta, or to an infant via the colostrum; or by artificial means such as by the administration of immune globulins.

7. Active immunization may be achieved by administration of one immunogen or a combination of immunogens.

8. The incubation period of a disease and the rapidity with which protective antibody titers develop influence both the efficacy of vaccination and the anamnestic effect of a booster injection.

9. The site of administration of a vaccine may be of great importance; many routes of immunization lead to the synthesis predominantly of serum IgM and IgG; oral administration of some vaccines leads to the induction of secretory IgA in the digestive tract.

10. Immunoprophylaxis has had striking success against subsequent infection; immunotherapy has had limited success in infectious diseases.

REFERENCES

Allen JE, Maizels RM (1997): Th1–Th2: reliable paradigm or dangerous dogma. *Immunol Today* 18:387.

Anonymous (1999): Recommended Childhood Immunization Schedule —United States, 1999. *JAMA*, 281:601.

Buckley RH, Schiff RI (1991): The use of intravenous immune globulin in immunodeficiency diseases. *N Engl J Med* 325:110.

Casadevall A, Scharff MD (1994): "Serum therapy" revisited: animal models of infection and the development of passive antibody therapy. *Antimicrob Agents Chemother* 38:1695.

Deitsch KW, Moxon ER, Wellems TE (1997): Shared themes of antigenic variation and virulence in bacterial, protozoal, and fungal infections. *Microbiol Molec Biol Rev* 61:283.

Doller PC (1993): Vaccination of adults against travel-related infectious diseases, and new developments in vaccines. *Infection* 21:1.

Gardner P, Schaffner W (1993): Immunization of adults. *N Engl J Med* 328:1252.

Lai WC, Bennett M. (1998): DNA vaccines. *Crit Rev Immunol* 18:449.

Pirofski L. Casadevall A (1998): The use of licenced vaccines for active immunization of the immunocompromised host. *Clin Microbiol Rev* 11:1.

Rabinovich NR, McInnes P, Klein DL, Hall BF (1994): Vaccine technologies: view to the future. *Science* 265:1401.

REVIEW QUESTIONS

For each question, choose the ONE BEST answer or completion.

1. The usual sequence of events in the development of an effective immune response to a viral infection is
   - A) interferon secretion, antibody synthesis, cellular immune response, NK cell ADCC.
   - B) antibody synthesis, interferon secretion, NK cell ADCC, cellular immune response.
   - C) NK cell ADCC, interferon secretion, antibody synthesis, cellular immune response
   - D) interferon secretion, cellular immune response, antibody synthesis, NK cell ADCC.
   - E) cellular immune response, interferon secretion, antibody synthesis, NK cell ADCC.

2. Differences between gram-positive and gram-negative bacteria include
   - A) staining with crystal violet.
   - B) ability of complement to lyse cells.
   - C) thickness of the peptidoglycan layer.
   - D) endotoxin in the cell walls of gram-negative bacteria.
   - E) All of the above.

3. Antigenic variation is a mechanism of immune evasion that results in
   - A) interference with attachment to host receptors.
   - B) induction of immune suppression.
   - C) alterations in important surface antigens such that escape variants arise as a result of immune selection.
   - D) mutations in surface antigens.
   - E) destruction of antigens by proteolytic enzymes

4. The best way to provide immunologic protection against tetanus neonatorum (of the newborn) is to
   - A) inject the infant with human tetanus antitoxin.
   - B) inject the newborn with tetanus toxoid.
   - C) inject the mother with toxoid within 72 hours of the birth of her child.
   - D) immunize the mother with tetanus toxoid before or early in pregnancy.
   - E) give the child antitoxin and toxoid for both passive and active immunization.

5. Active, durable immunization against poliomyelitis can be accomplished by oral administration of attenuated vaccine (Sabin) or by parenteral injection of inactivated (Salk) vaccine. These vaccines are equally effective in preventing disease because
   - A) both induce adequate IgA at the intestinal mucosa, the site of entry of the virus.
   - B) antibody in the serum protects against the viremia that leads to disease.

   C) viral antigen attaches to the anterior horn cells in the spinal cord, preventing attachment of virulent virus.

   D) both vaccines induce formation of interferon.

   E) both vaccines establish a mild infection that can lead to formation of antibody.

6. The administration of vaccines is not without hazard. Of the following, which is least likely to affect adversely an immunocompromised host?

   A) measles vaccine

   B) pneumococcal vaccine

   C) bacille Calmette-Guérin

   D) mumps vaccine

   E) Sabin poliomyelitis vaccine

7. The administration of foreign (e.g., equine) antitoxin for passive protection in humans can lead to serum sickness, which is characterized by all of the following *except*

   A) production by host of antibody to foreign antibody.

   B) onset in 24–48 hours.

   C) use of homologous antitoxin.

   D) deposition of antigen–antibody complexes at various sites in the host.

   E) although delayed, the reaction is not a cell-mediated, delayed, type IV immune response.

8. The pneumococcal polysaccharide vaccine should be administered to all *except*

   A) individuals with chronic cardiorespiratory disease.

   B) elderly (over 60 years of age) persons.

   C) children (under 2 years of age).

   D) persons with chronic renal failure.

   E) individuals with sickle-cell disease.

9. The following statements about human immune serum globulin (ISG) are true *except*:

   A) The source is human placenta.

   B) The globulins are obtained by precipitation with cold ethanol.

   C) The concentration of IgG is more than 10-fold greater than in plasma.

   D) IgA and IgM are present in concentrations slightly lower than in plasma.

   E) The ethanol precipitation does not render preparation of globulin free of hepatitis virus.

Answers to Review Questions

1. *D* The usual sequence of events in the host immune response to a viral infection is interferon secretion, cellular immune response, antibody synthesis, NK cell ADCC. Interferon is produced early in the course of viral infection and serves to slow the infection of adjoining cells. Cellular immune responses in the form of cytotoxic CD8 T cells occur early in viral infection and usually precede the appearance of serum-neutralizing antibody or NK-cell-mediated ADCC (which requires specific antibody).

2. *E* Differences between gram-positive and gram-negative bacteria include staining with crystal violet. Gram-negative cells can be lysed by complement but gram-positive cells are complement-resistant because of a thick peptidoglycan layer. Gram-negative bacteria have endotoxin in their cell walls that can cause hemodynamic compromise and septic shock in patients with gram-negative sepsis. Gram-positive bacteria lack endotoxin but have teichoic acids that are immunogenic.

3. *C* Antigenic variation is common to many pathogens and is a mechanism by which they are able to escape the immune system. Antigenic variation can be the result of various mechanisms including mutation, changes in surface protein expression, and natural variation among strains such as occurs in the pneumococci. The potential of a microorganism for antigenic variation is a major consideration in vaccine design.

4. *D* The simplest and most effective way to protect the newborn infant against exotoxic disease, such as tetanus and diphtheria, is to induce antibody in the mother. The antitoxic IgG passing through the placenta will provide the necessary protection. While tetanus antitoxin could be used to provide short-term passive protection, it would be more costly and require an otherwise unnecessary and painful injection. Injection of toxoid in the mother within 72 hours of delivery of the child would not allow time for induction of antibody. While antitoxin and toxoid could provide immediate passive and future active protection, the latter would have to be accompanied by future injections of toxoid and the former is expensive; both would require undesirable injections.

5. *B* Both attenuated and inactivated vaccines lead to formation of circulating antibody, which would provide protection by intercepting the infecting virus before it reaches the target tissue in the central nervous system. While the Sabin vaccine induces mucosal gut IgA that may intercept virus at the portal of entry, the parenterally injected Salk vaccine is not effective in inducing mucosal IgA. Viral antigen in the vaccine might attach to the anterior horn cells in the nervous system, but it probably would not provide durable immunity. Induction of interferon would represent potentially only brief protection. Only the Sabin vaccine, being attenuated and "live," would induce a mild infection.

6. *B* The pneumococcal vaccine consists of capsular polysaccharides from *Streptococcus pneumoniae* and represents a nonviable vaccine, which cannot lead to infection. Measles, mumps, and Sabin polio vaccines contain attenuated viruses, and BCG is an attenuated bacterium. These attenuated organisms are capable of proliferating in the human host. The normal host limits their replication, but the immunocompromised host may not be able to do so, and progressive infection may occur.

7. *B* The reactions that constitute serum sickness follow administration of the foreign substance within 6–12 days. During this time, the host produces antibody that reacts with the foreign substance(s), which persists in the host and leads to antigen–antibody complexes that can be deposited in joints, lymph nodes, skin, and elsewhere. The manifestation of the immune reaction, although appearing later, nevertheless are classified as type III rather than cell-mediated, delayed (type IV) hypersensitivity because they involve antibodies rather than T cells.

8. *C* Children under 2 years of age do not respond adequately to immunization with pure bacterial capsule polysaccharide vaccine. Therefore, vaccinating them may be useless. The various other individuals listed are particularly vulnerable to infection with *Streptococcus pneumoniae*. While some of them may mount a suboptimal response to the vaccine, they should nevertheless be vaccinated.

9. *E* The potential hazard of hepatitis viruses in human plasma is overcome by the separation of ethanol-precipitated globulins. The concentration of IgG is about 16,500 mg/dl, compared with 1200 mg/dl in plasma. Whereas the IgG thus becomes highly concentrated in ISG, IgA and IgM are relatively depleted, and their concentration in the ethanol-precipitated ISG is close to their original concentration in the plasma.

GLOSSARY

accessory cell A cell required to initiate immune response, often used to describe antigen-presenting cell (see also ANTIGEN-PRESENTING CELL).

acquired immune response See ADAPTIVE IMMUNE RESPONSE.

activation-induced cell death See APOPTOSIS.

acute-phase proteins A series of proteins, found in the blood shortly after the onset of an infection, that participate in the early phases of host defense against infection.

adaptive immune response The response of antigen-specific lymphocytes to antigen including the development of immunologic memory; also known as acquired immune response.

ADCC See ANTIBODY-DEPENDENT, CELL-MEDIATED CYTOTOXITY.

adhesion molecules Mediate the binding of one cell to other cells or to extracellular matrix proteins, integrins, selectins, and members of the immunoglobulin gene superfamily. These molecules are important in the operation of the immune system.

adjuvant A substance, given with antigen, that enhances the response to the injected antigen.

adoptive transfer The transfer of the capacity to make an immune response by transplantation of immunocompetent cells.

affinity A measure of the binding constant of a single antigen combining site with a monovalent antigenic determinant.

agglutination The aggregation of particulate antigen by antibodies. Applies to red blood cells as well as to bacteria and inert particles covered with antigen.

alleles Two or more alternate forms of a gene that occupy the same position or locus on a specific chromosome.

allelic exclusion The ability of heterozygous lymphoid cells to produce only one allelic form of antigen-specific receptor (Ig or TCR) when they have the genetic endowment to produce both. Genes other than those for the antigen-specific receptors are usually expressed codominantly.

allergen An antigen responsible for producing allergic reactions by inducing IgE synthesis.

allergy A term covering immune reactions to nonpathogenic antigens, which lead to inflammation and deleterious effects in the host.

allogeneic Genetically dissimilar within the same species.

allograft A tissue transplant (graft) between two genetically nonidentical members of a species.

allotypes Antigenic determinants that are present in allelic (alternate) forms. When used in association with immunoglobulin, allotypes describe allelic variants of immunoglobulins detected by antibodies raised between members of the same species.

alternate complement pathway The mechanism of complement activation that does not involve activation of the C1-C4-C2 pathway by antigen–antibody complexes, and begins with the activation of C3.

anamnestic Literally, means "does not forget"; it is used to describe immunologic memory, which leads to a rapid increase in response after reexposure to antigen.

anaphylatoxin Substance capable of releasing histamine from mast cells and basophils.

anaphylaxis Immediate hypersensitivity response to antigenic challenge, mediated by IgE and mast cells. It is a life-threatening allergic reaction, caused by the release of pharmacologically active agents.

anergy A state of antigen-specific nonresponsiveness in which a T or B cell is present but functionally unable to respond to antigen.

antibody Serum protein formed in response to immunization; antibodies are generally defined in terms of their specific binding to the immunizing antigen.

antibody-dependent, cell-mediated cytotoxicity (ADCC) A phenomenon in which target cells, coated with antibody, are destroyed by specialized killer cells (NK cells and macrophages), which bear receptors for the Fc portion of the coating antibody (Fc receptors). These receptors allow the killer cells to bind to the antibody-coated target.

antigen Any foreign material that is specifically bound by antibody or lymphocytes; also used loosely to describe materials used for immunization. Compare with IMMUNOGEN.

antigen-binding site The part of an immunoglobulin molecule or T-cell receptor that binds antigen specifically.

antigenic determinant A single antigenic site or epitope on a complex antigenic molecule or particle.

antigen presentation The display of antigen as peptide fragments bound to MHC molecules on the surface of a cell; T cells recognize antigen only when it is presented in this way.

antigen-presenting cell (APC) A specialized type of cell, bearing cell-surface class II MHC (see MAJOR HISTOCOMPATIBILITY COMPLEX) molecules, involved in processing and presentation of antigen to T cells.

APC See ANTIGEN-PRESENTING CELL.

antigen processing The degradation of proteins into peptides that can bind to MHC molecules for presentation to T cells. All protein antigens must be processed into peptides before they can be presented by MHC molecules.

antigen receptor The specific antigen-binding receptor on T or B lymphocytes; these receptors are transcribed and translated from rearrangements and translocation of V, D, and J genes.

antiserum (plural: **antisera**) The fluid component of clotted blood from an immune individual that contains a heterogeneous collection of antibodies against the molecule used for immunization. Such antibodies bind the antigen used for immunization. Each has its own structure, its own epitope on the antigen, and its own set of cross-reactions. This heterogeneity makes each antiserum unique.

apoptosis A form of programmed cell death caused by activation of endogenous molecules leading to the fragmentation of DNA.

Arthus reaction A hypersensitivity reaction produced by local formation of antigen–antibody aggregates that activate the complement cascade and cause thrombosis, hemorrhage, and acute inflammation.

atopy A term used to describe IgE-mediated allergic responses in humans, usually showing a genetic predisposition.

autochthonous Pertaining to self.

autograft A tissue transplant from one area to another on a single individual.

autoimmunity An immune response to self tissues or components. Such an immune response may have pathologic consequences leading to autoimmune diseases.

autologous Derived from the same individual, self.

avidity The summation of multiple affinities, for example, when a polyvalent antibody binds to a polyvalent antigen.

BALT See BRONCHUS-ASSOCIATED LYMPHOID TISSUE.

basophils White blood cells containing granules that stain with basic dyes. They are thought to have a function similar to mast cells.

B cell See B LYMPHOCYTE.

BCR B-cell receptors. See B LYMPHOCYTE.

Bence-Jones protein Dimers of immunoglobulin light chains in the urine of patients with multiple myeloma.

blocking antibody A functional term for an antibody molecule capable of blocking the interaction of antigen with other antibodies or with cells.

B lymphocyte (B cell) The precursors of antibody-forming plasma cell; expresses immunoglobulin on its surface.

bone marrow The site of hematopoiesis, in which stem cells give rise to the cellular elements of blood, including red blood cells, monocytes, polymorphonuclear leukocytes, platelets, and lymphocytes.

bronchus-associated lymphoid tissue (BALT) Secondary lymphoid organs connected to the bronchial tree.

bursa of Fabricius Site of development of B cells in birds; an outpouching of the cloaca.

CAM Cell-surface adhesion molecule. See ADHESION MOLECULES.

carcinoembryonic antigen (CEA) Antigen present during embryonic development that normally is not expressed in the adult but reappears in malignant cells.

carrier A large immunogenic molecule or particle to which a hapten or other non-immunogenic, epitope-bearing molecule may attach, allowing it to become immunogenic.

CD See CLUSTER OF DIFFERENTIATION and Appendix.

CDR See COMPLEMENTARITY-DETERMINING REGIONS.

CEA See CARCINOEMBRYONIC ANTIGEN.

cell-mediated cytotoxicity (CMC) Killing (lysis) of a target cell by an effector lymphocyte.

cell-mediated immunity (CMI) Immune reaction mediated by T cells, in contrast to humoral immunity, which is antibody-mediated. Also referred to as DELAYED-TYPE HYPERSENSITIVITY.

chemokines Small cytokines of relatively low molecular weight, released by a variety of cells, and involved in the migration and activation primarily of phagocytic cells and lymphocytes. They have a central role in inflammatory responses.

chemotaxis Migration of cells along a concentration gradient of an attractant.

chimera A mythical animal possessing the head of a lion, the body of a goat, and the tail of a snake. Refers to an individual containing cellular components derived from another genetically distinct individual.

classical complement pathway The mechanism of complement activation initiated by antigen–antibody aggregates and proceeding by way of C1 to C9.

class I, II, and III MHC molecules See MAJOR HISTOCOMPATIBILITY COMPLEX (MHC).

class switch See ISOTYPE SWITCH.

class II-associated invariant chain peptide (CLIP) A peptide of variable length cleaved from the invariant chain by proteases. CLIP remains associated with the class II MHC molecules in an unstable form until it is removed by the HLA–DM protein.

clonal deletion The loss of lymphocytes of a particular specificity due to contact with either self or foreign antigen.

clonal selection theory The prevalent concept that specificity and diversity of an immune response are the result of selection by antigen of specifically reactive clones from a large repertoire of preformed lymphocytes, each with individual specificities.

cluster of differentiation (CD) Cluster of antigens with which antibodies react that characterize cell-surface molecules.

combinatorial joining The joining of segments of DNA to generate essentially new genetic information, as occurs with Ig and TCR genes during the development of B and T cells. Combinatorial joining allows multiple opportunities for two sets of genes to combine in different ways.

complement A series of serum proteins involved in the mediation of immune reactions. The complement cascade is triggered classically by the interaction of antibody with specific antigen.

complementarity-determining regions (CDRs) Parts of immunoglobulins and T-cell receptors that determine their specificity and make contact with specific ligand. The CDRs are the most variable part of the molecule and contribute to the diversity of these molecules. There are three such regions (CDR1, CDR2, and CDR3) in each V domain.

complement receptors (CR) Cell-surface proteins on various cells that recognize and bind complement proteins that have bound pathogens or other antigens. CR on phagocytes allow them to identify pathogens coated with complement proteins for uptake and destruction. Complement receptors include CR1, the receptor for C1q, CR2, CR3, and CR4.

complete Freund's adjuvant (CFA) See FREUND'S COMPLETE ADJUVANT.

conformational epitopes Discontinuous epitopes on a protein antigen that are formed from several separate regions in the primary sequence of a protein when brought together by protein folding. Antibodies that bind conformational epitopes bind only native-folded proteins.

congenic (also coisogenic) Describes two individuals who differ only in the genes at a particular locus and are identical at all other loci.

constant region (C region) The invariant carboxyl-terminal portion of an immunoglobulin or TCR molecule, as distinct from the variable region at the amino terminus of the chain.

contact hypersensitivity A form of delayed-type hypersensitivity (type IV) in which T cells respond to antigens that are introduced by contact with the skin. Poison ivy hypersensitivity is a contact hypersensitivity reaction due to T-cell responses to the chemical antigen pentadecacatechal in poison ivy leaves.

convertase An enzymatic activity that converts a complement protein into its reactive form by cleaving it. Generation of the C3/C5 convertase is the pivotal event in complement activation.

Coombs test A test named for its originator, R.R.A. Coombs, used to detect antibodies by addition of an anti-immunoglobulin antibody.

CR See COMPLEMENT RECEPTORS.

C region See CONSTANT REGION.

cross-reactivity The ability of an antibody, specific for one antigen, to react with a second antigen; a measure of relatedness between two different antigenic substances.

CTLA-4 The high-affinity receptor for B7 molecules expressed on T cells.

cyclophosphamide An alkylating agent that is used as an immunosuppressive drug which acts by killing rapidly dividing cells, including lymphocytes proliferating in response to antigen.

cyclosporin A An immunosuppressive drug that inhibits signaling in T cells thus preventing T-cell activation and effector function. It acts by binding to cyclophilin to create a complex that binds to and inactivates the serine/threonine phosphatase calcineurin.

cytokine receptors Cellular receptors for cytokines. Binding of the cytokine to the cytokine receptor stimulates signal transduction resulting in new activities in the cell, such as growth, differentiation, or death.

cytokines Soluble substances secreted by cells, which have a variety of effects on other cells.

cytotoxic T cells T cells that can kill other cells. Most cytotoxic T cells are MHC class 1-restricted $CD8^+$ T cells, but $CD4^+$ T cells can also kill target cells in some cases.

D gene A small segment of immunoglobulin heavy-chain and T-cell receptor DNA, coding for the third hypervariable region of most receptors.

delayed-type hypersensitivity (DTH) A form of cell-mediated immunity elicited by antigen present in the skin. The reaction is mediated by $CD4^+$ T_H1 cells and involves release of cytokines and recruitment of monocytes and macrophages. It is called "delayed-type" because the reaction appears hours to days (usually 24–48 hours) after antigen is injected.

dendritic cells Interdigitating reticular cells, derived from bone-marrow precursors, that are found in T-cell areas of lymphoid tissues. They have a branched or dendritic morphology and are the most potent stimulators of T-cell responses. Dendritic cells present in nonlymphoid tissues do not appear to stimulate T-cell responses until they are activated and migrate to lymphoid tissues.

desensitization A procedure in which an allergic individual is exposed to increasing doses of allergen with the goal of inhibiting their allergic reactions. The mechanism responsible for this effect probably involves shifting the response from $CD4^+$ T_H2 to T_H1 cells and thus changing the antibody produced from IgE to IgG.

determinant Part of the antigen molecule that binds to an antibody-combining site or to a receptor on T cells; also termed epitope (see HAPTEN and EPITOPE).

differentiation antigen A cell-surface antigenic determinant found only on cells of a certain lineage and at a particular developmental stage; used as an immunologic market.

diversity gene segments see D GENE.

domain A compact segment of an immunoglobulin or TCR chain, made up of amino acids around an S-S bond.

DP, DQ, and DR molecules MHC class II molecules of humans found on B cells and antigen-presenting cells.

DTH See DELAYED-TYPE HYPERSENSITIVITY.

ECAM Endothelial cell adhesion molecule. See ADHESION MOLECULES.

effector cells Lymphocytes that can mediate the removal of pathogens or antigens from the body without the need for further differentiation. Effectors are distinct from naive lymphocytes, which must proliferate and differentiate before they can mediate effector functions. They are also distinct from memory cells which must differentiate and sometimes proliferate before they become effector cells.

ELISA See ENZYME-LINKED IMMUNOSORBENT ASSAY.

endogenous pyrogens Cytokines (e.g. IL-1, TNF_α) that can induce a rise in body temperature. They are distinct form exogenous substances such as endotoxin from gram-negative bacteria that induce fever by triggering endogenous pyrogen synthesis.

endotoxins Bacterial toxins that are released when bacterial cells are damaged or destroyed. The most important endotoxin is the lipopolysaccharide of gram-negative bacteria, which induces cytokine synthesis.

enzyme-linked immunosorbent assay (ELISA) An assay in which an enzyme is linked to an antibody and a colored substrate is used to measure the activity of bound enzyme and hence the amount of bound antibody.

eosinophils White blood cells thought to be important in defense against parasitic infections.

epitope An alternative term for antigenic determinant.

exon The region of DNA coding for a protein or a segment of a protein.

F(ab')$_2$ A fragment of an antibody containing two antigen-binding sites; generated by cleavage of the antibody molecule with the enzyme pepsin, which cuts at the hinge region C-terminally to the inter-heavy-chain disulfide bond.

Fab Fragment of antibody containing one antigen-binding site; generated by cleavage of the antibody with the enzyme papain, which cuts at the hinge region N-terminally to the inter-heavy-chain disulfide bond and generates two Fab fragments from one antibody molecule.

FACS see FLUORESCENCE-ACTIVATED CELL SORTER.

Fas A member of the TNF receptor family that is expressed on certain cells and makes them susceptible to killing by cells expressing Fas ligand. Binding of Fas ligand to Fas triggers apoptosis in the Fas-bearing cells.

Fc Fragment of antibody without antigen-binding sites, generated by cleavage with papain; the Fc fragment contains the C-terminal domains of the domains of the immunoglobulin heavy chains.

Fc receptor (FcR) A receptor on a cell surface with specific binding affinity for the Fc portion of an antibody molecule. Fc receptors are found on many types of cells.

FITC See fluorescein isothiocyanate.

FK506 (or tacrolimus) An immunosuppressive polypeptide drug that inactivates T cells by inhibiting signal transduction from the T cell receptor.

fluorescein isothiocyanate (FITC) A fluorescent dye which emits a yellow-green color and can be conjugated to antibody or other proteins.

fluorescence-activated cell sorter (FACS) An instrument that uses a laser to differentially deflect cells bound to fluorochrome-linked antibodies thus sorting the cells into fluorescent-positive and fluorescent-negative populations.

fluorescent antibody An antibody coupled with a fluorescent dye, used to detect antigen on cells, tissues, or microorganisms.

follicular dendritic cells Cells within lymphoid follicles which are crucial in selecting antigen-binding B cells during antibody responses. Their origin is uncertain. They have Fc receptors that are not internalized by receptor-mediated endocytosis and thus hold antigen–antibody complexes on their surface for long periods.

Freund's complete adjuvant An oil containing killed mycobacteria and an emulsifier, which, when emulsified with an immunogen in aqueous solution, enhances the immune response to that immunogen after injection. Termed *incomplete Freund's adjuvant* if mycobacteria are not included.

GALT See GUT-ASSOCIATED LYMPHOID TISSUE.

gene knockout Jargon for gene disruption by homologous recombination.

genotype All the genes possessed by an individual; in practice it refers to the particular alleles present at the loci in question.

germinal centers Secondary lymphoid structures that are sites of intense B-cell proliferation, selection, maturation, and death during antibody responses. They form around follicular dendritic cell networks after migration of B cells into lymphoid follicles.

germ line Refers to genes in germ cells as opposed to somatic cells. In immunology, it refers to genes in their unrearranged state rather than those rearranged for production of immunoglobulin or TCR molecules.

graft-versus-host reaction (GVH) The pathologic consequences of a response generally initiated by transplanted immunocompetent T lymphocytes into an allogeneic, immunologically incompetent host. The host is unable to reject the grafted T cells and becomes their target.

granuloma An organized structure in the form of a mass of mononuclear cells at the site of a persisting inflammation; the cells are mostly macrophages with some T lymphocytes at the periphery. It is a typical delayed hypersensitivity reaction that is persistent due to the continuous presence of a foreign body or infection.

gut-associated lymphoid tissue (GALT) Lymphoid tissue situated in the gastrointestinal mucosa and submucosa which constitutes the gastrointestinal immune system. GALT is present in the Peyer's patches, appendix, and tonsils.

GVH See GRAFT VERSUS HOST REACTION.

H-2 complex The major histocompatibility complex situated on chromosome 17 of the mouse; contains subregions K, I, D, and L.

haplotype A particular combination of closely linked genes on a chromosome inherited from one parent.

hapten A compound, usually of low molecular weight, that is not itself immunogenic but that, after conjugation to a carrier protein or cells, becomes immunogenic and induces antibody, which can bind the hapten alone in the absence of carrier.

HAT Hypoxanthine-aminopterin-thymidine.

H chain See HEAVY CHAIN.

heavy chain (H chain) The larger of the two types of chains that comprise a normal immunoglobulin or antibody molecule.

helper T cells A class of T cells that helps trigger B cells to make antibody against thymus-dependent antigens. Helper T cells also help in the differentiation of other T cells such as cytotoxic T cells.

hematopoiesis The generation of the cellular elements of blood, including the red blood cells, leukocytes, and platelets.

heterophile antigen A cross-reacting antigen that appears in widely ranging species such as humans and bacteria.

HEV See HIGH ENDOTHELIAL VENULES.

high endothelial venules (HEV) Specialized venules found in lymphoid tissues. Lymphocytes migrate from blood into lymphoid tissues by attaching to and migrating across the high endothelial cells of these vessels.

hinge region A flexible, open segment of an antibody molecule that allows bending of the molecule. The hinge region is located between Fab and Fc and is susceptible to enzymatic cleavage.

histamine A vasoactive amine stored in mast cell granules which is released by antigen binding to IgE molecules on mast cells causing dilation of local blood vessels and smooth muscle contraction. Histamine release produces some of the symptoms of immediate hypersensitivity reactions.

histocompatibility Literally, the ability of tissues to get along; in immunology, it means identity in all transplantation antigens. These antigens, in turn, are collectively referred to as histocompatibility antigens.

HIV See HUMAN IMMUNODEFICIENCY VIRUS.

HLA See HUMAN LEUKOCYTE ANTIGEN.

human immunodeficiency virus (HIV) Retrovirus that infects human CD4$^+$ cells and causes AIDS.

Human Leukocyte Antigen (HLA) The human major histocompatibility complex; contains the genes coding for the polymorphic MHC class I and II class molecules and many other important genes.

humanization Refers to the genetic engineering by which mouse V(D)J region genes defining a particular antigenic specificity are combined with human genes coding for the rest of the Ig molecule. Results in an antibody with a mouse-defined antigenic specificity but with human effector characteristics. Humanization reduces the immunogenicity of a mouse Ig in humans, making it more effective as an in vivo treatment than a completely mouse molecule.

humoral immunity refers to immune responses that involve antibody (contrast with cell-mediated immunity: T-cell responses in the absence of antibody). Can be transferred to another individual using antibody-containing serum.

hybridoma An immortalized hybrid cell resulting from the in vitro fusion of an antibody-secreting B cell with a myeloma; it secretes antibody without stimulation and proliferates continuously, both in vivo and in vitro. The term is also used for a hybrid T cell resulting from the fusion of a T lymphocyte with a thymoma (a malignant T cell); the T-cell hybridoma proliferates continuously and secretes cytokines upon activation by antigen and APC.

hyperacute graft rejection Rapid (minutes to hours) rejection of a graft mediated by preformed antibodies of the host reacting with the graft.

hypersensitivity State of reactivity to antigen that is greater than normal; denotes a deleterious rather than a protective outcome. Type I: IgE-mediated; type II: antibody-specific for a cellular antigen triggers the complement cascade; type III: antigen–antibody complexes deposit in tissues and activate complement; type IV: T-cell mediated.

hypervariable regions Portions of the light and heavy immunoglobulin chains that are highly variable in amino acid sequence from one immunoglobulin molecule to another, and that together constitute the antigen-binding site of an antibody molecule. Also, portions of the T-cell receptor that constitute the antigen-binding site. (see COMPLEMENTARITY-DETERMINING REGION).

Ia (I region-associated) An older term for mouse MHC class II genes and molecules; comprise I-A and I-E.

IDC See INTERDIGITATING DENDRITIC CELLS.

idiotype The combined antigenic determinants (idiotopes) expressed in the variable region of antibodies of an individual that are directed at a particular antigen.

Ig See IMMUNOGLOBULIN.

IL See INTERLEUKINS.

immature B cell IgM$^+$IgD$^+$ cell in the B cell lineage; easily tolerized by exposure to antigen.

immediate-type hypersensitivity (Type I) hypersensitivity reaction occurring within minutes after the interaction of antigen and IgE antibody.

immune adherence The adherence of particulate antigen coated with C3b to cells expressing C3b receptors; results in enhanced phagocytosis of bacteria by macrophages.

immune complex Molecules formed by the interaction of a soluble (that is, non-particulate) antigen with antibody molecules. Large immune complexes are cleared rapidly, but smaller complexes formed in antigen excess may deposit in tissues resulting in tissue damage.

immune modulators Substances that control the level of the immune response.

immunity The general term for resistance to a pathogen.

immunodeficiency Decrease in immune response that results from absence or defect of some component of the immune system.

immunodiffusion Identifies antigen or antibody by the formation of antigen–antibody complexes in a gel.

immunogen A substance capable of inducing an immune response (as well as reacting with the products of an immune response). Compare with antigen.

immunoglobulin (Ig) A general term for all antibody molecules: IgM, IgD, IgG, IgA, IgE; each Ig unit is made up of two heavy chains and two light chains and has two antigen-binding sites.

immunoglobulin superfamily Proteins involved in cellular recognition and interaction that are structurally and genetically related to immunoglobulins.

immunoreceptor tyrosine-based activation motif (ITAM) A pattern of amino acids in the cytoplasmic tail of many transmembrane receptor molecules, including Igα and Igβ and CD3 chains, which are phosphorylated and then associate with intracellular molecules as an early consequence of cell activation.

immunoreceptor tyrosine-based inhibitory motif (ITIM) A pattern of amino acids in the cytoplasmic tail of transmembrane molecules, such as CD32, which binds phosphatases. Once bound, the phosphatase removes phosphate groups from tyrosine residues in the ITAMs of other membrane molecules, and thus negatively regulates cell activation.

inflammation An acute or chronic response to tissue injury or infection involving accumulation of leukocytes, plasma proteins, and fluid.

innate immunity The antigen-nonspecific mechanisms involved in the early phase of resistance to a pathogen, which include phagocytic cells, cytokines, and complement; not expanded by repeat stimulation with the pathogen.

integrins A family of two-chain cell-surface adhesion molecules found on leukocytes; important in the adhesion of APC and lymphocytes, and in leukocyte migration into tissues.

intercellular adhesion molecules (ICAMs) 1, 2, and 3 Adhesion molecules on the surface of several cell types, including antigen-presenting cells and T cells that interact with integrins; members of the immunoglobulin superfamily.

interdigitating dendritic cells (IDC) Thymic bone marrow-derived cells which play a critical role in negative selection of developing thymocytes.

interferons (IFN) A group of proteins having antiviral activity and capable of enhancing and modifying the immune response.

interleukins (IL) Glycoproteins secreted by a variety of leukocytes that have effects on other leukocytes.

intron A segment of DNA that does not code for protein: the intervening sequence of nucleotides between coding sequences or exons.

isoelectric focusing Protein identification technique; proteins migrate in an electric field under a pH gradient to the pH at which their net charge is zero (their isoelectric point).

isograft Tissue transplanted between two genetically identical individuals (same as syngraft).

isohemagglutinins Naturally occurring IgM antibodies specific for the red blood cell antigens of the ABO blood groups; thought to result from immunization by bacteria in the gastrointestinal and respiratory tracts.

isotypes Also known as antibody classes. Antibodies that differ in the heavy chain constant regions: IgM, IgG, IgD, IgA and IgE. These differences result in distinct biological activities of the antibodies; distinguishable also on the basis of reaction with antisera raised in another species.

isotype switch The switch which occurs when a B cell stops secreting antibody of one isotype or class and starts producing antibody of a different isotype but with same antigenic specificity; involves joining rearranged VDJ gene unit to a different heavy-chain constant region gene.

ITAM See IMMUNORECEPTOR TYROSINE-BASED ACTIVATION MOTIF.

ITIM See IMMUNORECEPTOR TYROSINE-BASED INHIBITION MOTIF.

JAK See JANUS KINASES.

Janus kinases (JAK) Tyrosine kinases activated by cytokines binding to their cellular receptors.

J chain (joining chain) A polypeptide involved in the polymerization of immunoglobulin molecules IgM and IgA.

J gene A gene segment coding for the J or joining segment in immunoglobulin or T-cell receptor; in Ig light chains and TCR α and γ, a V gene segment rearranges to a J segment; in Ig heavy chains and TCR β and δ, a D gene segment rearranges to a J segment.

killer inhibitory receptor (KIR) a receptor expressed on NK cells that binds to class I MHC molecules on target cells; ligation of class I MHC inhibits the signaling that would otherwise lead to target cell killing.

killer T cell A T cell that kills a target cell expressing foreign antigen bound to MHC molecules on the surface of the target cell. Also called cytotoxic T cell.

KIR See KILLER INHIBITORY RECEPTOR.

LAK cells See LYMPHOKINE-ACTIVATED KILLER CELLS.

Langerhans cell Cell of the monocyte/dendritic cell family that takes up and processes antigens in the epidermal layer of the skin; migrates through lymphatics to lymph nodes draining the site of exposure to antigen, where it differentiates into a dendritic cell.

L chain See LIGHT CHAIN.

leukemia Uncontrolled proliferation of a malignant leukocyte.

leukocytes White blood cells; comprise monocytes/macrophages, lymphocytes and polymorphonuclear cells.

ligand A molecule or part of a molecule that binds to a receptor.

ligation The binding of a molecule or a part of a molecule to a receptor.

light chain (L chain) The light chain of the immunoglobulin molecule; occurs in two forms: κ or λ.

linked recognition The requirement for the T helper and B cell involved in the antibody response to a thymus-dependent antigen to interact with different epitopes physically linked in the same antigen.

lipopolysaccharide (LPS) Components of gram-negative bacteria cell walls; also known as endotoxin.

LPS See LIPOPOLYSACCHARIDE.

lymph Extracellular fluid that bathes tissues; contains tissue products, antigens, antibodies and cells (predominantly lymphocytes).

lymphatic system System of vessels through which lymph travels, and which includes organized structures—lymph nodes—at the intersection of vessels. Three major functions: to concentrate antigen from all parts of the body into a few lymphoid organs; to circulate lymphocytes through lymphoid organs so that antigen can interact with rare antigen-specific cells; and to carry products of the immune response (antibody and effector cells) to the bloodstream and tissues.

lymph nodes Secondary lymphoid organs, in which mature B and T lymphocytes respond to free antigen, or antigen associated with APC, brought in via lymphatic vessels.

lymphocytes Express antigen-specific receptors. Small leukocyte with virtually no cytoplasm, found in blood, tissues, and lymphoid organs such as lymph nodes, spleen, and Peyer's patches. Responsible for specificity, diversity, memory, and self–nonself discrimination.

lymphokine A cytokine secreted by lymphocytes.

lymphokine-activated killer (LAK) cells The heterogeneous population of lymphocytes, including NK cells, derived from the in vitro cytokine-driven activation of peripheral blood lymphocytes from a tumor-bearing patient.

lymphoma Lymphocyte tumors in lymphoid or other tissues; not generally found in the blood.

macrophages Large phagocytic leukocytes found in tissues; derived from blood monocytes.

major histocompatibility complex (MHC) A cluster of genes encoding polymorphic cell-surface molecules (MHC class I and class II) that are involved in interactions with T cells. These molecules also play a major role in transplantation rejection. Several other nonpolymorphic proteins are encoded in this region.

MALT See MUCOSAL-ASSOCIATED LYMPHOID TISSUE.

mast cell Bone-marrow derived granule-containing cell found in connective tissues; releases mediators such as histamine and cytokines following cell activation; plays a major role in allergic responses.

mature B cell B cells with IgM and IgD on their surface.

membrane attack complex Terminal components of the complement cascade (C7–C9) which form a pore on the surface of a target cell, resulting in cell damage or death.

memory In the immune system denotes that a second interaction with antigen leads to a more effective and more rapid response than the first interaction (primary response).

MHC See MAJOR HISTOCOMPATIBILITY COMPLEX.

MHC class I molecule A molecule encoded by genes of the MHC that participates in antigen presentation to $CD8^+$ (cytotoxic) T cells.

MHC class II molecule A molecule encoded by genes of the MHC that participates in antigen presentation to $CD4^+$ T cells.

MHC restriction The property of T lymphocytes to respond only when they are presented with the appropriate antigen in association with either self MHC class I or class II molecules.

minor histocompatibility antigens Antigens encoded outside the MHC which stimulate graft rejection, but not as rapidly as MHC molecules.

mitogen A substance that stimulates the proliferation of many different clones of lymphocytes.

mixed lymphocyte reaction (MLR) Proliferative response occurring when leukocytes from two individuals are mixed in vitro; T cells from one individual (the responder) are activated by MHC antigens expressed by APC of the other individual (the stimulator).

MLR See MIXED LYMPHOCYTE REACTION.

molecular mimicry Identity or similarity of epitopes expressed by a pathogen and by a self molecule; may explain how autoimmune responses develop.

monoclonal Means derived from a single clone, the progeny of a single cell. Generally refers to a population of T cells, B cells, or antibody that is homogeneous, and reactive with the same specificity toward an epitope.

monocyte Phagocytic leukocyte found in the blood; precursor to tissue macrophage.

motif A pattern of amino acids in the sequence of a molecule critical for the binding of a ligand.

mucosal-associated lymphoid tissue (MALT) System that connects lymphoid structures found in the gastrointestinal and respiratory tracts; includes tonsils, appendix, and Peyer's patches of the small intestine.

multiple sclerosis Disease of the central nervous system believed to be autoimmune in nature, in which an inflammatory response results in demyelination and loss of neurologic function.

myasthenia gravis Autoimmune disease in which antibody specific for the acetylcholine receptor expressed in muscle blocks function at the neuromuscular junction.

myeloma A tumor of plasma cells, generally secreting a single monoclonal immunoglobulin.

natural killer (NK) cells Large granular lymphocyte-like cells that kill various tumor cells in vitro and may play a role in resistance to tumors; also participate in ADCC; derived from the lymphoid progenitor but distinct from T and B lymphocytes —they do not exhibit antigenic specificity, and their number does not increase by immunization.

negative selection Step in development of B and T cells at which cells with potential reactivity to self molecules are functionally inactivated.

neutralization The ability of an antibody to block or inhibit the effects of a virus.

NK cells See NATURAL KILLER CELLS.

opsonization The coating of a particle such as a bacterium with antibody and/or a complement component (an opsonin) that leads to enhanced phagocytosis by phagocytic cells.

paracortical area (or paracortex) The T-cell area of the lymph node.

passive cutaneous anaphylaxis (PCA) The passive transfer of anaphylactic sensitivity by intradermal injection of serum from a sensitive donor.

passive hemagglutination Technique for measuring antibody, in which antigen-coated red blood cells are agglutinated by adding antibody specific for the antigen.

passive immunization Immunization of an individual by the transfer of antibody synthesized in another individual.

pathogen An agent which causes disease.

PCA See PASSIVE CUTANEOUS ANAPHYLAXIS.

PCR See POLYMERASE CHAIN REACTION.

perforin A molecule synthesized by cytotoxic T cells and NK cells that polymerizes on the surface of a target cell and creates a pore in the membrane, resulting in target cell death.

peripheral lymphoid organs Lymphoid organs other than the thymus; include spleen, lymph nodes, and mucosal associated lymphoid tissue.

peripheral tolerance Tolerance induced in mature lymphocytes outside the thymus.

Peyer's patches Clusters of lymphocytes distributed in the lining of the small intestine.

PHA See PHYTOHEMAGGLUTININ.

phagocytosis The engulfment of a particle or a microorganism by leukocytes such as macrophages and neutrophils.

phenotype The physical expression of an individual's genotype.

phosphatase Enzyme that removes phosphate groups from proteins.

phospholipase C gamma (PLC-γ) Enzyme involved in T-cell and B-cell activation pathways; splits phosphatidylinositol bisphosphate (PIP$_2$) into diacylglycerol (DAG) and inositol triphosphate (IP$_3$) leading to the activation of two major signaling pathways.

phytohemagglutinin (PHA) A mitogen that polyclonally activates T cells.

pinocytosis Ingestion of liquid or very small particles by vesicle formation in a cell.

plasma Fluid component of unclotted blood.

plasma cell The antibody-producing end-stage of B-cell differentiation.

platelets Bone-marrow derived cells crucial in blood clotting.

PMN leukocytes See POLYMORPHONUCLEAR LEUKOCYTES.

pokeweed mitogen A mitogen that polyclonally activates B cells.

polyclonal activator A substance that induces activation of many individual clones of either T or B cells. See MITOGEN.

poly-Ig receptor Binds to IgA at one surface of an epithelial cell, transports it through the cell, and releases it at the opposite lumenal surface; the IgA can then participate in protecting the mucosal system.

polymerase chain reaction (PCR) Produces large amounts of DNA from a sequence by repeated cycles of synthesis.

polymorphonuclear leukocytes (PMN) Leukocytes containing cytoplasmic granules with characteristic multilobed nucleus; three major types: neutrophils, eosinophils, and basophils.

polymorphism Literally, having many shapes; in genetics, the existence of multiple alleles at a particular genetic locus resulting in variants of the gene and product among different members of the species.

positive selection The process by which developing B and T cells receive signals in the primary lymphoid organ in which they are developing to continue their differentiation; in the absence of these signals the cells die.

pre-B cell Cell in the B cell lineage which has rearranged heavy but not light chain genes; expresses surrogate light chains and μ heavy chain at its surface in conjunction with Igα and Igβ; all these molecules comprise the pre-B cell receptor (pre-BCR).

precipitin reaction The mixing of soluble antigen and antibody at different proportions that can result in the precipitation of insoluble antigen-antibody complexes.

pre-T cell Cell in T-lymphocyte differentiation in the thymus that has rearranged TCR β genes and expresses TCR β polypeptide on the surface with the molecule pTα (gp33), forming the pre-T-cell receptor.

primary follicle Region of a secondary lymphoid organ containing predominantly unstimulated B lymphocytes; develops into a germinal center following antigen stimulation.

primary lymphoid organs Organs in which the early stages of T- and B-lymphocyte differentiation take place and antigen-specific receptors are first expressed.

primary response The immune response resulting from first encounter with antigen; generally small, with a long induction phase or lag period, and generates immunologic memory. In the primary B-cell response, mainly IgM antibodies are made.

priming The activation of naive lymphocytes by exposure to antigen.

pro-B cell Earliest stage of B cell differentiation in which a heavy chain D-gene segment rearranges to a J-gene segment.

programmed cell death See APOPTOSIS.

properdin (factor P) A positive regulator of the alternative pathway of complement activation; stabilizes C3bBb.

prophylaxis Protection.

proteasome Multiprotein cytoplasmic complex, which catabolizes proteins to 8–9 amino acid peptides.

protein kinase C Enzyme activated by calcium and diacylglycerol during T- and B-lymphocyte activation.

protooncogenes Cellular genes regulating growth control; mutation or aberrant expression can lead to malignant transformation of the cell.

provirus DNA form of a retrovirus integrated into the host DNA.

pseudogene Sequence of DNA resembling a gene but containing codons that prevent transcription into full-length RNA species.

pyogenic Refers to the generation of pus at the sites of response to bacteria with large capsules.

pyrogen A substance that causes fever.

radioallergosorbent test (RAST) A solid-phase radioimmunoassay for detecting IgE antibody specific for a particular allergen.

radioimmunoassay (RIA) A technique for measuring the level of a biologic substance in a sample, by measuring the binding of antigen to radioactively labeled antibody (or vice versa).

RAG-1 and RAG-2 (recombination activating genes) Genes and their products which are critically involved in V(D)J recombination in B and T cells.

rapamycin An immunosuppressive agent used to prevent transplantation rejection; blocks cytokine production.

receptor Generally a transmembrane molecule that binds to a ligand on the exterior surface of the cell, leading to biochemical changes inside the cell.

receptor editing Process by which the rearranged genes of a cell in the B-cell lineage may undergo a secondary rearrangement, generating a different antigenic specificity.

recombination See V(D)J RECOMBINATION.

recombination activating genes See RAG-1 AND RAG-2.

repertoire The complete library of antigenic specificities generated by either B or T lymphocytes to respond to foreign antigen.

RES See RETICULOENDOTHELIAL SYSTEM.

reticuloendothelial system (RES) A general term for the network of phagocytic cells.

reverse transcriptase Enzyme which transcribes the RNA genome of a retrovirus into DNA; used in molecular biology to convert RNA into complementary DNA (cDNA).

rheumatoid arthritis Autoimmune, inflammatory disease of the joints.

rheumatoid factor An autoantibody (usually IgM) that reacts with the individual's own IgG; present in rheumatoid arthritis.

SCID See SEVERE COMBINED IMMUNE DEFICIENCY DISEASE.

secondary lymphoid organs Organs in which antigen-driven proliferation and differentiation of mature B and T lymphocytes take place following antigen recognition.

second set rejection Accelerated rejection of an allograft in a primed recipient.

secretory component Cleaved component of the poly-Ig receptor that attaches to dimeric IgA and protects it from proteolytic cleavage as it is transported through an epithelial cell.

selectins A family of cell-surface adhesion molecules found on leukocytes and endothelial cells; bind to sugars on glycoproteins.

sensitization Prior immunization by antigen; generally used for first encounter with allergen.

sepsis Infection of the bloodstream.

serology Use of antibodies to detect antigens.

serum Residual fluid derived from clotted blood; contains antibodies.

serum sickness A type III hypersensitivity reaction resulting from deposition of circulating, soluble, antigen–antibody complexes leading to complement and neutrophil activation in tissues such as the kidney; typically induced following therapy with large doses of antibody from a foreign source, such as monoclonal antibodies made in mice (originally, by treating patients with horse serum).

severe combined immune deficiency (SCID) Disease resulting from early block in differentiation pathways of both B and T lymphocytes.

signal transducers and activators of transcription (STATs) Intracellular proteins phosphorylated by Janus kinases as a consequence of cytokine–cytokine receptor engagement.

signal transduction Processes involved in transmitting the signal received on the outer surface of the cell (e.g., by antigen binding to its receptor) into the nucleus of the cell, which lead to altered gene expression.

SLE See SYSTEMIC LUPUS ERYTHEMATOSUS.

slow-reacting substance of anaphylaxis (SRS-A) A group of leukotrienes released by mast cells during anaphylaxis that induces a prolonged contraction of smooth muscle.

somatic gene conversion nonreciprocal exchange of sequences between genes: part of the donor gene or genes is "copied" into an acceptor gene, but only the acceptor gene is altered; mechanism for generating diverse Ig repertoire in many nonhuman species.

somatic hypermutation Change in the variable region sequence of an antibody produced by a B cell following antigenic stimulation, resulting in increased antibody affinity for antigen.

spleen Largest of the secondary lymphoid organs; traps and concentrates foreign substances carried in the blood; composed of white pulp, rich in lymphoid cells, and red pulp, which contains many erythrocytes and macrophages.

STATs See SIGNAL TRANSDUCERS AND ACTIVATORS OF TRANSCRIPTION.

strain Set of animals (particularly mice and rats) in which every animal is bred to be genetically identical.

superantigen A molecule that activates all T cells with a particular $V\beta$ gene segment, irrespective of their $V\alpha$ expression.

suppression A mechanism for producing a specific state of immunologic unresponsiveness by which one cell or its products inhibits the function of another.

surrogate light chains Nonrearranging chains ($V\lambda5$ and V preB) expressed in conjunction with μ chain in the pre-B cell; form part of the pre-BCR.

switch region Region of B cell heavy chain DNA at which recombination occurs in antigen-stimulated cell; allows isotype switch (e.g., IgM to IgE).

syngeneic Literally, genetically identical; e.g., monozygotic twins or mice of the same strain.

syngraft Same as isograft.

systemic lupus erythematosus (SLE) An autoimmune disease which affects many organs of the body, and causes fever and joint pain. Patients produce high levels of antibodies against the components of cell nuclei, particularly DNA, and form circulating soluble antigen-antibody complexes. These complexes deposit in tissues such as the kidney, activate the complement cascade, and result in tissue damage.

TAP-1 and TAP-2 Molecules that selectively transport peptides from the cytoplasm to the endoplasmic reticulum of cells for binding to MHC class I molecules.

target A cell killed by one of the body's killer cells, such as a CTL or NK cell.

Tc cell T cytotoxic cell.

T-cell receptor (TCR) A two-chain structure on T cells that binds antigen: $\alpha\beta$ on the major set of T cells, $\gamma\delta$ on the minor set of T cells. The TCR complex comprises the antigen-binding chains associated at the cell surface with the signal transduction molecules CD3 plus ζ (zeta) or η (eta).

T cells The set of lymphocytes whose differentiation requires the thymus.

TCR See T-CELL RECEPTOR.

T-dependent antigen An immunogen that requires T helper cells to interact with B cells in order to induce antibody synthesis.

terminal deoxynucleotidyl transferase (TdT) Enzyme that inserts nontemplated nucleotides at the junctions of V, D, and J gene segments of Ig and TCR locus DNA; these N-nucleotides increase the diversity of antigen-specific receptors.

T_H1 A subset of CD4$^+$ T cells that synthesizes the cytokines IL-2, IFN-γ, and TNF-β; these cytokines activate NK cells, macrophages, and CD8$^+$ T-cells.

T_H2 A subset of CD4$^+$ T cells which synthesizes the cytokines IL-4, IL-5, IL-10, and IL-13; these cytokines predominate in the response to allergens and parasites (B-cell class switching to IgE, and eosinophil activation).

thymocytes T cells differentiating in the thymus.

thymus The primary lymphoid organ for T-cell differentiation, comprising an outer cortex and inner medulla; developing thymocytes interact with epithelial cells and bone marrow derived macrophages and interdigitating dendritic cells in the thymus.

TIL See TUMOR INFILTRATING LYMPHOCYTE.

T-independent antigen An immunogen that induces antibody synthesis in the absence of T cells or their products; antibodies synthesized generally only of the IgM isotype, and no memory response.

titer Used generally as an empirical measure of the avidity of an antibody; it is the reciprocal of the last dilution of a titration giving a measurable effect; e.g., if the last dilution of an antibody giving significant agglutination is 1:128, the titer is 128.

TNF See TUMOR NECROSIS FACTOR.

tolerance Antigen-specific unresponsiveness of B or T cells.

toxic shock syndrome The systemic reaction produced by the toxin derived from the bacterium *Staphylococcus aureus*; the toxin acts as a superantigen, which activates a high proportion of CD4$^+$ T cells to produce cytokines.

toxoid A nontoxic derivative of a toxin used as an immunogen for the induction of antibodies capable of cross-reacting with the toxin.

transplantation Grafting solid tissue (such as a kidney or heart) or cells (particularly bone marrow) from one individual to another. See ALLOGRAFT and XENOGRAFT.

tuberculin test Antigens derived the organism causing tuberculosis are injected subcutaneously; individuals who have been exposed to the organism and those who have been previously vaccinated with BCG develop a delayed hypersensitivity response at the injection site 24–48 hours later.

tumor infiltrating lymphocyte (TIL) Mononuclear cells derived from the inflammatory infiltrate of solid tumors.

tumor necrosis factor (TNF) A cytokine with various actions including the selective killing of tumor cells; toxicity may be the result of the production of free radicals following the binding of high-affinity cell surface receptors.

tumor-specific transplantation antigen (TSTA) Antigens uniquely expressed by certain tumor cells.

tyrosine kinases A family of enzymes which phosphorylates proteins on tyrosine residues, a critical step in lymphocyte activation. The key tyrosine kinases in T-cell activation are Lck, Fyn, and ZAP-70; those in B-cell activation are Blk, Fyn, Lyn, and Syk.

unresponsiveness Inability to respond to antigenic stimulus. Unresponsiveness may be specific for a particular antigen (see TOLERANCE), or broadly nonspecific as a result of damage to the entire immune system, for example, after whole-body irradiation.

vaccination Any protective immunization against a pathogen. Originally referred to immunization against smallpox with the less virulent cowpox (vaccinia) virus.

variable (V) regions The N-terminal portion of an Ig or TCR which contains the antigen-binding region of the molecule; V regions are formed by the recombination of V(D) and J gene segments.

V(D)J recombination Mechanism for generating antigen-specific receptors of T and B cells; it involves the joining of V, D, and J gene segments mediated by the enzyme complex V(D)J recombinase, and products of the RAG-1 and 2 genes.

virion A complete virus particle.

virus An organism comprising a protein coat and DNA or RNA genome; it requires a host cell for replication.

V regions See VARIABLE REGIONS.

Western blotting A technique to identify a specific protein in a mixture; proteins separated by gel electrophoresis are blotted onto a nitrocellulose membrane, and the protein of interest is detected by adding radiolabeled antibody specific for the protein.

wheal and flare Itchy reaction at skin site where antigen is injected into an allergic individual; characterized by erythema (redness due to dilation of blood vessels) and edema (swelling produced by release of serum into tissue).

xenogeneic Originating from a foreign species.

xenograft A tissue transplantation between individuals belonging to two different species.

X-linked agammaglobulinemia Disease in boys manifesting as absence of mature B cells; due to defective tyrosine kinase btk, B cell differentiation does not progress beyond pre-B cell.

X-linked hyper-IgM syndrome Disease in boys manifesting as inability to synthesize Ig isotypes other than IgM; result of defect in either CD40 or CD154.

ZAP-70 A T-cell specific tyrosine kinase involved in T cell activation.

Partial List of CD Antigens

CD antigen	Other names	Cellular expression	Function/comments	Ligand
CD1		Langerhans cells, dendritic cells, B cells, thymocytes	MHC class I-like molecule, associated with β2-microglobulin	Glycolipids
CD2	LFA-2	T cells, NK cells	T-cell adhesion molecule	CD58
CD3	T3	T cells	TCR signal transduction	
CD4	T4	Thymocytes, T_H1 and T_H2 T cells, monocytes, macrophages	TCR coreceptor, signal transduction	MHC class II, HIV-1 and HIV-2 gp120
CD5	Tp67 T1	B-cell subsets, T cells	Expression on B cells associated with polyreactivity	
CD8		T-cell subsets, cytotoxic T cells	TCR coreceptor, signal transduction	MHC class I
CD11a	LFA-1	Leukocytes	Adhesion molecule	ICAM 1, 2, 3
CD18		Leukocytes	Associates with CD11a, b, c, and d	
CD19		B cells	B-cell signal transduction	
CD20		B cells	Ca^{2+} channel in B-cell activation	
CD21	CR2	B cells, follicular dendritic cells	Involved in B-cell activation	EBV and complement (c3d)
CD25	TAC	Activated T cells, B cells	IL-2 receptor (α-chain)	IL-2
CD28	Tp44	T-cell subsets	T-cell costimulator molecule	B7 (CD80 and CD86)

CD antigen	Other names	Cellular expression	Function/comments	Ligand
CD32	FcγR II	Monocytes, granulocytes, B cells, eosinophils	Low-affinity receptor for IgG	Aggregated IgG and antigen–antibody complexes
CD34		Endothelial cells, hematopoietic precursors	Marker for early stem cells	L-selectin (CD62L)
CD40		B cells, macrophages, dendritic cells	Involved in T cell interactions with APCs and class switching; receptor for costimulatory signals	CD40L (CD154)
CD44	Pgp-1, H-CAM	Leukocytes, erythrocytes	Lymphocyte adhesion to HEV	Hyaluronic acid
CD50	ICAM-3	Broad (not on endothelial cells)	Adhesion molecule	LFA-1
CD54	ICAM-1	Broad	Adhesion molecule	CD11a, CD18, rhinovirus
CD55	Decay accelerating factor (DAF)	Broad	Causes dissociation of amplification convertases of complement cascade	C3b, CD97
CD58	LFA-3	Leukocytes, endothelial cells, epithelial cells, fibroblasts	Adhesion molecule	CD2
CD62L	L-Selectin, MEL-14	B cells, T cells, monocytes, NK cells	T-cell adhesion to HEV	CD34
CD74	Invariant chain	B cells, macrophages, monocytes, activated T cells	Associated with MHC class II in endoplasmic reticulum	
CD79a	Igα	B cells	Signal transduction molecules, components of B cell receptor	
CD79b	Igβ			
CD80	B7.1	B cells, macrophages, dendritic cells	Costimulatory molecule on APC	CD28, CTLA-4
CD81	Target of antipro-liferative antibody (TAPA-1)	Broad	Associates with CD19 and CD21 on B cells to form B-cell co-receptor	
CD86	B7.2	Activated B cells, macrophages, dendritic cells	Costimulatory molecule on APC	CD28, CTLA-4
CD95	Fas, Apo-1	Activated T and B cells, NK cells	Induces apoptosis following ligation with Fas ligand (CD95L)	TNF-like Fas ligand (CD95L)
CD97	GR1	Granulocytes, macrophages, activated T and B cells	Counterreceptor for CD55	CD55

CD antigen	Other names	Cellular expression	Function/comments	Ligand
CD102	ICAM-2	Endothelial cells, resting lymphocytes, platelets	Adhesion molecule	CD11a (LFA-1)
CD152	CTLA-4	Activated T cells	Negative regulator for T-cell activation	B7.1 (CD80) and B7.2 (CD86)
CD154	CD40L	Activated T cells	Ligation with CD40 on B cells induces B-cell proliferation and class switching	CD40

INDEX